Professional Nursing
Concepts & Challenges

Professional Nursing
Concepts & Challenges

5th Edition

KAY KITTRELL CHITTY, RN, EdD
Adjunct Faculty
College of Nursing
Medical University of South Carolina
Charleston, South Carolina

BETH PERRY BLACK, RN, PhD
Assistant Professor
School of Nursing
University of North Carolina at Chapel Hill
Chapel Hill, North Carolina

With 81 illustrations

SAUNDERS

ELSEVIER

SAUNDERS
ELSEVIER

11830 Westline Industrial Drive
St. Louis, Missouri 63146

Notice

Neither the Publisher nor the Authors assume any responsibility for any loss or injury and/or damage to persons or property arising out of or related to any use of the material contained in this book. It is the responsibility of the treating practitioner, relying on independent expertise and knowledge of the patient, to determine the best treatment and method of application for the patient.

The Publisher

Previous editions copyrighted © 2005, 2001, 1997, 1993 by W. B. Saunders Company

Library of Congress Control Number: 2007921987

Senior Editor: Yvonne Alexopoulos
Senior Developmental Editor: Lisa P. Newton
Publishing Services Manager: Deborah L. Vogel
Senior Project Manager: Ann E. Rogers
Design Direction: Amy Buxton

Printed in United States of America

Last digit is the print number: 9 8 7 6 5 4 3 2

The fifth edition of this book is dedicated to my parents, who empowered me to believe in myself, and to my husband, who is proud of me for doing so.

~~KKC

This edition is dedicated to my husband Tal and daughters Mandy and Kylie who have been wonderful, supportive companions in everything that I do, and to Mom and Dad who showed me how to live life with hope even when the odds seemed long.

~~BPB

CONTRIBUTORS

Beverly B. Foster, RN, PhD, BSN, MN, MPH
Clinical Associate Professor and Undergraduate
    Program Director
University of North Carolina at Chapel Hill
Chapel Hill, North Carolina

Brandi M. Hamlin, RN, MSN
Adjunct Faculty
University of North Carolina at Chapel Hill
School of Nursing
Chapel Hill, North Carolina

Judith K. Leavitt, RN, MEd, FAAN
Health Policy Consultant
Barnardsville, North Carolina

Shielda G. Rodgers, RN, PhD
Clinical Associate Professor
University of North Carolina at Chapel Hill
School of Nursing
Chapel Hill, North Carolina

R E V I E W E R S

Judith Sims Billings, RN, PhD
Assistant Dean
UNMC College of Nursing Kearney
Kearney, Nebraska

Barbara Carranti, RN, MS
LeMoyne University/Syracuse University
Syracuse, New York

Susan Gaston, RN, PhD
Director, School of Nursing
The University of Tulsa
Tulsa, Oklahoma

Paula Kopp, RN, MSN
Instructor, School of Nursing
The University of Southern Mississippi
Gulf Park Campus
Long Beach, Mississippi

Susan Lofton, RN, MSN, PhD
Professor of Nursing
University of Mississippi
School of Nursing
Jackson, Mississippi

Nancy MacMullen, BSN, MSN, PhD
University Professor
Department of Nursing
Governors State University
University Park, Illinois

Lois Schoener, RN, DNSc
Director, Nurse Education
Elmira College
Elmira, New York

Robi Thomas, RN, MS, AOCN, CHPN
Assistant Professor
Chairperson—Grand Rapids
McAuley School of Nursing
University of Detroit Mercy
Grand Rapids, Michigan

Janet P. Tracy, RN, PhD
Professor of Nursing
William Paterson University
Wayne, New Jersey

Mary E. Weyer, EdD, APN, CS
Associate Professor
Department of Nursing
Elmhurst College
Elmhurst, Illinois

STUDENT REVIEWERS

Beth Clark Ardila
Moss Point, Mississippi

Takiyah Banks
Glendale Heights, Illinois

Barbara Bowes
Nurse Manager
Baldwinsville, New York

Kathryn Danby
Horseheads, New York

Richard E. Jay, Jr
Alma, Nebraska

Rose Leahy
Bay St. Louis, Mississippi

Erin N. Pettera
North Platte, Nebraska

Johanna Pierce
New York, New York

Hollis (Tripp) Purviance, III, RN, C, BSN
Brandon, Mississippi

Robyn Starosta
Brookfield, Illinois

Mary Jo Vona
Camillus, New York

Steven Wybenga
San Francisco, California

Professions exist to serve society. When society changes, professions must also change. So it is with nursing. To maintain our relevance and dynamism today, professional nurses must possess skills that are more complex than previously have been required in the history of the nursing profession.

To be effective, nurses must master more information than ever before available about human health and disease; they must be good leaders and good team members; they must think critically and creatively; they must communicate and collaborate with a diverse array of patients, families, and health care colleagues; they must be caring and businesslike; they must grapple with practical, ethical, and legal dilemmas not dreamed of even a decade ago; and they must practice their profession in both traditional and nontraditional settings. To be an effective professional nurse today poses a significant challenge.

The fifth edition of this text is designed to assist students to understand what it means to be a professional nurse; to appreciate the history of nursing; to understand and prize nursing's values, standards, and ethics; to recognize and deal effectively with the social and economic factors that influence how the profession is practiced; and to appreciate the need to be lifelong learners and contributing members of the nursing profession. This edition addresses concepts underlying the elements of the American Association of Colleges of Nursing's latest (1998) document, The Essentials of Baccalaureate Education for Professional Nursing Practice.

Feedback from users of earlier editions revealed that this text is used in RN to BSN "bridge" courses, in early courses in generic baccalaureate curricula, and as a resource for practicing nurses and graduate students. An increasing number of students in nursing programs are seeking second undergraduate degrees, such as mid-life adults seeking a career change and others who bring considerable experience to the learning situation. Accordingly, every effort has been made to present material that is comprehensive enough to challenge users at all levels without overwhelming the novice. The text has been designed to be "student friendly," and care has been taken to keep jargon to a minimum yet to provide a comprehensive glossary to assist in developing and refining a professional vocabulary. The visual features of the book have been carefully improved with today's visual learner in mind.

In addition to being revised and updated, the fifth edition has been substantially reorganized. The order of the chapters has changed and content has been combined to eliminate redundancy and streamline the text. There are now 16 chapters instead of 22 in order to better synchronize with the number of weeks in a semester.

We undertook this reorganization with some trepidation, realizing that this will require some revision of course syllabi. A great deal of work is required in these revisions. With the demands on college and university faculty today, this is a lot to ask. Therefore, in order to assist in revision of course syllabi, we have included the new textbook plan below. This should help you find content that has been relocated in this edition and simplify the revision of your syllabus.

The lists of key terms have been removed from the first page of each chapter. Terms are highlighted in the text itself, as in previous editions. All terms in boldface print are in the Glossary. In addition, basic terms that may aid general student understanding have been added to the Glossary, even if they were not used in the book. We hope this will be valuable to students in introductory courses.

Content in every chapter has been streamlined and excessive detail has been removed. Photographs, illustrations, and other forms of visual interest have been added, as have real life scenarios, personal viewpoints, and thought-provoking questions. The stand-alone feature that enables chapters to be read in any order remains a feature of the fifth edition. We realize that faculty may wish to teach the content in a different order and that the order that works best in one curriculum may not work in others.

In spite of changes, faculty who used the book before will find that this edition feels and looks familiar, with many of the successful features maintained and updated. Self-assessment exercises were retained and expanded in this revision. Research Notes, now titled Evidence-Based Practice Notes, have been expanded in keeping with the profession's progress. Critical Thinking Exercises have been expanded, a new feature, Cultural Challenges, has been added to a number of chapters, and the content on cultural care has been expanded and enhanced. Clinical examples have been increased.

The Instructor's Manual has been revised by Kay Chitty, Beth Black, and Valerie Schluter based on user feedback to contain activities for both small and large groups. It contains in-class and out-of-class activities designed to enhance students' learning and to enrich classroom experiences. The Instructor's Manual also includes chapter outlines, chapter objectives, suggested readings, and a comprehensive test bank. Contact your sales representative or call our Sales Support Team at 1-800-222-9570 for further information.

As with earlier editions, it continues to be our heartfelt hope that the students and faculty who use this new edition will find it even more stimulating, enjoyable, and enlightening than the first four editions and that it will continue to contribute to the positive development of our profession.

Key to Finding Fourth Edition Content in the Fifth Edition

FOURTH EDITION Chapter	FIFTH EDITION Chapter
1 History	2 History and Social Context
2 Educational Patterns	7 Educational Patterns
3 Social Context	2 History and Social Context
4 Professional Associations	15 Political Activism
5 Nursing Today	1 Nursing Today
6 Professionalization	3 Professionalization
7 Defining Nursing	6 Becoming a Nurse
8 Socialization	6 Becoming a Nurse
9 Philosophies	12 Conceptual and Philosophical Bases
10 Major Concepts	12 Conceptual and Philosophical Bases
11 Nursing Theory	13 Nursing Theory
12 Research	11 Science of Nursing
13 Health Care Delivery System	14 Health Care Delivery System
14 Nursing Roles	14 Health Care Delivery System
15 Critical Thinking	8 Critical Thinking
16 Finance	14 Health Care Delivery System
17 Illness and Culture	10 Illness and Culture
18 Communication/Collaboration	9 Communication/Collaboration
19 Nursing Ethics	5 Ethical Aspects of Nursing
20 Legal Aspects	4 Legal Aspects
21 Political Action	15 Political Activism
21 Future Challenges	16 Future Challenges

Kay K. Chitty/Beth P. Black

ACKNOWLEDGMENTS

The successful completion of any major project brings a sense both of accomplishment and of relief. The completion of the fifth edition of *Professional Nursing: Concepts and Challenges* also brings overwhelming gratitude to the many individuals who participated in what has truly been a great team effort:

- To the faculty who used earlier editions and provided us their suggestions for revisions
- To students who send e-mails, expressing their gratitude for an interesting and readable textbook while offering ideas for improvement
- To the reference librarians at the Medical University of South Carolina for their unselfish donation of time, talents, and energy
- To Stephen Wybenga who shared his balanced insights about being a man in a female-dominated profession
- To the many nurses who shared their experiences and perceptions in interviews
- To all who assisted in gathering photographs— Shielda Rodgers, Pam Auchmuty, Nell Hodgson Woodruff School of Nursing at Emory University, the Washington State Nurses Association, the American Nurses Association, Edward J. Halloran, and Explore America Tours

Special thanks are due the contributors to this edition, who took on this extra responsibility in spite of already over-full personal and professional lives. Their recompense will not be tangible, for academia is sadly lacking in rewards for textbook writing. In an odd twist of values, publishing a research article in a scholarly journal that will be read by few and used by even fewer is seen as more desirable in today's colleges and universities than writing a textbook that has the potential to influence thousands of future professional nurses. In spite of this obstacle, these contributors rose to the occasion. Their love of the nursing profession and commitment to its hopeful future will serve as their remuneration. We are deeply indebted to them all.

CONTENTS

16 NURSING'S FUTURE CHALLENGES, 421

Kay Kittrell Chitty

Professional Nursing
Concepts & Challenges

Nursing Today

Kay Kittrell Chitty

Learning Outcomes

After studying this chapter, students will be able to:

- Describe the "average" registered nurse of today.
- Identify the broad range of settings in which today's registered nurses practice.
- Discuss emerging practice opportunities for nurses.

- Cite similarities and differences among nursing roles in various practice settings.
- Explain the roles of advanced practice nurses and the preparation required to assume these roles.

What is the profile of the "typical" registered nurse today? Is there an average registered nurse? Where do nurses work? What do they do? What type of preparation is required for various roles? How have new health care technologies and pressures to control health care costs affected nurses and nursing practice? As health care changes and nursing evolves to meet new challenges, the answers to these questions also change.

Far-reaching economic and social changes in the United States have profoundly affected the way health care is provided. Many of these changes have opened avenues to new and exciting employment opportunities for nurses. This chapter provides an overview of the registered nurse (RN) population in the United States and briefly presents a selection of employment options available to nurses today in hospital and community settings. Integrated into this chapter are interviews

with several nurses who describe their work and the rewards and challenges of their positions.

CURRENT STATUS OF NURSING IN THE UNITED STATES

To provide current information about practicing nurses, the federal government has conducted national surveys of actively licensed registered nurses in the United States every 4 years since the late 1970s. The most recent survey was conducted in March 2004. Data from this survey were published in 2005 by the U.S. Department of Health and Human Services, Division of Nursing, in a document titled *Preliminary Findings: 2004 National Sample Survey of Registered Nurses*. This document and information provided by the American Nurses Association (ANA), the National League for Nursing (NLN), and the American

Association of Colleges of Nursing provide a comprehensive look at the characteristics of registered nurses today.

Numbers

Registered nurses represent the largest group of health care providers in the United States. More than 2.9 million individuals held licenses as registered nurses in 2004, but only 2.4 million (83.2 percent) of these individuals were actively working in nursing. The remainder of the registered nurse population (16.8 percent) was either not working at all or working in fields other than nursing. Figures also indicated that less than two thirds (58.3 percent) of employed registered

nurses worked full-time, whereas almost one fourth (24.8 percent) worked part-time. The total number of licensed RNs working full-time within nursing, therefore, is far lower than the 2.9 million figure indicates, as shown in Figure 1-1.

Gender

Not surprisingly, the Division of Nursing's 2004 survey also showed that most registered nurses were women. Among employed RNs, only 5.7 percent were men. This figure seems to indicate a leveling off of the proportion of men in nursing, since the 2000 percentage was 5.4 percent and the 1996 percentage was also 5.4 percent. Even though the percentage of men in nursing has stabilized

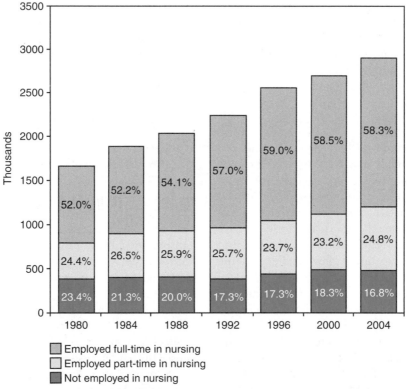

Figure 1-1

Registered nurse population by employment status, 1980-2004. (Data from U.S. Department of Health and Human Services, Health Resources and Services Administration: *Preliminary findings: 2004 national sample survey of registered nurses*, Washington, DC, 2005, Government Printing Office, p 1 [website]: http://bhpr.hrsa.gov/healthworkforce/reports/rnpopulation/preliminaryfindings.htm.)

for the time being, the number of men is still growing at a rate faster than that for the total registered nurse population. This is attributable to the fact that males accounted for 9.7 percent of all baccalaureate graduates in 2005 and 9.4 percent and 7.2 percent, respectively, of master's and doctoral program graduates (American Association of Colleges of Nursing, 2006).

In terms of absolute numbers, the 2004 survey revealed that there were 18,398 more male RNs in 2004 (when there were 161,300) than there were in 2000 (when there were 146,902). In addition, anecdotal reports from nursing faculty indicate that larger numbers of men are currently in the educational pipeline. The historic status of nursing as a female-dominated profession could eventually change as more male graduates of basic nursing programs enter the workforce.

Race and Ethnicity

As of 2004, the total registered nurse population was overwhelmingly composed of white, non-Hispanic individuals (88.4 percent). The 2004 National Sample Survey showed that distribution by ethnic/racial backgrounds of the 10.6 percent nonwhite employed registered nurses included African-American, 4.6 percent; Asian/Pacific Islander, 3.3 percent; Hispanic, 1.8 percent; and Native American/Alaskan Native, 0.4 percent. The remainder (1.5 percent) reported two or more racial backgrounds.

Despite efforts to recruit and retain nonwhites in the nursing profession, the percentages in each nonwhite category decreased between 2000 and 2004. This indicates that nursing still has a long way to go before the racial/ethnic composition of the profession more accurately reflects that of American society as a whole. This disparity can easily be seen when nursing's percentages are compared with those of the country overall, reported by the U.S. Census Bureau in July 2004 to be 67.9 percent white and 32.1 percent non-white. Figure 1-2 compares the racial/ethnic distribution of registered nurses with that of the United States population.

There is better news on the horizon for minorities in nursing, however. The AACN's 2005-2006 data show nearly 24 percent of undergraduate enrollees were from racial and ethnic minorities (American Association of Colleges of Nursing, 2006). The racial and ethnic composition of the nursing profession will change as these students graduate and begin practice.

Age

With respect to age, the registered nurse population is similar to the rest of American society: It is getting older. This "graying" of the workforce can be illustrated by comparing 1980 statistics with those from 2004. In 1980 the average age of all registered nurses was 40.3 years. This figure rose to 45.2 years by 2000, and increased to 46.8 years in 2004. The percent of nurses more than 54 years of age rose to 25.5 percent in 2004, up from 24.3 percent in 2000 and 17.2 percent in 1980. With new nurses entering practice each year, the average age might be expected to remain the same or decline. Many new nurses are beginning second careers, however, and are significantly older than the typical college graduate. Only 9.1 percent of newly licensed registered nurses in 2000 were younger than age 30, and this number dropped to 8.1 percent in 2004 (Figure 1-3).

Marital Status

The marital status of nurses has also been studied. In 2004 70.5 percent of nurses were married, 18.1 percent were widowed/divorced/separated, and 9.2 percent had never been married. Only 52.1 percent of employed nurses had children at home, with 28.3 percent of those children reportedly less than 6 years of age. Registered nurses who were part of a two-parent family with children younger than 6 years were more likely to work part-time than any other group.

Education

Nursing has more levels of initial preparation than most professions because of the variety of educational pathways that one can take to become a registered nurse. In 2004 of the 2,909,467 licensed registered nurses, 17.1 percent had diplomas as their highest nursing-related educational preparation; 33.7 percent held associate

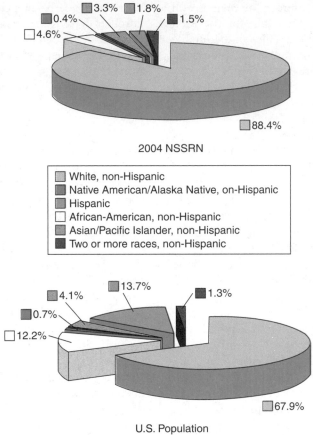

Figure 1-2

Distribution of registered nurses and the U.S. population by racial/ethnic background, 2004. (Data from U.S. Department of Health and Human Services, Health Resources and Services Administration: *Preliminary findings: 2004 national sample survey of registered nurses*, Washington, DC, 2005, Government Printing Office, p 4 [website]: http://bhpr.hrsa.gov/healthworkforce/reports/rnpopulation/preliminaryfindings.htm.)

degrees; 34.2 percent had baccalaureate degrees; and 13 percent held master's or doctoral degrees (U.S. Department of Health and Human Services, 2005). These figures represent slight declines in the numbers of diploma-educated nurses and associate degree–prepared nurses and slight increases in the number of nurses with baccalaureate and higher degrees since 2000. Figure 1-4 illustrates trends in the initial educational preparation of registered nurses in the United States from 1980 to 2004. One must note, however, that initial preparation is only part of

the educational picture for nurses because "increasing numbers of registered nurses receive baccalaureate and master's degrees, even if their initial preparation for nursing was an associate degree or diploma" (USDHHS, 2005).

Foreign-educated nurses

Approximately 3.5 percent (100,791) of RNs practicing in the United States in 2004 completed their basic nursing education outside the United States and its territories. About half of these (50.2 percent) were from the Philippines, 20.2 percent

Figure 1-3
Age distribution of the registered nurse population, 1980-2004. (Data from U.S. Department of Health and Human Services, Health Resources and Services Administration: *Preliminary findings: 2004 national sample survey of registered nurses*, Washington, DC, 2005, Government Printing Office, p 3 [website]: http://bhpr.hrsa.gov/healthworkforce/reports/rnpopulation/preliminaryfindings.htm.)

from Canada, and 8.4 percent from the United Kingdom, followed by Nigeria, Ireland, India, Hong Kong, Jamaica, Israel, and South Korea. Foreign-educated nurses cited all 50 states and the District of Columbia as their principal nursing practice location. The largest number reported working in California (25.5 percent), followed by Florida (9.6 percent), New York (9.3 percent), Texas (6.7 percent), and New Jersey (6.1 percent). The educational levels achieved by foreign-educated nurses exceed those of native-born American nurses with more than half (59.9 percent) having baccalaureate or higher degrees.

Two percent reported being doctorally prepared and more than 2 percent were advance practice nurses (APNs). More than two thirds (68.5 percent) are multilingual (U.S. Department of Health and Human Services, 2005).

Employment Opportunities for Nurses

As members of the largest health care profession in the United States, nurses practice in diverse settings such as hospitals, clinics, offices, homes, schools, workplaces, extended care facilities, the military, community centers, nursing homes, children's camps, and homeless shelters, among

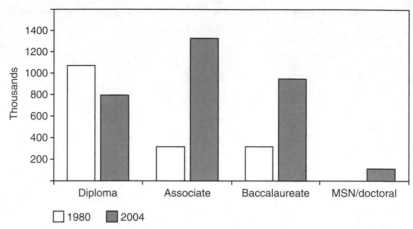

Figure 1-4
Trends in initial nursing preparation of the registered nurse population, 1980-2004. (Data from U.S. Department of Health and Human Services, Health Resources and Services Administration: *Preliminary findings: 2004 national sample survey of registered nurses,* Washington, DC, 2005, Government Printing Office, p 2 [website]: http://bhpr.hrsa.gov/healthworkforce/reports/rnpopulation/preliminaryfindings.htm.)

others. Increasingly, as state nurse practice acts are revised to cover independent advanced practice roles, registered nurses also work in private practice. Nurses in nurse-based practice must have advanced degrees or specialized education, training, and certification.

In 2004 hospitals remained the primary work-site for registered nurses (reported by 56.2 percent of those employed, down from 59.1 percent in 2000). After more than a decade of steady growth in numbers, employment in community health/public health settings, such as state or local health departments, home health services, community health centers, student health, occupational health, and faith community nursing, fell from an all-time high of 18.2 percent in 2000 to 14.9 percent of registered nurses in 2004. **Ambulatory care settings,** such as physician-based practices, nurse-based practices, free-standing emergency and surgical centers, or health maintenance organizations (HMOs), accounted for 11.5 percent. An additional 6.3 percent worked in nursing homes or **extended care** facilities. The remainder of employed registered nurses worked in settings such as schools of nursing; nursing associations; local, state, or federal governmental agencies; state

boards of nursing; or insurance companies (U.S. Department of Health and Human Services, 2005).

Not all nurses provide direct patient care as the primary part of their roles. A small but important group of nurses spend the majority of their time conducting research, teaching undergraduate and graduate students, managing companies as chief executives, and consulting with health care organizations. Nurses who have advanced levels of education, such as master's and doctoral degrees, are prepared to become researchers, educators, administrators, and advanced practice nurses, including nurse practitioners, clinical nurse specialists, certified nurse-midwives, and certified registered nurse anesthetists. These advanced practice roles are discussed in greater detail later in this chapter.

In deciding which of the many available practice options to select, nurses should consider several salient points: educational preparation required; their special talents, likes, and dislikes; and whether their preparation, talents, and preferences are a good match with the employment opportunities under consideration. Although a majority of nurses are employed in hospitals, many others are pursuing challenges elsewhere.

Numerous new opportunities and roles are being developed that use nurses' skills in different and exciting ways. What follows are descriptions of a sampling of the broad range of settings in which nurses now practice. In some instances, nurses are interviewed. It must be stressed that these areas represent only a sampling of the growing variety of opportunities available.

Hospital-based nursing

Nursing care originated and was practiced informally in home and community settings and moved into hospitals only within the last 150 years. Hospitals vary widely in size, comprehensiveness of services offered, and geographic location. In general, nurses in hospitals work with patients who have medical or surgical conditions, with sick children, with women and their newborns, with cancer patients, and with people who have had severe traumas or burns.

Within hospitals, nurses work in various units, such as in operating suites or emergency departments, in coronary and other special care units, on step-down or progressive care units, and in many other capacities. In addition to providing direct patient care, they serve as educators, managers, and administrators who teach or supervise others and establish the direction of nursing hospital-wide. A number of generalist and specialist certification opportunities are appropriate for hospital-based nurses, including medical-surgical nurse, pediatric nurse, perinatal nurse, acute care nurse practitioner, gerontological nurse, psychiatric and mental health nurse, nursing administration, nursing administration–advanced, nursing continuing education or staff development nurse, and informatics nurse. There is perhaps no other single work setting that offers so much employment variety to nurses as do hospitals.

The educational credentials required of registered nurses practicing in hospitals can range from associate degrees and diplomas to doctoral degrees. Generally, entry-level positions require only RN licensure. Many hospitals require nurses to hold baccalaureate degrees to advance on the clinical ladder or to assume management positions. A **clinical coordinator,** who is responsible for the management of more than one unit, is generally expected to have a master's degree.

Most new nurses choose to work in acute care hospitals initially to gain experience in organizing and delivering patient care to multiple patients. For many, staff nursing is extremely gratifying, and they continue in this role for their entire careers. Others pursue additional education, often provided by the hospital, in order to work in specialty units such as coronary care. Although specialty units usually require clinical experience and advanced training, some hospitals do allow exceptional new graduates to work in these units.

Some nurses find that management is their strength. **Nurse managers,** formerly called head nurses, are in charge of all activities on their units, including patient care, continuous quality improvement, personnel selection and evaluation, and resource management. Being a nurse manager in a hospital today is somewhat like running a business, and nurses need an entrepreneurial spirit and knowledge of business and financial principles to be most effective in this role.

Most nurses in hospitals provide direct patient care. In the past, it was necessary for nurses to assume administrative or management roles to be promoted or receive salary increases. Such positions removed them from bedside care. Today, in hospitals with clinical ladder programs, nurses no longer must make that choice; clinical ladder programs allow nurses to progress while staying in direct patient care roles.

A **clinical ladder** is a multiple-step program that begins with entry-level staff nurse positions. As nurses gain experience, participate in continuing education, demonstrate clinical competence, pursue formal education, and become certified, they are eligible to move up the rungs of the ladder.

At the top of most clinical ladders are **clinical nurse specialists (CNSs),** who are nurses with master's degrees in specialized areas of nursing, such as oncology. The role varies but generally includes responsibility for serving as a clinical mentor and role model for other nurses, as well as setting standards for nursing care on one or more particular units. The oncology clinical specialist, for example, works with the nurses on the oncology unit to help them stay informed of the latest research and skills useful in the care of patients with cancer. The clinical specialist is a resource person for the unit and often provides direct care to patients or families with particularly difficult or complex problems, establishes nursing protocols, and is responsible for ensuring that nurses adhere to high standards of care.

Salaries and responsibilities increase at the upper levels of clinical ladders. The clinical ladder concept benefits nurses by allowing them to advance while still working directly with patients. Hospitals also benefit by retaining experienced clinical nurses in direct patient care, thus improving the quality of nursing care throughout the hospital. Research has demonstrated that patient outcomes are more positive for patients cared for by baccalaureate (or higher) prepared registered nurses. The Evidence-Based Practice Note below describes a landmark study reported in the

 EVIDENCE-BASED PRACTICE
note

Several University of Pennsylvania researchers, led by distinguished nurse-researcher Dr. Linda Aiken, noted growing evidence suggesting "that nurse staffing affects the quality of care in hospitals, but little is known about whether the educational composition of registered nurses (RNs) in hospitals is related to patient outcomes." They wondered if the proportion of a hospital's staff of baccalaureate- or higher degree–prepared RNs contributed to improved patient outcomes. To answer this question, they undertook a large analysis of outcome data for 232,342 general, orthopedic, and vascular surgery patients discharged from 168 Pennsylvania hospitals over a 19-month period. They used statistical methods to control for risk factors such as age, sex, emergency or routine surgeries, type of surgery, preexisting conditions, surgeon qualifications, size of hospital, and other factors. Their findings were riveting: "To our knowledge, this study provides the first empirical evidence that hospitals' employment of nurses with BSN and higher degrees is associated with improved patient outcomes. Our findings indicate that surgical patients cared for in hospitals in which higher proportions of

direct-care RNs held bachelor's degrees experienced a substantial survival advantage over those treated in hospitals in which fewer staff nurses has BSN or higher degrees. Similarly, surgical patients experiencing serious complications during hospitalization were significantly more likely to survive in hospitals with a higher proportion of nurses with baccalaureate education" (p. 1621). Noting that fewer than half of all hospital staff nurses nationally are prepared at the baccalaureate level or higher, and citing the nursing shortage as a complicating factor, this group of researchers recommended "placing greater emphasis in national nurse workforce planning on policies to alter the educational composition of the future nurse workforce toward a greater proportion with baccalaureate or higher education as well as ensuring the adequacy of the overall supply" (p. 1623). They concluded that improved public financing of nursing education and increased employers' efforts to recruit and retain highly prepared bedside nurses could lead to substantial improvements in quality of care.

From Aiken LH et al: Educational levels of hospital nurses and surgical patient mortality, *JAMA* 290(12):1617-1623, 2003.

Journal of the American Medical Association (JAMA) comparing surgical patient outcomes and educational levels of nurses.

One of the greatest drawbacks to hospital nursing in the past was the necessity for nurses to work rigid schedules, which usually included evenings, nights, weekends, and holidays. Although hospital nurses still must work a fair share of undesirable times, **flexible staffing** is becoming the norm. Today, nurses on a particular unit often negotiate with one another and establish their own schedules to meet personal needs while still ensuring that appropriate patient care is provided.

Each hospital nursing role has its own unique characteristics. In the following profile, a registered nurse discusses his role as a bedside nurse in a burn unit:

> A burn nurse has to be gentle, strong, and patient enough to go slow. You must be confident enough to work alone; you must believe that what you're doing is in the patient's best interest because some of the procedures hurt far worse than anyone can imagine. Every burn is unique and a challenge. Fifteen years ago, the prognosis for surviving an extensive burn was not good, but with today's techniques for fluid replacement and the development of effective antibiotics, many patients are surviving the first few critical days. During the long hours of one-on-one care you really get to know your patient. There is nothing more rewarding.

When the "fit" between nurses and their role requirements is good, nursing is a gratifying profession, as an oncology nurse demonstrates in discussing her role:

> Being an oncology nurse and working with people with potentially terminal illnesses brings you close to patients and their families. The family room for our patients and their families is very homelike. Families bring food in and have dinner with their loved one right here. Working with dying patients is a tall order. You must be able to support the family and the patient through many stages of the dying process, including anger and depression. Experiencing cancer is always traumatic, with the diagnosis, the treatment, and the struggle to cope. But today's statistics show that more people survive cancer. Because of research and early detection, being diagnosed with cancer is no longer the automatic death sentence it used to be. I love getting involved with patients and their families and feel that I can contribute to their positive mental attitude, which can impact their disease process, or hold their hand and help them to die with dignity. They cry, I cry—it is part of my nursing, and I would have it no other way.

These are only two of the many possible roles nurses in hospital settings may choose. Although brief, these descriptions convey a flavor of the responsibility, complexity, and fulfillment to be found in hospital-based nursing (Figure 1-5).

Community health nursing

Lillian Wald is credited with initiating community health nursing when she established the Henry Street Settlement in New York City. **Community health nursing** today is a broad field encompassing areas formerly known as public health nursing and home health nursing. Community health nurses work in ambulatory

Figure 1-5
Hospital staff nurses work closely with the families of patients, as well as with the patients themselves. (*Courtesy Memorial Health Care Systems, Chattanooga, Tennessee.*)

clinics, health departments, hospices, and a variety of other community-based settings, including homes, where they provide nursing care to home-bound patients.

Community health nurses may work for either government or private agencies. Those working for public health departments provide care in clinics, schools, retirement communities, and other community settings. They focus on improving the overall health of communities by planning and implementing health programs, as well as delivering care for those with chronic health problems. These community health nurses provide educational programs in health maintenance, disease prevention, nutrition, and child care, among others. They conduct immunization clinics and health screenings and work with teachers, parents, physicians, and community leaders toward a healthier community.

Many health departments also have a home health component. Since 1980 there has been a tremendous increase in the number of public and private agencies providing home health services, a form of community health nursing. In fact, home health care is a growing segment of the health care industry (Figure 1-6). Many home health nurses predict that most health care services in the future will be provided in the home.

Home health care has traditionally been, and will continue to be, nursing's "turf." Home health nurses across the United States provide quality care in the most cost-effective and, for patients, comfortable setting possible—the home. Patients cared for at home today tend to be more seriously ill than ever; this is largely because of early hospital discharges in efforts to control costs. As a result, more high-technology equipment is being used in the home. Equipment and procedures formerly unheard of outside of hospital settings, such as ventilators, intravenous pumps, and administration of chemotherapy and total parenteral nutrition (TPN), are routinely encountered in home care today.

Home health nurses must possess up-to-date nursing knowledge and be secure in their own nursing skills, because they do not have the

Figure 1-6
Home health nursing is a major component of the health care industry. *(Courtesy Memorial Health Care Systems, Chattanooga, Tennessee.)*

immediate backup of more experienced nurses as they might in a hospital setting. These nurses must have strong assessment and communication skills. They must make independent judgments and be able to recognize patients' and families' teaching needs. Home health nurses must also know their limits and seek help when the patient's needs are beyond the scope of their abilities. A registered nurse working in home health relates her experience:

> I have always found a tremendous reward in working with the terminally ill and the elderly, and I get a great deal of contact with this particular population working in home health. One patient I cared for developed a pressure ulcer while at home. I was able to assess the patient's physiological needs as well as teach the family how to care for their loved one to prevent future skin breakdown. Within a few weeks the skin looked good, and the family felt important and involved. To me this is real nursing.

Community health nursing is growing as more and more nursing care is delivered outside the walls of hospitals. The American Nurses Credentialing Center offers certification in both community health and home health nursing at the generalist and clinical specialist levels. The increase in demand for nurses to work in a variety of community settings is expected to increase for the foreseeable future.

Nurse entrepreneurs

Some nurses are highly creative people who like finding new forms of expression and are challenged by the risks of starting a new enterprise. Such nurses may make good nurse entrepreneurs.

Similar to an entrepreneur in any field, a **nurse entrepreneur** identifies a need and creates a service to meet the identified need. Nurse entrepreneurs enjoy the **autonomy** (independent functioning) that is derived from owning and operating their own health-related businesses. Groups of nurses, some of whom are faculty members in schools of nursing, have opened nurse-managed centers to provide direct care to clients. Nurse entrepreneurs are self-employed as consultants to hospitals, nursing homes, and schools of nursing. Others have started nurse-based practices and carry their own caseloads of patients with physical or emotional needs. They are sometimes involved in presenting educational workshops and seminars. Some nurses establish their own apparel businesses, which provide articles of clothing for premature babies or physically challenged individuals. Others own and operate their own health equipment companies, health insurance agencies, and home health agencies. In today's burgeoning health care environment, there is no limit to the opportunities available to nurses with the entrepreneurial spirit. Here are a few comments from one such entrepreneur, the chief executive officer of a privately owned home health agency:

> I enjoy working for myself. I know that my success or failure in my business is up to me. Having your own home health agency is a lot of work. You have to be very organized, manage other people effec-

tively, and have excellent communication skills. You cannot be afraid to say no to the people. There is nothing better than the feeling I get when a family calls to say our nurses have made a difference in their loved one's life, but I also have to take the calls of complaint about my agency. Those are tough.

Increasingly, nurses are taking the business of health care into their own hands. They seem to agree that the opportunity to create their own companies has never been better. One such company offers nursing care for mothers, babies, and children. This company's emphasis is the care of women whose pregnancies may be complicated by diabetes, hypertension, or multiple births. The registered nurse founder described the services offered by her company:

> Our main specialty is managing high-risk pregnancies and high-risk newborns. Home care for these individuals is a boon not only to the patients themselves, but also to hospitals, insurance companies, and doctors. With the trend toward shorter hospital stays, risks are minimized if skilled maternity nurses are on hand to provide patients with specialty care in their homes.

As with almost any endeavor, disadvantages come with owning a small business. There is the risk of losing your investment if the business is unsuccessful. Fluctuations in income are common, especially in the early months, and regular paychecks may become a memory, at least in the beginning. A certain amount of pressure is created because of the total responsibility for meeting deadlines and paying bills, salaries, and taxes, but there is great opportunity as well.

In addition to financial incentives, there are intangible rewards in entrepreneurship. For some people, the autonomy and freedom to control their own practice are more than enough to compensate for the increased pressure and initial uncertainty.

With rapid changes occurring daily in the health care system, new and exciting possibilities abound. Alert nurses who possess creativity, initiative, and business savvy have tremendous opportunities as entrepreneurs. The Evidence-

Based Practice Note below describes the work of a pioneering nurse entrepreneur.

Office-based nursing

Nurses who are employed in medical office settings work in tandem with physicians or nurse practitioners and their patients. Office-based nursing activities include performing health assessments, drawing blood, giving immunizations, administering medications, and providing health teaching. Nurses in office settings also act as liaisons between patients and physicians or NPs. They amplify and clarify orders for patients, as well as provide emotional support to anxious patients. They may visit hospitalized patients, and some assist in surgery. Often, these nurses

EVIDENCE-BASED PRACTICE
note

Kathleen Vollman is a master's prepared critical care nurse practicing in Detroit, Michigan. In the early 1980s she observed that about 60 to 70 percent of her patients with acute respiratory distress syndrome (ARDS) died from a lack of oxygen. Attempts to oxygenate them with ventilators often further injured their lungs. Inspired by an article on animal research left in the break room by a pulmonologist, Kathleen began to think about positioning patients for maximum oxygenation.

First, she tried turning her patients with ARDS from side to back to side every 30 minutes, as had been done in the animal study. She took blood gas readings in each position and developed a schedule for each patient based on that person's unique responses. Patients seemed to do better when she used this simple, noninvasive, independent nursing function of positioning.

Encouraged by her patients' responses, she read more research studies and found two articles dealing with the beneficial effect of prone (face down) positioning on gas exchange. She tried this with positive results but encountered problems turning very ill patients into the prone position. Solving this problem became the subject of her master's research.

Kathleen and a relative who is a mechanical engineer developed a turning frame and tested it on healthy people in a simulated critical care environment. After testing, the device was modified twice and then tested with ARDS patients. Data were collected for over 10 months and showed the usefulness of the frame in improving oxygenation of these critically ill patients. Kathleen has since won several research awards and has patented her device. She licensed the device to a major manufacturer of hospital beds, and now the Vollman Prone Positioner is marketed internationally. The device costs $2,000 and can be reused after disinfecting. Kathleen serves as a consultant to the company on the marketing of the device and the education of those who will use it. She is listed in *Who's Who of American Inventors*.

Kathleen Vollman's story is an example of how a practicing nurse, making an observation and thinking creatively through possible solutions, became a researcher, an inventor, and ultimately, an entrepreneur. This is not an overnight success story, however; it has been nearly 25 years since Kathleen made her initial observations. She continues her research in prone positioning science today. You can read more about Kathleen Vollman's entrepreneurial activities online (www.vollman.com).

From Vollman KM: My search to help patients breathe, *Reflections* 25(2):16-18, 1999; Vollman KM, Bander JL: Improved oxygenation utilizing a prone positioner in patients with acute respiratory distress syndrome, *Intensive Care Med* 22:1105-1111, 1996; Vollman KM: Nurse entrepreneurship: taking an invention from birth to the marketplace, *Clin Nurse Specialist* 18(2):68-71, 2004.

supervise other office workers, such as practical nurses, nurse aides, scheduling clerks, and record clerks. Educational requirements, hours of work, and specific responsibilities vary, depending on the preferences of the employer.

A registered nurse who works for a group of three nephrologists describes a typical day:

> I first make rounds independently on patients in the dialysis center, making sure that they are tolerating the dialysis procedure and answering questions regarding their treatments and diets. I then make rounds with one of the physicians in the hospital as he visits patients and orders new treatments. The afternoon is spent in the office assessing patients as they come for their physician's visit. I may draw blood for a diagnostic test on one patient and do patient teaching regarding diet to another. No 2 days are alike, and that is what I love about this position. I have a sense of independence but still have daily patient contact.

Registered nurses considering employment in office settings need good communication skills, because a large part of their responsibilities includes communicating with patients, families, employers, pharmacists, and hospital admitting clerks. They should be careful to inquire about the specifics of the position because office practice nursing roles may range from routine task performance to the challenging, multifaceted functions described by the nurse interviewed above.

Occupational health nursing

Many large companies today employ occupational health nurses to provide basic health care services, health education, screenings, and emergency treatment to company employees at the workplace. Corporate executives have long known that good employee health reduces absenteeism, insurance costs, and worker errors, thereby improving company profitability. Occupational health nurses represent an important investment by companies. They are often asked to serve as consultants on health matters within the company. These nurses may participate in health-related policy development, such as policies governing employee smoking or family leaves (formerly limited to maternity leaves). Depending on the size of the company, the occupational health nurse may be the only health professional employed in a company and therefore may have a good deal of autonomy.

The minimum educational requirement for nurses in occupational health roles is licensure; however, the American Association of Occupational Health Nurses (AAOHN) recommends a baccalaureate degree. Occupational health nurses must possess knowledge and skills that enable them to perform routine physical assessments, including vision and hearing screenings, for all employees. Good interpersonal skills to provide counseling and referrals for lifestyle problems, such as stress or substance abuse, are a bonus for these nurses. They must also know first aid and cardiopulmonary resuscitation (CPR). If employed in a heavy industrial setting where burns or traumas are a risk, they must have special training in those medical emergencies.

Occupational health nurses also have responsibilities for identifying health risks in the entire work environment. They must be able to assess the environment for potential safety hazards and work with management to eliminate or reduce them. They need a working knowledge of governmental regulations, such as the requirements of the Occupational Safety and Health Administration (OSHA), and must ensure that the company is complying with regulations. They may instruct new workers in the effective use of protective devices such as safety glasses and noise canceling devices. These nurses also need to understand workers' compensation regulations and coordinate the care of injured workers with the treating physician.

Nurses in occupational settings have to be confident in their nursing skills, be effective communicators with both employees and managers, be able to motivate employees to adopt healthier habits, and be able to function independently in providing care. Certification for occupational health nurses is available through the American Board for Occupational Health Nurses (ABOHN).

Military nursing

Military nurses practice in peacetime and wartime settings in the army, navy, and air force. They may serve on active duty or in the reserves. They serve as staff nurses and supervisors in all major medical specialties. Both general and advanced practice opportunities are available in military nursing, and the settings in which these nurses practice have state-of-the-art technologies.

Military nurses often find themselves with broader responsibilities and scope of practice than do civilian nurses due to the demands of nursing "in the field," on aircraft, or onboard ship. Previous critical care, surgery, or trauma care experience is very desirable but not required. Military nurses are required to have a BSN for active duty. They enter active duty as officers and must be between the ages of 21 and 46 1/2 when they begin active duty.

A major benefit of military nursing is the opportunity for advanced education. Military nurses are encouraged to seek advanced degrees, and support is provided during schooling. The military pays for tuition, books, moving expenses, and even salary for nurses obtaining advanced degrees. This allows the student to focus on his/her studies. Nurses with advanced degrees are eligible for promotion in rank at an accelerated pace.

Travel and change are integral to military nursing, so these nurses must enjoy both. Military nurses in the reserves must be committed to readiness; they must be ready to go at a moment's notice. All military nurses may be called on for global wartime duty. These nurses take great pride in the fact that they are providing care to our fighting forces in every theatre of operations.

An active reserve nurse recently wrote, "Events of 9/11 were the catalyst that made me realize that the right thing for me to do was to return to the military and merge that with my nursing career as an emergency nurse in the Army Nurse Corps" (Hardin, 2006). To learn more about military nursing, you can read an excellent article, "Esprit de Nurse Corps" by Barbara Barzoloski-O'Connor, in the online magazine *Nursing Spectrum*. This article can be found at http://community.nursingspectrum.com/MagazineArticles/article.cfm?AID=1560.

School nursing

According to the National Association of School Nurses (2006), "School nursing is a specialized practice of professional nursing that advances the well-being, academic success, and life-long achievement of students." A **school nurse** should enjoy working with children, their families, teachers, school administrators, and parent-teacher organizations.

Although many states have well-developed school nurse programs, others do not. Very few states achieve the federally recommended ratio of 1:750 (a recommended minimum number of 1 school nurse for every 750 students). In fact, a number of states have up to 10,000 students under the care of 1 school nurse (U.S. Department of Health and Human Services, 2001). With such high ratios, it is difficult to imagine how children in these states can be deriving substantial health benefits from the school nurse program.

Health care futurists believe that school nursing is the wave of the future. In medically underserved areas and with the number of uninsured families increasing, the role of school nurse is sometimes expanded to include members of the school child's immediate family. Obviously, this requires many more school nurses—along with willingness by state and local school boards to pay them. Without adequate qualified staffing, the nation's children cannot receive the full benefits of school nurse programs. The News Note on p. 15 describes the impact of the school nurse shortage on school children.

Most school systems require nurses to have a minimum of a baccalaureate degree in nursing, whereas some school districts have higher educational requirements. Prior experience working with children is also usually required. School health has become a specialty in its own right, and in states where school health is a priority, graduate programs in school health nursing have been established. The National Board for Certification of School Nurses (NBCSN) is the official certifying body for school nurses.

School nurses need a working knowledge of human growth and development to detect *newsnote* *School Nurse Shortage Is Cause for Concern—How Bad Is It?*

Thousands of children with asthma, attention deficit disorder, food allergies, injuries from accidents, and other health problems rely on teachers, school secretaries, or parent volunteers because there are not enough school nurses.

- More than 3.5 million school children take medications at school, including 200 types of prescription drugs.
- It is estimated that every 30 minutes of the school day a student suffers an injury significant enough to cause him or her to miss a half-day or more of school.
- Approximately two students per classroom suffer from asthma. During the 2002 school year, American students lost about 14.7 million school days to asthma.
- Allergies to peanuts doubled from 1997 to 2002.
- Students with diabetes, seizures, cerebral palsy, cystic fibrosis, and other serious disorders are in regular classroom situations with no one to monitor their medical conditions.
- A 1999 ruling by the U.S. Supreme Court requires public schools to provide care for students with disabilities. This means that someone must know how to use devices such as tracheostomy tubes, ventilators, feeding pumps, and catheters.

In spite of the increasing demands for health care services in public schools, the number of school nurses is declining around the nation.

- In 3 years the Dearborn, Michigan, public schools cut school nurses at 32 schools from 9 nurses to only 5. They now depend on school secretaries to take care of minor health problems.
- Three of the seven school nurses in Baldwin County, Georgia, were laid off in 2005 because of lack of money.
- The number of California schools with full-time nurses fell from 7 percent in 1998 to 5 percent in 2003.
- In Florida schools during 2003-2004, 6007 calls were made to 911 for injuries or illness because no school nurse was available.

Children's advocates underscore the urgency of the situation. "Schools without nurses are putting children in harm's way," says William Sears, a pediatrician and author of more than 30 books on child care. "If we can't afford school nurses, we've got our priorities skewed." U.S. Representative Lois Capps, a Democrat from California and former school nurse, agrees. She worries "that staff members at schools without nurses might fail to spot illnesses among students" or be unable to respond during emergencies. "It's a ticking time bomb," she says.

From Horovitz B, McCoy K: Nurse shortage puts school kids at risk, *USA Today*, Dec 14, 2005, p A-1.

developmental problems early and refer children to appropriate therapists. Counseling skills are important because many children turn to the school nurse as counselor. School nurses keep records of children's required immunizations and are responsible for ensuring that immunizations are current. When an outbreak of a childhood communicable disease occurs, school nurses edu-

cate parents, teachers, and students about treatment and prevention of disease transmission.

Although the essentially well child is the focus of the school nurse's work, the practice of mainstreaming has brought many chronically ill, injured, developmentally delayed, and physically challenged students into regular school classrooms. School nurses must work closely with families, teachers, and the community to provide these children with the special care they need while at school—and these needs can be significant.

School nurses work closely with teachers to incorporate health concepts into the curriculum. They endorse the teaching of basic hygiene, such as hand washing following bathroom use and dental hygiene. School nurses encourage the inclusion of age-appropriate nutritional information in school curricula and healthful foods in cafeteria and vending machine choices. They conduct vision and hearing screenings and make referrals to qualified physicians or other health care providers when routine screenings identify problems outside the nurses' scope of practice.

School nurses must be prepared to handle both routine illnesses of children and adolescents and emergencies. One of their major concerns is safety. Accidents are the leading cause of death in children of all ages, yet accidents are preventable. Prevention includes both protection from obvious hazards and education of teachers, parents, and students about how to avoid accidents. School nurses work with teachers, school bus drivers, cafeteria workers, and other school employees to provide the safest possible environment. When accidents occur, first aid for minor injuries and emergency care for more severe ones are additional skills school nurses use. Detection of evidence of child neglect and abuse is a sensitive but essential aspect of school nursing. School violence or bullying can also result in injury, absenteeism, and anxiety.

School nursing is a complex and multifaceted field that is constantly expanding. It represents a challenge for those nurses who choose it as a career.

Hospice and palliative care nursing

Hospice and palliative care nursing is a rapidly developing specialty in nursing dedicated to improving the experience of seriously ill and dying patients and their families. It was initiated as a result of a $28 million study by the Robert Wood Johnson Foundation in the mid-1990s. This study found that there were significant problems associated with the care of seriously ill and dying patients. The problems reported included poor communication, continued aggressive treatment after treatment was no longer effective, and high levels of pain. The study pointed out the "overriding need to change the kind of care dying Americans receive" (Last Acts Task Force, 1998, p. 109).

According to the ANA document *Scope and Standards of Hospice and Palliative Care Nursing Practice,* "Hospice and palliative care nursing reflects a holistic philosophy of care implemented across the life span and across diverse health settings . . . . The goal of hospice and palliative nursing is to promote the patient's quality of life through the relief of suffering along the illness trajectory, through the death of the patient, and into the bereavement period of the family" (ANA, 2002, p. 1). The ANA (2002) identified three major precepts underlying hospice and end-of-life care:

■ Persons are living until the moment of death.
■ Coordinated care should be offered by a variety of professionals, with attention to the physical, psychological, social, and spiritual needs of patients and their families.
■ Care should be sensitive to patient/family diversity or cultural beliefs.

Nursing curricula traditionally have not included extensive content to prepare nurses to deal effectively with dying patients and their families. The American Association of Colleges of Nursing (AACN) used the three precepts identified above to develop a document titled "Peaceful Death." This document identifies the competencies needed by baccalaureate nurses for palliative/hospice care and outlines where these competencies can fit into nursing curricula. You can review this document and other resources online (www.aacn.nche.edu/Publications/ deathfin.htm).

End-of-life care is largely the responsibility of nurses. In recognition of this fact, the ANA formulated a position statement regarding the promotion of comfort and relief of pain of dying patients, reinforcing the nurse's obligation to promote comfort and ensure aggressive efforts to relieve pain and suffering (American Nurses Association, 2003). This position statement can be found online (www.nursingworld.org/readroom/position/ethics/etpain.htm).

Hospice and palliative care nurses work in a variety of settings, including inpatient palliative/hospice units, free-standing residential hospices, community-based or home hospice programs, ambulatory palliative care programs, teams of consultants in palliative care, and skilled nursing facilities. Both generalist and advanced practice nurses work in palliative care. The certifying agency is the National Board for the Certification of Hospice and Palliative Nurses (NBCHPN). By 2004 more than 7400 registered nurses had become certified hospice and palliative nurses.

With the aging population, end-of-life needs are expected to increase. Every nurse, not just specialists in hospice and palliative care, should be familiar with the precepts of palliative and end-of-life nursing care.

Case management nursing

Case management is a dynamic, challenging, and growing field in nursing, having evolved in the mid-1980s as a way of managing health care costs and patient **length of stay (LOS).** It involves systematic collaboration with patients, their significant others, and their health care providers to coordinate high-quality health care services in a cost-effective manner with positive patient outcomes. Another aspect of nursing case management includes decreasing fragmentation and duplication of care (Tahan, Huber, and Downey, 2006). The case manager is the person responsible for this process, and although registered nurses are not the only professionals who act as case managers, they are uniquely prepared for this role. Because of their broad educational backgrounds, skill in arranging and providing patient education and referrals, orientation toward holistic care and health promotion, and communication and interpersonal skills, nurses are particularly well suited for case management.

Depending on the case management model being used—and there are many—the nursing case manager may follow the patient from the diagnostic phase through hospitalization, rehabilitation, and back to home care. Through careful planning, every step of the patient's care can be coordinated in a timely manner.

One key to making case management work is the use of critical paths that include specific time lines and standard treatment protocols. A **critical path** is an abbreviated version of the case management plan and is used for daily decision making about patient care. It lists key nursing and medical interventions that should occur within a certain time line to ensure positive patient outcomes. Case management is considered successful if the patient is well enough for discharge within the length of stay directed by the diagnostic-related grouping. A sample critical path can be found on the Evolve website (www.evolve.elsevier.com/Chitty/professional/).

Although there are challenges in making the transition from caregiver to case manager, both patient satisfaction and nurse satisfaction are high with the one-on-one relationship fostered with case management. Patients like the security of having one familiar person managing their care, and a nursing case manager has the satisfaction of coordinating a patient's care from beginning to end. Certification in nursing case management is offered by the American Nurses Credentialing Center. You may also hear case management nursing referred to as "care management nursing," a name more consistent with nursing's values.

Telehealth nursing

Telehealth is defined as "the removal of time and distance barriers for the delivery of health care services and related health care activities through telecommunication technology" (American Nurses Association, 1999, p. 1). **Telehealth nursing** is generally not a separate nursing role because few nurses use telehealth exclusively in their practices. Rather, it is most often found as a part of almost every other nursing role. At the most basic level, nurses have always used the telephone to communicate with physicians, patients, and other health care providers. Today's technologies have evolved far beyond the telephone to include bedside computers, interactive audio and video linkages, teleconferencing, real-time transmission of patients' diagnostic and clinical data, and more.

The use of telehealth expands access to health care for underserved populations and individuals in both urban and rural areas. It also serves to reduce the sense of professional isolation experienced by those who work in such areas and may assist in attracting and retaining health care professionals in remote areas (American Nurses Association, 1999).

Practical uses of telehealth technology include faxing a change in a patient's drug order; consulting by telephone with other care providers; accessing a lab report from a remote site with a wireless, handheld computer; counseling patients on medications, diet, activity, or other therapy over the telephone or computer; or participating in interactive video sessions such as an interdisciplinary team consultation about a complex patient issue. Although the fundamentals of basic nursing practice do not change because nurses use telehealth technologies, its use may require adaptation or modification of usual procedures. In addition, telenurses must develop competence in the use of each new type of telehealth technology, and these may change rapidly. The American Nurses Association identified *Competencies for Telehealth Technologies in Nursing* (1999) to assist nurses to evaluate and guide their practice.

Numerous legal and regulatory issues surround nursing care delivered through telehealth technologies. The *Online Journal of Nursing Issues* has posted a comprehensive article enumerating these (www.nursingworld.org/ojin/topic16/tpc16_3.htm). The American Association of Ambulatory Care Nurses (2004) has developed practice standards for this emerging specialty to define and describe telehealth nursing practice and outline expectations for the telehealth nurse.

You can learn more about telehealth, an area of growing interest in nursing and other health professions, as well as some controversy, from the Association of Telemedicine Service Providers (www.atsp.org), from the American Telemedicine Association (www.atmeda.org), and from the American Academy of Ambulatory Care Nursing (www.aaacn.org).

Faith community nursing

Interest in spirituality and its relation to wellness and healing in recent years prompted the development of a practice area known as **faith community nursing**. This area of nursing, formerly termed parish nursing, takes a holistic approach to healing that involves partnerships between congregations, their pastoral staffs, and health care providers. Since its development in the Chicago area in the 1980s by a hospital chaplain, Dr. Granger E. Westberg, faith community nursing has spread rapidly and now includes more than 5000 nurses in paid and volunteer positions across the country (Abuelouf, 1998). According to the American Nurses Association definition:

> Faith community nursing is the specialized practice of professional nursing that focuses on the intentional care of the spirit as part of the process of promoting holistic health and preventing or minimizing illness in a faith community (American Nurses Association, 2005, p. 1).

The spiritual dimension is central to faith community nursing practice. The nurse's own spiritual journey is an essential aspect of this nursing role. Faith community nursing is based on the belief that spiritual health is central to well-being and influences a person's entire being.

Faith community nurses serve as members of the ministry staff or clergy of a church or other faith community. They practice independently, within the legal scope of the individual state's nurse practice act. Roles of the faith community nurse include health educator and counselor, advocate for health services, referral agent, coordinator of volunteer health ministers, developer of support groups, and integrator of spiritual practices and health. The Interview on p. 19 provides a discussion with a faith community nurse who describes her calling and her practice.

As faith community nursing has evolved, so have the standards for minimum preparation for nurses entering the specialty. Present preferred preparation includes a baccalaureate or higher degree in nursing, including preparation in community nursing, experience as an RN using the nursing process, knowledge of the health care assets of the community, specialized knowledge of the spiritual beliefs and practices of the faith community, and knowledge and skills to implement *Faith Community Nursing: Scope and Standards of Practice* (American Nurses Association, 2005, p. 5). This document, which sets forth the responsibilities for which faith community nurses

 interv**iew**   *Amy Corder, RN, MSN, CRRN*

Faith Community Nurse

Interviewer: Describe a typical day in your practice.

Corder: There is no "typical" day. Every day is different, which is what I love about faith community nursing. There are many aspects of my work, a number of which are not usually thought of as nursing. I help the congregation understand the interaction and connection between body, mind, and spirit. This is important because unhealthy behaviors or emotions often affect us physically in harmful ways.

Interviewer: What is the focus of your practice?

Corder: One aspect is health maintenance, such as teaching nutrition and diet, dental health, medication management, blood pressure screenings, and the like. I also visit parishioners in their homes, mostly older adults. Recently I visited a lady with a stasis ulcer on her leg. After my assessment and much discussion, she agreed to let me make a referral to a wound specialist. I don't do invasive procedures like a home health nurse might do. My focus is in the role of teaching, counseling, supporting, and often just encouraging people about how to improve their lives physically, mentally, and spiritually both within the congregation and the community.

Interviewer: What has surprised you about faith community nursing?

Corder: It surprised me how much writing I do. I am frequently asked to write an article for a newsletter or a small local paper about my current programs or about what I do as a faith community nurse. I also make a lot of presentations, which takes some research. I sure didn't appreciate writing all of those papers in school, but now I'm glad because it gave me confidence in my writing and research skills.

Interviewer: How did you prepare yourself to be a faith community nurse?

Corder: By searching and establishing my own spiritual foundation and having an open mind and heart, in order to hear God's calling. Faith community nursing is a calling by God. I do not believe you can be totally effective in assisting others in discovering and improving their spirituality for better health unless you have achieved a certain amount of spiritual awareness within your own life. Education-wise, I have a BSN and a master's degree in gerontological nursing. I have primarily worked in the areas of rehabilitation nursing and long-term care, which has prepared me well for what I do.

Interviewer: What is the most challenging part of your work?

Corder: The most challenging part of my work is learning about the philosophy of health ministry and faith community nursing and applying it to my practice. Although faith community nursing has been around for 12 to 15 years, it is still a relatively new field. I am the first faith community nurse for my congregation, and there are fewer than a dozen other faith community nurses in our community, although that number is growing. This is an exciting time for our congregation as we explore the role of health ministry and faith community nursing together.

are accountable and reflects the values and priorities of the specialty, can be obtained from the American Nurses Association. Certification is not yet available for faith community nurses.

Informatics nursing

Another exciting specialty area evolving in nursing is nursing informatics (NI). The **informatics nurse** combines nursing science with information management science and computer science to manage information nurses need and to make that information accessible. This field encompasses the full range of activities that focus on information handling in nursing (American Nurses Association, 2001) and assists nurses to carry out the work of nursing efficiently and effectively. Because it "has been estimated that nurses spend as much as 50 percent of their time gathering, coordinating, and documenting information" (Meadows, 2002), it is easy to understand the potential benefits of streamlining this process. Benefits of clinical information systems include improved patient safety, reduction in variability of care, improved communication, improved clinical decision making, and increased efficiency of staff.

In contrast to computer science systems analysts, informatics nurses must clearly understand the information they handle and how other nurses will use it. Nursing knowledge is specialized and must be accessible by nurse users; otherwise, it is useless in improving patient care. Complex information systems are more likely to fail when end-users are not consulted during the planning and design process (American Nurses Association, 2001). Because they are nurses themselves, informatics nurses are best able to understand the needs of nurses who use the systems and can design them with the needs, skills, and time constraints of those nurses in mind.

Informatics nurses may work in clinical areas, ensuring that the direct caregiver nurse is provided with complete and accurate information about patients' health needs and nursing care requirements. They may also practice in non-clinical areas such as nursing education or administration, where they design ways to make information needed by teachers, students, and managers easily accessible. In addition to practicing in hospitals and universities, informatics nurses also work in the military, health maintenance organizations, and research settings.

All nurses must be prepared to use informatics to communicate, manage knowledge, mitigate error, and support decision making. This is considered so important that it is one of the five core competencies identified in the Institute of Medicine's 2003 report, *Health Professions Education: A Bridge to Quality*. Information technology can help nurses deliver more effective care in a number of ways. Some examples include computerizing a nursing document or system; writing a program to support nursing care of patients; developing an interactive video disc system for educational purposes; helping nurse managers develop systems to use nursing resources effectively (such as people, money, supplies); or designing systems to collect and aggregate clinical data so they can be analyzed to assess the cost and outcomes of nursing care.

As a minimum, nurses specializing in informatics should have a bachelor's degree in nursing and additional knowledge and experience in the field of informatics. Advanced practice in nursing informatics requires preparation at the graduate level in nursing (American Nurses Association, 2001). Certification for informatics nurses is available through the American Nurses Credentialing Center.

NURSING OPPORTUNITIES REQUIRING HIGHER DEGREES

Many registered nurses choose to pursue roles that require a master's degree, doctoral degree, or specialized education in a specific area. These roles include clinical nurse specialists, nurse managers, nurse executives in hospital settings, nurse educators (whether in clinical or academic settings), nurse anesthetists, nurse-midwives, and other advanced practice nurses.

Nurse Educators

In 2004, 48,666 registered nurses worked in nursing education (U.S. Department of Health and Human Services, 2005). These nurses teach in LPN/LVN programs, diploma programs, associate degree programs, baccalaureate and higher-degree programs, and programs preparing nursing assistants. Nurse educators in accredited schools of nursing offering a baccalaureate or higher degree must hold a minimum of a master's degree in nursing; in 2006 43.2 percent had doctoral degrees in nursing or other fields (National League for Nursing, 2006).

Most nursing faculty (95.9 percent) are women, and 10.7 percent are members of minority groups (National League for Nursing, 2006.). In 2005-2006 10.7 percent of master's students chose nursing education to prepare for a teaching role, compared with 3.5 percent in 2002-2003 (American Association of Colleges of Nursing, 2006). This represents an increase which, if continued, will reverse the downward trend of the past decade and may ameliorate concerns about a critical shortage of nursing faculty in the future.

Advanced Practice Nursing (APN)

Advanced practice nurse (APN) is an umbrella term applied to a registered nurse who has met advanced educational and clinical practice requirements beyond the 2 to 4 years of basic nursing education demanded of all registered nurses. Advanced practice nursing is growing rapidly, with approximately 240,461 of registered nurses (8.3 percent) in 2004 having the education and credentials to work as advanced practice nurses, up from 196,279 in 2000. This growth is spurred by several factors, including increased demand for primary care coupled with increased specialization of physicians and heightened demand for efficient and cost-effective treatment.

Patient acceptance of advanced practice nurses is high. A growing body of evidence is accumulating that confirms that advanced practice nurses deliver high-quality care, exceeding that delivered by physicians on several measures. It is estimated that 60 to 80 percent of primary and preventive care traditionally performed by physicians can be safely done by advanced practice nurses.

There are four categories of advanced practice nurses: nurse practitioner, clinical nurse specialist, certified nurse-midwife, and certified registered nurse anesthetist. Figure 1-7 shows the breakdown of advanced practice nurses by area of specialty in 2004.

Nurse practitioner (NP)

Opportunities for nurses in expanded roles in health care have created a boom in **nurse practitioner (NP)** education. There were 150 nurse practitioner education programs in 1992. By 2005 this number had risen to 334 (AACN, 2006). These programs grant master's degrees or postmaster's certificates and prepare nurses to sit for national certification examinations as nurse practitioners. The length of the programs varies, depending on prior education of the students. In 2004 there were 141,209 nurse practitioners in the United States. This figure includes the 14,699 who are also clinical nurse specialists (U.S. Department of Health and Human Services, 2005).

States vary in the amount of practice autonomy accorded to nurse practitioners. According to the annual survey conducted by *The Nurse Practitioner: The American Journal of Primary Health Care* (Phillips, 2006), there are 27 states in which the board of nursing has sole authority in NP scope of practice. In those states there are no statutory or regulatory requirements for physician collaboration, direction, or supervision. An additional 14 states require some physician collaboration. Physician supervision is required in 5 states. In 5 states, the scope of NP practice is determined jointly by the board of nursing and the board of medicine (Phillips, 2006). Nurse practitioners beginning practice in a new state should check the status of the advanced practice laws in that state before making firm commitments because some states still place limitations on NP independence.

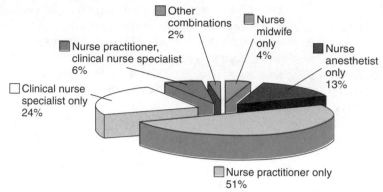

Figure 1-7
Advanced practice nurses by specialty area, March 2004. (Data from U.S. Department of Health and Human Services, Health Resources and Services Administration: *Preliminary findings: 2004 national sample survey of registered nurses*, Washington, DC, 2005, Government Printing Office, p 7 [website]: http://bhpr.hrsa.gov/healthworkforce/reports/rnpopulation/preliminaryfindings.htm.)

Nurse practitioners work in clinics, nursing homes, their own offices, or physicians' offices. Others work for hospitals, health maintenance organizations (HMOs), or private industry. Most nurse practitioners choose a specialty area such as adult, family, or pediatric health care. They are qualified to handle a wide range of basic health problems. These nurses can perform physical examinations, take medical histories, diagnose and treat common acute and chronic illnesses and injuries, order and interpret laboratory tests and x-ray films, and counsel and educate clients (Figure 1-8).

In 2006 nurse practitioners could legally write prescriptions in 37 states with some physician supervision, whereas in 13 states and the District of Columbia, nurse practitioners could prescribe independent of physician involvement (Phillips, 2006). Some NPs are independent practitioners and can be directly reimbursed by Medicare, Medicaid, and military and private insurers for their work.

Clinical nurse specialist (CNS)

Clinical nurse specialists (CNSs) work in a variety of settings, including hospitals, clinics, nursing homes, their own offices, private industry, home care, and health maintenance organizations.

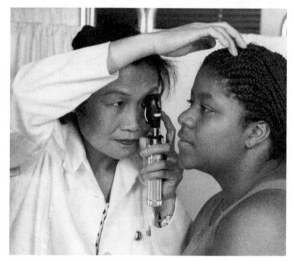

Figure 1-8
A nurse practitioner examines her patient. *(Photo by Fielding Freed.)*

These nurses hold advanced nursing degrees—master's or doctoral—and are qualified to handle a wide range of physical and mental health problems. They are experts in a particular field of clinical practice, such as mental health, gerontology, cardiac care, cancer care, community health, or neonatal health, and they perform health assessments, make diagnoses, deliver treatment, and develop quality control methods. Additionally, clinical nurse specialists work in consultation, research, education, and administration. Direct reimbursement to some clinical nurse specialists is possible through Medicare, Medicaid, and military and private insurers. In 2004 there were 72,521 clinical nurse specialists in the United States, including 14,689 who were both nurse practitioners and clinical nurse specialists (U.S. Department of Health and Human Services, 2005).

Certified nurse-midwife (CNM)

In 2004 there were an estimated 13,684 nurse-midwives in the United States (U.S. Department of Health and Human Services, 2005), 93.7 percent of whom are nationally certified. **Certified nurse-midwives (CNMs)** provide well-woman care and attend to or assist in childbirth in various settings, including hospitals, birthing centers, and homes. They are prepared in formal nurse-midwife courses of at least 9 months in length. Of the 43 nurse-midwife programs accredited by the American College of Nurse-Midwives, 39 offer a master's degree, accounting for an average of 1.5 years of specialized education beyond basic nursing education (American College of Nurse-Midwives, 2006).

Births attended by nurse-midwives are among the safest. According to the National Center for Health Statistics, certified nurse-midwives attended 310,342 births in 2003. This represented more than 10 percent of all spontaneous vaginal births in the United States in 2003 (Martin, Hamilton, Sutton et al, 2005). Historically, births attended by nurse-midwives have had half the national average rates for cesarean sections and higher rates of successful vaginal births after a previous cesarean, both considered measures of high-quality obstetrical care. A study published in the June 2003 edition of the *American Journal of Public Health* documents that "low-risk patients receiving collaborative midwifery care had birth success rates comparable to those who saw only

physicians, with fewer interventions, more options, and lower cost to the health care system" (Jackson, Lang, Swartz et al, 2003, p. 1003).

Certified nurse-midwives have the widest prescriptive rights of all advanced practice nurses. As of 2004, certified nurse-midwives were able to prescribe medication in 48 states and 3 jurisdictions, including the District of Columbia (American College of Nurse-Midwives, 2006).

Because of patient acceptance and a good safety record, deliveries attended by nurse-midwives have increased every year since 1975 (American College of Nurse-Midwives, 2006) and are expected to increase in the future.

Certified registered nurse anesthetist (CRNA)

There were 32,523 certified registered nurse anesthetists (CRNAs) in the United States in 2004 (U.S. Department of Health and Human Services, 2005). Nurse anesthetists administer about 65 percent of the more than 26 million anesthetics given to patients each year and are the only anesthesia providers in nearly one third of U.S. hospitals. Collaborating with physician anesthesiologists or often working independently, they are found in a variety of settings, including operating suites; obstetrical delivery rooms; the offices of dentists, podiatrists, ophthalmologists, and plastic surgeons; and ambulatory surgical facilities (American Association of Nurse Anesthetists, 2006).

To become a certified registered nurse anesthetist, nurses must complete 2 to 3 years of specialized education in a master's program beyond the required 4-year bachelor's degree. There are 99 accredited nurse anesthesia programs in the United States, ranging from 24 to 36 months in length. Nurse anesthetists must also meet national certification and recertification requirements. According to the American Association of Nurse Anesthetists, 49 percent of the nation's CRNAs are men, as compared with only 5.7 percent in all nursing fields (American Association of Nurse Anesthetists, 2006).

The safety of care delivered by CRNAs is well established. Although all anesthesia care today is safer than in the past, few specialists can claim, as nurse anesthetists can, that their professional liability premiums are 39 percent lower across the country than 15 years ago (American Association of Nurse Anesthetists, 2006).

Issues in advanced practice nursing

Each year in January, *The Nurse Practitioner: The American Journal of Primary Health Care* publishes an update on legislation affecting advanced practice nursing. Over the years, advances have been made toward removing the barriers to autonomous practice for advanced practice nurses (APNs) in many, but not all, states.

In the past, substantial barriers to APN autonomy existed because of the overlap between traditional medical and nursing functions. A decade ago, the picture was considerably less optimistic than it is now. The issue of APNs practicing autonomously was a politically charged arena, with organized medicine positioned firmly against all efforts of nurses to be recognized as independent health care providers receiving direct reimbursement for their services. Organized nursing, however, persevered. Nurses, through their professional associations, continued their efforts to change laws that limit the scope of nursing practice. Their efforts were aided by the fact that numerous published studies validated the safety, cost-efficiency, and high patient acceptance of APN care.

According to the 2006 *Nurse Practitioner* update (Phillips, 2006), both the public and legislators at state and national levels have begun to appreciate the role that advanced practice nurses have played in increasing the efficiency and availability of primary health care delivery while reducing costs. However, opposition to APN autonomy persists. Roadblocks to full practice autonomy continue, primarily because of the resistance of organized physicians in spite of positive patient outcome data. Although progress has been made, there remains the need for all APNs to continue to work with their professional organizations to promote legislation mandating full autonomy. Until the U.S. Congress approves legislation to provide primary health care for all citizens and makes provisions for advanced practice nurses to share fully in the provision of that care, the practice parameters of advanced practice nurses are at the mercy of the various state legislatures.

EMPLOYMENT OUTLOOK IN NURSING

The Bureau of Labor Statistics, a division of the U.S. Department of Labor, is confident about nursing's overall employment prospects in the near and distant future. According to the Bureau (U.S. Department of Labor, 2006), nurses can expect their employment opportunities to grow "much faster than the average" (meaning a 21 to 35 percent increase) through the year 2014. They estimate that during this time, 1.2 million RNs will be needed to meet growing patient needs and to replace retiring nurses. Registered nurses were second on the Bureau's list of the 30 occupations with the largest projected job growth in the years 2005-2014 (U.S. Department of Labor, 2006). Several factors are fueling this growth, including technological advances and the increasing emphasis on primary care. The aging of the nation's population also has a significant impact, because older people are more likely to require medical care. As aging nurses retire, many additional job openings will result.

Opportunities in hospitals, traditionally the largest employers of nurses, will grow more slowly than those in community-based sectors. The most rapid hospital-based growth is projected to occur in outpatient facilities, such as same-day surgery centers, rehabilitation programs, and outpatient cancer centers.

Home health care positions are expected to increase the fastest of all. This is in response to the expanding elderly population's needs and the preference for and cost-effectiveness of home care. Furthermore, technological advances are making it possible to bring increasingly complex treatments into the home.

Another expected area of high growth will occur in assisted living and nursing home care; this is primarily in response to the larger number of frail elderly in their 80s and 90s requiring long term care. As hospitals come under greater pressure to decrease the average patient length of stay (LOS), nursing home admissions will increase, as will growth in long-term rehabilitation units (U.S. Department of Labor, 2006).

An additional factor influencing employment patterns for registered nurses is the tendency for sophisticated medical procedures to be performed in physicians' offices, clinics, ambulatory surgical centers, and other outpatient settings. Registered nurses' expertise will be needed to care for patients undergoing procedures formerly performed only in hospital settings.

Advanced practice nurses can also expect to find themselves in higher demand for the foreseeable future. The evolution of integrated health care networks focusing on primary care and health maintenance and pressure for cost-effective care are ideal conditions for advanced nursing practice.

Nursing Salaries

Salaries in the nursing profession vary widely according to practice setting, level of preparation and credentials, experience, and region of the country. The latest survey of *The Registered Nurse Population: March 2004* (U.S. Department of Health and Human Services, 2005) showed positive signs in terms of salaries for registered nurses, however, the seventh annual nationwide survey conducted by the journal *Nursing 2006* indicated that salaries and benefits and leveled off in some regions (Mee, 2006).

Although salaries have generally increased nationwide, discussing salary trends from a national perspective is often misleading. For instance, salaries in urban areas are much higher than those in rural communities and so is the cost of living. Readers should bear this in mind when reviewing these figures. Regional salaries tend to be more realistic measures. Figure 1-9

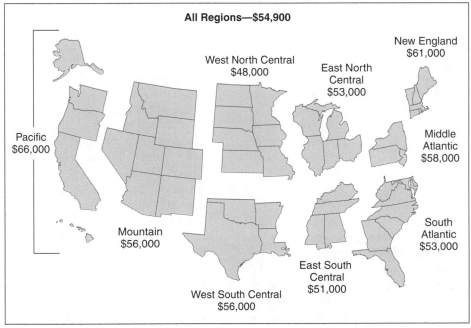

Figure 1-9
Average annual salaries of full-time registered nurses by region. (Data from Mee CL: Salary survey, *Nursing 2006* 36(10):46-51, 2006.)

shows the average annual salaries of staff nurses in each geographical area of the United States in January 2006. Regional variations are apparent. It should be noted that these figures do not include salaries of advanced practice nurses, whose earnings are higher than the averages shown for staff nurses.

Nationwide in 2005, the average salary of nurse practitioners was $74,812 (Tumolo and Rollet, 2005). For certified nurse-midwives, the average in 2004, the latest year for which figures are available, was $70,000 (American College of Nurse Midwives, 2004). Certified registered nurse anesthetists in 2004 averaged $140,000, the highest of any advanced practice specialty group (Horton, 2006). Clearly, additional preparation and responsibility increase earning potential.

Most of the wage growth for nurses appears early in their careers and tapers off in time. In 2000 staff RNs employed full-time in nursing who had been working for 5 years typically earned salaries 15 to 17 percent higher than those newly entering the field. However, these same nurses earned only 1 to 3 percent less than nurses who graduated 15 to 20 years earlier (U.S. Department of Health and Human Services, 2001). This decreased potential for salary improvements may account for nurses leaving patient care for additional education and/or other careers in nursing or outside the profession, an issue that must be addressed to improve retention in the profession.

SUMMARY OF *Key Points*

- There are more than 2.9 million registered nurses in the United States, and over 2.4 million are actively practicing. Fewer than 60 percent work full-time.
- Approximately 56.2 percent of working nurses are employed in hospitals, a traditional setting for nursing practice, but one that will see dramatic changes as health care in the United States continues to become more community-based.

- A continuing trend is the growth of opportunities for nurses in practice settings outside the traditional hospital.
- Increased use of advanced practice nurses as providers of primary care may be part of the solution to the U.S. health care crisis that is caused by the aging of the baby boom generation, the fast-growing group of frail elderly, technological advances, and cost-containment measures in the health care sector.
- Advanced practice nurses are capable of delivering high-quality care to many segments of the population not currently receiving health care or receiving substandard care.
- If the nation is to benefit from the services of advanced practice nurses, legal barriers to their practice must be removed through the political action of organized nursing and politically active nurses.
- Government projections are for the demand for nurses, including advanced practice nurses, to increase through the year 2014 and beyond.

CRITICAL THINKING QUESTIONS

1. What characteristics do today's nurses have in common, and in what ways do they differ?
2. Think of the areas of nursing that interest you most. How do your personal and professional qualifications compare with the characteristics needed in the roles discussed in this chapter?
3. Interview nurses in various practice settings, especially those not covered in this chapter. Find out how they prepared for their positions, what their daily activities are, and what they find most challenging and rewarding about their work.
4. Call the nurse recruiter or personnel office of a nearby hospital and inquire about salaries and other benefits for entry-level and advanced practice nursing positions. How do they compare with those listed in this chapter? Is there a clinical ladder program? How does it work?

5. Interview an advanced practice nurse working in your community. What does he or she see as the major barriers to practice?
6. Contact your state nurses' association to find out what legislative initiatives are being undertaken to remove barriers to full APRN practice in your state.

REFERENCES

Abuelouf A: Community health ministry: meeting many needs, *Tennessee Nurse* 61(6):22, 31, 1998.

Aiken LH, Clarke SP, Cheung RB et al: Educational levels of hospital nurses and surgical patient mortality, *JAMA* 290(12):1617-1623, 2003.

American Association of Ambulatory Care Nurses: *Telehealth nursing practice administration and practice standards,* ed 3, Pitman, NJ, 2004, American Association of Ambulatory Care Nurses.

American Association of Colleges of Nursing: *Enrollment and graduations in baccalaureate and graduate programs in nursing, 2005-2006,* Washington, DC, 2006, American Association of Colleges of Nursing.

American Association of Nurse Anesthetists: *Nurse anesthetists at a glance,* 2006 (website): http://www.aana.com/crna/ataglance.asp.

American College of Nurse-Midwives: Selected results of ACNM compensation and benefits survey, 2005 (website: http://www.midwife.org/siteFiles/education/ACNM_salary_survey_2005.pdf.

American College of Nurse-Midwives: *Basic facts about certified nurse-midwives,* 2006 (website): http://www.midwife.org/display.cfm?id=368.

American Nurses Association: *Competencies for telehealth technologies in nursing,* Washington, DC, 1999, American Nurses Association.

American Nurses Association: *Scope and standards of nursing informatics practice,* Washington, DC, 2001, American Nurses Association.

American Nurses Association: *Scope and standards of hospice and palliative care nursing practice,* Washington, DC, 2002, American Nurses Publishing.

American Nurses Association: Position statement on pain management and control of pain in dying patients, Washington, DC, 2003, (website): http://www.nursingworld.org/readroom/position/ethics/etpain.htm.

American Nurses Association [in collaboration with the Health Ministries Association]: *Faith Community Nursing: Scope and standards of practice,* Washington, DC, 2005, American Nurses Association.

American Nurses Association and National Association of School Nurses: *Scope and standards of school nursing practice,* Silver Spring, Md, 2005, American Nurses Association.

Hardin C: Personal communication, 2006.

Horovitz B, McCoy K: Nurse shortage puts school kids at risk, *USA Today,* Dec 14, 2005, p A-1.

Horton S: Personal communication, 2006.

Institute of Medicine: Health professions education: a bridge to quality, Washington, DC, 2003, National Academy of Sciences.

Jackson DJ, Lang JM, Swartz WH et al: Outcomes, safety, and resource utilization in a collaborative care birth center program, *Am J Public Health* 93(6):999-1006, 2003.

Last Acts Task Force: National policy statements on end of life care: precepts of palliative care, *J Palliative Med* 1(2):109-112, 1998.

Martin JA, Hamilton BE, Sutton PD et al: Births: final data for 2003, *National vital statistics reports,* 54:2, Hyattsville, Md, 2005, National Center for Health Statistics.

Meadows G: Nursing informatics: an evolving specialty, *Nurs Econ* 20(6):300-301, 2002.

Mee CL: Salary survey, *Nursing 2006* 36(10): 46-51, 2006.

National Association of School Nurses: *Definition of school nursing,* 2006 (website): http://www.nasn.org/Default.aspx?tabid=57.

National League for Nursing: Nurse educators 2006: a report of the faculty census survey of RN and graduate programs, New York, 2006, National League for Nursing.

Phillips SJ: Eighteenth annual legislative update: a comprehensive look at the legislative issues affecting advanced nursing practice, *Nurse Practitioner: Am J Prim Health Care* 31(1):6-11, 2006.

Tahan HA, Huber DL, Downey WT: Case managers' roles and functions, *Lippincott's Case Management* 11(1):4-22, 2006.

Tumolo J, Rollet J: 2005 Salary survey results: a place at the table, Advance for Nurse Practitioners (website): http://nurse-practitioners.advanceweb.com/common/editorial/editorial.aspx?CC=65135.

U.S. Department of Health and Human Services, Health Resources and Services Administration: The registered nurse population, March 2000: findings from the national sample survey of registered nurses, Washington, DC, 2001, Government Printing Office.

U.S. Department of Health and Human Services, Health Resources and Services Administration: *Projected supply, demand, and shortages of registered nurses: 2000-2020,* Washington, DC, 2002, Government Printing Office.

U.S. Department of Health and Human Services, Health Resources and Services Administration: *Preliminary findings: 2004 national sample survey of registered nurses,* Washington, DC, 2005, Government Printing Office.

U.S. Department of Labor, Bureau of Labor Statistics: *Occupational outlook handbook: 2006-07,* Washington, DC, 2006, Government Printing Office, (website): http://www.bls.gov/oco/ocos083.htm.

Vollman KM: My search to help patients breathe, *Reflections* 25(2):16-18, 1999.

Vollman KM: Nurse entrepreneurship: taking an invention from birth to the marketplace, *Clin Nurse Specialist* 18(2):68-71, 2004.

Vollman KM, Bander JL: Improved oxygenation utilizing a prone positioner in patients with acute respiratory distress syndrome, *Intensive Care Med* 22:1105-1111, 1996.

2

The History and Social Context of Nursing

Shielda Rodgers

HISTORICAL CONTEXT OF NURSING

The history of nursing has been tied to societal issues in every period of its development. From the work of Florence Nightingale in the Crimea in the mid-1800s to the present, the profession has been influenced by the social, political, and economic climate of the times as well as by technological advances and theoretical shifts in medicine and science. This chapter presents an overview of some of the highlights of nursing's history and several of its leaders as well as a discussion of current and past social forces that have shaped the discipline's course of development.

---

*The author wishes to acknowledge the contributions of Arlene W. Keeling and Kay K. Chitty in the preparation of this chapter.

Mid–Nineteenth-Century Nursing in England: The Influence of Florence Nightingale

Nursing's most notable early figure, **Florence Nightingale,** was born into the aristocratic social sphere of Victorian England in 1820. As a young woman, Nightingale (Figure 2-1) often felt stifled by her privileged and protected social position. As was customary at the time, aristocratic women visited and brought comfort to the sick and poor. The young Florence often accompanied her mother on these visits. At the age of 30, against her parents' wishes, Nightingale entered the nurses'

Figure 2-1
Florence Nightingale (1820-1910), founder of modern nursing. (*T. Cole, wood engraving, National Library of Medicine, Bethesda, Maryland.*)

training program in Kaiserswerth, Germany, where she spent 3 years learning the basics of nursing under the guidance of the Protestant deaconesses. She also studied under the Sisters of Charity in Paris.

On hearing of the horrible conditions suffered by the sick and wounded British soldiers in Turkey during the Crimean War, Nightingale took a small band of untrained women to the British hospital in Scutari. With great compassion and despite the opposition of military officers, Nightingale set about the task of organizing and cleaning the hospital and providing care to the wounded soldiers. Armed with excellent training in statistics, Nightingale gathered data on morbidity and mortality of the soldiers in Scutari. Using this supportive evidence, she effectively argued the case for reform of the entire British Army medical system.

Following the Crimean War, Nightingale founded the first training school for nurses at St. Thomas's Hospital in London (1860), which would become the model for nursing education in the United States. Perhaps her most famous publication is the 1859 *Notes on Nursing: What It Is and What It Is Not.* In this document Nightingale stated clearly for the first time that mastering a unique body of knowledge was required of those wishing to practice professional nursing (Nightingale, 1859).

Her publications, dedication to hospital reform, commitment to upgrading conditions for the sick and wounded in the military, and establishment of training schools for nurses all greatly affected the development of nursing in the United States as well as in her native England.

1861-1873: The American Civil War—An Impetus for "Trained Nursing"

At the onset of the Civil War there were no professional nurses available to tend the wounded and no organized system of medical care in either the Union or the Confederacy. Conditions on the battlefield and in military "hospitals" were horrible, with wounded and dying men lying in agony in filthy conditions (Young, 1959, p. 134).

Appeals for nurses were made, and women on both sides responded. Most significant perhaps was the response by the Catholic orders, particularly the Sisters of Charity, the Sisters of Mercy, and the Sisters of the Holy Cross, who had a long history of providing care for the sick (Wall, 1995). Doubtless the most skillful and devoted of the women who nursed in the Civil War, these religious sisters were highly disciplined, organized, and efficient.

On both the Union and the Confederate sides of the war, as well as on the war's Western Front, women arose to meet the needs of the sick and wounded. A number of leaders emerged, including Dorothea L. Dix, a long-time advocate for the mentally ill in pre-war years. She was appointed Superintendent of Women Nurses of the (Union) Army. In that position she was instrumental in creating a month-long training program at two New York hospitals for women who wished to serve. Thousands of women volunteered. Among the women who served the Union forces were several African-American women, including Sojourner Truth, a famous abolitionist, and Harriet Tubman, a former field slave who established the "underground railroad" and herself led numerous slaves to freedom. Another former slave, Susie King Taylor, first worked as a laundress but was called upon to assist as a nurse. She is noted for teaching soldiers, African-American and white, how to read and write.

Mary Ann ("Mother") Bickerdyke, an uneducated, widowed housekeeper known locally for her nursing ability, was sent to the Western Front to investigate the situation in the hospital camp at Cairo, Illinois, where she found appalling conditions. Bickerdyke had no official authority and was opposed by the camp surgeons, but this did not deter her efforts to bring order out of chaos and create clean, if not sanitary, conditions. Even though she was not a formally trained nurse she provided much needed nursing services and deserves her place in history.

Clara Barton is another well-known nursing pioneer. Barton, a Massachusetts woman who worked as a copyist in the U.S. Patent Office, began an independent campaign to provide relief for the soldiers. Appealing to the nation for supplies of woolen shirts, blankets, towels, lanterns, camp kettles, and other necessities (Barton, 1862), she established her own system of distribution, refusing to enlist in the military nurse corps headed by Dorothea Dix (Oates, 1994). Barton took a leave of absence from her patent job, and traveled to Culpeper, Virginia. At the scene of the battle, she set up a makeshift field hospital and cared for the wounded and dying. During this battle, Barton gained her famous title, "Angel of the Battlefield." Her efforts did not end with the war. Barton went on to found an organization whose name is synonymous with compassionate service: the American Red Cross.

The women of the South also responded by demonstrating a vast outpouring of support for their soldiers. Until the last months of 1861 and early 1862, Confederate hospitals were staffed by female volunteers or wounded soldiers. When the Confederate government assumed control, several women were appointed as superintendents of hospitals. Superintendent Sallie Thompkins, who had earlier established a private hospital in Richmond, Virginia, was commissioned a "captain of Cavalry, unassigned" by Confederate President Davis, and was the only woman in the Confederacy to hold military rank.

While thousands of women supported the war effort, only a few were appointed as matrons of hospitals. One of the earliest to be placed in charge was Phoebe Pember. Before her September 1862 assignment to Chimborazo Hospital, a sprawling government-run institution on the western boundary of Richmond, Virginia, the care was provided by "sick or wounded men, convalescing and placed in that position, however ignorant they might be—until strong enough for field duty" (Pember, 1959, p. 18).

The Civil War, for all of its destruction and horror, helped to advance the cause of professional nursing as these leaders, even though largely untrained, demonstrated dramatic improvements in care. The success in the reform of military hospitals would open the doors for reform of civilian hospital facilities throughout the country (Rosenberg, 1987).

1869-1900: Formal Education and Training Schools for Nurses

The move toward formal education and training for nurses grew following the Civil War. Support was garnered from physicians as well as the United States Sanitary Commission. At the American Medical Association meeting of 1869, Dr. Samuel Gross, chair of the Committee on the Training of Nurses, put forth three proposals regarding nursing training. The most important of these was the recommendation that large hospitals begin the process of developing training schools for nurses. Simultaneously, members of the United States Sanitary Commission, who had served during the war and learned its lessons, began to lobby for the creation of nursing schools (Donahue, 1996). Support for their efforts gained momentum as advocates of social reform reported the shockingly inadequate conditions that existed in many hospitals.

The first training schools for nurses and the feminization of nursing

The first three American training schools for nurses, modeled after Nightingale's famous school at St. Thomas's Hospital in London, opened in 1873. The so-called "famous trio" consisted of Bellevue Training School for Nurses in New York City, Connecticut Training School for Nurses in New Haven, and the Boston Training School for Nurses at Massachusetts General Hospital in Boston (Donahue, 1996). The first trained nurse in the United States, **Linda Richards,** graduated 1 year later.

The widely held Victorian belief in women's innate sensitivity and high morals led to the early requirement that applicants to these programs be female, for it was thought that only these feminine qualities could improve the quality of nursing care. Thus sensitivity, breeding, intelligence, and "ladylike" behavior, including submission to authority, were highly desired personal characteristics for applicants. The feminization of the profession took root with the accompanying effect of discrimination against men. The number of training schools increased steadily during the last decades of the nineteenth century, and by 1900 they played a critical role in providing hospitals with a stable, subservient, female workforce, as hospitals came to be staffed primarily by students (Figure 2-2).

Some schools in the North admitted a token number of African-American students to their programs. The training school at the New England Hospital for Women and Children agreed to admit one African-American and one Jewish student in each of their classes if they met all entrance qualifications. **Mary Eliza Mahoney** (Figure 2-3), the first African-American professionally educated nurse, received her training there. Historical Note 2-1 provides more information about Mahoney.

Figure 2-2
Nurses training in the bacteriological lab at Bellevue Hospital, New York City, circa 1900. (*The Bettman Archive, New York.*)

The development of separate schools for African-Americans seeking to become nurses soon emerged out of a necessity to provide care to the African-American population in a segregated American society. The first program established exclusively for training of African-American

Figure 2-3
Mary Eliza Mahoney (1845-1926), the first trained African-American nurse in the United States.

women in nursing was established at the Atlanta Baptist Female Seminary (later Spelman Seminary, now Spelman College) in Atlanta, Georgia, in 1886. This program was 2 years long and led to a diploma in nursing. Spelman closed its program in 1928 after graduating 117 nurses (Carnegie, 1995).

Male students were not allowed in the early nursing schools. The earliest school established exclusively for the training of men in nursing was the School for Male Nurses at the New York City Training School, established in 1886. The Mills College of Nursing at Bellevue Hospital was the second male school, founded in 1888. In 1898 the Alexian Brothers Hospital in Chicago established a nursing school to train males. They opened a second school in 1928 in St. Louis. These events are significant to nursing as they emphasize the separation of females and males that was common in this era.

The beginning of professional organizations for nurses

The 1893 Chicago World's Fair was an unlikely setting for a turning point in nursing's history. Several influential nursing leaders of the century, including Isabel Hampton (Robb), Lavinia Lloyd Dock, and Bedford Fenwick of Great Britain, gathered to share ideas and discuss issues pertaining

---

🏛 *Historical* NOTE 2-1

Mary Eliza Mahoney (1845-1926) is known as the first educated, professionally trained African-American nurse. She began her nursing training at the New England Hospital for Women and Children at age 33. An inscription in records from the New England Hospital reads "Mary E. Mahoney, first coloured girl admitted" (Miller, 1986, p. 19). The course of study was rigorous and being admitted was highly competitive. When Ms. Mahoney applied, there were 40 applicants; 18 were accepted for a probationary period, only half of those (9) were kept after probation, and only 3 received the diploma. Mahoney was one of the three. As was common in her day, her practice mainly consisted of private duty nursing with families in the Boston area. To celebrate her accomplishments and her status as the first African-American professional nurse, the Mary Mahoney Award was established by the National Association of Colored Graduate Nurses (NACGN) in 1935 with the first award given in 1936. This organization was later blended with the American Nurses Association. ■

to nursing education. Isabel Hampton (Robb) presented a paper "protesting the lack of uniformity in nursing school curricula and the inadequacy of nursing education." A paper by Florence Nightingale on the need for scientific training of nurses was read. Also at this event the precursor to the National League for Nursing, the American Society of Superintendents of Training Schools for Nurses, was formed to address issues in nursing education. The society changed its name in 1912 to the National League of Nursing Education (NLNE) and in 1952 became the **National League for Nursing (NLN).** This World's Fair had indeed been a pivotal point in nursing history.

In 1896 Isabel Hampton Robb founded the Nurses' Associated Alumnae of the United States and Canada, which in 1911 became officially known as the **American Nurses Association (ANA).** The initial mission of this group was to enhance collaboration among practicing nurses and educators.

At the close of the decade, in 1899, this same group of American nursing leaders, along with nursing leaders from abroad, collaborated with Bedford Fenwick of Britain to found the **International Council of Nurses (ICN).** The ICN was dedicated to uniting nursing organizations of all nations, and, fittingly, the first meeting was held at the World Exposition in Buffalo, New York, in 1901. At that meeting, a major topic of discussion was one that would dramatically change the practice of nursing: state registration of nurses.

Initially, minority group nurses were excluded from the ANA. After 1916, African-American nurses were admitted to membership through their state association but southern states and the District of Columbia barred their membership. African-American nurses recognized the need for their own professional organization to deal with the challenges they faced. Martha Franklin sent 1500 letters to African-American nurses and nursing schools across the country to gather support for this idea (Carnegie, 1995). In response, the **National Association for Colored Graduate Nurses** was formed in 1908 in New York with the

objectives of achieving higher professional standards, breaking down discriminatory practices faced by "Negro" nurses in schools of nursing and nursing organizations, and developing leadership among African-American nurses. The group dissolved in 1951 after deciding it had met these objectives and following the ANA's commitment of full support of minority groups as well as abolishment of discrimination in all aspects of the profession.

Visiting nursing: The Henry Street settlement

Early in the twentieth century, the young profession of nursing was called upon to address the ills caused by the influx of large numbers of immigrants who came seeking work in the factories of the Northeast. Because of poverty and overcrowded, primitive living conditions in inner city tenements, infectious disease became a serious problem. The **Henry Street Settlement** was established on New York's Lower East Side to address some of these problems. Its founder, Lillian Wald, obtained financial assistance from private sources and began what is considered the first formalized public health nursing practice. Her colleague Lavinia Dock (Figure 2-4) assisted Wald at the Henry Street Settlement. Services provided by visiting nurses and through clinic visits included caring for well babies, treating minor illnesses, preventing disease transmission, and providing health education to the neighborhood (Cherry and Jacob, 2005). Historical Note 2-2 describes another pioneering nurse, Margaret Sanger, whose work was inspired by the plight of immigrant women on the Lower East Side.

"A successful experiment": African-American clinic nursing in New York City

Tuberculosis was a major health problem in the teeming slums of the newly developing cities. Dr. Edward T. Devine, president of the Charity Organization Society, noted the high incidence of tuberculosis among New York City's African-American population. Aware of racial barriers and cultural resistance to seeking medical care, Dr. Devine determined that a "Negro" district

Figure 2-4
Lavinia Lloyd Dock (1858-1956), one of nursing's greatest early leaders, a radical feminist, and zealous suffragist. (*Reproduced with permission of the Special Collections, Milbank Memorial Library, Teachers College, Columbia University.*)

Historical NOTE 2-2

Margaret Sanger, a nurse who worked on the Lower East Side of New York City in 1912, was struck by the lack of knowledge of immigrant women about pregnancy and contraception. After witnessing the death of Sadie Sachs from a self-attempted abortion, Sanger was inspired to action by the tragedy and became determined to teach women about birth control. A radical activist in her early years, Sanger devoted the remainder of her life to the birth control movement and became a national figure in that cause (Kennedy, 1970). ■

Figure 2-5
Jessie Sleet Scales, a visionary African-American nurse, was among the first to bring community health nursing principles to the slums of New York City around 1900. (*Reproduced with permission of the E. M. Carnegie Collection, Archives of Hampton University.*)

nurse should be hired to work in the African-American community to persuade people to accept treatment. Jessie Sleet Scales (Figure 2-5), an African-American nurse who had been trained at Providence Hospital in Chicago, a hospital exclusively for "colored people," was chosen to work on a trial basis. Her report to the Charity Organization Society was published in the

American Journal of Nursing in 1901, titled "A Successful Experiment":

> I beg to render to you a report of the work done by me as a district nurse among the colored people of New York City during the months of October and November … I have visited forty-one families and made 156 calls in connection with these families, caring for nine cases of consumption, four cases of peritonitis, two cases of chickenpox, two cases of cancer, one case of diphtheria, two cases of heart disease, two cases of tumor, one case of gastric catarrh, two cases of pneumonia, four cases of rheumatism, and two cases of scalp wound. I have given baths, applied poultices, dressed wounds, washed and dressed newborn babies, cared for mothers … (Sleet, 1901, p. 729).

Jessie Sleet Scales later recommended to Lillian Wald that Elizabeth Tyler, a graduate of Freedmen's Hospital Training School for Nurses, work with African-American patients at the Henry Street Settlement. Working within the confines of a racist society, she and Tyler established the Stillman House, a branch of the Henry Street Settlement serving "colored people" in a small store on West 61st Street. For community health nursing, the addition of these pioneer African-American nurses to the ranks of the Henry Street Settlement signified activism, expansion, and growth. Despite the ever-present racial barriers and deplorable living and health conditions, these courageous young women succeeded in providing excellent nursing care to underserved families with spiraling health care needs.

War again creates the need for nurses: Spanish-American War—1898

In 1898 the United States Congress declared war on Spain, and once again, nursing had a major role to play. A physician, Anita M. McGee, rather than a nurse, was appointed head of the Hospital Corps, a group formed to recruit nurses. Encouraged by Isabel Hampton Robb and the fledgling Nurses' Associated Alumnae of the United States and Canada, McGee initially wanted only graduates of nurse training schools in the Hospital Corps

(Wall, 1995). It soon became apparent that this requirement could not be met. The typhoid fever epidemic created a greater need than anticipated, and as a result, others, including the Sisters of the Holy Cross and untrained African-American nurses who had had typhoid fever in the past, were accepted for service (Wall, 1995). Namahyyoke Curtis was employed as a contract nurse by the War Department during the Spanish-American War, making her the first trained African-American nurse in this capacity. This marked the first attempt to use only trained nurses in war, thereby setting the stage for the development of a permanent Army Nurse Corps (1901) and Navy Nurse Corps (1908) (Figure 2-6).

1900-1917: A Young Profession Faces New Challenges

A key event during this decade was the publication of the first edition of the *American Journal of Nursing* in October 1900. Those working to bring this project to fruition included nurse leaders Isabel Hampton Robb, Mary Adelaide Nutting, Lavinia L. Dock, Sophia Palmer, and Mary E. Davis. Sophia Palmer, director of nursing at

Figure 2-6

Red Cross nursing in the Spanish-American War, circa 1898. Nurses on deck of the hospital ship "Relief" near Cuba. (*National Library of Medicine, Bethesda, Maryland.*)

Rochester City Hospital, New York, was appointed as the first editor, with "the aim of the editors to present month by month the most useful facts, the most progressive thought and the latest news that the profession has to offer in the most attractive form that can be secured" (Palmer, 1900, p. 64). A second event of wide-sweeping importance was the institution of state licensure, which also occurred during the first decade of the twentieth century.

State licensure: A milestone for the profession

Early efforts at licensure were not well received. Following an educational campaign, the International Council of Nurses passed a resolution asking each country and state to provide for licensure of their nurses. As a result, state legislatures in North Carolina, New Jersey, New York, and Virginia passed what was termed **permissive licensure laws** for nursing in 1903. Nurses did not have to be registered to practice, but could not use the title of registered nurse unless they were registered. By 1923 all states required examinations for permissive licensure but these exams were not standardized (Cherry and Jacob, 2005). During the 1930s New York became the first state to have mandatory licensure with the mandate not taking full effect until 1947. In 1950 the National League for Nursing assumed responsibility for administering the first nation-wide State Board Test Pool Examination.

1917-1919: The Flu Epidemic and World War I Bring New Challenges to a Young Profession

Two significant events coincided in 1917 to challenge nursing: the United States entered World War I, and an influenza epidemic swept the country. The concept of using trained female nurses to care for soldiers had been proved in earlier wars; therefore when the United States entered the war in Europe, the **National Committee on Nursing** was formed (Dock and Stewart, 1920). This committee was chaired by Mary Adelaide Nutting, professor of Nursing and Health at Columbia University, and included Jane A. Delano, director of Nursing in the American Red Cross, among others. Charged with supplying an adequate number of trained nurses to U.S. Army hospitals abroad, the committee initiated a national publicity campaign to recruit young women to enter nurses training (Figure 2-7), established the Army School of Nursing with Annie Goodrich as dean, introduced college women to nursing in the Vassar Training Camp for Nurses, and began widespread public education in home nursing and hygiene through Red Cross nursing. Historical Note 2-3 describes the impact of the influenza epidemic on the nation and the profession.

Figure 2-7

A World War I Red Cross nursing poster, 1918. "Not one shall be left behind!" by James Montgomery Flagg, is typical of World War I recruitment posters. Nurses answered the call in record numbers. (*Collection of the Library of Congress.*)

On the home front, the flu epidemic of 1917 to 1919 increased the public's awareness of the necessity of public health nursing. Across the nation, the public health service, American Red Cross, and Visiting Nursing Associations mobilized to provide care for the thousands of citizens struck with influenza. In spring 1919, the second wave of the flu epidemic struck the East Coast and swept across the country. Although not as lethal as the first, the flu epidemic closed businesses, schools, and churches and increased demands for nursing services.

Figure 2-8
Mary Breckinridge, founder of the Frontier Nursing Service, on her way to visit patients in rural Kentucky. *(Used with permission of the Frontier Nursing Service, Wendover, Ky.)*

1920-1930: The Young Profession Makes Strides

By the time World War I ended, nursing had demonstrated its ability both to provide care to the war-wounded and to respond effectively to the influenza epidemic at home. In 1920 Congress passed a bill that provided nurses with military rank (Dock and Stewart, 1920). The 1920s also saw increased use of hospitals and an acceptance of the scientific basis of medicine.

Two other noteworthy events of the decade included the publication of the Goldmark Report, a study of nursing education (discussed in Chapter 7) that advocated the establishment of collegiate schools of nursing rather than hospital-based diploma programs, and establishment of programs in rural midwifery.

The Frontier Nursing Service

In 1925 Mary Breckinridge, a nurse and midwife, established the Kentucky Committee for Mothers and Babies, later to be known as the **Frontier Nursing Service (FNS)**. This service provided the first organized midwifery program in the United States. Nurses of the FNS worked in isolated rural areas in the Appalachian Mountains. They traveled by horseback to serve the health needs of the poverty-stricken mountain people (Figure 2-8).

FNS nurses delivered babies, provided prenatal and postnatal care, educated mothers and their families about nutrition and hygiene, and cared for the sick. Through this rural midwifery service, Breckinridge demonstrated that nurses could play a significant role in providing primary rural health care.

1931-1945: The Profession Responds to the Great Depression and World War II

With hospitals largely staffed by nursing students, most graduate nurses worked as private duty nurses in patients' homes. This changed with the Great Depression because many families could no longer afford nursing services. This forced many nurses into unemployment. In 1933 President Franklin D. Roosevelt established the Civil Works Administration (CWA) in which nurses participated by providing rural and school health services. They also took part in specific projects, such as conducting health surveys on communicable disease and nutrition of children (Fitzpatrick, 1975). Hospitals were affected by the economic plunge and were forced to close their schools of nursing. As a result, they no longer had a reliable, inexpensive student workforce just at the time there was a dramatic increase in the number of patients who needed charity care. The solution soon became apparent: unemployed graduate nurses, willing to work for minimum pay, were recruited to work in the hospitals rather than in private duty. This change in how hospitals were staffed had lasting implications for the profession.

The Social Security Act of 1935, another part of President Roosevelt's plans to bring the nation out of the Depression, enhanced the practice of public health nursing. One of its stated purposes was to strengthen public health services and to provide medical care for crippled children and the blind. With monies from this act, public health nursing became the major avenue for the provision of care to dependent mothers and children, the blind, and crippled children (Cherry and Jacob, 2005).

World War II: New opportunities for nursing

With the advent of World War II the nation's military once again found itself without an adequate supply of nurses. In response Congress enacted legislation to provide 1 million dollars for nursing education. The military and collegiate programs of nursing formed an alliance to train student nurses in what was known as the **Cadet Nurse Corps.** Students received tuition, books, a stipend, and a uniform in return for a promise to serve as nurses for the duration of the war in either civilian or military hospitals, the Indian Health Service, or public health facilities (Robinson and Perry, 2001). Approximately 124,000 nurses volunteered, graduated, and were certified for military services in the Army and Navy Nurse Corps during the years 1943-1948. Despite the segregation of the time, African-American collegiate programs as well as the National Association of Colored Graduate Nurses were active participants in the Cadet Nurse Corps.

1945-1960: The Rise of Hospitals— Bureaucracy, Science, and Shortages

After the war, further progress toward professionalization was made. In 1947 military nurses were awarded full commissioned officer status in both the Army and the Navy Nurse Corps, and segregation of African-American nurses was ended. Julie O. Flikke was the first nurse to be promoted to the rank of colonel in the U.S. Army. In 1954 men were allowed to enter the military nursing corps.

In 1946 the Hill-Burton Act was enacted, providing funds to construct hospitals and leading to a surge in the growth of new facilities. This rapid expansion in the number of hospital beds resulted in an acute shortage of nurses and increasingly difficult working conditions. Long hours, inadequate salaries, and increasing patient loads made many nurses unhappy with their jobs, and threats of strikes and collective bargaining ensued.

In response to the shortages, "team nursing" was introduced. Team nursing involved the provision of care to a group of patients by a team of care providers. Although efficient, the method fragmented patient care and removed the registered nurse from the bedside. See Chapter 14 for a description of team nursing. Another response to the shortage was the institution of the associate degree nursing program, discussed in more detail in Chapter 7. As nursing continued to search for its identity, it focused on the scientific bases for nursing practice. Clinical nursing research began in earnest, and the *Journal of Nursing Research* was first published.

1961-1985: New Roles for Nurses

Two 1965 amendments to the Social Security Act, designed to ensure access to health care for elderly, poor, and disabled Americans, resulted in the establishment of Medicare and Medicaid. Soon after, hospitals began to rely heavily on reimbursements from Medicare and Medicaid. Because the majority of the care for the sick was taking place in hospitals rather than homes, the hospital setting became the preferred place of employment for nurses. This gave rise to new opportunities and roles for nurses.

The 1960s were the era of specialty care and clinical specialization for nurses. The successful development of the clinical specialist role in psychiatric nursing—combined with the proliferation of intensive care units and technological advances of the period—fostered the growth of clinical specialization in many areas of nursing, including cardiac-thoracic surgery and coronary care. The increase in medical specialization, along with the concurrent shortage of primary care physicians and the public demand for improved access to health care that grew out of President Johnson's "Great Society" reforms, fostered the emergence of the nurse practitioner (NP) in primary care. In 1971 Idaho became the first state to recognize diagnosis and treatment as part of the legal scope of practice for nurse practitioners.

Nursing in Vietnam

War, this time in Vietnam, again provided nurses with opportunities to stretch the boundaries of the discipline. The Vietnam War occurred in jungles not easily accessed by rescue workers or medics and without clearly drawn lines of combat. Mobile hospital units were set up in the jungles, where nurses often worked without the direct supervision of physicians as they fought to save lives of the wounded. They performed emergency procedures such as tracheotomies and chest tube insertions, never before executed by nurses. They also had to deal with the lack of support on home soil, where the Vietnam War was controversial and often the cause for widespread protests. The trauma of the battlefield would be intensified by this lack of support at home, and many nurses suffered posttraumatic stress disorder (PTSD), as did the returning soldiers.

1986-2006: Challenges for Nursing: Managed Care, Technology, Diversity, Terrorism

With the advent of managed care in the late 1980s and the resulting emphasis on health care reform as a way to continue to cut the costs of medical care, nursing was caught up in the whirlwind of change. Determined to take a proactive stance in the reform effort, the nursing profession wrote its *Agenda for Health Care Reform* in 1992. The plan for reform was comprehensive and focused on restructuring the health care system in the United States to reduce costs and improve access to care. When health care reform did not pass in Congress in the early days of the Clinton administration, insurance companies nevertheless demanded accountability for costs. The system of diagnostic-related groups (DRGs) and managed care were instituted in efforts to improve quality of care within the context of reducing costs. This era is marked by attempts to obtain third-party reimbursement for advanced practice nurses in both primary and acute care.

Another major event of the past 20 years was the influx of technology in health care. Electronic medical records became the norm, with computers at the bedside. Other technological advances keep patients alive who previously would have succumbed to their illnesses, creating new ethical challenges for nurses.

Today's nurse is all too aware of the challenges of the global community in which the threats of war, bioterrorism, and emerging epidemics, such as avian flu, are a reality. The profession is now called upon to educate nurses and others on how to treat those suffering from new maladies, including the physical and psychological scars of war wounds and homeland terrorist acts.

More than ever, we recognize the need for culturally sensitive care. With the immigration of large numbers of Latinos into the United States in recent years, nurses must address the unique health care needs of this immigrant population in the face of significant language barriers. As a result, diversity training becomes a must for the nursing workforce to ensure that nurses provide culturally competent and meaningful care. Nurses must work with a diverse nursing staff as well as with diverse patient populations. And sadly, with the return of soldiers from Middle East conflicts, especially the Iraq war, new health concerns secondary to war may emerge.

The nursing profession cannot meet the challenges of the future without an accurate understanding of its past. Cognizant of their heritage, nurses look to meet the challenges of the present and plan for the future.

SOCIAL CONTEXT OF NURSING

From its beginning nursing has been impacted by the societal practices and values of each age. This social context has shaped nurses' attitudes, nursing practice, attitudes of the public, and professionalization of the discipline over the years. The social context also influences who chooses nursing as a career.

As you read this section, think about what drew you into the profession of nursing. What is the story of your individual journey into nursing? One nurse's story is found in the Critical Thinking Challenge 2-1. As you read her story, identify factors that influenced her choice of career. Then think of your own story and identify social forces that have influenced your career choice. Spend a few minutes now to reflect on your own individual journey toward nursing.

Several social factors that have influenced the development of professional nursing will be explored in this section, including:

- The fact that nursing is a female-dominated profession
- Technological advances
- The entry of men into the profession
- **Demographics** (population trends) in the nation
- The public's image of nursing
- Recurring shortages of adequate numbers of nurses

Traditional Socialization of Women

Socialization is the process whereby values and expectations are transmitted from generation to generation. Parents and others in a child's sphere of influence teach lessons about appropriate gender roles and behavior, both intentionally and unintentionally. As a result, gender role stereotyping is commonplace. **Stereotypes** are biased attitudes developed through interactions with family, friends, and others in an individual's social and cultural system. **Gender role stereotypes** are those biases or prejudices that portray how men and women "ought" to behave in society or within their cultural group. Some common gender role stereotypes of women identified by Cummings (1995) are found in Box 2-1.

Gender role stereotyping can be subtle. It begins early in life and can easily be overlooked unless one is attuned to the forms in which it can occur. For example, girls are always given dolls for play but rarely does a parent buy a girl a toy toolbox or a Tonka truck. Boys may have a favorite

---

CRITICAL THINKING *Challenge 2-1*

One Nurse's Journey into Nursing

Instructions: Analyze the story below and determine some of the factors that influenced this nurse's choice of a career. What assumptions did she make about the profession before entering it? Were her assumptions accurate or inaccurate? How would her assumptions hold up today?

"During childhood I had taken care of wounded dogs and played nurse to numerous dolls. I watched as my grandmother made cough syrup with tree bark, applied snuff to wasp bites, and practiced a variety of other healing treatments for our extended family. But maybe my real fascination for nursing can be attributed to my neighbor who was a nurse. During the summers

or other times when school was out I watched her leave for work in her crisp white uniform, white hose and white shoes. When I was in fourth grade she came and talked to our class about health. Throughout my years in school I was an excellent student but never considered any other career. My algebra and trigonometry teacher tried relentlessly to steer me to major in math since that was my favorite subject in school, but for the life of me I could not fathom how a career in math could be exciting or challenging. And so it was that I entered a baccalaureate program in nursing following high school graduation."

stuffed animal but not a doll. The Evidence-Based Practice Note below describes a study of popular children's television programs that analyzed gender messages aimed at 1-year-old through 5-year-old children.

The Female Role

Historically in Western culture, girls learn to be "feminine," which has traditionally meant passive, dependent, affectionate, emotional, and expressive. They learned that beauty and charm make one desirable to men—and that catching a man is a major life goal. This is considered an **androcentric,** or male-centered, cultural bias. Women have generally been socialized to avoid risk-taking and conflict, to acquiesce to authority, to be submissive, and to seek out careers that were suitable to their female characteristics, such as teaching or nursing. As women have demanded their rightful place in all arenas, some of the myths of the feminine mystique have been dispelled. Although there have been major changes in the female role over the decades, many people

EVIDENCE-BASED PRACTICE

note

Kimberly Powell and Lori Abels are researchers who examined children's television programs to assess the manner in which gender roles were presented. They defined sex-role as "a set of activities deemed appropriate for one sex but not the other" and sex-role stereotypes as existing when "actions are thought of as simply masculine or feminine and tend to be resistant to change" (p. 14). Powell and Abels decided to focus on two popular television programs aimed at preschool (ages 2 to 5) children—*Barney & Friends* and *Teletubbies*—for gendered themes, characteristics, and messages within the programs. For a theme to be identified, both researchers must have spotted it and it had to appear in at least half the episodes, which they viewed separately to avoid influencing each other.

After studying 10 episodes of each program, these researchers found that gendered messages and behaviors were presented in a number of ways. For example, female characters were usually followers; they looked feminine, that is, small or petite; they were underrepresented in the occupations portrayed; they played feminine roles such as caretaker or peacemaker; and they were shown in activities such as braiding hair, cooking, and washing dishes. Male characters were usually leaders; appeared in a variety of masculine occupations and roles, such as playing basketball, driving a bulldozer, or building a wall; were larger physically; and were stereotypically male in appearance. Socially, males were active and females passive.

The researchers concluded that both programs did well at opening up acceptable behavior choices for boys, such as being cooperative and social, yet they maintained sex-role stereotypes such as caretaker and follower for girls. They made three suggestions for improving gender representation in preschool television programs:

1. Depict women as construction workers or men as child care providers to present children with more options in learning what men and women can do.
2. Alternate males and females as leaders.
3. Design some programs that show females in action with males observing, or better yet, all working together and equally active.

Powell KA, Abels L: Sex-role stereotypes in TV programs aimed at the preschool audience: an analysis of Teletubbies and Barney & Friends, *Women Language* 25(2):14-22, 2002.

Mother
- Subrogates own needs
- Freely gives advice
- Becomes the peacemaker
- Fosters dependence
- Is passive, wants recognition

Iron Maiden
- Is competitive versus collaborative
- Possesses the ability to "be in charge"
- Gives critical feedback
- Sets rigid interpersonal boundaries
- Can be unapproachable

Superwoman
- Demands perfection
- Will not delegate
- Overcommits her time
- Assumes multiple roles
- Feels isolated, not supported

Based on Cummings SH: Attila the Hun versus Attila the hen: gender socialization of the American nurse, *Nurs Admin Q* 19(2):25, 1995.

have held on to their prejudices regarding these feminine "traits."

Female stereotyping in nursing

It is difficult to separate the traditional women's history from a profession that has been traditionally occupied by women. When nursing as a profession began in the mid-1800s, the most common roles assumed by women were within their families and involved caring for others, maintaining a household, and pleasing their husbands. Respectable women did not work outside the home for money, but rather relied on their husbands or families for support. The first formal schools of nursing in the United States were developed to attract these "respectable women" into nursing, which was designed to increase the value society put on nursing. Stereotyping of

women also included the notion that women were intellectually inferior to men and hence women were not called upon to make decisions or think. This type of stereotyping was an impetus for the type of training that nurses received, basically task oriented, and this form of instruction persisted for many years.

As nursing education moved into the academic setting, these trends and stereotypes were slowly whittled away. However, similar to other traditionally female professions such as teaching and social work, nursing has been plagued with low status and low pay. Although men are entering nursing and many boundaries have been broken, some challenges continue in this area because of the **paternalistic** nature of the health care environment.

Nursing, Feminism, and Women's Movements

The goals of feminist movements and the nursing profession would seem to be aligned; however, this is not necessarily true. Nursing, feminism, and women's movements have had an uneasy relationship. Contemporary feminists have criticized nursing leaders, past and present, for failing to change the culture of nursing to a feminist one. For example, the relatively young American Nurses Association (ANA) refused to endorse women's **suffrage** until 1915, although the fight for women's suffrage (right to vote) had been going on for the previous 40 years. Decades later, the ANA chose not to endorse the passage of the Equal Rights Amendment (ERA) until the late 1970s, citing the belief that biological differences between men and women demanded special legislative attention that the more generic ERA did not address. Feminists who favored the passage of the ERA, even though it was imperfect, believed this reasoning was specious.

It is not surprising then that nursing has been viewed by some feminists as a traditional and even oppressive female occupation. The health care environment historically has been one in which male physicians and male chief executive officers have dictated to female nursing administrators. These men made decisions for and about nurses with little input from them, reinforcing the notion that females did not know what was best for them. Nursing leaders have aligned themselves with agencies and individuals that they believed were in the best position to assist them to accomplish their agenda. Unfortunately, rarely were these individuals female, nor were agencies led by females. Many nurses have inadvertently contributed to the divide between nursing and women's movements by passively looking to others outside nursing to improve conditions in nursing rather than working with other nurses to strengthen the profession from within.

Nursing and the women's movement

The women's movement that began in the 1960s has had a profound effect on society and has both hurt and helped the nursing profession. As women of the 1960s and 1970s sought career opportunities beyond the traditional female ones of teaching and nursing, bright and able women who formerly might have become nurses pursued careers in accounting, architecture, engineering, computer science, and a variety of other fields. This meant that nursing faced more competition for students than it once did because of the heightened interest in other careers by young women.

When women can freely choose any professional field of study, they often seek opportunities that may offer more competitive salaries, better schedules, and a more exciting career trajectory. An interesting recent phenomenon has occurred, however. Across the United States nursing programs are seeing an increasing number of applicants who have degrees in other areas or who have had careers in other disciplines such as school teachers, attorneys, engineers, computer programmers, accountants, businesspeople, and other health-related occupations. The current appeal of nursing to both men and women in this category seems to be related to the fact that a career in nursing can provide economic and job security. A more significant reason for this trend is that in spite of a vast number of career choices

now available to men and women, nursing's appeal is strong to people of both genders who want to make a difference in the lives of others.

The women's movement helped nursing by bringing economic issues such as low salaries and poor working conditions into the open. The movement provoked a conscious awareness that equality and autonomy for women were inherent rights, not privileges, and stimulated the passage of legislation to ensure those rights.

Nursing also benefited from the women's movement in more subtle ways. As nursing students were increasingly educated in colleges and universities, they were exposed to campus activism, protest, and organizations that were trying to change the status of women. Learning informal lessons about power and how to bring about change had a positive effect on students, who later used this knowledge to improve the status of nursing.

Despite these positive directions, the nursing profession was slow to internalize the women's movement messages of self-determination and commitment. Feminism and women's movements have helped nurses learn that women can be autonomous and assertive. With the firm commitment of all its members, male and female, to lifelong full participation, nursing can grow to its maximum potential, expand opportunities for its members, give voice to all its members, male and female, and ultimately contribute to the advancement of society at large. Even individuals who do not consider themselves feminists can agree that these are important goals for nursing.

Men in Nursing

Men are not new to the profession of nursing. During the eleventh, twelfth, and thirteenth centuries in Europe they supplied much of the nursing care, often within the authority of military religious orders. It was not until late in the nineteenth century that nursing became a predominantly female profession.

Florence Nightingale played a crucial role in this turn of events by asserting that nursing was a female discipline. She worked hard to establish nursing as a worthy career for respectable women and largely ignored the historical contributions of men. The male role as she saw it was confined to supplying physical strength, such as lifting, moving, or controlling patients, when needed. To compound the issue, the early schools for training nurses in the United States did not admit males, establishing an early tradition of discrimination in the profession. An exception was the field of psychiatric nursing, a field that in the early days often required physical stamina and strength. It was therefore considered an appropriate field for men.

In 1901 when the U.S. Congress created the Army Nurse Corps, and then a few years later the Navy Nurse Corps, men were excluded from participation. Male nurses who entered the military did so as "privates in the Army or as pharmacist's mates third class in the Navy with the result being that male nurses employed in the military service had no official status" (Kalisch and Kalisch, 2005). Even in times of war these men were not allowed to practice as nurses but rather were given jobs that any other male was assigned to perform, such as driving trucks or operating heavy equipment. The ANA House of Delegates in 1942 drafted a resolution to be sent to the Surgeons General of the Army and the Navy asking them to allow male members of the ANA to serve as nurses. However, this effort met with continued resistance. It was not until 1955 that the first male received a commission as a nurse.

Because of the lack of training programs and the gender restrictions placed on military nurses, it was difficult for men to enter nursing before World War II. In the school year 1939-1940 the four all-male nursing schools had a total enrollment of 212 and there were 62 coeducational schools (Kalisch and Kalisch, 2005). After World War II, the GI Bill helped to increase the number of male nursing students by providing funding for education. Military corpsmen entered nursing schools in large numbers, as they have following every major military conflict since World War II.

Current trends

The total number of men practicing nursing rose from 79,557 in 1992 to 113,683 in 1996, which represented an increase of nearly 70 percent in only 4 years. This trend did not continue, however, because the March 2000 survey by the Division of Nursing of the U.S. Department of Health and Human Services (U.S. Department of Health and Human Services, 2001) revealed that approximately 146,902 of the 2,694,540 RNs in this country were men. Although the number of men in nursing was considerably higher in 2000, overall growth in the numbers of registered nurses meant that men represented exactly the same percentage, 5.4 percent, as in 1996. Preliminary findings of the National Sample Survey of Registered Nurses for 2004 (U.S. Department of Health and Human Services, 2005) indicate that only a slight increase (5.7%) in the percentage of male nurses has occurred (Figure 2-9).

The number of men in nursing is expected to rise as currently enrolled students graduate. An American Association of Colleges of Nursing (AACN) survey in 2003 revealed that 8.4% of respondents enrolled in undergraduate programs

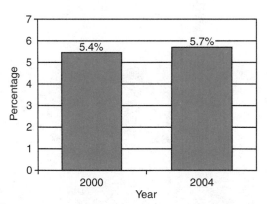

Figure 2-9
Men still comprise a small percentage of the total RN population, with a slight increase from 2000 to 2004. (*Data from U.S. Department of Health and Human Services, Division of Nursing:* The registered nurse population, March 2004: national sample survey of registered nurses, preliminary findings, *Washington, DC, 2005, Government Printing Office, p 8.*)

were men. The male nurse, when compared with his female counterpart, is likely to be younger, to be employed full-time in nursing, to have more non-nursing education, and to have chosen nursing as a second career. Their motivations for entering nursing, however, are similar to those of their female counterparts (Figure 2-10). A recent survey of men asked respondents to rate why they entered nursing using a 5-point scale with 5 being the most important. Hart (2005) reported that the top three reasons were a desire to help people (4.24), the perception that nursing is a growth profession with many career paths (4.0), and the desire to have a stable career (3.67).

The American Assembly for Men in Nursing (AAMN)

The American Assembly for Men in Nursing (AAMN) was founded in 1974 with the stated purpose of providing "a framework for nurses, as a group, to meet, to discuss and influence factors which affect men as nurses" (AAMN, 2003). The organization's objectives are as follows (AAMN, 2003):

- Encourage men of all ages to become nurses and join together with all nurses in strengthening and humanizing health care.

Figure 2-10
In spite of their small numbers, men in nursing play an important role in the profession.

- Support men who are nurses to grow professionally and demonstrate to one another and to society the increasing contributions being made by men within the nursing profession.
- Advocate for continued research, education, and dissemination of information about men's health issues, men in nursing, and nursing knowledge at the local and national levels.
- Support members' full participation in the nursing profession and its organizations and use this assembly for the limited objectives stated above.

The fact that the members of this group thought a separate organization was necessary to achieve their objectives raises the following question: "Have men in nursing suffered discrimination because of their gender?"

Attitudes toward men in nursing

Men interested in health care historically became physicians, and later dentists or physical therapists, whereas women became nurses. Because nursing is a traditionally female-dominated profession, men in the profession may have their masculinity called into question. Although the pervasive homophobia in our society and the belief that nursing is strictly a feminine profession may be changing, these attitudes are still pervasive enough to affect the decisions of young men making career choices.

Several issues face the men who do choose nursing. They often feel role strain—an emotional reaction that may be felt by a person in a profession that has a social structure dominated by members of the opposite sex. For men raised in the androcentric American culture, unaccustomed to anti-male gender discrimination, this can create anxiety and discontent. Another issue men face is lack of public awareness that men can be as well suited for nursing as women. Patients as well as people in general commonly assume that a man delivering health care is either a physician or a medical student. One common myth surrounding men in nursing is that they wanted to be physicians but were not intelligent enough to get into medical school.

Male nurses may experience discrimination from practicing nurses, physicians, and the public. Female nurses often ask male counterparts for assistance only when lifting and turning patients, emphasizing physical strength rather than professional expertise. It is all too common for male students to find themselves unwelcome in prenatal clinics, delivery rooms, and other settings in which male physicians have free access. This type of behavior poses a problem for clinical faculty, who must make every attempt to advocate for the student or find other clinical experiences. Even female patients on regular medical or surgical services may refuse to have the male student perform basic skills such as insertion of an indwelling catheter or giving a bath. In Box 2-2 a man who is a junior nursing student in a large university reflects on his experiences, some of which parallel the examples presented earlier.

Being a male in the nursing profession may have a positive side, however. Williams (1995) discussed some of what she termed "hidden advantages" for men in nursing. She asserted that men are preferred in hiring because of their strength and a perceived potential for better leadership. She speculated that because of their "renegade status" in a female-dominated profession, men are given more respect and encouraged to increase their education and enter the most prestigious specializations. Many male physicians tend to treat male nurses as equals, as do men in management positions, rarely being disrespectful in their interactions.

Williams also reported that men tend to earn more money than their female counterparts in nursing. A study in 2002 revealed that male nurses do earn about 12 percent more than female nurses, but identifying the reasons for this disparity from among the countless possible variables has proven difficult (Sex Discrimination, 2002). Some speculate that part of this difference is that a majority of men work in specialty areas that pay more, such as intensive care units, burn units, and emergency departments.

Much remains to be done to attract more men to nursing. Schools of nursing must take a proactive approach to recruiting qualified applicants and creating an environment where men feel welcome and not isolated. Male professors can serve as role models and provide a supportive environment to male students. Textbooks and journals, as well as school of nursing publications, should portray males in pictures, and refrain from automatic use of "she" when referring to the nurse. Figure 2-11 is an example of a recruitment advertisement featuring gender diversity in nursing.

Box 2-2 | Reflections of a Man in Nursing

"Like many other students, I chose nursing because I wanted to help others and have a rewarding career. When I began to tell family and friends, my decision was met with resistance. I quickly became conscious of the influence social norms had in genderizing nursing. Male nurses are generally respected among other nurses; it's oftentimes patients and other health care providers who view nursing as a job only capable by females.

A few months ago, I overheard a local radio disc jockey state that he would refuse care by a male nurse. In my experiences, I've had patients refuse a male nurse in the room during their delivery while allowing a male obstetrician to remain present. I suppose that some believe males lack the nurturing and caring presence synonymous with nursing.

As nurses gain more autonomy and the discipline shifts towards a specialized form of health care it is likely attitudes towards male nurses will change as well. While males and other minorities alike continue to make names for themselves they will inspire others who once may not have considered this career, leaving the profession no choice but to diversify."

The comments of a junior nursing student, May 2006.

Whether men in nursing experience disadvantages or advantages or some of both, one thing is certain: The increasing number of men in nursing will make the profession diverse, which should be seen as a positive trend. All members of the profession should recognize that both "feminine" and "masculine" qualities and abilities, however they are defined, are needed to strengthen the profession and to provide holistic care to individuals.

Male trailblazers in nursing

Considering how few men are nurses, they have made considerable impact on the profession. The earliest recorded male nurse was James Derham, an African-American slave who worked as a nurse in 1783 in New Orleans. With his earnings he was able to buy his freedom. Later he studied medicine and practiced as a physician after traveling north to Philadelphia.

Male nurses struggled in their early attempts to be recognized in the military. Edward Lyon, a nurse anesthetist from Kings Park, New York, was the first male nurse commissioned as a second lieutenant in the U.S. Army Nurse Corps on October 10, 1955. A recent achievement was that of General Bill Bester, who became the first male nurse to be promoted to Chief Nurse of the Army in 2000 and the first man to head any of the three branches of the military nurse corps.

Luther P. Christman is considered a pioneer in nursing who has made a significant impact on the profession. Dr. Christman was the first man to be named dean of a nursing school in the United States. As dean at Vanderbilt University in Nashville, Tennessee, he was the first to employ African-American women faculty at the university. Throughout his career he has championed the recruitment of men into nursing and the elevation of the profession through his commitment to education, including expanded nursing roles such as the clinical nurse specialist. Dr. Christman was the founder of both the National Student Nurses Association and the American Association for Men in Nursing. The American Nurses Association honored him with a Hall of Fame Award in 2004 (American Nurses Association, 2004).

Randolph Rasch, another professor at Vanderbilt University, accomplished many "firsts." He was the first African-American man to earn a PhD in nursing. His degree was awarded in 1988 from the University of Texas at Austin. He was also the first African-American man to graduate from the nursing program at Andrews University in Berrien Springs, Michigan, and the first African-American male public health nurse in Michigan. Rasch stated that he had thought about attending medical school but he liked nursing's holistic approach to patient care. His research is in the area of HIV/AIDS and men's health issues (Williams, 2006).

Figure 2-11
An example of an advertisement that depicts men in nursing in a favorable way. *(Reprinted with permission from Johnson & Johnson, The Campaign for Nursing's Future.)*

Image of Nursing

The images of nurses seen in advertisements and on television shows may be the first impression that people have of nursing. First impressions based on media images affect public attitudes toward the profession. While the public's view of nursing has changed over time, most people do not appreciate the complexity and range of today's professional nursing role.

Uniforms and caps: where did they go?

Some speculate that a part of nursing's identity problem is attributable to the disappearance of the traditional mode of dress. A wide array of health care personnel attend to any given patient, with no distinct way of distinguishing who is a registered nurse. Gone are the traditional white caps and uniforms of yesteryear that made nurses instantly identifiable. Instead, nurses and other health care workers don role-blurring scrubs in a variety of colors and patterns and in which everybody looks alike. A stethoscope might signify that the wearer is a nurse, but stethoscopes are also used by many other types of personnel. Identification badges carry titles, but are difficult to see.

Caps were originally worn by nurses to cover the long hair that was the style for women in Victorian times. They quickly became a symbol of the profession. In the United States each school had a unique cap that was instantly recognizable. Nursing schools held capping ceremonies during which they presented caps to students as a symbol of their progress toward graduation. The cap saw its demise in the late 1960s through the 1970s. Many nurses were glad to see the cap disappear, believing it was part of the stereotypical image the public held of nursing.

There has recently been some movement toward reestablishing identifiable dress norms for professional nurses. The News Note below describes one hospital's attempts to redesign nursing attire with the assistance of a fashionable sportswear designer.

Formal or informal styles of address?

Another area affecting the image of nursing is the manner in which health professionals address one another. Nurses in most agencies refer to themselves by first name, for example: "Good morning, my name is Nia and I'm going to be your nurse for today." Physicians usually introduce themselves by title and last name, for example: "I am Doctor White." If formal titles are used for physicians, should they not be used for nurses? Nurses have reported being uncomfortable with this practice, thinking that it establishes a formality that could interfere with the nurse-patient relationship. Gordon (2005) in an informal survey of approximately 30 lay people found that the respondents did not think it would be odd for nurses to refer to themselves more formally. Nursing educators could take the lead in restoring more professional modes of address as a norm during educational experiences.

The public's perception of nurses: Surveys

In spite of internal and external challenges facing the nursing profession, "nurses are generally well thought of by the public and their image is very positive" (Ulmer, 2000). Results of a Harris poll in July 2000, which surveyed more than 1000 people about their attitudes toward nursing, showed the

 news note

After investing large sums of money in redecorating the hospital, administrators at Valley Hospital in Ridgewood, New Jersey, engaged New York clothing designer Yeohlee Teng to create attractive clothing for the more than 1000 Valley Hospital nurses. One goal was to make it possible for patients to distinguish nurses from the other hospital employees. Following 8 months of meetings, design reviews, fabric selections, and workroom fittings, Yeohlee, as she is known professionally, presented muslin prototypes of the new designs to a group of hospital managers and nurses. As nurses modeled one new uniform after another to the assembled group, each was critiqued for function, fit, comfort, and general appeal. In the end, the nurses remained convinced that scrubs were still the most practical, comfortable, and popular choice for nurses at Valley Hospital, disappointing both administrators and the designer.

Seabrook J: The white dress: what should nurses wear? *The New Yorker* 78(4):122-128, 2002.

following results: 92 percent trusted information given by nurses and 85 percent would be "pleased" if their child became a nurse (Ulrich, 2003). The accuracy of this high public regard was reinforced by annual Gallup polls from 1999 to 2005. Nurses came out on top of these polls on honesty and ethics in the professions surveyed. In six of the last seven years since the nursing profession was added to the poll, nursing has rated number 1. The only exception was in 2001, when nursing ranked second to firefighters in the wake of the September 11 attacks.

Influence of the media on nursing's image

The influence of the media's portrayals of nurses is extremely powerful, and this causes great concern for nursing because the image portrayed has often been negative and demeaning. Nurses have variously been portrayed as angels of mercy, handmaidens to physicians, sex symbols, unintelligent bimbos, battle-axes, or sadistic torturers.

Television shows in hospital settings have proliferated in recent years with few of them depicting nurses in a realistic fashion. In many shows nurses are only background figures, rarely displaying their thinking skills.

Some nurses appear to be undisturbed by these images. For example, a senior nursing student commented, "I see the television shows as entertainment, and only entertainment. I know what nurses do and I think that most people in the public understand that these portrayals are not realistic. Physicians are also portrayed quite negatively in the shows, especially *Grey's Anatomy*." The Center for Nursing Advocacy in its Golden Lamp Awards for 2005 identified six episodes of *Grey's Anatomy* as one of the year's worst portrayals of nursing (Image of Nursing, 2006). Even if some individual nurses are not concerned about how the profession is portrayed in the media, the profession as a whole needs to be concerned.

Initiatives to improve nursing's image in the media

Foundations, corporations, and nursing groups have undertaken initiatives to analyze and/or improve nursing's image in the media. Three major initiatives are discussed here.

The Woodhull Study on Nursing and the Media

A comprehensive study of nursing in the print media was conducted in September 1997 by 17 students and 3 faculty coordinators from the University of Rochester (New York) School of Nursing (URSN). In this study, sponsored by Sigma Theta Tau International (STTI) and URSN, students examined approximately 20,000 articles from 16 newspapers, magazines, and trade publications. The **Woodhull Study on Nursing and the Media**, as it was called, was named in honor of the late Nancy Woodhull, a founding editor of *USA Today*. Woodhull became an advocate of nursing following her diagnosis of lung cancer, when she was impressed with the comprehensive nursing care she received. She suggested the study and assisted in the design of the survey after she became concerned about the absence of media attention to nurses and nursing.

In December 1997 the students presented their findings and recommendations to a mixed audience of nurses and national media representatives at the STTI Biennial Convention. The key finding was, "Nurses and the nursing profession are essentially invisible to the media and, consequently, to the American public" (Sigma Theta Tau International, 1998, p. 8). The purpose of the Woodhull Study, its major findings, and strategies to guide the nursing profession's collective response are found in Box 2-3.

The Johnson & Johnson campaign

Johnson & Johnson, the giant health care corporation, began a $20 million campaign, the Campaign for Nursing's Future, in 2002 "to enhance the image of the nursing profession, recruit new nurses and educators, and to retain nurses currently in the system" (Donelan, Buerhaus, Ulrich et al, 2005). This campaign included initiatives in print media, television advertising, student scholarships, fund raising, and research. Half of the money allotted to the campaign through 2006

Box **2-3** **The Woodhull Study at a Glance: Purpose, Findings, and Recommendations**

Purpose of the Study

The Woodhull study was designed to survey and analyze the portrayal of health care and nursing in U.S. newspapers, news magazines, and health care industry trade publications.

Key Study Findings

Nurses and the nursing profession are essentially invisible in media coverage of health care and, consequently, to the American public.

1. Nurses were cited only 4 percent of the time in the more than 2000 health-related articles gathered from 16 major news publications.
2. The few references to nurses or nursing that did occur were simply mentioned in passing.
3. In many of the stories, nurses and nursing would have been sources more germane to the story subject matter than the references selected.
4. Health care industry publications were no more likely to take advantage of nursing expertise, focusing more attention on bottom-line issues such as business or policy.

Key Study Recommendations

1. Both media and nursing should take more proactive roles in establishing an ongoing dialogue.
2. The often-repeated advice in media articles and advertisements to "consult your doctor" ignores the role of nurses in health care and needs to be changed to "consult your primary health care provider."
3. Journalists should distinguish researchers with doctoral degrees from medical doctors to add clarity to health care coverage.
4. To provide comprehensive coverage of health care, the media should include information by and about nurses.
5. It is essential to distinguish health care from medicine as subject matter in the media.

Adapted from Sigma Theta Tau International: *The Woodhull study on nursing and the media: health care's invisible partner*, Indianapolis, Ind, 1998, Sigma Theta Tau International-Center Nursing Press.

was spent on publications such as posters, videos, and pamphlets as well as television advertisement. Part of the company's efforts are also focused on increasing the number of individuals choosing nursing careers through recruitment and retention of nursing students. The campaign's website, http://www.Discovernursing.com, is popular among nursing students and prospective students. This campaign also is aimed at children through its cartoon characters, called "the Nursing Gang," who were placed on book covers distributed to children across the United States. Some of the accomplishments listed in Johnson & Johnson's progress report were the following:

- 2 million unique visitors visited the website.
- 46% of young people ages 18-24 recalled seeing the national advertising.
- 8 million pieces of recruitment materials were distributed free of charge.
- 97% of high schools surveyed used the materials.
- 84% of nursing schools who used the materials experienced an increase in applications and/or enrollments.
- More than 500 student scholarships, more than 100 renewable faculty fellowships, and greater than 100 grants to nursing schools were established and/or awarded (Smith, 2005).

A survey of nursing students, chief nursing officers, and registered nurses (Donelan et al, 2005) found that the campaign had positive effects for nursing. Participants in this study reported significant awareness of the advertisements and the website. Even though the campaign is ongoing and the total impact has not been evaluated, early reports indicate that the positive impact will be far-reaching. This landmark effort by a major American corporation provides a stimulus to the nursing profession to partner with other entities to continue the quest for an accurate image of professional nursing, thereby addressing the nursing shortage.

The Center for Nursing Advocacy

In 2001 a group of graduate students at Johns Hopkins University School of Nursing formed The Center for Nursing Advocacy. Among other concerns, they believed that the inadequate and inaccurate portrayal of nurses in the media contributed to public misconceptions about the profession and thereby to the nursing shortage. Since forming, they have engaged in a number of campaigns to improve nursing's image, including commissioning a script for a pilot of a nurse-centered hospital-based television show. To learn more about this organization, visit their website (http://www.nursingadvocacy.org/about_us/about_us.html).

Box 2-4 presents a checklist for monitoring media images of nurses and nursing. Use this checklist as you view television, watch movies, read books and newspapers, and look at advertisements. Then take action:

■ Write letters to those responsible for negative nursing images on television and in films.
■ Write to the companies that sponsor television programs with negative images of nurses.
■ Write letters to the editors of publications that present nursing in a less than favorable light.
■ Boycott programs, films, and products that promote negative images of nurses and nursing.

In the final analysis, it is the professional responsibility of each and every nurse to reinforce positive images of nursing and, equally as important, to speak out against negative ones. Nurses cannot and should not attribute their image problems to any other group, including physicians or the media. The nursing profession has the major responsibility for improving its own image. The major avenue for changing the image occurs one nurse-patient encounter at a time, where nurses demonstrate what it is nurses do and look and behave professionally. Additionally, organizations such as the American Nurses Association can enhance nursing's image by offering services as consultants to media and setting professional standards.

Social Phenomena Affecting Nursing

Over the course of American nursing history, nurses have responded as individuals and as a profession to wars, poverty, epidemics, women's movements, and other social phenomena. Contemporary nursing also seeks to respond as a profession to social changes that shape our nation and the world.

Although not an exhaustive list, five major social phenomena have been identified for discussion: the aging population, the rise of **consumerism,** increasing cultural diversity, technological advances, and violence.

Aging of America

Persons in America are living longer because of more sophisticated health care and better lives in general. The increase in this population (ages 65 and older) has been steady and dramatic (Figure 2-12). The number of people 75 years of age or older in 2020—well within the working lives of most of today's nursing students—is expected to reach 21.8 million. The very old (>85) represent the fastest growing segment of the total population. In contrast, the number of 35- to 44-year-old Americans is expected to decline from 44.7 million in 2000 to 39.6 million by 2020. This phenomenon is often referred to as "the graying of America."

People older than age 75 are more likely than younger people to be poor, widowed, female,

Box **2-4** **Checklist for Monitoring Media Images of Nurses and Nursing**

Prominence in the Plot
1. Are nurse characters seen in leading or supportive roles?
2. Are nurse characters shown taking an active part in the proceedings, or are they shown primarily in the background (e.g., handing instruments, carrying trays, pushing wheelchairs)?
3. To what extent are nurse characters shown in professional roles, engaged in nursing practice?
4. Do nurse characters or other characters provide the actual nursing care?
5. In scenes with nonnursing professionals (e.g., physicians, hospital administrators), who does most of the talking?

Demographics
6. Does the portrayal show that men, as well as women, may aspire to a career in nursing?
7. Are nurse characters shown to be of varying ages?
8. Are some nurse characters single and others married?

Personality Traits
9. Are nurse characters portrayed as:

a. Intelligent	e. Sophisticated	i. Nurturant
b. Rational	f. Problem solvers	j. Empathic
c. Confident	g. Assertive	k. Sincere
d. Ambitious	h. Powerful	l. Kind

10. If other health care providers are included in the program, what differences are seen in their personality traits as compared with nurse characters?
11. When nurse characters exhibit personality traits 9a through 9h listed above, do such portrayals show them to be abnormal in some way?

Primary Values
12. Do nurse characters exhibit values for:

a. Service to others, humanism	b. Scholarship, achievement

13. If other health care providers are included in the program, what differences are seen in their primary values as compared with nurse characters?
14. When nurse characters exhibit the primary values of scholarship and achievement, do such portrayals show them to be abnormal in some way?

Sex Objects
15. Are nurse characters portrayed as sex objects?
16. Are nurse characters referred to in sexually demeaning terms?
17. Are nurse characters presented as appealing because of their physical attractiveness or "cuteness" as opposed to their intellectual capacity, professional commitment, or skill?

Continued

Box 2-4 Checklist for Monitoring Media Images of Nurses and Nursing—cont'd

Role of the Nurse

18. Is the profession of nursing shown to be an attractive and fulfilling long-term career?
19. Is the work of the nurse characters shown to be creative and exciting?

Career Orientation

20. How important is the career of nursing to the nurse character portrayed?
21. How does this compare with other professionals depicted in the program?

Professional Competence

22. Are nurse characters praised for their professional capabilities by other characters?
23. Do nurse characters praise other professionals?
24. Do nurse characters exhibit autonomous judgment in professional matters?
25. Is there a gratuitous message that a nurse's role in health care is a supportive rather than central one?
26. Do nurse characters positively influence patient/family welfare?
27. Are nurse characters shown harming or acting to the detriment of patients?
28. How does the professional competence of nurse characters compare with the professional competence of other health care providers?
29. When nurse characters exhibit professional competence, are they shown to be abnormal in some way?

Education

30. Who actually teaches the nursing students?
31. Who appears to be in charge of nursing education?
32. Is there evidence that the practice of nursing requires special knowledge and skills?
33. What is actually taught to nursing students?

Administration

34. Are any roles filled by nurse administrators or managers, or are all nurse characters shown as staff nurses or students?
35. Is there evidence of an administrative hierarchy in nursing, or are nurses shown answering to physicians or hospital administrators?
36. Are nurse characters shown turning to other nurses for assistance, or are they depicted as relying on a physician or other character (generally male) for guidance, strength, or rescuing?

Overall Assessment and Comments

37. Overall, is this a positive or negative portrayal of nursing? Why or why not?

From *The Changing Image of the Nurse* by Kalisch and Kalisch, ©1987. Adapted by permission of Prentice-Hall, Upper Saddle River, NJ.

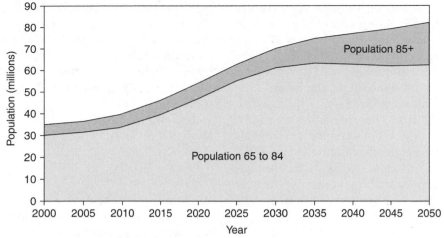

Figure 2-12
Population projections, ages 65 to 84 and ages 85 and over: 2000-2050. *(From U.S. Department of Health and Human Services, Health Resources and Services Administration:* Projected supply, demand, and shortages of registered nurses: 2000-2020, *Washington, DC, 2002, Government Printing Office.)*

living alone, and suffering from chronic conditions such as arthritis, hypertension, and heart disease. As a consequence of these and other factors, this age-group uses a disproportionately higher share of health services than other age-groups, with people older than 65 having twice as many contacts with the health care system as those younger than 65 (U.S. Department of Health and Human Services, 2002).

The oldest "baby boomers," those Americans born between 1946 and 1964, will create a bulge in the aging population between the years 2010 and 2030. As these postwar babies age, their large numbers are expected to create an additional strain on the health care system. Up until this point in the history of the United States, the elderly population has always been vastly outnumbered by younger people. The disproportion between healthy, young adults and more fragile elderly adults expected in the next 20 years will create stress on the economic and social systems of our nation. The graying of America will have a profound impact on the health care system and the nursing profession, stretching an already-challenged capacity to provide adequate medical and nursing care.

The nursing profession has responded to the aging population by increasing courses offered in gerontological nursing to prepare nurses to care for elders more effectively. Most nursing programs have basic content on nursing care of the elderly integrated into the curriculum, and many baccalaureate programs have free-standing gerontology courses for their undergraduates. Gerontological nursing is now considered a specialty, as evidenced by certification at the generalist, specialist, and nurse practitioner levels offered by the American Nurses Credentialing Center. Colleges of nursing offer master's-level preparation for gerontological clinical specialists and nurse practitioners. In spite of these responses, much remains to be done to prepare nurses for the dramatic increase in the number of aging patients they will encounter in the next few decades.

Consumer movement

Since the 1960s there has been a movement by consumers to make all businesses, including the health care system, more accountable for their actions. The American public, fueled by the principles of **consumerism**, criticized the dehumanization of health care. This led to the development in 1972 of the American Hospital Association's (AHA) document "A Patient's Bill of Rights," which guaranteed certain rights and privileges to every hospitalized patient. "A Patient's Bill of Rights" was revised in 1992, and in 2003 the AHA replaced it with a five-page brochure titled "The Patient Care Partnership: Understanding Expectations, Rights, and Responsibilities." These brochures are meant to simplify and make more accessible the essentials of the former Patient's Bill of Rights and are available in several languages free of charge through the AHA (http://www.hospitalconnect.com:80/aha/ptcommunication/partnership/partnership/index.html).

Until the AHA's "A Patient's Bill of Rights" was published, the prevailing attitude in health care was that providers knew best, and good patients simply followed directions without asking questions. This is known as **medical paternalism**.

The rise of consumerism in health care led to the involvement of consumers in pressing Congress for legislation protecting the public from inadequate care, experimental drugs, poor nutrition, and many other health-related issues. Consumer groups have demanded controls on spiraling health care costs and gained participation on boards of health, planning agencies, accrediting bodies, and professional licensing boards. Most state boards of nursing have at least one consumer member. Consumers must actively participate in the health care system, be responsible for their own health maintenance, and demand high quality and cost-effectiveness.

The 106th United States Congress, responding to the reaction of health care consumers to limited choices and restrictions brought about by managed care, debated a Federal Patient's Bill of Rights. This document, the result of lobbying efforts of nursing organizations, consumers, organized medicine, the American Association of Retired Persons (AARP), and many others, was designed to ensure that every American had a basic level of care.

As expected, the 107th Congress revisited patient protections. After many months, much debate, and innumerable modifications, the McCain/Edwards/Kennedy Bipartisan Patient Protection Act (S. 1052) was passed by the United States Senate on June 29, 2001. A similar bill, also with numerous modifications, the Ganske/Dingle/Norwood Bipartisan Patient Protection Act (H.R. 2563), passed the House of Representatives on August 2, 2001. As of the press date of this book, federal patient protection provisions had not yet been passed by the United States Congress.

Cultural diversity

Unquestionably, the diverse cultures that now call the United States home have affected the health care delivery system. In eras past, immigrants were most often from European and Asian countries and frequently found themselves in cultural enclaves within major cities. While descendants of Africans are seen as part of the "diverse culture" of America, one must remember that the early Africans did not enter the country as immigrants but rather as merchandise. Modern day African-Americans' perceptions of the health care system are rooted in their unique history and pose challenges to health care providers.

The 1990s saw a massive influx of Latinos from Mexico and other South American countries into the United States. People from other lands often have different values, health beliefs, and health practices, as well as some diseases already well-controlled in the United States. Instead of blending, as in a melting pot, individuals from other countries are increasingly appreciated for the uniqueness and flavor they bring to life in the United States, and many prefer to preserve their own cultural heritage rather than becoming "Americanized."

The exact number of persons in the various racial/ethnic groups is difficult to pinpoint. Identifying by race does not necessarily capture all the different cultures that may have migrated from a country. The concept of race as used by the U.S. Census Bureau depends on "self-identification by respondents; that is, the individual's perception of his/her racial identity" (U.S. Bureau of the Census, 2002, p. 5). A problem with this method is that biracial people are forced to identify themselves as either one race or the other, which introduces inaccuracy into the data.

The population of most minority racial/ethnic groups in the United States is growing. In 2002 the total population was 284,797,000. Of this number, non-Hispanic whites were the largest group with 196,219,000, or 68.9 percent of the total. The second largest and fastest growing minority group were persons of Hispanic origin, with 36,972,000, or 13 percent. Next in size was the African-American population, numbering 36,247,000, or 12.7 percent. Asians numbered 10,983,000 (3.9 percent) followed by Native Americans at 2,726,000 (less than 1 percent). The group identified as "other," which includes anyone who does not mark one of the five major categories on the census form, was reported at 4,552,000, or 1.6 percent of the total population (U.S. Bureau of the Census, 2002).

It is expected that the historically dominant Anglo-American (white) culture will become a minority group by the middle of the twenty-first century. This represents a radical change in the historical demographics and attitudes of the nation. Nursing must also change to meet the requirements of the ethnic groups they serve.

Diversity in the profession

In order to meet the challenge of an increasingly diverse population entering the health care system, the nursing profession needs to educate all of its nurses to be culturally competent. The number of nurses from minority groups has never been equivalent to their percentage in the total population. Even though the numbers are growing, they are not keeping pace with the population growth of racial/ethnic minorities. In 2000 minorities represented only 12 percent of all registered nurses, up from 10 percent in 1996 but still far less than the percentage of minorities in the overall population, which stood at 30 percent in 2000 (U.S. Department of Health and Human Services, 2001). A more recent report indicates that African-Americans, Hispanic Americans, and Native Americans make up approximately 25 percent of the U.S. population but only 9 percent of its nurses (Maxwell, 2005). Preliminary findings from the 2004 National Sample Survey of Registered Nurses show that ethnic minority group nurses comprise 10.6 percent of the total number of registered nurses, as shown in Chapter 1, Figure 1-2, on page 4. Managers, educators, and other nursing leaders will require training so they can be culturally competent leaders for nurses and students who may have backgrounds different from their own.

A comprehensive governmental assessment of racial/ethnic diversity within nursing was presented in a report to the Secretary of Health and Human Services and Congress in 2000 by the National Advisory Council on Nurse Education and Practice (NACNEP). Titled "A National Agenda for Nursing Workforce Racial/Ethnic Diversity," this document presented challenges to achieving diversity and recommended goals and actions that could serve as a national action agenda to address those challenges. The report is available at no charge from the Health Resources and Services Administration (http://ask.hrsa.gov/detail.cfm?PubID=BHP00082). A summary of the document is online (http://www.bhpr.hrsa.gov/nursing/nacnep/divrepex.htm).

Attention to the development of culturally competent nurses has become an integral part of all progressive nursing education programs and is likely to become an even stronger influence in the future. Nurses cannot know every detail regarding every culture that they encounter; rather nurses must be educated on how to perform individualized care that includes assessment of a patient's culture. Johnson (2005) stated that "cultural competency occurs when nurses know what health and illness mean to patients in the context of their cultural heritage" (p. 53). You will learn more about cultural competence in Chapter 10.

Technological Advances

Advances in biomedical technology and information technology have had a major impact on the practice of nursing. Since the early 1950s, health care has been increasingly supported by advances in technology, and the hospital business has become a major technologically based industry.

Types of technology

Technology seen in health care can be grouped into three major categories: biomedical, information, and knowledge (Yoder-Wise, 2003).

Biomedical technology involves complex machines or implantable devices used in patient care settings for a variety of reasons—for example, pacemakers, internal automated defibrillators, insulin pumps, artificial organs, and various invasive monitoring systems such as those used to measure intracranial pressure. This form of technology affects nursing practice because nurses assume responsibility for monitoring the data generated from these machines and for assessing the safety and effectiveness of implantable equipment in relation to patient well-being. In many instances the nurse is called upon to react to the data and revise the plan of care based on the data received.

Information technology (IT) refers to a variety of computer-based applications used to communicate, store, manage, retrieve, and process information. Nurses assumed much of the responsibility for data entry and retrieval with the advent of this technology. Computers are common on nursing units and at the bedside, and most hospitals have at least some degree of computerization of the medical records.

In some health care organizations, nursing information systems are handheld, allowing nurses to enter and access data about the patient directly from the patient's side, whether in an inpatient, outpatient, or home setting. This type of technology allows for more timely documentation of care, and because documentation is done at the time of care, the information is likely to be more accurate. Data that are stored electronically are also more convenient, because data can be accessed by any other care provider at any time, as opposed to the hard copy chart that only one person can view or use at a time.

This convenience can come at the expense of patient privacy, and the privacy and confidentiality of patient information is both an ethical and a legal issue. **The Health Insurance Portability and Accountability Act (HIPAA)** of 1996 is legislation designed to protect patients' health care information from misuse. A more complete discussion of HIPAA's provisions is found in Chapter 4.

Knowledge technology is described as "technology of the mind." It involves the use of computer systems to transform information into knowledge and to generate new knowledge. Through the creation of "expert systems," this form of technology assists nurses with clinical judgments about patient management problems. An example of knowledge technology includes medication administration carts that prompt the nurse for data needed before giving a particular medication. Nurse clinicians and nurse leaders should play a role in programming these devices to maximize their effectiveness in improving nursing care and patient outcomes. Human simulation mannequin are gaining popularity in schools of nursing. They make it possible to simulate a clinical event such as a cardiac arrest or pneumothorax, allowing the student to practice clinical assessment and intervention skills. One of the benefits of computerized expert systems is that they can provide practice in decision making for novice nurses and nurses who may be working outside their area of expertise without increased risk to a patient (Figure 2-13).

High-tech versus high-touch nursing care

As technology becomes more pervasive, some may wonder if the compassionate, personalized care for the patient will disappear. Technological advances now allow nurses to monitor their patients' conditions on computer screens at remote sites. Without even seeing the patient, nurses can gather large amounts of information and make nursing decisions based on that information. As nurses rely more on technology, they may actually spend less time with the patient, creating dissatisfaction on the part of patients and families.

There is a very real risk that the effectiveness of a nurse's practice may be diminished if the nurse cannot integrate the information technology into

Figure 2-13
Advanced technology is used to enhance clinical decision making in novices. Here students use a human simulator in a lab setting to refine their skills. *(Photo courtesy of the University of North Carolina at Chapel Hill School of Nursing.)*

Figure 2-14
In high-tech environments the nurse must remember the significance of human touch in healing and in demonstrating care and compassion. *(Courtesy Emory University.)*

his or her practice in a seamless fashion, as opposed to allowing it to be the focus of their care and becoming a distraction. It cannot be overemphasized that nurses must actively guard against ignoring patients' needs for human interaction as a result of attention to technology (Figure 2-14).

Successfully combining technology and caring requires sensitivity to patients' physical, emotional, and spiritual needs. This has always been a part of nursing's skill set. This type of emotional connectivity has been termed **emotional intelligence** (Simpson and Keegan, 2003).

Violence in America

Violence has become widespread in America, and the results have had a profound impact on the health care system. Caring for the victims may include care in the emergency department, on surgical floors, in trauma units, or in psychiatric units. In addition, the nurse may be called upon to enter the legal system as a result of an encounter with the victim. Nurses are increasingly affected, both personally and professionally, by the prevalence of violence. Nurses should be concerned not only with patients who have been

victims of violence but also with the possibility of violence in the workplace. Despite overwhelming media attention to the problem and congressional debates about gun control, violence continues to be an ugly reality in the lives of many Americans. Perhaps this is because the root causes of violence are complex, multiple, and not readily changeable.

The Surgeon General's workshop: 1985

Official concerns about violence in America were brought to the attention of the public as early as 1985 when the Surgeon General of the United States identified violence as a major public health issue (Cron, 1986). The resulting Surgeon General's Workshop on Violence and Public Health, held in 1985, brought together more than 100 health professionals to discuss violence-related issues. Since then, thousands of research studies have been conducted and millions of dollars have been spent in attempts to understand violent behavior, its causes and effects, and effective interventions. Violence cannot be eradicated through classroom education, legislation, or changes to nursing curricula, because it is rooted in a deeper societal ill. Root causes for violence are too complex for simple solutions. One only has to read any newspaper on any given day to know that little progress has been made in the 21 years since the Surgeon General's Workshop.

Causes and types of societal violence

Violence has been linked with poverty, family breakdown, racism, poor education, substance abuse, ready availability of weapons, the media, video games, pop culture, and a culture of tolerance for violence. Social programs aimed at reducing violence have for the most part failed, mainly because of the complexity of identifying the cause. Intervening in these problems has proved to be politically, economically, and strategically overwhelming; thus the violence continues. In this section three major types of violence are discussed: sexual assault, domestic abuse, and other assaults with weapons, such as knives and guns. The untold physical and emotional damage wrought by these crimes has a profound effect not only on victims but also on nursing practice.

Sexual assault. Sexual assault rates are rising disproportionately to the overall crime rate. The National Institute of Justice estimates that there are more than 1 million sexual assaults each year, two thirds of which go unreported (American Medical Association, 1996). Victims of sexual assault are usually, but not always, women, with men comprising only 5 percent of the victims. Contrary to some beliefs that have linked sexual assault with lower socioeconomic levels, sexual assault occurs at all socioeconomic levels, educational levels, religious denominations, and even in gay/lesbian relationships. Because of the influx of the victims into emergency departments, the **sexual assault nurse examiner (SANE)** has been created to prepare nurses to interview sexual assault victims in a sensitive manner while treating their injuries and collecting forensic evidence needed to prosecute perpetrators successfully. Children and the elderly are also increasingly victims of sexual assault. The needs of child victims of sexual assault are extraordinary; sexual violence against children can be life-threatening as well as psychologically devastating. In addition to the psychological and physical components of abuse, the victim must make decisions regarding the legal ramifications of being a victim of a crime.

Domestic abuse. It is estimated that between 850,000 and 1.5 million women are assaulted by their domestic partners annually (Bureau of Justice, 1999; Centers for Disease Control, 2000). Domestic abuse most often occurs to powerless or vulnerable groups such as young women, children, and the elderly. The rate of children dying as a result of maltreatment in the home in 2000 was 1.71 percent per 100,000 children (U.S. Department of Health and Human Services, 2000). Many others are neglected, physically or sexually abused, or psychologically abused. A National Elder Abuse Incidence Study conducted in 1996 found that 551,011 elders, defined as those age 60 or older, were victims of abuse, neglect, and/or self-neglect (National Center on Elder Abuse, 2003). Dealing with battered women (and men) or the elderly creates the need for nurses to be aware of subtle signs of abuse that victims are often unwilling to report for fear of reprisal. Nurses' physical assessment and interviewing skills allow them to determine whether the injuries seen are consistent with the injury being reported or might indicate abuse. Nurses are in a position to detect abuse even when the patient has been admitted for other reasons. Failure to report suspected abuse can result in legal action against the nurse.

Assaults with weapons. Possession of guns by young Americans has become widespread in rural as well as urban areas in the United States. As a result assaults with weapons have become a societal issue and a major concern for the health care system, especially for emergency departments and trauma units. This onslaught of violence is primarily among young men, and in many instances can be correlated with gang activity. These assaults are the leading cause of spinal cord injuries and emergency ostomy procedures in emergency departments. The impact on nursing has been significant. Nurses have required additional training in the care of these victims during acute stages as well as the unique challenges posed by long-term rehabilitation.

A professional response to violent crime

In addition to becoming clinically proficient in caring for the physical needs of victims of violence, nurses must meet the emotional and psychiatric needs of these patients.

How has nursing responded? An obvious and needed response is to include content on violence in nursing curricula. The American Association of Colleges of Nursing recommends that all nursing programs address the issue and suggests the following content:

1. Acknowledgment of the scope of the problem
2. Assessment skills related to the identification and documentation of abuse and its health effects
3. Interventions to reduce vulnerability and increase safety, especially of women, children, and elders
4. Cultural competence in dealing with violence as a health care problem
5. Legal and ethical issues in treating and reporting violence
6. Activities to prevent domestic violence (American Association of Colleges of Nursing, 1999, p. 2)

Nurses must also take individual initiatives to address the problem. Attendance at continuing education programs can enhance the information received in basic nursing education. The Nursing Network on Violence and Abuse International (NNVAI) advocates this approach. The response to the new health problems created by violence is evident in the emergence of new nursing roles such as sexual assault nurse examiner, expert witness, spinal cord injury specialist, and safety consultant. Despite these initial efforts, much remains to be done.

Violence in the workplace against nurses

Violence in the health care workplace is on the rise and becoming a worldwide problem. The National Institute for Occupational Safety and Health (NIOSH) has defined workplace violence as any physical assault, threatening behavior, or verbal abuse occurring in the work setting: "It includes but is not limited to beatings, stabbings, suicides, shootings, rapes, near homicides, psychological trauma such as threats, obscene phone calls, an intimidating presence, and harassment of any nature such as being followed, sworn at or shouted at" (OSHA, 1996, p. 1). Workplace violence may be committed by strangers, patients, co-workers, or the victim's personal acquaintances.

The emergency department has become the target of efforts to curb violence against nurses by outsiders. On occasion perpetrators of violent crimes follow their victim to the treatment facility. When the violence continues, nurses may become innocent victims. In addition to the emergency department, common settings for violence include psychiatric facilities, waiting rooms, and on home visits. The type of assault ranges from threats, slaps, kicks, and shoves, to injuries from weapons. Many of these assaults result in serious injury, and in some instances death. The incidence of theft of drugs from hospitals by those seeking drugs for street use has also risen, placing nurses in harm's way.

Although it is not always the case, violence against nurses tends to follow a pattern of nonverbal threatening behavior that escalates to verbal threats or harassment and continues on to actual physical violence. A classic case of escalating levels of violent behavior can, in retrospect, be seen in the behavior of Robert Flores, the University of Arizona College of Nursing student who killed three nursing faculty members and then himself in October 2002. Fellow students and other faculty later reported that his behavior had followed a pattern of increasing threat (Gassen, 2002) as he experienced difficulty passing nursing courses.

Most incidents of workplace violence against nurses do not end as tragically as the Flores case in Arizona, but clearly, violence toward nurses in the workplace is a cause for concern for individual nurses as well as the profession as a whole.

Imbalance in Supply and Demand for Nurses

There is nothing new about periodic imbalances between the number of nurses working and available nursing positions. Over many decades there have been rare, brief periods of oversupply of nurses and more frequent and longer-lasting nursing shortages. By far the more common concern is an inadequate supply of registered nurses to meet the health care needs of the nation.

External and internal causes of nursing shortages

The term "nursing shortage" is misleading because actual shortages are usually confined to institutional settings such as hospitals and nursing homes. Causes of shortages may be seen as either external or internal. Internal causes include salary issues, long hours, increased responsibility for unlicensed workers, and significant responsibility with little authority. External causes include changes in demand for nursing services, the increasing age of the American population, greater **acuity** (degree of illness) of hospitalized individuals, public perceptions of nursing as a profession, and ever-widening career options for women.

Historical efforts to manage nursing shortages

In the past, each time a shortage of registered nurses became acute, two solutions were tried: (1) increase the supply of nurses and (2) create a less trained worker to supplement the number of nurses. Practical nursing programs, which produce graduates in only 1 year, were created to meet civilian and military needs of the United States during World War II. The nursing shortage of the 1950s stimulated a desire to shorten basic RN programs, and 2-year associate degree programs were the result. In the 1960s shortages led to the creation of the position of unit manager; this manager was expected to take over certain tasks to relieve nurses, who could then concentrate on providing patient care. The 1970s produced other new positions, such as emergency medical technicians (EMTs), physician's assistants, respiratory therapists, and others who took on various aspects of patient care formerly performed by nurses. The shortage of nurses in the late 1980s resulted in a proposal by the American

Medical Association to create yet another "nurse extender" called the registered care technician. However, this initiative was short-lived as nurses responded quickly and negatively, with nurse leaders stating that nurses could not be responsible for direct caregivers that nurses had not trained.

Another method of increasing the supply of nurses is to import them from other English-speaking countries. Nurses from the United Kingdom, Australia, New Zealand, certain Caribbean islands, South Africa, and the Philippines are targeted for recruitment. Companies have been established to prepare them to take the NCLEX-RN successfully in order to practice in this country. Regardless of what American nurses think of this practice, it is widespread, profitable for companies, and continues today.

As mentioned earlier, shortages are often limited to certain geographic areas or specialties. In those cases, redistributing already-licensed RNs can be seen as a solution. Many agencies specialize in providing nurses for short-term assignments, often called "traveling nurses." The American Hospital Association reported in 2003 that 56 percent of hospitals surveyed were using traveling or agency nurses—at great expense—to fill vacancies (Joint Commission on Accreditation of Healthcare Organizations, 2003).

The current shortage

The current nursing shortage, which began in 2000, is deepening and will continue to do so for the foreseeable future (Figure 2-15). Explaining why there is a shortage is complex. Like many issues in nursing there is no simple explanation and the issue is multifaceted. What is known is that the shortage exists and is more crucial in traditional settings such as hospitals and long term care facilities. One reason for the shortage is an increased demand for nurses because of the growth in total population, especially an aging population that has extensive health care needs. The shortage is also compounded by the fact that the nursing workforce is aging and the number of new entrants to the profession is not keeping

Figure 2-15

National supply and demand projections for FTE registered nurses, 2000-2020. In 2000 the national supply of FTE (full-time equivalent) registered nurses was estimated at 1.89 million, whereas the demand was estimated at 2 million, a shortage of 110,000, or 6 percent. Based on what is known about trends in the supply of RNs and the anticipated demand, the shortage is expected to grow relatively slowly until 2010, by which time it will have reached 12 percent. At that point, demand will begin to exceed supply at an accelerated rate, and by 2015 the shortage will have almost quadrupled to 20 percent. If not addressed, and if current trends continue, the shortage is projected to grow to 29 percent by 2020. Factors driving the growth in demand include an 18 percent increase in population, a larger proportion of elderly persons, and medical advances that heighten the need for nurses. *(From U.S. Department of Health and Human Services, Health Resources and Services Administration:* Projected supply, demand, and shortages of registered nurses: 2000-2020, *Washington, DC, 2002, Government Printing Office, pp 2-3.)*

pace with the numbers who are exiting. The 2004 National Sample Survey of Registered Nurses identified three factors that seem to be contributing to the aging of the RN workforce:

- A decline in the total number of nursing school graduates
- The higher average age of recent graduates
- The aging of the entire existing pool of licensed nurses

Shortages are sometimes blamed on the phenomenon of nurses leaving hospital work for nonhospital nursing positions, such as in the insurance industry or in pharmaceutical sales. In spite of the fact that in 2004 8.5 percent of licensed nurses were estimated to be employed in fields other than hospitals, long-term care, nursing education, public health, or ambulatory care, hospitals employ nearly the same proportion of the total pool of registered nurses, 56 percent, as they did in 2000, when they employed 59 percent. The total number of RNs working in hospitals was greater than in 2000 even though the overall percentage was constant. This is attributable to several factors.

- More nursing care hours per capita are being provided to hospitalized patients today because of a higher acuity of their illnesses and needs that demand more time.
- Technological advances in medical care have created the need for special care units, staffed with specialized nurses. In these units, because patients are critically ill, one nurse can safely care for only one or two patients.
- Advances in technology prolong lives of chronically ill patients, which in turn creates more need for long-term nursing care.
- Cost-containment measures have caused hospital consolidations, downsizing, and reengineering. The result is more patients in fewer hospitals staffed with reduced numbers of personnel.

Initiatives to provide a stable supply of RNs

Recognizing that dramatic swings in the supply of and demand for registered nurses harm the profession, jeopardize patient care, and are costly to nurses and their employers, organizations inside and outside of nursing have called for mechanisms to ensure more even distribution of the workforce. Here are four major initiatives making an impact:

- The Robert Wood Johnson Foundation (RWJF), a private foundation that funds innovative health care initiatives, has committed tens of millions of dollars to pursuing programs that help nursing schools, hospitals, and other health care agencies create regional workforce development systems. This initiative is named "Colleagues in Caring."
- Johnson & Johnson's "Campaign for Nursing's Future," was mentioned earlier. J&J is working in partnership with the National Student Nurses Association (NSNA), the National League for Nursing (NLN), the American Nurses Association (ANA), the Association of Nurse Executives (AONE), and Sigma Theta Tau International Honor Society of Nursing.
- The federal government is also involved in the effort. On August 1, 2002, President Bush signed into law the Nurse Reinvestment Act, which provided for a number of meaningful incentives to bring more nurses into the profession.
- The American Nurses Credentialing Center (ANCC) Magnet Recognition Program is a model for employers to earn the designation "employer of choice" by implementing a model program designed to attract and retain nurses in acute hospital settings.

Numerous other initiatives by nursing associations, colleges of nursing, and states are also underway. To learn more about the four efforts described above, visit Evolve for WebLinks related to the content of this chapter: http://evolve. elsevier.com/Chitty/professional/.

The impact of nursing's shortage on patient outcomes

The foremost researcher on the topic of nursing shortage and its effect on patient outcomes is Peter Buerhaus (Buerhaus, 2005). Two national surveys in 2002 and 2004 by Buerhaus (Buerhaus et al, 2005a) examined the impact of the nursing shortage on patient outcomes and quality of care. Findings from these surveys indicate that hospital nurses and nursing officers believe that a shortage of registered nurses presents a major problem for the quality of patient care (Buerhaus et al, 2005b). A 2004 study by Buerhaus et al. (2005b) found 62 percent of nurses in 2002 and 67 percent in 2004 believed that the nursing shortage created problems in early detection of patient complications; 68 percent of 2002 participants and 71 percent of 2004 participants identified the ability of nurses to maintain patient safety was a problem. Overwhelmingly, both groups felt that the shortage had impacted the amount of time the nurse could spend with patients (93 percent and 92 percent, respectively). The gap between a desirable level of care and the care these nurses were able to provide created both stress and **moral distress.**

Clearly hospitals and other agencies employing nurses are faced with one of the most significant shortages of nursing's history. Nursing leaders and employers need to examine and evaluate the working environment as a contributor to the shortage. Consumers—individual patients and third-party payers—will no longer tolerate poor patient outcomes. Simply increasing the numbers of nurses that receive licenses through fast track programs or importing nurses from other countries does not increase the long-term number of practicing nurses. Attention needs to be given to factors within work environments that cause nurses to work fewer hours or leave nursing entirely. Some of these include salary structure, benefits, and the status of nurses in the hospital (Buerhaus et al, 2005a). Other factors include heavy patient assignments, inability to complete the work required in the allotted time, and increased stress in the work environment.

To date there are no clear-cut solutions to the problem of periodic imbalances in the supply of and demand for nurses. With dramatic demographic changes on the horizon, however, shortages are likely to remain a recurring theme for the immediate future.

SUMMARY OF *Key Points*

- In 1860 Florence Nightingale founded a school for nurses at St. Thomas's Hospital, London, that became the model for nursing education in the United States.
- Formal educational programs for U.S. nurses were established in 1873.
- The period between the 1873 World's Fair and 1908 marked a time of organizing for nurses. During that time the forerunners of the National League for Nursing (NLN), the American Nurses Association (ANA), the International Council of Nurses (ICN), and the National Association for Colored Graduate Nurses were formed.
- The initiation of state licensure in 1903 heralded standardization of nursing education programs that, until this time, had varied widely.
- The establishment of the Henry Street Settlement and the rise of community health nursing played a major role in the widespread public acceptance of nurses, particularly African-American nurses.
- World War I and the influenza epidemic of 1917-1919 created a strong demand for nursing services. Many nursing schools were opened in response, mostly in hospitals.
- The Great Depression and World War II created new opportunities for nurses, including the Cadet Nurse Corps, which added 179,000 new registered nurses to the profession by the end of the war, but denied membership to men.
- Since World War II, hospital expansion, technological advances, and social changes have created new and progressively autonomous roles for nurses, especially advanced practice nurses.

- Social trends that have affected nursing include feminism, the women's movement, the consumer movement, the "graying of America," cultural diversity, men in nursing, violence, and technological advances in health care and information management.
- Numerous nurses from ethnically diverse groups and men have made major contributions to the development of the profession of nursing.
- Individual nurses must take direct action when nursing is presented in an unfavorable light in the media.
- The number of men in nursing is gradually increasing.
- Consumers, aided by information available on the Internet, are becoming more aware and demanding that they be treated as equal members of the health care team.
- Nurses are expected to become culturally competent in order to meet the needs of an increasingly diverse population of both patients and colleagues.
- Nurses must not forget the art of nursing that involves compassionate care despite the presence of a dizzying array of technology.
- Imbalances in the supply of and demand for nurses arise periodically because of changes in society and in health care itself. A number of ongoing initiatives have been designed to ensure an adequate supply of registered nurses, yet shortages continue.

REFERENCES

American Assembly of Men in Nursing: *Purpose and objectives,* 2003 (website): http://www.aamn.org.

American Association of Colleges of Nursing: 1999 position statement on violence as a public health problem, 1999 (website): http://aacn.nche.edu/Publications/positions/violence.htm.

American Association of Colleges of Nursing: *Annual state of the schools,* 2002 (website): http://www.aacn.nche.edu/Media/annualreport02.pdf.

American Medical Association: *Facts about sexual abuse,* 1996 (website): www.acep.org/2.614.0.html.

American Nurses Association: *2004 hall of fame awards,* 2004 (website): http://nursingworld.org/hof/christman.pdf.

Barton C: *Diary: the papers of Clara Barton (1812-1912),* Washington, DC, 1862, Library of Congress, Manuscript Division.

Buerhaus PI: Six-part series on the state of the RN workforce in the United States, *Nurs Economics* 23(2):58-60, 2005.

CRITICAL THINKING QUESTIONS

1. Florence Nightingale is often credited with being the first nurse researcher. Why do you think this is so?
2. Discuss the significance of the events that occurred during the Chicago World's Fair, 1893, to the advancement of the nursing profession.
3. Do you agree with the view that nursing is inevitably tied to the greater issues of the women's movement throughout the world? Why or why not? How has this attitude affected the entry of men into nursing?
4. Wars have often been the driving force in creating social change. How have wars influenced the profession of nursing?
5. What role did the military have in integrating the profession of nursing for African-Americans and other minorities?
6. Discuss the role the military played in perpetuating discriminatory practices against men in nursing.
7. Explain how being a female-dominated profession has affected the development of the nursing profession.
8. Describe your ideal nurse. What social stereotypes does your description reveal? Does your "ideal nurse" belong to a particular gender, race, ethnic group, or generation?
9. What positive and negative impact has the consumer movement had on health care in the United States? How do you reflect consumerism when using the health care system?
10. Why is a bill of rights necessary in health care? Examine the document found at the following website and give a rationale for each "right" listed (www.hospitalconnect.com:80/aha/ptcommunication/index.html).
11. List three social factors that have the potential to stimulate or squelch interest in nursing as a profession and explain their impact. Recommend ways the profession can capitalize on or combat each factor you listed.
12. If everyone in a health care setting dresses alike, how does this impact nursing's image? In addition to attire, what would you recommend as an appropriate or acceptable look for nurses? Be sure to address hair, makeup, facial hair for men, jewelry, piercings, and tattoos.
13. The nursing shortage is projected to worsen in the next few years. Discuss the reasons for the deepening of this shortage and strategies to address it.

Buerhaus PI, Donelan K, Ulrich BT et al: Is the shortage of hospital registered nurses getting better or worse? Findings from two recent national surveys of RNs, *Nurs Economics* 23(2):61-71, 96, 2005a.

Buerhaus PI, Donelan K, Ulrich BT et al: Hospital RNs' and CNOs' perceptions of the impact of the nursing shortage on the quality of care, *Nurs Economic$* 23(5):214-221, 2005b.

Bureau of Justice: *Intimate partner violence and age of victim, 1993-1999,* 1999 (website): http://www.ojp.usdoj.gov/bjs/abstract/ipva99.htm.

Carnegie ME: *The path we tread: blacks in nursing, 1854-1994,* Philadelphia, 1995, JB Lippincott.

Centers for Disease Control and Prevention: *Intimate partner violence fact sheet,* 2000 (website): http://www.cdc.giv/ncipc/dvp/dvam/htm.

Cherry B, Jacob S: *Contemporary nursing: issues, trends and management,* St Louis, 2005, Mosby.

Cron T: The Surgeon General's workshop on violence and public health: review of recommendations, *Pub Health Rep* 101:8-14, 1986.

Cummings SH: Attila the Hun versus Attila the hen: gender socialization of the American nurse, *Nurs Admin Quart* 19(2):19-29, 1995.

Dock LL, Stewart IM: *A short history of nursing,* New York, 1920, Putnam.

Donahue MP: *Nursing: the finest art: an illustrated history,* ed 2, Philadelphia, 1996, Mosby.

Donelan K, Buerhaus PI, Ulrich BT et al: Awareness and perceptions of the Johnson & Johnson Campaign for nursing's future: views from nursing students, RNs, and CNOs, *Nurs Economic$* 23(4):150-156, 180, 2005.

Fitzpatrick ML: Nursing and the Great Depression, *Am J Nurs* 75(12):2188-2190, 1975.

Gassen SG: Flores on the edge for years, *Arizona Daily Star,* Nov 26, 2002 (website): http://www.azstar-net.com/specialreports/21126FLORES.html.

Gordon S: *Nursing against the odds: how health care cost cutting, media stereotypes and medical hubris undermine nurses and patient care,* Ithaca, NY, 2005, Cornell University Press.

Hart KA: What do men in nursing really want? *Nursing* 35(11):46-48, 2005.

Image of nursing: media portrayals, cheers, and jeers, *Nursing* 36(3):33, 2006.

Johnson LD: The role of cultural competency in eliminating health disparities, *Minority Nurse: 52-55,* Winter 2005.

Joint Commission on Accreditation of Healthcare Organizations: *Quick statistics on the nursing shortage,* 2003 (website): http://www.jcaho.org/News?Room/Press?Kits/quick?statistics?on?the?nursing?shortage.htm.

Kalisch PA, Kalisch BJ: *The changing image of the nurse,* Reading, Mass, 1987, Addison-Wesley.

Kalisch PA, Kalisch BJ: *American nursing: a history,* Philadelphia, 2005, Lippincott Williams & Wilkins.

Kalist D: The gender earnings gap in the RN labor market, *Nurs Economics* 20(4):155-162, 2002.

Kennedy D: *Birth control in America: the career of Margaret Sanger,* New Haven, 1970, Yale University Press.

Maxwell M: It's not just black and white: how diverse is your workforce?, *Nurs Economics* 23(3):139-140, 2005.

Miller HS: *America's first black professional nurse,* Atlanta, 1986, Wright Publishing.

National Center on Elder Abuse: *The basics: major types of elder abuse,* 2003 (website): http://www.elder-abusecenter.org/basic/index.html.

Nightingale F: *Notes on nursing: what it is and what it is not,* Reprint, Philadelphia, 1946, JB Lippincott (originally published in 1859).

Oates SB: *A woman of valor,* New York, 1994, The Free Press.

Occupational Safety and Health Administration: *Protecting community workers against violence,* Fact sheet No. OSHA 96-53, Washington, DC, 1996, Government Printing Office.

Palmer S: The editor, *Am J Nurs* 1(1):64, 1900.

Pember PY: *A Southern woman's story,* Atlanta, 1959, Bill Wiley.

Petry L: The U.S. Cadet Nurse Corps: a summing up, *Am J Nurs* 45(12):1027-1028, 1945.

Powell KA, Abels L: Sex-role stereotypes in TV programs aimed at the preschool audience: an analysis of Teletubbies and Barney & Friends, *Women Language* 25(2):14-22, 2002.

Robinson TM, Perry PM: *Cadet nurse stories: the call for and response of women during World War II,* Indianapolis, 2001, Sigma Theta Tau International-Center Nursing Press.

Rosenberg CE: *The care of strangers,* New York, 1987, Basic Books.

Seabrook J: The white dress: what should nurses wear? *The New Yorker* 78(4):122-128, 2002.

Sigma Theta Tau International: *The Woodhull Study on nursing and the media: health care's invisible partner,* Indianapolis, IN, 1998, Sigma Theta Tau International-Center Nursing Press.

Simpson RL, Keegan AJ: How connected are you? Emotional intelligence in a high-tech world, *Nurs Admin Quart* 26(2):80-86, 2003.

Sleet J: A successful experiment, *Am J Nurs* 2:729, 1901.

Smith A: J & J's campaign for nursing's future: the gift that keeps on giving, *Nurs Economics* 23(4):199-200, 2005.

Ulmer BC: The image of nursing, *AORN J* 71(6):26-27, 2000.

Ulrich B: A matter of trust, *NurseWeek,* 2003 (website): http://www.nurseweek.com/ednote/03/121803_ca_sc_print.html.

U.S. Bureau of the Census: *Statistical abstract of the United States: 2002,* ed 122, Washington, DC, 2002, Government Printing Office.

U.S. Department of Health and Human Services, Children's Bureau: *Child maltreatment 2000,* Chapter 1, 2000 (website): http://www.acf.hhs.gov/programs/cb/publications/cm00/ chapterone.htm.

U.S. Department of Health and Human Services, Division of Nursing: *The registered nurse population, March 2000: findings from the national sample survey of registered nurses,* Washington, DC, 2001, Government Printing Office.

U.S. Department of Health and Human Services, Division of Nursing: *The registered nurse population, March 2004: national sample survey of registered nurses, preliminary findings,* Washington, DC, 2005, Government Printing Office.

U.S. Department of Health and Human Services, Health Resources and Services Administration: *Projected supply, demand, and shortages of registered nurses:*

2000-2020, Washington, DC, 2002, Government Printing Office.

Wall BM: Courage to care: the Sisters of the Holy Cross in the Spanish-American War, *Nurs Hist Rev* 3:55-77, 1995.

Williams CL: Hidden advantages for men in nursing, *Nurs Admin Quart* 19(2):63-70, 1995.

Williams D: *Nurse, teacher, trailblazer,* 2006 (website): http://www.minoritynurse.com/features/other/03-15-05a.html.

Yoder-Wise P: *Leading and managing in nursing,* St Louis, 2003, Mosby.

Young A: *The women and the crisis: women of the North in the Civil War,* New York, 1959, McDowell, Obolensky.

The Professionalization of Nursing

Kay Kittrell Chitty

Learning Outcomes

After studying this chapter, students will be able to:

- Identify the characteristics of a profession.
- Distinguish between the characteristics of professions and occupations.
- Describe how professions evolve.
- Evaluate nursing's position on the professionalism continuum.
- Explain the elements of nursing's contract with society.

- Recognize characteristic behaviors that exemplify professional nurses.
- Describe outcomes of professional nursing practice.
- Assess themselves in the development of professional conduct.

What is a profession, and who can be called a professional? These terms are used loosely in everyday conversation. Historically, only medicine, law, and the ministry were considered professions. Today, however, **professional** is a term commonly used to identify many types of people, ranging from athletes to pharmacists. Are all these individuals professionals? Is the value of the term professional diminished when it is used indiscriminately to describe any work done by any group? Does possession of a license to practice as a registered nurse make a person a professional nurse? Knowledge, skills, and expertise are part of being a professional. As you will see in this chapter, there are many other criteria to be examined in a discussion of what contributes to **professionalism** in general and in nursing specifically.

HISTORICAL REVIEW: CHARACTERISTICS OF A PROFESSION

For nearly a century scholars have grappled with the meaning of **profession**. They have generally agreed that a profession is an occupational group with a set of attitudes or behaviors, or both. In this section we will briefly review several definitions by scholars through the years and identify major similarities.

Abraham Flexner

Every serious study of professions must begin with a tribute to Abraham Flexner. In the early 1900s, the Carnegie Foundation issued a series of papers about professional schools. The first of these reports was based on sociologist Abraham Flexner's 1910 study of medical education (Flexner,

1910). The **Flexner Report,** as it became known, is a classic piece of educational literature that provided the impetus for the much-needed reform of medical education.

Flexner went on to study other disciplines and later, in a paper about social work, published a list of criteria that he believed were characteristic of all true professions (Flexner, 1915). Flexner's work has stood the test of time. Since his original criteria were published, they have been widely used as a benchmark for determining the status of various occupations in terms of professionalism and have had a profound influence on professional education in several disciplines, including nursing (see Critical Thinking Challenge 3-1).

Flexner's criteria stipulate that a profession:

1. Is basically intellectual (as opposed to physical) and is accompanied by a high degree of individual responsibility.
2. Is based on a body of knowledge that can be learned and is refreshed and refined through research. (Today, this is known as evidence-based practice.)
3. Is practical, in addition to being theoretical.
4. Can be taught through a process of highly specialized professional education.
5. Has a strong internal organization of members and a well-developed group consciousness.

6. Has practitioners who are motivated by altruism (the desire to help others) and who are responsive to public interests (Figure 3-1).

Since 1915, other authorities have identified criteria for professions, building on but varying slightly from Flexner's.

Richard H. Hall

Another sociologist, Richard H. Hall, published a seminal work on professionalism in 1968. Hall described a professional model that classified attributes such as educational qualifications, professional organizations, and sense of calling. He identified five indicators of an individual's attitude toward professionalism (1968):

1. Use of a professional organization as a primary point of reference
2. Belief in the value of public service
3. Belief in self-regulation
4. Commitment to a profession that goes beyond economic incentives
5. A sense of autonomy in practice

Hall recommended that each profession needed to develop its own methods of measuring

Figure 3-1
According to experts, professionals are motivated by altruism, a desire to help others. (*Courtesy Medical University of South Carolina.*)

CRITICAL THINKING *Challenge 3-1*

Are We There Yet? Nursing as a Profession

Feminists in nursing have expressed concern that traditional definitions of the profession, such as Flexner's, are incomplete because they embody only the masculine worldview. They believe that adhering to traditional criteria for professions has had the effect of relegating nursing, teaching, social work, and other female-dominated fields to the status of "semiprofessions." Explore this idea in a class or small group discussion, remembering to respect viewpoints different from your own.

professionalism that recognize the uniqueness of that discipline.

Contemporary Conceptualizations of Profession

Individuals and groups continue attempts to identify what professionals believe, think, and do. Muller (1998) indicated that "professionalism involves the application of knowledge and skills, a high standard of practice, leadership, self-regulation, professional commitment, social values, and service-directed activity."

A pharmacy profession task force spent 5 years studying and promoting pharmacy student professionalism (Task Force on Professionalism, 2000). They reached back into the history of professional development in the broad sense, reviewing the work of numerous scholars. From this review they distilled a list of 10 common characteristics of the members of a profession:

1. Prolonged specialized training in a body of abstract knowledge
2. A service orientation
3. An ideology based on the original faith professed by members
4. An ethic that is binding on the practitioners
5. A body of knowledge unique to the members
6. A set of skills that forms the technique of the profession
7. A guild of those entitled to practice the profession
8. Authority granted by society in the form of licensure or certification
9. A recognized setting in which the profession is practiced
10. A theory of societal benefits derived from the ideology

Major Similarities

As you see, authorities have not always agreed about the number of criteria and the types of behaviors and characteristics of professions. A review of a variety of publications on this topic, however, reveals that there are three criteria that consistently appear: service/altruism, specialized knowledge, and autonomy/ethics (Flexner, 1915;

Hall, 1968, 1982; Carr-Saunders and Wilson, 1933; Adams, Miller, and Beck, 1996; Huber, 2000).

1. Service implies a sense of calling to the discipline, a sense of mission, and a responsibility to the public.
2. Knowledge implies specialized education, including both theoretical knowledge and techniques or skills.
3. Practice autonomy implies having control over one's own practice. It also implies having a code of ethics governing standards of conduct within the profession (Huber, 2000).

After nearly a century of study, contemplation, and deliberation, there is still no clear-cut consensus about what constitutes a profession, nor is there likely to be. Occupational groups are constantly pushing to become more professional and to receive public acknowledgment of their professional status. As they do so, conceptions of profession change.

THE EVOLUTION FROM OCCUPATION TO PROFESSION

Professions usually evolved from occupations that originally consisted of tasks but developed more specialized educational pathways and publicly legitimized status. The established professions, such as law, medicine, and the ministry, generally followed a typical developmental pattern of stages that occurred sequentially. First, practitioners performed full-time work in the discipline. They then determined work standards, identified a body of knowledge, and established educational programs in institutions of higher learning. Next, they promoted organization into effective occupational associations. Then they worked toward legal protection that limited practice of their unique skills by outsiders. Finally, they established codes of ethics (Carr-Saunders and Wilson, 1933). This process can be termed **professionalization.**

Another analysis of the evolution from occupation to profession was done by Houle (1980). He identified a number of characteristics that indicate that an occupational group is moving along the continuum toward professional status. First is the definition of the group's mission and foundations of practice. Then comes mastery of theoretical knowledge, development of the capacity to solve problems, the use of practical knowledge, and self-enhancement (continued learning and development). Finally, Houle identified nine characteristics that indicate that an occupation is developing a **collective identity** or group identification, which is necessary for professions. These include formal training, credentialing, creation of a subculture, legal right to practice, public acceptance, ethical practice, discipline of incompetent/unethical practitioners, relationship to other practitioners, and relationship to users of services.

The term **occupation** is often used interchangeably with *profession*, but their definitions differ. *Webster's New World Dictionary* (1996) defines occupation as "what occupies, or engages, one's time; business; employment." In this discussion we define profession as "a calling, vocation, or form of employment that provides a needed service to society and possesses characteristics of expertise, autonomy, long academic preparation, commitment, and responsibility" (Huber, 2000, p. 34).

There is widespread, overall agreement that a profession is different from an occupation in at least two major ways—preparation and commitment.

Professional Preparation

Professional preparation usually takes place in a college or university setting. Preparation is prolonged to include instruction in the specialized body of knowledge and techniques of the profession. Professional preparation includes more than knowledge and skills, however. It also includes orientation to the beliefs, values, and attitudes expected of the members of the profession. Standards of practice and ethical considerations are also included. These components of professional education are part of the process of socialization into a profession and are discussed in Chapter 6. According to Miller (1985), preparation enables

professional practitioners to act in a logical, rational manner rather than relying on intuition or trial and error. An ever-expanding base of knowledge in all disciplines complicates the challenges of professional preparation.

The belief that there are "core competencies" that should be included in all health professional education was suggested by the Institute of Medicine in 2003 following study by a task force of over 150 health professionals of all disciplines in a Health Professions Education Summit. The report issued following this summit identified five core competencies that all students of health professions should acquire (Greiner and Knebel, 2003).

1. Provide patient-centered care.
2. Work in interdisciplinary teams.
3. Employ evidence-based practice.
4. Apply quality improvement principles.
5. Utilize informatics.

The Evidence-Based Practice Note on p. 73 describes a study that examined nursing students' beliefs about what it means to be a professional.

Professional Commitment

Professionals' commitment to their profession is strong. They derive much of their personal identification from their work and consider it an integral part of their lives. People engaging in a profession often consider it their "calling." Historically, professionals' commitment to their profession has transcended their expectation of material reward. Although people may readily change occupations, it is less common for people to change professions. Several critical differences between occupations and professions are summarized in Table 3-1.

BARRIERS TO PROFESSIONALISM IN NURSING

As a group, nurses must strive to reduce the barriers to professionalization. The first step in that process is developing an awareness of those barriers. Several major barriers will be discussed here.

EVIDENCE-BASED PRACTICE

note

Three professors at a Tennessee university sought to understand how students develop professional identity. They conducted a qualitative, existential-phenomenological study of baccalaureate students to determine their ideas of what it means to be a professional. Sixty-nine nursing students at various levels of education were asked to describe specific experiences in which they "felt professional." The researchers analyzed these figural (outstanding) experiences for common patterns or themes. Three interrelated themes were identified: belonging, knowing, and affirmation.

■ An example of belonging: "I knew ... that I had acted as a professional and knowledgeable nurse and even though that man died, the team did everything they could to keep him alive and I was a team member. It was a satisfying moment."

■ An example of knowing: "For myself, my nursing knowledge and actions make me a professional. However, when this nursing knowledge is applied and the client and family express their appreciation of my nursing efforts, then I feel professional."

■ An example of affirmation: "I had one family who just couldn't believe I was in nursing school. They stated that I was so 'professional and caring' and that I was a 'great nurse.' Then I said, 'Well, I'm not a nurse yet; I'll be graduating in one year.' That made me feel like I was actually a nurse."

The researchers suggested that courses encouraging students to reflect on the meaning of the profession and being a professional should be offered early in the curriculum. They stated their belief that "developing a sense of professionalism is equally important as knowledge and skills."

From Secrest J, Norwood BR, Keatley VM: "I was actually a nurse": the meaning of professionalism for baccalaureate nursing students, *J Nurs Educ* 42(2):77-82, 2003.

Table 3-1 COMPARISON OF CHARACTERISTICS OF OCCUPATIONS AND PROFESSIONS

Occupation	Profession
Training may occur on the job.	Education takes place in a college or university.
Length of training varies.	Education is prolonged.
Work is largely manual.	Work involves mental creativity.
Decision making is guided largely by experience or by trial and error.	Decision making is based largely on science or theoretical constructs.
Values, beliefs, and ethics are not prominent features of preparation.	Values, beliefs, and ethics are an integral part of preparation.
Commitment and personal identification vary.	Commitment and personal identification are strong.
Workers are supervised.	Workers are autonomous.
People often change jobs.	People are unlikely to change professions.
Material reward is main motivation.	Commitment transcends material reward.
Accountability rests primarily with employer.	Accountability rests with individual.

Variability in Educational Preparation

The most obvious barrier to nursing's achievement of professional status is the variability of educational backgrounds of its practitioners. There is no other profession that allows entry into practice at less than the baccalaureate level. To the contrary, many professions, such as law, medicine, and physical therapy, require postgraduate preparation for professional practice. Because professional status and power increase with education, a legitimate question is, "How can nursing take its place as a peer among the professions when most nurses currently in practice do not hold the baccalaureate degree?" The differentiation between professional nursing and technical nursing is a challenging issue that has not yet been resolved. Educational diversity within nursing has slowed the progress toward acceptance of the baccalaureate or higher degree as the prerequisite for professional practice. Lack of resolution of these differences threatens to undermine nursing's continued steady development as a profession (Christman, 1998). This is a painful issue for nurses, creating division and anger whenever it is discussed. For the profession as a whole to progress, we must move beyond personal feelings to look objectively at how nursing stacks up when compared with other groups—groups to whom we wish to be compared—and adjust our aims accordingly.

Gender Issues

Although gender was not identified as a criterion by any of the scholars of professionalism, it plays a major role in the perceived value of female-dominated professions such as teaching, social work, and nursing. Although the number of men in nursing is gradually increasing, a gender balance may never be achieved. This will continue to be a hindrance, because of the persistent prevalence of outmoded thinking and the resultant devaluing of "women's work" in our society.

Historical Influences

Nursing's historical connections with religious orders and the military continue to have influence, both positive and negative, today. Aspects that have become liabilities with the passage of time include unquestioning obedience, which runs counter to the professional values of autonomy and self-determination, and altruism, which mitigates against the fair economic valuation of the work of nursing. Nurses should be aware that unquestioning obedience stifles the creative thinking and problem solving required for professional practice. Similar to other helping professionals, nurses must resist pressures to feel guilty or greedy for expecting to be paid well for their complex and demanding work.

External Conflicts

As nurses have become more highly educated and able to provide services that were formerly part of medical practice, conflicts with medicine have inevitably arisen. Much of the power, influence, and resources of organized nursing has gone toward lobbying efforts in state legislatures to ensure that the legal scope of nursing practice is protected and appropriately enhanced. These efforts should and will continue on the professional association level. On the personal level, however, nurses must strive for collaboration, not competition, with physicians and other health personnel with whom they work. Nurses must demonstrate their unique knowledge, expertise, and skills so that professional autonomy can be exercised within the various bureaucratic organizations in which they work.

Internal Conflicts

Professional nursing's power is fragmented by subgroups and dissention. Rivalry among diploma-educated, associate degree–educated, and baccalaureate-educated nurses saps the vitality of the profession. The proliferation of nursing organizations (see a list of nursing organizations at www.nurse.org/orgs.shtml) and competition among them for members also diminish nursing's potential. Less than 10 percent of the 2.9 million registered nurses in the United States are members of the ANA, the largest professional nursing organization. The fact that most nurses are not members of any professional organization impairs nursing's ability to govern itself, set standards, and use its collective power to lobby effectively for positive changes in health care. These are major challenges for nursing if it is to realize its potential collective professional power and autonomy.

NURSING'S PATHWAY TO PROFESSIONALISM

Nursing's pathway to professionalism has not been smooth. For decades an ongoing subject for discussion in nursing circles has been the following question: "Is nursing a profession?" Much has been spoken and written on both sides of this issue over the years. Nursing sociologists do not all agree that nursing is a profession. Some believe that it is, at best, an emerging profession. Others cite the progress nursing has made toward meeting the commonly accepted criteria for full-fledged professional status. Still others believe that nursing leaders, by embracing the masculine orientation to professionalism embodied in the work of Flexner and others, have supported the existing patriarchal order, thereby prolonging the subordination of nursing to male-dominated professions such as medicine (Wuest, 1994). Let us look critically now at various criteria and nursing's status in relation to them.

Bixler and Bixlers' Criteria

Roy and Genevieve Bixler, a husband and wife team of nonnurses who were advocates and supporters of nursing, first wrote about the status of nursing as a profession in 1945. In 1959 they again appraised nursing according to their original seven criteria, noting the progress made (Bixler and Bixler, 1959). Their criteria included the following:

1. "A profession utilizes in its practice a well-defined and well-organized body of specialized knowledge which is on the intellectual level of higher learning" (p. 1142).
2. "A profession constantly enlarges the body of knowledge it uses and improves its techniques of education and service by the use of the scientific method" (p. 1143).

3. "A profession entrusts the education of its practitioners to institutions of higher education" (p. 1144).
4. "A profession applies its body of knowledge in practical services which are vital to human and social welfare" (p. 1145).
5. "A profession functions autonomously in the formulation of professional policy and in the control of professional activity thereby" (p. 1145).
6. "A profession attracts individuals of intellectual and personal qualities who exalt service above personal gain and who recognize their chosen occupation as a life work" (p. 1146).
7. "A profession strives to compensate its practitioners by providing freedom of action, opportunity for continuous professional growth, and economic security" (p. 1146).

Kelly's Criteria

Lucie Kelly, RN, PhD, FAAN, is an outstanding nurse writer, teacher, and influential leader. She was editor of the journal *Nursing Outlook* and president of Sigma Theta Tau International Honor Society of Nursing, among many career highlights. Dr. Kelly has spent much of her nursing career exploring the dimensions of professional nursing. She compiled the following set of eight characteristics of a profession many years ago (Kelly, 1981, p. 157), but they remain relevant today:

1. The services provided are vital to humanity and the welfare of society.
2. There is a special body of knowledge that is continually enlarged through research.
3. The services involve intellectual activities; individual responsibility (**accountability**) is a strong feature.
4. Practitioners are educated in institutions of higher learning.
5. Practitioners are relatively independent and control their own policies and activities (**autonomy**).
6. Practitioners are motivated by service (altruism) and consider their work an important component of their lives.

7. There is a code of ethics to guide the decisions and conduct of practitioners.
8. There is an organization (**association**) that encourages and supports high standards of practice.

Let us examine how well contemporary nursing fulfills these eight characteristics.

"The services provided are vital to humanity and the welfare of society"

If random students were asked why they chose nursing, most would reply, "To help people." Certainly nursing is a service that is essential to the well-being of people and to society as a whole. Nursing promotes the maintenance and restoration of health of individuals, groups, and communities. The goal of nursing is to assist others to attain the highest level of wellness of which they are capable. **Caring**—meaning nurturing and helping others—is a basic component of professional nursing.

"There is a special body of knowledge that is continually enlarged through research"

In the past, nursing was based on principles borrowed from the physical and social sciences and other disciplines. Today, however, there is a body of knowledge that is uniquely nursing's own. Although this was not always so, the amount of investigation and analysis of nursing care has expanded rapidly in the past 30 years. Nursing theory development is also proceeding swiftly. Nursing is no longer based on trial and error but increasingly relies on theory development and research as a basis for practice. We call the reliance on research as a basis for nursing practice **evidence-based practice**. You will learn more about theory, research, and evidence-based practice later in this book.

"The services involve intellectual activities; individual responsibility (accountability) is a strong feature"

Nursing developed and refined its own unique approach to practice, called the nursing process. The nursing process is essentially a cognitive (mental) activity that requires both critical and creative thinking and serves as the basis for providing nursing care. The profession is now engaged in an ongoing effort to identify and standardize nursing diagnoses, interventions, and outcomes, all of which are parts of the nursing process.

Individual accountability in nursing has become the hallmark of practice. Accountability, according to the American Nurses Association's (ANA) *Code of Ethics for Nurses* (2001), is being answerable to someone for something one has done. Provision 4 of the Code states, "The nurse is responsible and accountable for individual nursing practice and determines the appropriate delegation of tasks consistent with the nurse's obligation to provide optimum patient care" (p. 5). Through legal opinions and court cases, society has demonstrated that it, too, holds nurses individually responsible for their actions as well as for those of unlicensed personnel under their supervision.

"Practitioners are educated in institutions of higher learning"

As presented in Chapter 7, the first university-based nursing program began in 1909 at the University of Minnesota. Several studies, including Esther Lucille Brown's 1948 report, *Nursing for the Future*, called for nursing education to be based in universities and colleges (Brown, 1948). Another milestone was the 1965 position paper of the ANA, which called for all nursing education to take place in institutions of higher education (American Nurses Association, 1965).

The majority of programs offering basic nursing education are now associate degree and baccalaureate programs located in colleges and universities. There are growing numbers of master's and doctoral programs in nursing, although the number of graduates is small compared with other health professions.

"Practitioners are relatively independent and control their own policies and activities (autonomy)"

Autonomy, or control over one's practice, is another controversial area for nursing. Although many nursing actions are independent, most nurses are employed in hospitals, where authority resides in one's position. One's place in the hierarchy, rather than expertise, confers or denies power and status. Physicians are widely regarded as gatekeepers, and their authorization or supervision is required before many activities can occur. Nurse practice acts in many states reinforce nursing's tenuous self-determination by requiring that nurses perform certain actions only when authorized by supervising physicians or hospital protocols.

There are at least three groups that have historically attempted to control nursing practice: organized medicine, health service administration, and organized nursing. Both the medical profession and health service administration have attempted to maintain control of nursing because they believe it is in their best interest to keep nurses dependent on them. Both are well organized, well funded, and have powerful lobbies at state and national levels. This is a major challenge to full autonomy for nurses.

"Practitioners are motivated by service (altruism) and consider their work an important component of their lives"

As a group, nurses are dedicated to the ideal of service to others, also known as **altruism.** This ideal has sometimes become intertwined with economic issues and historically has been exploited by employers of nurses. No one questions the right of other professionals to charge reasonable fees for the services they render; when nurses want higher salaries, however, others sometimes call their altruism into question. Nurses must take responsibility for their own financial well-being and for the health of the profession. This will, in turn, ensure its continued attractiveness to those who might choose nursing as a career. If there are to be adequate numbers of nurses to meet society's needs, salaries must be comparable with those in competing disciplines. Being motivated by salary does nothing to diminish a nurse's altruism or professionalism.

Another issue, consideration of work as a primary component of life, has been a thornier problem for nurses. Commitment to a career is not a value equally shared by all nurses. Some still regard nursing as a job and drop in and out of practice depending on economic and family needs. This approach, although appealing to many nurses and conducive to traditional family management, has retarded the development of professional attitudes and behaviors for the profession as a whole.

"There is a code of ethics to guide the decisions and conduct of practitioners"

An ethical code does not stipulate how an individual should act in a specific situation; rather, it provides professional standards and a framework for decision making. The trust placed in the nursing profession by the public requires that nurses act with integrity. To aid them in doing so, both the International Council of Nurses (ICN) and the ANA, among others, have established codes of nursing ethics through which profession-wide standards of practice are established, promoted, and refined. The *Code of Ethics for Nurses*, which will be discussed later in the chapter, can be found on the inside back cover of this text.

In 1893 long before these codes were written, "The Florence Nightingale Pledge" (Box 3-1) was created by a committee headed by Lystra Eggert Gretter and presented to the Farrand Training School for Nurses located at Harper Hospital in Detroit, Michigan (Dock and Stewart, 1920). Its similarities to the medical profession's Hippocratic Oath are obvious. The Nightingale Pledge can be considered nursing's first code of ethics. It is presented here not only for its historic value but also because it established the roots for our current code.

"There is an organization (association) that encourages and supports high standards of practice"

As will be discussed in Chapter 15, a number of professional associations have been formed to promote the improvement of the nursing profession. Among these is the ANA, which all registered nurses are eligible to join. According to its bylaws, the purposes of the ANA are to work for the improvement of health standards and the availability of health care services for all people, to foster high standards of nursing, and to stimulate and promote the professional development of nurses and advance their economic and general welfare (Figure 3-2; American Nurses Association, 1997). The ANA is also the official voice of nursing and therefore is the primary advocate for nursing interests in general. As mentioned earlier, fewer than 1 of 10 nurses belongs to this official professional organization. The political power that could be derived from the unified efforts of 2.9 million registered nurses nationwide would be impressive; sadly, that goal has not yet been realized.

Miller's Wheel of Professionalism in Nursing

Using commonalities she detected in the work of sociologists and nursing leaders, as well as statements from *Nursing's Social Policy Statement* and *Code of Ethics for Nurses*, Miller (1985; Adams and Miller, 2001) created a model (or visual expression) to conceptualize nursing professionalism. She titled this model the Wheel of Professionalism (Figure 3-3).

In Miller's wheel, the center represents the essential foundation of nursing education in an institution of higher learning. According to Adams et al. (1996), "Each of the eight spokes represents other behaviors deemed necessary in maintaining or increasing nurses' professionalism. They are competence and continuing education; adherence

Figure 3-2
Professionals belong to associations that encourage and support ethical standards of practice. (*Courtesy Tennessee Nurses Association.*)

Box 3-1 The Florence Nightingale Pledge

I solemnly pledge myself before God and in the presence of this assembly to pass my life in purity and to practice my profession faithfully.

I will abstain from whatever is deleterious and mischievous, and will not take or knowingly administer any harmful drug. I will do all in my power to maintain and elevate the standard of my profession, and will hold in confidence all personal matters committed to my keeping and all family affairs coming to my knowledge in the practice of my calling.

With loyalty will I endeavor to aid the physician in his work and devote myself to the welfare of those committed to my care.

From Dock LL, Stewart IM: *A short history of nursing*, New York, 1920, Putnam.

Figure 3-3
The Wheel of Professionalism in nursing. (*Copyright 1984 Barbara Kemp Miller.*)

to the code of ethics; participation in the primary and referent professional organization, i.e., ANA and state constituent member association; publication and communication; orientation toward community services; theory and research development and utilization; and self-regulation and autonomy" (p. 79). To test the wheel model, Adams and Miller devised their own instrument, Professionalism in Nursing Behaviors Inventory, which was revised and tested. Research continues to refine this instrument, which is to be used by nurses themselves to evaluate their professional growth.

Standards Established by the Profession Itself

Any exploration of nursing's development as a profession would be incomplete without a discussion of two major documents that guide all nurses in their professional commitments. These are *Nursing's Social Policy Statement* (American Nurses Association, 2003) and the *Code of Ethics for Nurses with Interpretive Statements* (American Nurses Association, 2001).

Nursing's Social Policy Statement: a contract with society

Although criteria for professions vary, all professions have one criterion in common: an obligation to the recipients of their services. Nursing, therefore, has an obligation to those who receive nursing care. The nature of the social contract between the members of the nursing profession and society is summarized in *Nursing's Social Policy Statement*. This document, last revised in 2003, is the result of several years of work by literally hundreds of nurses. It serves "as a framework for understanding professional nursing's relationship with society and nursing's obligation to those who receive professional nursing care" (p. 1). Here is part of what *Nursing's Social Policy Statement* has to say about nursing as a profession:

> Professional nursing, like other professions, is an essential part of the society from which it grew and within which it continues to evolve. Professional nursing is dynamic, rather than static, reflecting the changing nature of societal need. Professional

nursing can be said to be "owned by society in the sense that a profession acquires recognition, relevance, and even meaning in terms of its relationship to that society, its culture and institutions, and its other members" (American Nurses Association, 2003, pp. 1-2).

Nursing's Social Policy Statement is only 15 pages in length; yet it addresses a broad array of topics of concern that occur when nursing intersects with the society it serves. Topics include the following: the social context of nursing; values and assumptions undergirding the statement; a definition of nursing; the knowledge base for nursing practice; the scope of both basic and advanced nursing practice; and the professional, legal, and self-regulation of nursing practice. A careful reading of this brief document will provide the reader with the essence of nursing's professionalism. (It is available from American Nurses Publishing; see References.)

The *Code of Ethics for Nurses*

As you will recall, most of the early scholars attempting to define profession mentioned ethical behavior as a hallmark of a profession. In fact, a code of ethics is generally considered a tool that guides a group toward professional self-definition and provides evidence of professional legitimacy.

A **code of ethics** is a written, public document that reminds practitioners and the public they serve of the specific responsibilities and obligations accepted by the profession's practitioners. Since the inception of formalized education for nurses, the practice of nursing has been guided by ethical standards promoted first by Florence Nightingale and thereafter by nursing groups. The *Code of Ethics for Nurses* has been modified over the years as nursing and its social context have evolved. It is intended to guide the practice of registered nurses in all practice settings with all types of clients. The most recent version, *Code of Ethics for Nurses with Interpretive Statements,* was approved in 2001.

There are nine provisions in the 2001 *Code*, each of which is accompanied by interpretive statements intended to clarify the provision. The first three provisions describe "the fundamental values and commitments of the nurse; the next three address boundaries of duty and loyalty; and the last three address aspects of duties beyond individual patient encounters" (p. 2). Read the provisions of the *Code of Ethics for Nurses* on the inside back cover of this text. The entire document, including interpretive statements, is available for review online (http://nursingworld.org/ethics/code/protected_nwcoe303.htm).

Today's health care environment often presents challenges to nurses' ethics. Cost-conscious hospitals, managed care plans, and staffing insufficiencies created by both economic factors and nursing shortages are just a few of the many strains on nursing practice (Hook, 2001). The *Code* exists to strengthen and guide nurses' decision making as they navigate the troubled waters that now exist in many practice settings. The *Code* empowers nurses to maintain their focus on the patient as the center of health care.

Current concerns about professionalism in nursing have arisen in the last few years as some nurses seem to have become more nurse-centered than patient-centered. Is nursing losing its patient-centered focus? Patients and their families have reported that "nursing has changed" and identified conduct by nurses that is at odds with their perceptions of "what nurses do." This has caused concerned nurses to think deeply about the profession and where it is going (Roberts, 2005). Regardless of the responsibility and workloads of today's nurses, the fact remains that nurses are paid to take care of patients and their loved ones (Cooper, 2005). Nursing has long prided itself as being the health care profession that cares. Certainly the behaviors exhibited by an individual nurse reflect the character and values of that individual and can enhance patient well-being and patient outcomes. You can assess your patient-centered focus using the self-assessment exercise found in Box 3-2.

COLLEGIALITY AS AN ATTRIBUTE OF THE PROFESSIONAL NURSE

A sometimes overlooked but increasingly important aspect of professionalism in nursing is collegiality. The promotion of collaboration,

---

Box 3-2 Self-Assessment: Am I a Patient-Centered Nurse?

1. Do I refrain from talking about myself and my problems to patients and their families?
2. Do I always introduce myself to patients and families when I first meet them?
3. When a patient or family member approaches me, do I immediately acknowledge them and turn my attention to them as soon as possible?
4. Do I really listen when patients and family members attempt to express a problem or concern?
5. Do I clarify patients' reasons for refusing medications or treatments without becoming defensive or taking the refusal personally?
6. Do I give prompt attention to all my patients, even those who are "difficult"?
7. Do I make every effort to be pleasant and polite to patients, family members, co-workers, and students, even when I am having a bad day?
8. Do I explain procedures to patients and take every opportunity to educate them about their medications and conditions?
9. Am I am alert to patient anxiety and attempt to "talk them through" anxiety-laden procedures?
10. Do I project high self-regard through my professional image, which includes tidy hair style, clean and polished shoes, neat uniform, short nails, and conservative makeup/grooming?
11. Do I recognize that I am accountable for both my actions and my omissions?
12. Do I take every opportunity to learn, grow, and enhance my competence as a nurse?

Adapted from Cooper PG: A call for a return to patient-centered care, *Nurs Forum* 40(3):73-74, 2005.

cooperation, and recognition of interdependence among members of the nursing profession is the essence of **collegiality.** Professional nurses demonstrate collegiality by sharing with, supporting, assisting, and counseling other nurses and nursing students. These behaviors can be seen when nurses, for example, take part in professional organizations, mentor less experienced nurses, willingly serve as role models for nursing students, welcome learners and their instructors in the practice setting, assist researchers with data gathering, publish in professional literature, and support peer-assistance programs for impaired nurses.

The value placed on collegiality as a professional attribute can be seen in the ANA's 2004 publication *Nursing's Social Policy Statement,* which includes collegiality as one of nine standards of professional performance. The practice of nursing would be enhanced if the commitment nurses feel toward their patients was equaled by their commitment to one another and to nurturing the next generation of professional nurses.

An article titled "Being Good and Doing Good" by Bruhn (2001) outlines 12 points on professionalism, a number of which serve as reminders of the value of collegiality (Box 3-3).

NEED FOR A NEW PARADIGM

As society and health care have become more complex, perhaps the time has come to shift away from a rigid conceptualization of profession toward viewing the achievement of professional status as a dynamic, ongoing process. Huber (2000) recommends that we view professionalization as a continuum from nonprofessional to semiprofessional to professional, related to the degree to which an occupational group is characterized by the achievement of identified professional criteria. Instead of asking, "Is nursing a profession?" it may be more fruitful to ask, "How is nursing progressing in the dynamic process of professionalization?" or "Where on the professional continuum is nursing right now?" Although

---

| Box **3-3** | **Points on Professionalism** |

- Be civil—Treat people with respect. You do not have to like or agree with a person to treat him or her as you would want to be treated.
- Be ethical—Stand up for personal and professional standards. Do what is right, not what is expected.
- Be honest—Be forthright; do not participate in gossip and rumor.
- Be the best—Strive to be better than good.
- Be consistent—Behavior should coincide with values and beliefs.
- Be a communicator—Invite ideas, opinions, and feedback from patients and colleagues.
- Be accountable—Do what you say you will do. Take responsibility for your own actions.
- Be collaborative—Work in partnership with others for the benefit of patients.
- Be forgiving—Everyone makes mistakes; give people a fair chance.
- Be current—Keep knowledge and skills up to date.
- Be involved—Be active at local, state, and national levels.
- Be a model—What a person says and does reflects on his or her profession.
- Be responsible for self—Take responsibility for your own learning needs and be assertive in making them known to teachers and mentors.
- Be prepared—Do assignments for classes and prepare for labs and clinicals in advance, brushing up on skills if needed.

From Bruhn JG: Being good and doing good: the culture of professionalism in the health professions, *Health Care Manag* 19(4):47-58, 2001; and Cheyne D: Take responsibility for your learning needs, *Nurs Standard* 20(7):88, 2005.

barriers remain, some of which were identified earlier in this chapter, nursing has made a great deal of progress in the past few decades and is poised to continue that progress in the future.

To summarize this discussion of professionalism in nursing, read Critical Thinking Challenge 3-2 and identify the professional behaviors exhibited in the case study presented.

CRITICAL THINKING *Challenge 3-2*

Identifying Professional Nursing Behaviors

Instructions: If being a professional nurse is different from practicing the occupation of nursing, there must be certain behaviors that differentiate the two. Read the case study below; then, using various criteria for professions presented in this chapter and the Code of Ethics for Nurses, *identify professional behaviors exhibited by Joan. For each behavior you identify, state which source or document, such as the* Code *or* Social Policy Statement, *promotes that behavior.*

Joan is a 32-year-old married mother of two. She graduated from River City College of Nursing at the age of 26 and has been practicing since her graduation. Her first position was as a staff nurse at Providence Hospital, a 300-bed private hospital. Nursing administration at Providence encourages nurses to provide individualized nursing care while protecting the dignity and autonomy of each patient and family. She chose Providence because the hospital's philosophy of nursing paralleled her own. Another reason Joan selected this hospital was that she wanted to practice oncology (cancer) nursing, and there is an oncology unit at Providence.

Each day Joan uses the nursing process in caring for her patients and in dealing with their families. That means she assesses their condition, plans and implements their care, and evaluates the care she has given. Then she documents what she has done in each patient's database in the accepted format. She communicates clearly to the other members of the nursing staff and to the other health care professionals involved in the care of the patients on her unit but refuses to discuss her patients with others not involved in their direct care.

After 2 years as a staff nurse, Joan accepted a position as a team leader. This means that now she takes responsibility not only for her own practice but also for that of licensed practical nurses and nursing assistants on her team. To do this effectively, she stays abreast of changes in her state's nurse practice act and Providence Hospital's policies and procedures. In addition, she updates her knowledge by reading current journals and research periodicals. She makes it a policy to attend at least two nursing conferences each year to stay on top of trends. She belongs to her professional organization and participates as an active member. She finds that this is another source of the latest information on professional issues.

Joan looks forward to working with the nursing students at Providence Hospital. She remembers when she was a student and how a word from a practicing nurse could make or break her day. Of course, students do mean extra work, but she sees this as a part of her role and patiently provides the guidance they need, even when she is busy.

In the course of her daily work, Joan sometimes has a question about certain procedures. She is not embarrassed to seek help from more experienced nurses, from textbooks, or from other health professionals. Sometimes she offers suggestions to the head nurse and the oncology clinical nurse specialist about possible research questions and participates in gathering data when the unit takes on a research study.

Providence Hospital uses a shared governance model, which means nurses serve on committees that develop and interpret nursing policies and procedures. Joan serves on two committees and chairs another. Right now the hospital is preparing a self-study for an upcoming accreditation, so the meetings are frequent. Instead of complaining about the meetings, Joan prepares and organizes her portion of the

Continued

<u>CRITICAL THINKING</u> *Challenge 3-2*

Identifying Professional Nursing Behaviors—Cont'd

meeting so that everyone's time is used most effectively. She has to delegate some of her patient care responsibilities to others while she is attending meetings. Because she has taken the time to know the other workers' skills and abilities, she does not worry about what happens while she is gone and asks for a full report when she returns to her unit.

At the end of the day when Joan goes home, she occasionally gets a call from a friend with a health-related question or a request to give a neighbor's child an allergy injection. Although she is tired, she recognizes that in the eyes of others, she represents the nursing profession. She is proud to be trusted and respected for her knowledge, skills, and dedication. Helping others through nursing care is something Joan has wanted to do since she was small, and she finds it very fulfilling.

Lately, Joan has recognized in herself some troubling signs: She has been irritable and impatient with family and co-workers and generally out of sorts. She has gained weight and is exercising less than usual. She wonders whether working with terminally ill patients and their families is the source of her stress. Joan's husband has suggested that she take "a break" from nursing and stay home with the children, but after talking it over with her nurse manager, she has decided to ask for assignment to different nursing responsibilities for a while. She knows that she needs to be her own advocate and take care of herself. Next week she will begin a 3-month stint in outpatient surgery, where she believes the emotional intensity will be a bit lower.

SUMMARY OF *Key Points*

- Commitment to a profession is different from having a job or an occupation.
- A review of scholarly writing about professions reveals that there are several characteristics that all professions have in common.
- A body of knowledge, specialized education, service to society, accountability, autonomy, and ethical standards are a few of the hallmarks of professions.
- The feminist perspective includes the belief that the emphasis on professionalism has not helped nursing and has prevented nurses from appreciating, valuing, exploring, and refining the feminine caring experience (Wuest, 1994).
- Although nursing has a briefer history than some traditional professions and is still dealing

with autonomy, preparation, and commitment issues, great progress has been made in moving nursing along the professionalization continuum.
- An awareness of the characteristics of professions and professional behavior helps nurses assume leadership in continuing progress toward professionalism.
- *Nursing's Social Policy Statement* is considered nursing's contract with society.
- Being a professional is a dynamic process, not a condition or state of being.
- Professional growth begins during professional education and evolves throughout the different stages of nurses' careers.

CRITICAL THINKING QUESTIONS

1. What is the relationship between training and education?
2. On a scale of 1 to 10, rate nursing on each of the criteria for professions identified by two of the following: Flexner, Hall, Bixler and Bixler, and Kelly.
3. Describe at least five characteristic behaviors of professional nurses.
4. Discuss the Nightingale Pledge (see Box 3-1) as a historical document, as an ethical statement, and as a reflection of Florence Nightingale's social and cultural environment. What value does this document have for today's nurse?
5. Using Miller's Wheel of Professionalism, identify specific activities that fit under each of the "spokes." How might a novice nurse's behaviors in relation to each spoke differ from those of a seasoned practitioner? Where does evidence-based practice fit into this model?
6. How might nursing be different today if all its practitioners viewed it as their profession rather than a job?

REFERENCES

Adams D, Miller BK: Professionalism in nursing behaviors of nurse practitioners, *J Prof Nurs* 17(4):203-210, 2001.

Adams D, Miller BK, Beck L: Professionalism behaviors of hospital nurse executives and middle managers in 10 western states, *West J Nurs Res* 18(1):77-89, 1996.

American Nurses Association: *Educational preparation for nurse practitioners and assistants to nurses: a position paper,* Kansas City, Mo, 1965, American Nurses Association.

American Nurses Association: *Association bylaws,* Kansas City, Mo, 1997, American Nurses Association.

American Nurses Association: *Code of ethics for nurses with interpretive statements,* Washington, DC, 2001, American Nurses Publishing.

American Nurses Association: *Nursing: scope and standards of practice,* Washington, DC, 2003 (website): nursesbooks.org.

American Nurses Association: *Nursing's social policy statement,* ed 2, Washington, DC, 2004 (website): nursesbooks.org.

Bixler GK, Bixler RW: The professional status of nursing, *Am J Nurs* 59(8):1142-1147, 1959.

Brown EL: *Nursing for the future,* New York, 1948, Russell Sage Foundation.

Bruhn JG: Being good and doing good: the culture of professionalism in the health professions, *Health Care Manag* 19(4):47-58, 2001.

Carr-Saunders AM, Wilson PA: *The professions,* Oxford, 1933, Clarendon Press.

Cheyne D: Take responsibility for your learning needs, *Nurs Standard* 20(7):88, 2005.

Christman L: Who is a nurse? *Image: J Nurs Scholar* 30(3):211-214, 1998.

Cooper PG: A call for a return to patient-centered care, *Nurs Forum* 40(3):73-74, 2005.

Dock LL, Stewart IM: *A short history of nursing,* New York, 1920, Putnam.

Flexner A: *Medical education in the United States and Canada: a report to the Carnegie Foundation for the advancement of teaching,* Bethesda, Md, 1910, Science & Health Publications.

Flexner A: Is social work a profession? *School Soc* 1(26):901, 1915.

Greiner AC, Knebel E, editors: *Health professions education: a bridge to quality,* Washington, DC, 2003, Institute of Medicine, National Academies Press.

Hall RH: Professionalization and bureaucratization, *Am Sociol Rev* 33:92-104, 1968.

Hall RH: The professionals, employed professionals, and the professional association. In *Professionalism and the empowerment of nursing,* Kansas City, Mo, 1982, American Nurses Association.

Hook K: Empowered caring and the code of ethics, *ANA Ethics & Human Rights Issues Update* 1(2), 2001 (website): www.nursingworld.org/ethics/update/vol1no2a.htm.

Houle C: *Continuing learning in the professions,* San Francisco, Calif, 1980, Jossey-Bass.

Huber D: *Leadership and nursing care management,* Philadelphia, 2000, WB Saunders.

Kelly L: *Dimensions of professional nursing,* ed 4, New York, 1981, Macmillan.

Miller BK: Just what is a professional? *Nurs Success Today* 2(4):21-27, 1985.

Muller M: *Nursing dynamics,* ed 2, Sandton, South Africa, 1998, Heinemann.

Roberts D: Competence and professionalism, *Med Surg Nurs* 14(4):211, 2005.

Secrest J, Norwood BR, Keatley VM: "I was actually a nurse": the meaning of professionalism for baccalaureate nursing students, *J Nurs Ed* 42(2):77-82, 2003.

Task Force on Professionalism: White paper on pharmacy student professionalism, *J Am Pharm Assoc* 40(1):96-100, 2000.

Webster's new world dictionary, New York, 1996, Simon & Schuster.

Wuest J: Professionalism and the evolution of nursing as a discipline: a feminist perspective, *J Prof Nurs* 19(6):357-367, 1994.

4

Legal Aspects of Nursing

Beverly B. Foster and Virginia Trotter Betts

Learning Outcomes

After studying this chapter, students will be able to:

- Describe the components of a model nurse practice act.
- Discuss the authority of state boards of nursing.
- Explain the conditions that must be present for malpractice to occur.

- Identify nursing concerns related to delegation, assault and battery, informed consent, and confidentiality.
- Describe strategies nurses can use to protect their patients, thereby protecting themselves from legal actions.

Professional nurses have many complex and intertwined relationships with the law that are important to identify and understand. The legal aspect of nursing is an area that is both extremely important and constantly changing. Therefore nursing education programs sometimes offer required or elective courses in law as applied to nursing. "Nursing and the law" is also one of the most popular continuing education topics for nurses. This chapter highlights key legal issues that affect professional nurses. It is essential to maintain a working knowledge of the law as it relates to professional nursing practice, even more critical now in a time of an expanding scope of practice. Nurses who do not understand and stay abreast of the changes in laws and regulations that govern nursing practice may find themselves with an increased exposure to liability and also be

involved in disciplinary measures, fines, or litigation (Aiken, 2004).

AMERICAN LEGAL SYSTEM

The purpose of the law in the United States is found in the Preamble to the U.S. Constitution: to ensure order, protect the individual person, resolve disputes, and promote the general welfare. To achieve these broad objectives, the law concerns itself with the legal relationships between persons and the government.

All law in the United States flows from the U.S. Constitution and must conform to its principles. The Constitution provides for division of powers through the establishment of three branches of government: judicial, executive, and legislative. The chief functions of the judicial branch are to resolve legal disputes, interpret statutory laws, and amend the common law. The executive branch implements laws through governmental agencies. The legislative branch may delegate authority to governmental agencies, which in turn create rules, regulations, and programs to meet the intent of a statute. The legislative branch creates statutory laws and speaks most directly for the people. Figure 4-1 depicts the sources of law in the United States.

The word **law** is defined as rules of conduct that are authored and enforced by formal authorities, and hold people accountable for compliance (Helm, 2003). Law encompasses the actions of the legislative branch in enacting statutes, the executive branch in administering the statutes through rules, and the judicial branch in interpreting statutes and rules.

Three major types of laws govern American society: common law, statutory law, and administrative law. United States law evolved from centuries-old English **common law.** Common law is decisional or judge-made law. Every time a judge makes a legal decision, the body of common law expands.

In addition to common law, there are **statutory laws,** which are laws established through formal legislative processes. Every time the U.S. Congress or a state legislature passes legislation, the body of statutory law expands.

Administrative laws result when the legislative branch of a government delegates authority to governmental agencies to create laws that meet the intent of a statute. Both federal and state administrative laws have the force and effect of statutory law.

As important as it is to understand the sources and types of law, it is equally important to know how laws can be violated. A necessary distinction is the difference between civil and criminal law. **Civil law** recognizes and enforces the rights of individuals, such as disputes over legal rights or duties of individuals in relation to one another. An example of a civil case is a child custody dispute. In civil cases, the party judged responsible for the harm may be required to pay compensation to the injured party. In contrast, **criminal law** involves public concerns regarding an individual's unlawful behavior that threatens society, such as murder or possession of illegal substances. The criminal court system both defines what constitutes a crime and may also mandate specific punishments (Aiken, 2004). Individuals convicted of criminal charges usually pay through the loss

Figure 4-1
Sources of law in the United States.

of some degree of their freedom, ranging from probation to imprisonment. They may also be required to pay monetary fines. Administrative cases result when a person violates the regulations and rules established by administrative law, such as when a nurse or physician practices without a valid license. Punishment may involve having a license revoked or suspended or being placed on probation. In egregious cases, imprisonment may be required.

Professional nurses need to be aware of a wide array of legal issues. Nurses must be particularly aware of the statutory authority governing nursing practice, the executive authority of state boards of nursing, the civil law areas of torts, privacy rights, and the evolving common law related to health care. The remainder of this chapter focuses on these key areas.

NURSING AS A PRACTICE DISCIPLINE

The practice parameters of disciplines such as nursing, medicine, dentistry, law, and many others are established by state legislation and are regulated by the individual states through regulatory agencies and boards. These boards are established by state legislation and are given statutory authority by state legislatures to enforce professional practice acts. The practitioners of these disciplines cannot legally practice without a license.

The purpose of licensing certain professions is to protect the public health, safety, and welfare. The statute that defines and controls nursing is called a **nurse practice act.** All 50 states and several U.S. territories have nurse practice acts passed by their legislatures. These acts are administered and enforced through regulatory bodies known as **state boards of nursing.**

Statutory Authority of State Nurse Practice Acts

Nurses, as health care providers, have certain rights, responsibilities, and recognitions through various state laws, or statutes. The nurse practice act in each state accomplishes at least four objectives:

1. Defines the practice of professional nursing
2. Sets the minimum educational qualifications and other requirements for licensure
3. Determines the legal titles and abbreviations nurses may use
4. Provides for disciplinary action of licensees for certain causes

In many states, nurse practice acts also define the responsibilities and authorities of the state board of nursing (National Council of State Boards of Nursing, 2006). Thus the nurse practice act of the state in which nurses practice is the most important statutory law affecting nursing practice within the bounds of that state (Figure 4-2).

Once the law regarding nursing practice is established or amended by the legislature, the legislative branch delegates authority to enforce the law to an executive agency, usually the state board of nursing. State boards of nursing are responsible for enforcing the nurse practice acts in the various states. The state board of nursing publicizes rules and regulations that expand the law. The statutory law plus the rules and regulations propagated by the state board of nursing give full meaning to the nurse practice act in each state.

Figure 4-2
In addition to the nurse practice act for your state, *Nursing's Social Policy Statement, Scope and Standards of Practice,* and *Code of Ethics for Nurses* represent the cornerstones of legal practice. Every professional nurse should have current copies of these documents and be familiar with their contents. *(Photo by Kay Chitty.)*

Nurse practice acts are revised from time to time to keep up with new developments in health care and changes in nursing practice. State nurses' associations are usually instrumental in lobbying for appropriate updating of nurse practice acts.

Because of the importance of practice acts to professional nurses, both the American Nurses Association (ANA) and the National Council of State Boards of Nursing (NCSBN) have developed suggested language for the content of state nurse practice acts. The ANA's *Model Practice Act* was published in 1996 to guide state nurses associations seeking revisions in their nurse practice acts (American Nurses Association, 1996). The guidelines encourage consideration of the many issues inherent in a nurse practice act and the political realities of each state's legislative and regulatory processes. Through this document, the ANA recognizes the great importance of the nurse practice act and urges that the following content be included:

1. A clear differentiation between advanced and generalist nursing practice
2. Authority for boards of nursing to regulate advanced nursing practice, including authority for prescription writing
3. Authority for boards of nursing to oversee unlicensed assistive personnel
4. Clarification of the nurse's responsibility for delegation to and supervision of other personnel
5. Support for mandatory licensure for nurses while retaining sufficient flexibility to accommodate the changing nature of nursing practice

The ANA document provides a broad definition of the practice of professional nursing and appropriate professional practice activities. It incorporates aspects of technical nursing practice and identifies technical activities (American Nurses Association, 1996).

The model nurse practice act guidelines recognize the baccalaureate degree with a major in nursing (bachelor of science in nursing, or BSN) as the minimum educational credential for the professional nurse. There has been extensive debate about the need to change the minimum educational qualifications for professional nursing practice. In the early 1980s and again in 1995, the ANA reaffirmed its long-standing position that the baccalaureate degree should be the minimum educational qualification for professional nursing practice and the associate degree the minimum educational qualification for technical nursing practice. Although a number of states support the BSN as the minimum entry into practice requirement, no states currently require it.

The NCSBN's *Model Nurse Practice Act* and *Model Nursing Administrative Rules* (National Council of State Boards of Nursing, 2004) are comprehensive documents developed to guide the states, and are available online at www.ncbon.org/regulation/index.asp. The NCSBN began development of model regulations in 1982, with subsequent revisions in 1988 and 1993 to 1994. NCSBN describes the current model, in its third major revision, as both a standard toward which states may strive as well as a reflection of the current and changing regulatory and health care system environments. Discussions over the past 20 years at the national level, facilitated by both NCSBN and ANA, have brought a national perspective on nursing regulation to the state level, fostered dialogue and the development of more consistent standards across state lines, and provided increased protection for the public (Mikos, 2004).

Executive Authority of State Boards of Nursing

Both federal and state laws provide for the executive branch of government to administer and implement laws. The state executive, or governor, generally delegates the responsibility for administering the nurse practice act to an executive agency—the state board of nursing. In most states, the state board of nursing consists of registered nurses (RNs), licensed practical nurses (LPNs), and consumers (members of the general public), all of whom are generally appointed to the board by the governor.

The state board of nursing's authority is limited. It can adopt rules that clarify general provisions of the nurse practice act, but it does not have the authority to enlarge the law.

State boards of nursing usually have three functions:

1. Quasi-executive—authority to administer the nurse practice act
2. Quasi-legislative—authority to adopt rules necessary to implement the act
3. Quasi-judicial—authority to deny, suspend, or revoke a license or to otherwise discipline a licensee or to deny an application for licensure

Each of these functions is as broad or as limited as the state legislature specifies in the nurse practice act and related laws.

State boards of nursing may be independent agencies in the executive branch of state government or part of a department or bureau such as a department of licensure and regulation. Some state boards have authority to carry out the nurse practice act without review of their actions by other state officials. Others must recommend action to another department or bureau and receive approval of the recommendation before the decision is finalized.

Licensing Powers

The **licensure** process is a police power of the state that, through the legislative branch, determines what groups are to be licensed and the limitations of such licenses. Licensure laws may be either mandatory or permissive. A mandatory law requires any person who practices the profession or occupation to be licensed. A permissive law protects the use of the title granted in the law but does not prohibit persons from practicing the profession or occupation if they do not use the title. All states now have a mandatory licensure law for the practice of nursing in order to safeguard the public.

Just as the state has the power to issue a nursing license based on established criteria, so does it retain the power to discipline a licensee for performing professional functions in a manner that is dangerous to patients or the general public. Discipline may include sanctions such as license suspension or revocation arising from unsafe, uninformed, or impaired practice by the nurse licensee. Sadly, the most common reason nurses are disciplined by state boards of nursing is for practicing while impaired (under the influence of a substance).

Historically, the nursing profession has demonstrated a commitment to the rehabilitation of nurses whose practice is below standard because of impairment by psychological dysfunction or substance abuse and misuse. In 1990 the ANA published suggested state legislation that included a *Nursing Disciplinary Diversion Act* (American Nurses Association, 1990). This publication recommended a diversion procedure, such as a peer assistance program to combat substance abuse, as a voluntary alternative to the traditional disciplinary actions of suspension or revocation of a license. In a NCSBN survey of boards of nursing (NCSBN, 2006), nearly all responding boards had nondisciplinary alternative programs (disciplinary diversion processes) to assist chemically impaired nurses to return to safe nursing practice. Additionally, over half the boards also provided alternative programs for psychiatric and mental health problems, and one third had provisions for physical or other health problems.

In most states, state boards of nursing have the authority to enforce minimum criteria for nursing education programs. The practice act usually stipulates that an applicant for licensure must graduate from a state-approved nursing education program as a prerequisite to being admitted to the licensure examination. This means that schools of nursing must have state approval to operate. State approval requirements are generally less stringent than are national accreditation standards. Schools may voluntarily seek national accreditation to demonstrate that they meet higher than minimal standards. Although many other professions and occupations require graduation from a nationally accredited educational program as a prerequisite of licensure, only state approval is currently required in nursing. Some states are currently undertaking rule changes to require national accreditation of programs as a component of state approval.

Licensure Examinations

Since 1944 most state boards of nursing have participated in a cooperative effort to assist in the interstate mobility of nurses, both registered nurses and licensed practical nurses. Because nurse licensure examinations are national examinations, they facilitate this system, called **licensure by endorsement.** Endorsement means that registered nurses and licensed practical nurses (or licensed vocational nurses [LVNs]) are free to practice in other states without having to take another licensing examination. If they submit proof of licensure in another state and pay a licensure fee, they can receive licensure in the new state by endorsement. Licensure by endorsement is not available to all practice disciplines. Nursing's plan serves as a national model for other licensed professions and occupations.

Until 1978 the national nursing licensing examination was developed by the ANA's Council of State Boards of Nursing, and the National League for Nursing served as the testing service. In 1978 the National Council of State Boards of Nursing (NCSBN) was established and continued the activities of the ANA Council of State Boards. Through the NCSBN, each state participates in the licensing process through test plan and item development, periodic validation of the exam content with current practice, and adoption of a minimum passing score.

The nurse licensure examinations are called the National Council Licensure Examination for Registered Nurses (NCLEX-RN) and the National Council Licensure Examination for Practical Nurses (NCLEX-PN). The test was traditionally administered by paper and pencil; however, the state boards of nursing and the NCSBN began administering them by computerized adaptive testing (CAT) in 1994. The test plan for the NCLEX-RN licensure examination, which is updated periodically, provides for the examination to measure critical thinking and nursing competence in all phases of the nursing process. The test plan can be reviewed at the NCSBN website at https://www.ncsbn.org/454.htm.

Trends in Licensure: Nurse Licensure Compact

As society has become more mobile, need for a new regulatory approach to promote mobility of nurses while still protecting the public health, safety, and welfare has been identified. In response to this mobility, the increase in travel nursing, the increasing practice of telehealth (being physically present in one state while providing nursing care to a patient in another state through electronic means), and other regulatory pressures, the National Council of State Boards of Nursing developed and promoted a **mutual recognition model** for nursing licensure. The mutual recognition model allows a registered nurse to have one license (in the state of residency) yet practice in other compact member states without additional licenses. While practicing in another state, the nurse is subject to that state's laws, scope of practice, and discipline.

The concept of a single license for each nurse and the concomitant reduction of state barriers provides better protection for the public through improved tracking of nurses for disciplinary purposes and information sharing. See Box 4-1 for an example of effective cross-state communication to protect the public. Nursing workforce mobility during national or regional disasters is also increased (Hellquist and Spector, 2004).

Each state that wishes to participate in the compact must pass legislation enabling the board of nursing to enter into the interstate **Nurse Licensure Compact (NLC).** Utah, Texas, and Wisconsin were the first states to implement the compact on January 1, 2000. By March 31, 2006, 20 states had enacted this legislation and 2 states were pending (National Council of State Boards of Nursing, 2006). Nurses licensed in any state that has implemented the compact can practice in their own states as well as in any other compact state without applying for licensure by endorsement. Updated information about the status of states in relation to the compact can be found online at https://www.ncsbn.org/158.htm. Application of the compact model to advanced practice nurses is under discussion.

Box **4-1** **Nurse Licensure Compact Speeds Resolution of Disciplinary Issues**

A registered nurse licensed in Utah (a Nurse Licensure Compact [NLC] state) was being monitored by the Utah Board of Nursing for issues related to alcohol abuse. The nurse had accepted a position as a traveler with a hospital in Idaho (also a NLC state), where she worked under the privilege granted by her Utah license. The nurse arrived at her job in Idaho having consumed alcohol and, when confronted by her co-workers, admitted her impairment, which was subsequently confirmed through urine screen results. The nurse was sent home on administrative leave pending investigation by the hospital. The Idaho Board of Nursing was notified of the situation once the hospital had received the urine screen results. The Idaho Board contacted the Utah Board, which requested evidence of the alcohol use to initiate disciplinary action. The Idaho Board requested copies of the positive urine screen and hospital notes of the personnel incident, which were then faxed to the Utah Board. Within a week, the Utah Board had taken action to revoke this nurse's license, thereby denying her the privilege to practice in any other NLC state. This is an example of how provisions of the Nurse Licensure Compact assist boards of nursing to cooperate with each other in a timely way, affording enhanced protection of the public.

From Hellquist K, Spector N: A primer: the National Council of State Boards of Nursing nurse licensure compact, *JONA Health Care Law Ethics Regul* 6(4):86-89, 2004. Used with permission.

Exploration of the global perspective on nursing regulation is currently on the NCSBN agenda (Apple and Spector, 2005). Based on a demand from nurses educated abroad, the NCSBN began administering the NCLEX internationally to competent nurses applying for U.S. licensure in January 2005. The recruitment of nurses from outside the United States, particularly from poorer nations with their own high health care demands, is controversial (Dugger, 2006), with both legal and ethical considerations. Refer to Cultural Considerations Challenge 5-1 in Chapter 5 for a fuller discussion of the issues surrounding recruiting nurses from other countries to practice in the United States.

LEGAL RISKS IN PROFESSIONAL NURSING PRACTICE

Nurses make decisions daily that affect the well-being of their patients. Because they have access to personal information about patients and interact with them during stressful times, they are in positions of great responsibility and trust. Several areas of nursing practice—in particular, delegation, informed consent, and confidentiality —are fraught with legal risk. Nurses may also be charged with malpractice or assault and battery. In this section, we will discuss these areas of concern.

Malpractice

Malpractice lawsuits are on the rise and more nurses are being named defendants in these lawsuits (National Practitioner Data Bank, 2004). **Malpractice** is the greatest legal concern of health care practitioners. To understand malpractice, nurses must first understand the legal concepts of torts and negligence. **Torts** are civil wrongs against a person and may be either intentional or unintentional. For a tort to exist, there must be harm resulting from the action, but the harm may be physical, emotional, or economic. An intentional tort refers to willful acts that violate another person's rights or property.

Negligence is the failure to act as a reasonably prudent person would have acted in specific circumstances. For example, if in burning yard debris on a windy day a man sets fire to his neighbor's garage, the neighbor may charge negligence. A reasonably prudent person would not have started a yard fire on a windy day, and an injury (the burned garage) can be shown to be a direct result of his failure to act prudently. The differences between negligence and intentional torts are summarized in Table 4-1.

Malpractice is negligence applied to the acts of a professional. In other words, malpractice occurs when a professional fails to act as a reasonably prudent professional would have acted under specific circumstances. Malpractice is classified as

an unintentional tort. This means that it is not necessary to prove that the professional intended to be negligent. In malpractice, legal action may be based on the accused person doing things that should not have been done (commissions) and not doing things that should have been done (omissions).

When a patient brings a malpractice claim against a nurse defendant, evidence is presented to the jury to determine whether the elements of liability are present. At question is whether the nurse met the prevailing **standard of care.** The nursing standard of care is what the reasonably prudent nurse, under similar circumstances, would have done. It is a peer standard of care that reflects not excellence but a minimum standard of "do no harm." The nursing standard of care is decided by a jury on a case-by-case basis and is developed through use of **expert witness** testimony; documents, including national **standards of nursing practice;** the patient record; and other pertinent evidence such as the direct testimony of the patient, the nurse, and others. Box 4-2 illustrates the presumed failure of an RN to meet the local standard of care.

CRITICAL THINKING *Challenge*

You hear nursing colleagues discussing prevention of malpractice and you notice that some nurses are spending more time tending to patients' records than they are in providing care to patients. Think about how this emphasis on "defensive practice," that is, making sure that your patient's chart is perfect, may actually impede the delivery of safe care. As you think about this issue, consider what the purpose of charting is. How can you use the medical record to enhance the care of your patients? How might excessive charting harm you in a malpractice suit?

Table 4-1 DIFFERENCES BETWEEN NEGLIGENCE AND INTENTIONAL TORTS

Negligence	Intentional Torts*
INTENT	
May occur without any intent to act	Requires an intent to interfere with another's rights; a hostile motive not required
PROOF OF DAMAGES	
Requires proof of a specific injury	Proof of actual injury not required
DUTY OR STANDARDS OF CARE	
Relevant; usually involves expert witnesses	Not needed
CONSENT	
Not necessarily a defense	Always may be a defense

*Examples of intentional torts include defamation (libel or slander), invasion of privacy, assault and battery, false imprisonment, and intentional infliction of emotional distress.
From Aiken T: *Legal, ethical, and political issues in nursing*, Philadelphia, 2004, FA Davis.

Box **4-2** **Standards of Care: A Case Example**

An 8-month-old infant was brought to the emergency department (ED) by his parents with signifi-cant fever and dehydration. The family with the infant was Spanish speaking and included a family member trained in nursing in her home country. Intravenous (IV) fluids were ordered for rehydra-tion. Because of the need for the infant to be able to move from bed to the arms of her caregivers, the IV was set up before needle insertion with both regular and extension length tubing. The emergency department RN, a new nurse in her second year in the emergency department, failed to flush the line to clear air from the tubing, and then inserted the needle and began the infusion. This was noted by the family, and an unsuccessful attempt was made to alert the medical staff. The infant subsequently died from a significant air embolus confirmed on autopsy. The family reported the event to the local district attorney, who investigated the incident. In considering whether charges were to be brought against the nurse, the following standards of care were considered:

1. Hospital policy indicated an interpreter should have been called for communication with family.
2. Hospital policies and orientation competency guidelines, completed by this nurse, indicated flushing of an IV line was a required step in the process.
3. Local schools of nursing indicated flushing of an IV line was part of basic skills training, and current textbooks about fundamentals of nursing confirmed this content.
4. Other nurses in local EDs were interviewed and all reported that flushing of an IV line before insertion was standard practice.
5. The company manufacturing the IV tubing had visual and written instructions on the box indi-cating proper use of the product, including flushing of the line.

The prerequisite of a malpractice action is twofold: The defendant (nurse) has specialized knowledge and skills and through the practice of that specialized knowledge causes the plaintiff's (patient's) injury. For a plaintiff patient to prove that the nurse defendant is liable for the injury, all elements of a cause of action for negligence must be proved. These elements, the same for any pro-fessional accused of malpractice, are as follows:

1. The professional (nurse) has assumed the **duty of care** (responsibility for the patient's care).
2. The professional (nurse) breached the duty of care by failing to meet the standard of care.
3. The failure of the professional (nurse) to meet the standard of care was the **proximate cause** of the injury.
4. The injury is proved.

Setting forth all elements of a malpractice action requires a high degree of proof. Monetary damages are awarded when a patient plaintiff prevails. These awards are based on proven eco-nomic losses, such as time missed from work or out-of-pocket health care costs, and on remuner-ation for pain and suffering caused by the injury. In the case of a death, the next of kin can become the plaintiff on behalf of the deceased patient.

In the past, some malpractice lawsuits involved nurses, but the physician or hospital defendants were traditionally called on to pay damages even when the substandard care was provided by nurses. In these instances, physicians were impli-cated through the **"captain of the ship" doctrine.** This doctrine implies that the physician is ulti-mately in charge of all patient care and thus should be responsible financially. Hospitals were implicated through the legal theory of **respon-deat superior** (from Latin, meaning "let the master answer"), which attributes the acts of employees to their employer (Blumenreich, 2005). However, as nurses have obtained more creden-tials and their expertise, autonomy, and authority for nursing practice have increased, direct liabil-ity for nursing care has risen correspondingly.

Croke (2003) conducted a review of "more than 350 trial, appellate, and supreme court case summaries" (p. 56) from a variety of legal research sources and analyzed 253 cases that met the following criteria: A nurse was engaged in the practice of nursing as defined by his or her state's nurse practice act; a nurse was a defendant in a civil lawsuit as the result of an unintentional action (no criminal cases were considered); and a trial was held between 1995 and 2001.

Analysis revealed, not surprisingly, that the largest number of cases of reported negligence occurred in acute care hospitals (60 percent). Other settings included nursing homes/rehabil- itation/transitional care units (18 percent), psy- chiatric settings (8 percent), home health settings (2 percent), and physician offices (2 percent); also included were cases involving care by advanced practice nurses (9 percent).

This review identified six major categories of negligence resulting in malpractice lawsuits against nurses: failure to follow standards of care, failure to use equipment in a responsible manner, failure to communicate, failure to document, fai- lure to assess and monitor, and failure to act as a patient advocate. More details of Croke's analysis are presented in Box 4-3.

Some examples of malpractice that involved professional nurses were covered in the popular press. One such highly publicized case involved a number of nurses at a Massachusetts hospital who carried out a physician's faulty order and gave two different cancer patients overdoses of chemo- therapy (Trossman, 1999). Another example was an operating room nurse who failed to follow well- established hospital policy for identifying and preparing patients for surgery. This breach of pro- cedure resulted in the removal of one patient's only functioning kidney (*Holbrooks v. Duke Hospital, Inc.,* 305 SE^2 69, 1983). Although physicians and facilities were also involved in both of these cases, the nurses were named as codefendants because they too fell below the standard of care, and "but for" their actions, these serious injuries would not have occurred. Student nurse errors and omissions may also be considered by the courts as profes-

sional malpractice, not ordinary negligence, as in the case of a student administering nystatin intravenously rather than orally (*Legal Eagle Eye Newsletter for the Nursing Profession,* 2005).

The lesson to be learned from such malpractice cases is that professional nurses must carefully consider the legal implications of practice and be willing and capable of conforming to professional standards and all legal expectations. Among fac- tors leading to the increase in the number of mal- practice cases against nurses is delegation.

Delegation

Delegation—that is, "empowering one to act for another"—is an issue that carries great legal and safety implications in nursing practice. The ability to delegate has generally been reserved for profes- sionals because they hold licenses that sanction the entire scope of practice for a particular pro- fession. Professional nurses, for example, may delegate independent nursing activities (as well as medical functions that have been delegated to them) to other nursing personnel. State nurse practice acts do not give delegatory authority to licensed practical or vocational nurses.

It is critical to understand that professional nurses retain accountability for acts delegated to another person and are responsible for deter- mining that the delegated person (delegatee) is competent to perform the delegated act. Like- wise, the delegatee is responsible for carrying out the delegated act safely. The professional nurse remains legally liable, however, for the nursing acts delegated to others unless the delegatee is also a licensed professional whose scope includes the assigned act.

Delegatory acts must also be considered from the standpoint of their ethical implications. The ANA's *Code of Ethics for Nurses* states, "The nurse is responsible and accountable for individual nursing practice and determines the appropriate delegation of tasks consistent with the nurse's obligation to provide optimum patient care" (American Nurses Association, 2001, Section 4.4). An important related point is that nurses are ethically bound to refuse to perform acts that are

Box 4-3 Six Major Categories of Negligence That Result in Malpractice Lawsuits

1. **Failure to follow standards of care,** including failure to:
   - Perform a complete admission assessment or design a plan of care.
   - Adhere to standardized protocols or institutional policies and procedures (for example, using an improper injection site).
   - Follow a physician's verbal or written orders.
2. **Failure to use equipment in a responsible manner,** including failure to:
   - Follow the manufacturer's recommendations for operating equipment.
   - Check equipment for safety before use.
   - Place equipment properly during treatment.
   - Learn how equipment functions.
3. **Failure to communicate,** including failure to:
   - Notify a physician in a timely manner when conditions warrant it.
   - Listen to a patient's complaints and act on them.
   - Communicate effectively with a patient (for example, inadequate or ineffective communication of discharge instructions).
   - Seek higher medical authorization for a treatment.
4. **Failure to document,** including failure to note in the patient's medical record:
   - A patient's progress and response to treatment.
   - A patient's injuries.
   - Pertinent nursing assessment information (for example, drug allergies).
   - A physician's medical orders.
   - Information about telephone conversations with physicians, including time, content of communication between nurse and physician, and actions taken.
5. **Failure to assess and monitor,** including failure to:
   - Complete a shift assessment.
   - Implement a plan of care.
   - Observe a patient's ongoing progress.
   - Interpret a patient's signs and symptoms.
6. **Failure to act as a patient advocate,** including failure to:
   - Question discharge orders when a patient's condition warrants it.
   - Question incomplete or illegible medical orders.
   - Provide a safe environment.

Reprinted with permission from Croke EM: Nurses, negligence, and malpractice: an analysis based on more than 250 cases against nurses, *Am J Nurs* 103(9):54-63, 2003.

not within their area of expertise, even if a physician or hospital authority requests that they perform them.

Delegation is an important liability and one not fully appreciated by many practicing nurses. The professional nurse's primary legal and ethical consideration must be the patient's right to safe, effective nursing care. Box 4-4 contains an excerpt from the *Code of Ethics for Nurses* pertaining to delegation (American Nurses Association, 2001, Section 4.4).

Recognizing that registered nurses are ethically and legally accountable during acts of delegation, the National Council of State Boards of Nursing (NCSBN) published *Five Rights of Delegation* (1995). These five rights are the following:

Box **4-4** **American Nurses Association's** *Code of Ethics for Nurses* **Section 4.4 Delegation of Nursing Activities**

Because the nurse is accountable for the quality of nursing care given to patients, nurses are accountable for the assignment of nursing responsibilities to other nurses and the delegation of nursing care activities to other health care workers. While delegation and assignment are used here in a generic moral sense, it is understood that individual states may have a particular legal definition of these terms.

The nurse must make reasonable efforts to assess individual competence when assigning selected components of nursing care to other health care workers. This assessment involves evaluating the knowledge, skills, and experience of the individual to whom the care is assigned, the complexity of the assigned tasks, and the health status of the patient. The nurse is also responsible for monitoring the activities of these individuals and evaluating the quality of the care provided. Nurses may not delegate responsibilities such as assessment and evaluation; they may delegate tasks. The nurse must not knowingly assign or delegate to any member of the nursing team a task for which that person is not prepared or qualified. Employer policies or directives do not relieve the nurse of responsibility for making judgments about the delegation and assignment of nursing care tasks.

Nurses functioning in management or administrative roles have a particular responsibility to provide an environment that supports and facilitates appropriate assignment and delegation. This includes providing appropriate orientation to staff, assisting less experienced nurses in developing necessary skills and competencies, and establishing policies and procedures that protect both the patient and the nurse from the inappropriate assignment or delegation of nursing responsibilities, activities, or tasks.

Nurses functioning in educator or preceptor roles may have less direct relationships with patients. However, through assignment of nursing care activities to learners, they share responsibility and accountability for the care provided. It is imperative that the knowledge and skills of the learner be sufficient to provide the assigned nursing care and that appropriate supervision be provided to protect both the patient and the learner.

Reprinted with permission of American Nurses Association: *Code of ethics for nurses with interpretive statements*, Washington, DC, 2001, American Nurses Publishing, Section 4.4.

1. Right task: The task is appropriate for delegation in a specific care situation.
2. Right circumstances: The appropriateness of the patient's health status, care delivery setting, complexity of the activity and delegate's competency, available resources, and other relevant factors are considered.
3. Right person: The nurse can verify that the delegatee's competencies match the individual patient needs.
4. Right direction/communication: Clear, specific instructions are given, including the objective of the task, time frames, and expected results.
5. Right supervision/evaluation: Supervision and evaluation of the patient and the performance of the task are accomplished by the delegating nurse or other licensed nurse (National Council of State Boards of Nursing, 1995).

With the present nursing shortage, the use of unlicensed, assistive personnel has grown and further increased the nurse's liability related to delegation. NCSBN has developed a position paper on "Working with Others" (National Council of State Boards of Nursing, 2006) as well as model regulatory language. This paper and other additional information on delegation can be found on the National Council of State Boards of Nursing website at www.ncsbn.org.

In an attempt to further clarify issues of delegation, the American Nurses Association (2005a) also defined the responsibilities of the nurse when delegating to nursing assistive personnel. They reinforce the stance that the RN may delegate elements of care, but cannot delegate the nursing process itself. Further, they reaffirm that the judgment of the nurse is primary in determining the patients, environments, and care situations for safe delegation; and that the nurse remains responsible for evaluating the outcomes of nursing care.

Currently the most debated area of delegation involves the delegation of medication administration to unlicensed assistive personnel. In an exploratory study of board of nursing executives and practice specialists about medication administration for older adults in assisted living facilities, it was found that current practices vary across states, with 22 states permitting nurses to delegate at least some type of medication administration to assistive personnel. The majority of states that permit delegation also addressed the nurses' accountability in the relationship. In some states, however, nursing aides can be trained to administer medications outside the nurse delegation model (Reinhard, Young, Kane et al, 2006). This is a disturbing change that bears close scrutiny from the nursing profession.

Assault and Battery

Assault and battery is an intentional tort that is often the basis for legal action against a nurse defendant. **Assault** is a threat or an attempt to make bodily contact with another person without the person's consent. Assault precedes battery; it causes the person to fear that battery is about to occur. **Battery** is the assault carried out, the impermissible, unprivileged touching of one person by another. Actual harm may or may not occur as a result of assault and battery.

If, for example, a nurse threatens a patient with a vitamin injection if he does not eat his meals, the patient may charge assault. Actually giving the patient a vitamin injection against his will leaves the nurse open to charges of battery, even if there is a physician's order. It is important to remember that patients have the right to refuse treatment, even if the treatment would be in their best interest. Both by common law and by statute, **informed consent** is required in the health care context as a defense to battery (*42 United States Code* 1395 cc., 1990).

Informed Consent

All patients must be given an opportunity to grant informed consent before treatment unless there is a life-threatening emergency. Three major conditions of informed consent are the following:

1. Consent must be given voluntarily.
2. Consent must be given by an individual with the capacity and competence to understand.
3. The patient must be given enough information to be the ultimate decision maker.

Informed consent is a full, knowing authorization by the patient for care, treatment, and procedures and must include information about the risks, benefits, side effects, costs, and alternatives. Consumers of health care need a great deal of information and should be told everything that they would consider significant in making a treatment decision. This is a long-standing element of health care law (*Canterbury v. Spence,* 464 F^2 772, 1972).

For informed consent to be legally valid, elements of completeness, competency, and voluntariness are evaluated. **Completeness** refers to the quality of the information provided. **Competency** takes into account the capability of a particular patient to understand the information given and make a choice. **Voluntariness** refers to the freedom the patient has to accept or reject alternatives. In the case of patients who are minors, who are under the effects of drugs or alcohol (including preoperative medications), or who have other mental deficits, it is questionable that competency to consent exists. For example, a nurse was asked to obtain a signed consent for an endoscopic procedure from a patient with advanced dementia. In this situation, consent needs to be granted by the patient's spouse, next-of-kin, or court-ordered guardian or health care proxy (Garvis, 2005).

The role of nurses in informed consent, unless they are themselves primary providers, is to collaborate with the primary provider, most often a physician. A nurse may witness a patient's signing of informed consent documents but is not responsible for explaining the proposed treatment (Figure 4-3). The nurse is not responsible for evaluating whether the physician has truly explained the significant risks, benefits, and alternative treatments. However, professional nurses are responsible for determining that the elements for valid consent are in place, providing feedback if the patient wishes to change consent, and communicating the patient's need for further information to the primary provider.

CONFIDENTIALITY

Confidentiality is both a legal and an ethical concern in nursing practice. Confidentiality is the protection of private information gathered about a patient during the provision of health care services. The *Code of Ethics for Nurses* states, ". . . ? the nurse has a duty to maintain confidentiality of all patient information . . . . Only information pertinent to a patient's treatment and welfare is disclosed, and only to those

Figure 4-3

Professional nurses may be called on to witness a patient's signing of informed consent documents. The primary provider, however, is responsible for providing necessary information to the patient or legal guardian. *(From Leahy JM, Kizilay PE:* Foundations of nursing practice, *Philadelphia, 1998, WB Saunders.)*

directly involved with the patient's care. The nurse safeguards the client's right to privacy by judiciously protecting information of a confidential nature" (American Nurses Association, 2001, Section 3.2).

The *Code* acknowledges exceptions to the obligation of confidentiality. These include discussing the care of patients with others involved in their direct care, quality assurance activities, legally mandated disclosure to public health authorities, and information required by third-party payers (American Nurses Association, 2001). The *Code* also recognizes the need to disclose information without the patient's consent when the safety of innocent parties is in question (*Tarasoff v. Board of Regents of the University of California*, 551 P² 334, 1976).

The principle of confidentiality is protected by state and federal statutes, but there are exceptions and limitations. Although some professions have statutorily protected **privileged communication,** such as attorneys and priests, nurses are usually not included in such statutes. Thus nurses may be ordered by a court to share information without the patient's consent. It is essential for the professional nurse to understand these legal limitations.

In certain situations, through statute and common law, the antithesis of confidentiality has developed—the **duty to report** or disclose. These laws require nurses and other health professionals to report child abuse, gunshot wounds, certain communicable diseases, and threats toward third parties. These laws vary by state and may be the responsibility of institutions providing health care services and not of an individual practitioner. Nurses should be aware of these requirements, however, and make sure the appropriate supervisory person is informed.

The Health Insurance Portability and Accountability Act of 1996 (HIPAA)

The Health Insurance Portability and Accountability Act of 1996 (HIPAA) is the first-ever federal privacy standard governing protection of patients' medical records. The privacy provisions in the act began as a 337-word guideline, but as the final regulations were written, the provisions swelled to 101,000 words (Parker, 2003). HIPAA was designed, in part, to reinforce the protection of patient information as it is transmitted electronically, but the final act goes far beyond that goal. The new regulations protect medical records and other individually identifiable health information, whether on paper, in computers, or communicated orally.

HIPAA requires all health care providers, including doctors, hospitals, health plans, pharmacies, public health authorities, insurance companies, billing agencies, information systems sales and service providers, and others, to ensure the privacy and confidentiality of patients. Although passed in 1996, the confidentiality regulations were not implemented until April 2003 in order to give providers time to prepare the necessary safeguards and documents and to train workers in their use.

HIPAA regulations require several major patient protections:

- Patients are able to see and obtain copies of their medical records, generally within 30 days of their request, and to request corrections if they detect errors. Providers may charge patients for the cost of copying and mailing the records.
- Providers must give patients written notice describing the provider's information practices and explaining patients' rights. Patients must be asked to agree to these practices by signing or initialing the notice.
- Limitations are placed on the length of time records can be retrieved, what information can be shared, where it can be shared, and who can be present when it is shared.

A number of other protections are provided in this comprehensive federal legislation. The document can be viewed online at www.hhs.gov/news/facts/privacy.html.

In the early months following implementation of HIPAA requirements, doctors, nurses, hospitals, and other providers experienced confusion about which disclosures were allowed. Since the act makes provision for civil and criminal penalties, including stiff fines, for entities that misuse personal health information, health care professionals were understandably reluctant to talk to others about a patient, even when the other person was a family member or caregiver with a genuine need to know (Landro, 2003). The struggle to integrate HIPAA into clinical practice continues, and has prompted reflection on the impact on nursing (Flores and Dodier, 2005). It certainly has caused an increase in repetitive paperwork (Kumekawa, 2005). For many nurses, however, HIPAA is also an affirmation of our long-standing responsibility to our patients (Erickson and Millar, 2006). Analysis of HIPAA 2 years into implementation supported its role in the protection of patient privacy but noted the tremendous impact on the clinical environment, including high implementation costs (Harman, 2005). The U.S. Department of Health and Human Services, which was delegated the role of developing the regulations and rules of this law, provides extensive outreach, guidance, and technical assistance to providers online at www.hhs.gov/ocr/hipaa.

EVOLVING LEGAL ISSUES AND THE NURSE

Because of the dynamic nature of nursing and health care, legal issues affecting nursing practice are also evolving. Specific legal issues that illustrate the changing nature of nursing practice are related to role changes, supervision of assistive personnel, payment mechanisms, and issues associated with the implementation of the Patient Self-Determination Act. Each of these issues is briefly discussed in the following sections.

Role Changes in Health Care

Just as a nurse's knowledge base and the nurse's accountability for nursing practice have increased over time, so has the need to expand the **legal authority** for nursing practice. Even though the definitions and parameters of nursing outlined in nurse practice acts may seem to be an issue of concern only to nurses, this is not the case.

Nurses have found that as they worked through their constituent member (state nurses) associations to modify and update these acts, they met significant political resistance. This is due, in part, to the defensiveness of organized medicine, which often views an expansion of nurses' domain as a diminishment of physicians' roles or as a threat to physicians' economic base.

Professional nurses realize that it is important for a state nurse practice act to reflect nursing practice accurately and to keep up with changes in health care delivery as they occur. Otherwise, nurses have questionable legal basis for practice and are open to prosecution. Health care is becoming more specialized, so nursing specialties and subspecialties are increasing. Advanced practice nurses set the pace for evolving nursing practice, and the nurse practice act must support their ability to offer nursing services to consumers in various settings (Cady, 2003). Many functions defined as advanced practice have been absorbed into the statutory scope of professional nursing practice.

Historically, in some states, nurses in advanced practice, such as nurse-midwives, nurse practitioners, and nurses in private practice, have not been supported by timely changes in the nurse practice act. For example, nurses in a women's health practice in Missouri were sued for practicing medicine without a license. After intense litigation, their practice was supported by the Missouri Supreme Court. The court found "legislative intent" in the nurse practice act not to limit nursing practice except to protect the public. The nurses in question were well credentialed and were practicing with the knowledge and support of the Missouri Board of Nursing and the Missouri Nurses Association, so the safety of the public was not in question (*Sermchief v. Gonzales*, 660 SW^2 683, 1983).

This is only one example of the legal exposure nurses face when their state's nurse practice act is not updated periodically to support explicitly an expanded scope of practice. Working within the constituent member (state nurses) association to expand the evolving scope of nursing practice appropriately ensures the growth of the profession and increases the number of primary care providers needed by the public. Professional nurses must support their professional associations, which led the development of legislation that accurately reflects current nursing practice at all levels.

In an effort to promote national dialogue regarding advanced practice nurses and regulation, the NCSBN, in collaboration with the American Association of Colleges of Nursing and the National Organization of Nurse Practitioner Faculties, has developed a draft vision paper related to credentialing of advanced practice nurses. The draft paper is available to local boards of nursing for comment at this time (National Council of State Boards of Nursing, 2006). This document has evoked both comment and controversy, and work is continuing.

Prescriptive authority

An important role expansion for advanced practice nurses is prescriptive authority. **Prescriptive authority** is defined as the legal acknowledgment of prescription writing as an appropriate act of nursing practice. The ANA, the American Academy of Nurse Practitioners, and others support prescriptive authority for advanced practice nurses (APNs), as distinguished from generalist registered nurses.

Nurses should consider several questions about prescriptive authority: Does the state recognize prescriptive authority for nurses? If so, is the state board of nursing the state regulatory authority for this practice? Does the law require physician collaboration or supervision or written protocols? What are the parameters for prescribing controlled substances, if any?

In 2006 advanced practice nurses had some type of prescriptive authority in all 50 states. This authority ranged from completely independent authority with no collaborative requirements in 13 states and districts (Alaska, Arizona, Iowa, Maine, Montana, New Hampshire, New Mexico, Oregon, Utah, Washington, Wisconsin, and Wyoming, and in the District of Columbia), to 5 states (Alabama, Florida, Kentucky, Missouri, and Texas) where nurse practitioners can prescribe (excluding controlled substances) with some degree of physician involvement or delegation of prescription writing (Phillips, 2006). In the remaining states, nurse practitioners can prescribe (including controlled substances) with some degree of physician involvement or delegation of prescription writing (Phillips, 2006). Variation among states regarding physician involvement in APN practice has prompted nurses in Georgia to sustain a 15-year battle for more autonomy (Nelson, 2006).

Both generalist and advanced practice nurses must understand prescriptive authority of advanced practice in their states. Generalist nurses must know from whom they can accept medication orders, and APNs must stay within their legal scope of practice.

Supervision of unlicensed assistive personnel

Another evolving legal issue is the continued role expansion of **unlicensed assistive personnel** or limited licensed (licensed practical/vocational nurses) personnel within health care institutions. Nurse aides (i.e., unlicensed assistive personnel) are increasingly being substituted for nurses, thus creating greater risks to patients and increasing the liability of nurses, who supervise their work. Studies such as the one described in the accompanying Evidence-Based Practice Note indicate that lack of professional nurse supervision and the educational level of nurses themselves significantly affect patients, institutions, and nurses alike (Institute of Medicine, 1996; Buerhaus, Needleman, Mattke et al, 2002; Aiken, Clarke, Cheung et al, 2003).

The substitution of unlicensed personnel for registered nurses is a strategy used by health care facilities to hold down costs. Such substitution is ill-advised because it jeopardizes quality of care and places the registered nurse at increased risk for patient injury liability because of acts performed or omitted by unlicensed assistive personnel. It is questionable whether, in the long term, professional nursing care is actually more expensive than care provided by unlicensed personnel, who are less likely to provide patient teaching and recognize complications.

The licensure or state approval of assistive personnel is a complex and confounding issue that has relevance for registered nurses because professional nurses are legally responsible for the tasks performed by the assistive personnel they supervise. Having nationally standardized education and training for these workers would ensure nurses of a minimum level of competence in their co-workers. The NCSBN has developed the National Nurse Aide Assessment Program (NNAAP) examination, a test of both cognitive and skill performance to certify nurse aide competency. At present 23 states use the NNAAP for aide certification. See www.ncsbn.org/testing/index.asp for further details about this competency test. Whatever their preparation, it remains the responsibility of professional nurses to know the limitations of the assistive personnel under their supervision.

Payment mechanisms for nurses

Nurses are increasingly practicing in nontraditional roles and settings. Many professional nurses are both capable of and interested in offering nursing services as private practitioners, but payment mechanisms may limit such activities. Nurses are concerned about offering services for which consumers are unable to obtain reimbursement from their insurance carriers, and third-party reimbursement has traditionally been limited to care provided by physicians.

Over the years, nurses and their professional associations have supported state and federal legislation to provide direct and indirect payments to nurses for nursing services rendered. A major legislative victory in the 8-year fight to obtain direct reimbursement of advanced practice nurses came with the passage of the 1997 Balanced Budget Act. This legislation authorized nurse practitioners and clinical specialists, beginning in January 1998, to bill the Medicare program directly for nursing services furnished in any setting. It remains a regulatory challenge to

☼ EVIDENCE-BASED PRACTICE

note

An interdisciplinary group of Pennsylvania researchers, led by Linda Aiken, a doctorally prepared nurse from the University of Pennsylvania, was concerned about nurse understaffing and the resulting threats to patient safety in hospitals. The group members decided to study the educational composition of registered nurses (RNs) in relation to patient outcomes. Their objective was "to examine whether the proportion of hospital RNs educated at the baccalaureate level or higher is associated with risk-adjusted mortality and failure to rescue (deaths in surgical patients with serious complications)" (p. 1617).

The researchers analyzed outcome data for 232,342 general, orthopedic, and vascular surgery patients discharged from 168 nonfederal adult general Pennsylvania hospitals between April 1, 1998, and November 30, 1999. These figures were linked to data on educational composition, staffing, and other characteristics.

The percentage of RNs with a bachelor's or higher degree ranged from 0 percent to 77 percent in the various hospitals in the study. "After adjusting for patient characteristics and hospital structural characteristics (size, teaching status, level of technology), as well as for nurse staffing, nurse experience, and whether the patient's surgeon was board-certified, a 10 percent increase in the proportion of bedside nurses holding a bachelor's degree was associated with a 5 percent decrease in both the likelihood of patients dying within 30 days of admission and the odds of failure to rescue" (p. 1617).

These researchers concluded that significantly lower mortality and failure to rescue rates were found in hospitals with higher proportions of baccalaureate-prepared nurses. They recommended that investments in public funds be made to increase the number of baccalaureate nurses in order to substantially improve the quality of care in the nation.

Aiken LH, Clarke SP, Cheung RB et al: Educational levels of hospital nurses and surgical patient mortality, *J Am Med Assoc* 290(12):1617-1623, 2003.

devise a fair and equitable payment system for advanced practice nurses, whose scopes of practice vary from state to state.

This federal legislation became a model for commercial insurers. During the 1990s changes in state insurance laws were enacted in many states to achieve direct payment for nursing services from private insurance companies. This means that consumers of health care may choose to receive services from physicians, nurses, or other qualified health professionals and receive insurance reimbursement for the chosen professional's fees. Nurses are concerned that these changes are often not implemented or that nurses are paid less for services similar to those provided by other health care professionals who are paid at a higher rate.

Laws are often passed that are not implemented. This occurs when the group affected by the law (for example, the insurance industry) is unwilling to implement the changes and no "watchdog" agency is created to ensure that changes occur. For example, federal legislation was enacted requiring state Medicaid agencies to pay certain nurses (nurse practitioners, nurse-midwives, and nurse anesthetists) directly for services provided to Medicaid recipients. As with the laws affecting private insurers, these requirements have not been implemented in every state. Nurses may need to seek legal remedies to require implementation of policies mandated by federal law (*Nurse Midwifery Associates v. Hibbett,* 918 Fed² 605, 1990).

Following failed efforts to overhaul the entire health care system during the Clinton administration, health care finance nevertheless underwent dramatic changes. One significant change was from fee-for-service provider reimbursement to capitation. Additionally, many individual and group insurance plans changed from indemnity plans to **managed care plans,** such as health maintenance organizations (HMOs) and preferred provider organizations (PPOs). These shifts have posed new challenges for nurses, because they are often not included on HMO and PPO provider panels. As a result of these new challenges, the ANA and constituent member (state) associations are working to ensure that nurses are included on managed care panels, in "any willing provider" clauses, and in all federal insurance programs as appropriate providers of basic plan services.

Patient Self-Determination Act

Although the **Patient Self-Determination Act (PSDA)** became effective in 1991, more than 15 years later there remain many problems in its implementation. Nurses are in a position to help patients and families understand this law and how it can assist them to have the end-of-life care they prefer.

The PSDA applies to acute care and long term care facilities that receive Medicare and Medicaid funds. It encourages patients to consider which life-prolonging treatment options they desire and to document their preferences in case they should later become incapable of participating in the decision-making process. Written instructions recognized by state law that describe an individual's preferences in regard to medical intervention should the individual become incapacitated is called an **advance directive.**

This act was passed partly in response to the U.S. Supreme Court's decision in *Cruzan v. Director Missouri Department of Health* (110 Supreme Court 2841, 1990), which was viewed as limiting an individual's ability to direct health care when unable to do so. The PSDA requires

the health care facility to document whether the patient has completed an advance directive.

The PSDA's basic assumption is that each person has legal and moral rights to informed consent about medical treatments with a focus on the person's right to choose (the ethical principle of autonomy). The act does not create any new rights, and no patient is required to execute an advance directive.

According to the PSDA, acute care (hospitals) and long term care facilities must:

1. Provide written information to all adult patients about their rights under state law.
2. Ensure institutional compliance with state laws on advance directives.
3. Provide for education of staff and the community on advance directives.
4. Document in the medical record whether the patient has an advance directive.

The Agency for Health Care Policy Research reported that even when patients had advance directives in place, the directives were not guiding end-of-life care as legislators and advocates had anticipated. This was attributable to several factors: the patients were not considered hopelessly ill; the family members were not available, too overwhelmed to implement the patient's wishes, or disagreed with the patient's wishes; and the advance directive itself was not specific enough or did not cover pertinent clinical issues (Ditto, Danks, and Smucker, 2001). The nursing role with advance directives can often become a tangle of state and federal laws, hospital policies, and conflicting family desires (Ryan, 2004). Documentation of the existence of advance directives and use of them in planning care is an important patient advocacy role for nurses and is a legal requirement that needs careful implementation in clinical settings.

PREVENTING LEGAL PROBLEMS IN NURSING PRACTICE

Although the range of potential "hot spots" for health care litigation may seem enormous, the vast majority of nurses never encounter the legal system during their professional careers. This is because there are a number of effective strategies that professional nurses can use to limit the possibility of legal action. These will now be explored.

Practice in a Safe Setting

To be truly safe, facilities in which nurses work must be committed to safe patient care. The safest situation is one in which the agency:

1. Employs an appropriate number and skill mix of personnel to care adequately for the number of agency patients at all levels of acuity.
2. Has policies, procedures, and personnel practices that promote **quality improvement.**
3. Keeps equipment in good working order.
4. Provides orientation to new employees, supervises all levels of employees, and provides opportunities for employees to learn new procedures consistent with the level of health care services provided by the agency.

In addition to an active quality improvement program, each health care organization should have a **risk management** program. Risk management seeks to identify and eliminate potential safety hazards, thereby reducing patient and staff injuries. Common areas of risk include patient falls, failure to monitor, failure to ensure patient safety, improper performance of a treatment, failure to respond to a patient, medication errors, failure to follow agency procedure, improper technique, and failure to supervise treatment (Aiken, 2004).

In a nonrandom survey of nearly 5000 practicing nurses regarding patient safety in their worksites, 80 percent of the nurses believed that bedside nurses contribute to a culture of safety, while voicing concern that chronic understaffing impeded safe care (Manno, Hogan, Heberlein et al, 2006). In a desire to promote improvements in patient safety, the Joint Commission on Accreditation of Healthcare Organizations (JCAHO, 2005) adopted patient safety goals in 2005. These 14 goals identify significant ways in which patient safety can be enhanced through environmental, educational, practice, and policy changes. They can be reviewed online at http://www.jointcommission.org/PatientSafety/NationalPatientSafetyGoals.

Crossing the Quality Chasm: The IOM Health Care Quality Initiative

In 1996 the Institute of Medicine (IOM), an arm of the nonprofit National Academy of Science, launched "a concerted, ongoing effort focused on assessing and improving the nation's quality of care" (IOM, 2006). The IOM defines quality as, "the degree to which health services for individuals and populations increase the likelihood of desired health outcomes and are consistent with current professional knowledge" (IOM, 2006).

The first phase of this initiative documented a serious and pervasive quality problem in the nation's health care delivery system through an intensive review of the literature conducted by RAND. The second phase identified a vision for transformation of the health care system to "close the chasm between what we know to be good quality care and what actually exists in practice" (IOM, 2006). Two reports were released during the second phase: *To Err Is Human: Building a Safer Health System* (IOM, 1999) and *Crossing the Quality Chasm: The IOM Health Care Quality Initiative* (IOM, 2001). These reports stressed complete reform of the health system, not just "reform around the margins." *To Err Is Human* described how "tens of thousands of Americans die each year from medical errors and effectively put the issue of patient safety and quality on the radar screen of public and private policymakers" (IOM, 2006). *Crossing the Quality Chasm* described "broader quality issues and defined six aims—care should be safe, effective, patient-centered, timely, efficient and equitable" (IOM, 2006).

The third phase of the IOM effort continues and focuses on operationalizing the vision of the *Quality Chasm* report. The IOM, working in conjunction with representatives of many other professions, including nursing, hopes to create a more patient-responsive twenty-first century health system. During this phase, a series of topical reports have been published. Several of these are important for nursing, in particular: *Health Professions Education: A Bridge to Quality* (IOM, 2003) and *Transforming the Work Environment of Nurses* (IOM, 2004). These efforts, when combined with those of each professional nurse and each setting where nurses work, should create a safer, more effective health care system in which quality and safety have a high priority. Legal problems in nursing practice will thereby be minimized.

Communicate With Other Health Professionals, Patients, and Families

The professional nurse must have open and clear communication with nurses, physicians, and other health care professionals. Safe nurses trust their own assessments, inform physicians and others of changes in patients' conditions, and question unclear or inaccurate physicians' orders. A key aspect of communication essential in preventing legal problems is keeping good patient records. This written form of communication is called **documentation.**

The clinical record, particularly the nurse's notes, provides the core of evidence about each patient's nursing care. No matter how good the nursing care, if the nurse fails to document it in the clinical record, in the eyes of the law the care did not take place. Be sure to document accurately, in a timely manner, and concisely. Know the charting policies of your agency and your unit, particularly the acceptable abbreviations.

Current and descriptive documentation of patient care is essential, not only to provide quality care but also to protect the nurse. Assessments, plans, interventions, and evaluation of the patient's progress must be reflected in the patient's clinical record if malpractice is alleged. Nurses must also document telephone calls with patients, family members, physicians, and other health care providers.

If a patient is angry, noncompliant, or complaining, nurses should be even more careful to document thoroughly. Professional nurses recognize that establishing and maintaining good communication and rapport with patients and their families not only is an aspect of best practice but also is a means of protection from lawsuits.

Accountability for accurate documentation has increased in recent years because of the advent of electronic documentation and multiple uses of recorded data, such as reimbursement, research, and quality assurance audits. The importance of the patient record and the information therein as basis for safe practice remains (American Nurses Association, 2005b). Common documentation pitfalls to avoid include leaving gaps in data or entries, including subjective bias in notes, and deviating from agency policies and procedures for recording (Austin, 2006).

Meet the Standard of Care

The most important protective strategy for the nurse is to be a knowledgeable and safe practitioner and to meet the standard of care with all patients. Meeting the standard of care involves being technically competent, keeping up-to-date with health care innovations, being aware of peer expectations, and participating as an equal on the health care team.

Nurses must familiarize themselves with the policies and procedures of the agency in which they work and must not deviate from those policies. They must know how to use equipment properly and to know when that equipment is malfunctioning and in need of repair. They must keep up with trends in their area of practice through reading the professional literature and attending continuing education conferences and workshops. Professional nurses must use national standards of practice as parameters for caregiving, care planning, and care evaluation. The ANA has promulgated generic and specialty standards of nursing practice and published these in the document *Nursing: Scope and Standards of Practice* (2004). These national standards can be used by quality improvement programs in individual hospitals in establishing their own "local" standards of nursing care.

Continued competence is an issue the nursing profession has not uniformly addressed. At this time, different states have differing requirements for continuing education as a prerequisite for license renewal. The efficacy of continuing education mandates has been challenged (Smith, 2004). The NCSBN is conducting a study of continued competence through a practice analysis of core knowledge, skills, and abilities necessary beyond entry-level practice (National Council of State Boards of Nursing, 2005). An example of using creative methods of maintaining competency can be found on the North Carolina Board of Nursing's website: http://www.ncbon.org/prac-contcomp.asp. The wise nurse recognizes that continuing education and maintaining competence are essential to safe practice, whether or not they are state requirements.

In the final analysis, the best protection a nurse can have is to know the limits of his or her own education, expertise, and nurse practice act. Staying within those limits may sometimes require nurses to enlist assistance from more experienced nurses in order to meet the standard of care. This should be viewed as a learning opportunity and an indication of maturity rather than a failure or evidence of incompetence. Box 4-5 presents information about documents professional nurses should read, understand, and keep in their professional libraries to ensure that they meet the standard of care.

Carry and Understand Professional Liability Insurance

Despite the efforts of dedicated professionals, sometimes mistakes are made and, unfortunately, patients are injured. It is essential for nurses to carry professional liability insurance to protect their assets and income in case they are required to pay monetary compensation to an injured patient. Nursing students should also carry insurance, and most nursing education programs require that they do so. In addition to carrying the insurance, nurses must read and understand the provisions of their malpractice coverage.

Professional liability insurance policies vary. Generally, they provide up to $2 million coverage for a single incident and up to $4 million total. The amount of coverage depends on the nurse's specialty. Nurse-midwives, for example, pay much higher liability insurance premiums than do psychiatric nurses because a nurse-midwife's potential for being sued is greater. Look for a policy that has portable coverage and make sure that it covers court judgments, out-of-court settlements, legal fees, and court costs. Furthermore, a good policy covers incidents occurring anytime—as long as the incident took place while the policy was in force, even if you no longer carry the insurance (occurrence policy).

Professional liability insurance is available through most state nurses' associations, nursing students' associations, and private insurers. Group policies, such as those available through professional associations, are usually less expensive than individual policies and are an important benefit of association membership. Box 4-6 provides information about the two main types of professional liability policies.

Liability and the National Practitioner Data Bank

The Health Care Quality Improvement Act (Public Law 100-177) was passed by Congress in 1986. It established a **National Practitioner Data Bank (NPDB)** to encourage identification and discipline of health care practitioners who engage in unprofessional behavior. An additional purpose was to restrict the ability of those practitioners to move from state to state without disclosing problems of damaging or incompetent practice. The act requires that the following be reported to the National Data Bank:

- Any malpractice payments made on behalf of any licensed health practitioner
- Any licensure action taken by a licensing body
- Any clinical privilege suspension or revocation by a health care facility
- Any clinical society censorship action

The NPDB is maintained by the U.S. Department of Health and Human Services, Bureau of Health Professions, Division of Practitioner Data Banks. It affects nurses in two major ways:

1. Malpractice payments made on behalf of a nurse are reported to the NPDB and copied to the state board of nursing.
2. An inquiry to the NPDB is required when nurses apply for hospital privileges and is required every 2 years for renewal of hospital privileges.

Box **4-5** **Four Documents You Should Own**

Professional nurses are accountable for practicing within their scope of practice. In order to stay abreast of changes that may affect the scope of nursing practice, you should always have the latest revision of the following four documents. You must read and understand them and be mindful of their provisions as you practice.

1. A copy of the nurse practice act of the state in which you practice. The address of your state's board of nursing can be found on the Evolve website (www.evolve.elsevier.com/Chitty/professional/). Familiarity with the law in your state is a key safeguard against inadvertent overstepping your limits of practice while understanding the full set of responsibilities that your state requires you to fulfill as a professional registered nurse.

2. *Nursing's Social Policy Statement.* Available from the American Nurses Association (www.nursing-world.org), this short but important document lays out in concise language the most current definition of nursing; the knowledge base for nursing, including specialization and advanced practice roles; and the regulation of practice. It represents "an expression of the social contract between society and professional nursing" (p. v.) in this country. The ANA has taken the position that the scope of nursing practice should flow from the definition of nursing that is contained in this document. It therefore has considerable impact on the national scope of practice.

3. *Nursing: Scope and Standards of Practice.* Also published by the ANA, this document expands on the Social Policy Statement. It focuses on defining and delimiting clinical practice and its safe implementation. Scope and standards' statements, in conjunction with other documents, are widely used in legal cases to determine whether a nurse has met the "standard of care" in a particular case. In addition to this general document, the ANA has published standards for 21 specialized areas of practice, such as hospice and palliative care and gerontological, pediatric, neuroscience, vascular, and psychiatric–mental health nursing, among others.

4. *ANA's Code of Ethics for Nurses with Interpretive Statements.* This document is available for viewing only (www.nursingworld.org/ethics/code/protected_nwcoe303.htm) and may be purchased even if you are not yet a member of the American Nurses Association. It describes the nine ethical provisions that cover all aspects of nursing practice, found inside the back cover of this text. In addition, it adds a number of clarifying statements for each of the nine provisions. Knowledge of your professional organization's code of ethics is an important protection for you as you begin or continue your nursing practice.

According to the NPDB, "only about 1 out of 100 malpractice payment reports were for nurses" (National Practitioner Data Bank, 2004, p. 27). In 2004 the NPDB annual report stated that over the history of the database, registered nurses have been responsible for only 3139 malpractice payments. This constitutes only 1.2 percent of all malpractice payments made. Slightly less than two thirds of those payments were for nonspecialized registered nurses (62.7 percent). Just over one third of the claims were for advanced practice nurses. This includes nurse anesthetists, who were responsible for 20.7 percent of all nurse payments, and nurse-midwives, who were responsible for 9.2 percent of all nurse payments. Nurse practitioners accounted for 7.3 percent of all nurse payments.

The NPDB reported that problems with the monitoring of patients, implementing treatments, and medication problems have been responsible for the majority of payments for nonspecialized nurses, followed by obstetrical and surgical

Box **4-6** Basic Types of Professional Liability
          Insurance Policies

Occurrence Policies

Cover injuries that occur during the period
covered by the policy, whether or not the policy
is still in effect at the time the suit is brought.

Claims-Made Policies

Cover injuries only if the injury occurs within
the policy period and the claim is reported to
the insurance company during the policy period
or during the "tail." A tail is an uninterrupted
extension of the policy period and is also known
as the extending reporting endorsement.

Box **4-7** Guidelines for Preventing Legal
          Problems in Nursing Practice

- Practice safely in a safe setting.
- Communicate with other health professionals, patients, and—with patient's permission—family members. Document fully,
  carefully, and in a timely manner.
- Delegate wisely, remembering the five
  "rights" of delegation.
- Meet or exceed the standard of care by staying
  on top of new developments and skills.
- Carry professional liability insurance and
  know the specifics of the policy.
- Promote positive interpersonal relationships
  and a nondefensive manner while practicing
  caring, compassionate, holistic nursing care.

problems. In 2004 the median malpractice payment for all types of nurses was $100,000, and the
mean was $302,738 (National Practitioner Data
Bank, 2004).

Promote Positive Interpersonal Relationships

Even in the face of untoward outcomes from a
health care provider, it is usually only the dis-
gruntled patient that sues. Therefore the best
strategy for the professional nurse is prevention
of legal actions through positive interpersonal
relationships.

Prevention includes giving personalized,
concerned care; including the patient and the
family in planning and implementing care; and
promoting positive, open interpersonal relationships that communicate caring and compassion.
When confronted with angry patients or family
members, wise nurses avoid criticizing or blaming
other health care providers and maintain a concerned and nondefensive manner.

The professional nurse who is clinically competent and caring, communicates openly with
patients, and acknowledges the holism of the
patient is likely to prevent most legal problems.
Box 4-7 summarizes the important steps nurses
can take to avoid legal problems in professional
practice.

SUMMARY OF *Key Points*

- Nurses must recognize that the law is a system
  of rules that governs conduct and attaches consequences to certain behavior.
- Consequences include civil or criminal action
  or both.
- Nursing practice is limited by the definition of
  practice in the state nurse practice act and the
  qualifications for licensure to practice nursing
  in that state.
- The law is dynamic and must be responsive to
  society's needs.
- Broadening the scope of nursing practice has
  increased the possibility for legal actions
  involving nurses.
- Technological advances have increased concern
  about informed consent and patients' rights to
  direct the care they choose to receive or refuse.
- Many nurses possess inadequate knowledge of
  legal issues that affect nursing practice every
  day. These issues deserve increased attention by
  nurses in all areas of practice.

CRITICAL THINKING QUESTIONS

1. Using your state's nurse practice act, describe the scope of practice of the registered nurse. When was the last time the law was modified? Does it accurately reflect current nursing practice?
2. Read the section of the nurse practice act relating to advanced practice. What differences are identified between the scope of practice of the general registered nurse and that of the advanced practice nurse?
3. If a physician writes an order for an unusually high dose of a medication, what steps should the nurse take to ensure patient safety?
4. What are the liability issues for a nurse who fails to raise the side rails on a postoperative patient's bed if the patient is injured in a fall?
5. Explain the Patient Self-Determination Act to your family and friends. What questions do they have about an advance directive? Find out what the laws regarding advance directives are in your state.
6. When you are interviewing for a position, what questions should you ask to determine whether it is a legally safe setting in which to practice?
7. In your state, under what circumstances can a nurse who administers a medication causing an allergic reaction be found negligent?
8. Discuss the legal and ethical issues for a nurse who is asked by a nurse manager to help clear up a backlog of paperwork by postdating forms and signing off on equipment inspections that were not performed as required.

REFERENCES

Aiken LH, Clarke SP, Cheung RB et al: Educational levels of hospital nurses and surgical patient mortality, *J Am Med Assoc* 290(12):1617-1623, 2003.

Aiken T: *Legal, ethical and political issues in nursing,* Philadelphia, 2004, FA Davis.

American Nurses Association: *Suggested state legislation: nurse practice act, nursing disciplinary diversion act, prescriptive authority act,* Kansas City, Mo, 1990, American Nurses Association.

American Nurses Association: *Model practice act,* Washington, DC, 1996, American Nurses Publishing.

American Nurses Association: *Code of ethics for nurses with interpretive statements,* Washington, DC, 2001, American Nurses Publishing.

American Nurses Association: *Nursing: scope and standards of practice,* Washington, DC, 2004, American Nurses Publishing.

American Nurses Association: *Principles for delegation,* Silver Spring, Md, 2005a, American Nurses Publishing.

American Nurses Association: *Principles for documentation,* Silver Spring, Md, 2005b, American Nurses Publishing.

Apple K, Spector N: Global initiatives in regulation at National Council of State Boards of Nursing, *JONA Health Care Law Ethics Regul* 7(4):112-113, 2005.

Austin S: Ladies of the jury I present the nursing documentation, *Nursing2006* 36(1):56-64, 2006.

Blumenreich GA: Doctrine of corporate liability, *AANA J* 73(4):253-257, 2005.

Buerhaus PI, Needleman J, Mattke S et al: Strengthening hospital nursing, *Health Affairs* 21(5):123-132, 2002.

Cady RF: *Advanced practice nurse's legal handbook,* Philadelphia, 2003, Lippincott Williams & Wilkins.

Croke EM: Nurses, negligence and malpractice: an analysis based on more than 250 cases against nurses, *Am J Nurs* 103(9):54-63, 2003.

Ditto PH, Danks JH, Smucker WD: Advance directive as acts of communication, *Arch Intern Med* 161:421-430, 2001.

Dugger CW: US plan to lure nurses may hurt poor nations, *New York Times,* May 24, 2006.

Erickson JI, Millar S: Caring for patients while respecting their privacy: renewing our commitment, *ANA/Online J Issues Nurs,* downloaded 2006.

Flores JA, Dodier A: HIPAA: past, present and future implications for nurses, *Online J Issues Nurs* 10(2), 2005.

Garvis MS: Getting informed consent when competence is at issue, *RN* 68(8):68, 2005.

Harman LB: HIPAA: a few years later, *Online J Issues Nurse* 10(2), 2005.

Hellquist K, Spector N: A primer: the National Council of State Boards of Nursing nurse licensure compact, *JONA Health Care Law Ethics Regul* 6(4):86-89, 2004.

Helm A: *Nursing practice: sidestepping legal minefields,* Philadelphia, 2003, Lippincott Williams & Wilkins.

Institute of Medicine: *Nursing staff in hospitals and nursing homes: is it adequate?* Washington, DC, 1996, National Academies Press.

Institute of Medicine: *To err is human: building a safer health care system,* 1999 (website): www.iom.edu/CMS/8089.aspx.

Institute of Medicine: *Crossing the quality chasm: the IOM health care quality initiative,* 2001 (website): www.iom.edu/CMS/8089.aspx.

Institute of Medicine: Redesigning care delivery, 2003, www.iom.edu/CMS/8089.aspx.

Institute of Medicine: *Keeping patients safe: transforming the work environment of nurses,* 2004 (website): www.iom.edu/CMS/8089.aspx.

Institute of Medicine: *IOM health care quality initiative,* 2006 (website): www.iom.edu/CMS/8089.aspx.

Joint Commission on Accreditation of Healthcare Organizations: *National patient safety goals,* 2005 (website): www.jointcommission.org/PatientSafety.

Kumekawa J: Overview and summary: HIPAA: how our health care world has changed, *Online J Issues Nurs* 10(2), 2005.

Landro L: Health-privacy act poses problems, *The Wall Street Journal,* April 24, CCXLII(44):D-3, 2003.

Leahy JM, Kizilay PE: *Foundations of nursing practice,* Philadelphia, 1998, WB Saunders.

Legal Eagle Eye Newsletter for the Nursing Profession, Nov 2005, p 7.

Manno M, Hogan P, Heberlein V et al: Nursing2006 patient-safety survey report, *Nursing2006* 36(5):54-63, 2006.

Mikos CA: Inside the nurse practice act, *Nursing Manag* 35(9):20-24, 2004.

National Council of State Boards of Nursing: *Delegation,* 1995 (website): www.ncsbn.org/regulation/uap_delegation_documents_delegation.asp.

National Council of State Boards of Nursing: *Model nurse practice act,* 2004 (website): www.ncsbn.org/regulation/nursingpractice_nursing_practice_model_act_and_rules.asp.

National Council of State Boards of Nursing: Meeting the ongoing challenge of continued competence, 2005 (website): www.ncsbn.org/regulation/continued_competence.asp.

National Council of State Boards of Nursing: Working with others: a position paper, 2006 (website): www.ncsbn.org/pdfs/Working_with_Others.pdf.

National Practitioner Data Bank: *Annual report,* 2004 (website): www.npdb-hipdb.com/annualrpt.html.

Nelson R: The politics of prescribing, *Am J Nurs* 106(3):25-26, 2006.

Parker L: Medical-privacy law creates wide confusion, *USA Today,* October 17:1A-2A, 2003.

Phillips SJ: Eighteenth annual legislative update: a comprehensive look at the legislative issues affecting advanced nursing practice, *Am J Prim Health Care* 31(1):6-8, 11, 2006.

Reinhard SC, Young HM, Kane RA et al: Nurse delegation of medication administration for older adults in assisted living, *Nurs Outlook* 54:74-80, 2006.

Ryan B: Advance directives: your role, *RN* 67(5):59-62, 2004.

Smith JE: Exploring the efficacy of continuing education mandates, *JONA's Health Care Law Ethics Regul* 6(1):22-31, 2004.

Trossman S: ANA, MNA support Dana-Farber nurses facing disciplinary action, *Am Nurse* 31(2), 1999.

Ethical Aspects of Nursing

Shielda Rodgers*

Learning Outcomes

After studying this chapter, students will be able to:

- Differentiate between ethics, values, and morals.
- Discuss the relevance of a code of ethics for the profession of nursing.
- Identify and define basic ethical principles.
- Discuss the theoretical basis for ethical decision making central to resolving ethical dilemmas and moral development.
- Describe ethical dilemmas resulting from conflicts between patients, health care professionals, family members, and institutions.

- Identify a model for ethical decision making and discuss the steps of the model.
- Discuss the impact of ethical issues on nurses and other health care professionals.
- Discuss the concept of justice as an ethical principle in health care delivery.
- Recognize the ethical dilemma that impaired or incompetent colleagues present.
- Be familiar with the ethical dilemma of inappropriate technology use.

In today's health care environment, more than at any other time in history, nurses are faced with the challenges of ethical dilemmas created by the very nature of their work. Nurses must make decisions about the allocation of scarce resources, what and how much information to share with patients and their families, how to manage and deal with colleagues who are performing at less than optimal levels, and how to resolve conflicts between patient or family wishes and institutional policies. In order for nurses to manage this complex assortment of issues, as well as others,

an understanding of the theoretical basis for ethical decision making is required. Throughout nursing education and practice, nurses are called upon to exercise judgment when making clinical decisions. However, when nurses encounter dilemmas of an ethical nature, they need an ethical decision-making model that can be readily applied to the situation, and that works for the individual nurse in the context of his or her own value system. Box 5-1, "Letter to Nursing Students From a Nurse Practitioner," describes the importance of ethical decision-making skills in day-to-day nursing situations.

To understand ethics and its relationship to health care, the terms *morals, values, ethics,* and

*The author acknowledges the contributions of Pamela S. Chally and M. Catherine Hough in the preparation of this chapter.

Box **5-1** Letter to Nursing Students From a Nurse Practitioner

Dear Nursing Student,

As you begin your nursing education, your focus may be on competently performing tangible clinical skills that require psychomotor dexterity. Knowledge of ethical decision making skills and encountering ethical dilemmas may seem to be near the end of a long list of overwhelming responsibilities. However, a solid ethical decision making foundation will long outlast the initial anxiety associated with learning new psychomotor skills.

In your nursing career, regardless of your chosen practice location, you will routinely be faced with opportunities to develop your ethical decision making skills. What are some points to consider when developing these skills?

Take a critical look at yourself. Identify your values and beliefs. Are these values and beliefs firmly entrenched, or are you easily swayed toward change by outside pressure? Are you willing to take a firm advocacy stance on an issue you believe is correct? Are you just as willing to admit if you are wrong and learn from your experience? Are you comfortable with sensitive or confidential information placed in your possession? When necessary, can you take a neutral stance and avoid the temptation to give advice? Can you comfortably accept both personal praise and constructive criticism?

Like many of these questions, ethical dilemmas cannot always be answered by a simple "yes" or "no." Ethical dilemmas may occur at the individual, group or community level. Many of you will face these dilemmas on a routine basis. Some situations will be more obviously dramatic than others. You may be involved in supporting a patient or family through a "do not resuscitate" decision, the decision to terminate life support systems in a nonviable patient, or organ donation decisions. You may encounter a suicidal or homicidal patient who confides in no one else. You may encounter a chemically or otherwise impaired health care provider.

As you mature in your nursing experience, encountering and resolving ethical dilemmas to the best possible outcome can prove to be a personally rewarding experience for both you and those who benefit from your abilities. Do not avoid these ethical dilemmas. Instead, meet these challenges with confidence and professionalism using the principles of ethical decision making.

Best wishes as you continue your nursing education and in your future nursing career.

Sandra H. Carr, MN, ARNP

Courtesy Sandra H. Carr.

bioethics must first be clarified. It is important to recognize that philosophers and scholars have conflicting viewpoints on how to define these terms. In many writings, the terms *morals* and *ethics* are used interchangeably. For the purposes of this textbook, distinctions will be made between the two and the following definitions of terms are used. **Morals** are established rules of conduct to be used in situations where a decision about right and wrong must be made. Morals provide standards of behavior that guide the actions of an individual or social group. An example of a moral standard is "Good people do not lie." **Values,** on the other hand, are attitudes, ideals, or beliefs that one holds and uses to guide behavior. They are learned over time and are influenced by life experiences and culture. Values are freely chosen and indicate what the individual considers important, such as honesty.

Ethics is a term used to reflect what actions an individual should take. It is derived from the Greek term *ethos*, which means habits or customs.

Ethics are process-oriented and involve critical analysis of actions. If ethicists, people who study ethics, reflected on the moral statement "One should not lie," they would clarify definitions of lying and explore whether or not there are circumstances under which lying might be acceptable.

The application of ethical theories and principles to moral issues or problems in health care is called **bioethics.** Bioethics (also referred to as biomedical ethics) as an area of ethical inquiry came into existence around 1970, as the health care system began to give attention not only to treating and curing disease but also to patients' rights and a concern for the total patient. Bioethics is concerned with determining what should be done in a specific situation by applying ethical principles.

Advances in science and medicine, combined with the infusion of technology, have added to the growth of bioethics as a field of inquiry. These advances have allowed health care providers to save more lives and keep people alive that would have previously succumbed. While solving some problems, these advances often create ethical dilemmas for health care providers. For example, people are now kept "alive" even when there is no higher brain activity. Should they be kept alive under these circumstances just because we now have the technology to do so? This kind of issue requires that nurses be concerned with what should be done for patients under their care. It is important that actions be critically analyzed for their appropriateness because health care professionals possess a good deal of power over those in their care.

When nurses are faced with ethical dilemmas and there are constraints that limit their actions, they may experience **moral distress** (Hardingham, 2004). Moral distress is the pain or anguish affecting the mind, body, or relationships in response to a situation in which the person is aware of a moral problem, acknowledges moral responsibility, and makes a moral judgment about the correct action; yet, as a result of real or perceived constraints, participates in perceived moral wrongdoing (Nathaniel, 2002, p. 4).

An example of a situation creating moral distress follows:

> A nurse in the perioperative suite overhears his immediate supervisor tell a recovery room patient's wife, "You can ask them anything when they are coming out of anesthesia and they will tell you the truth; they can't help it." Later the wife emerges, terribly distraught, because of the response her husband gave to her question, "Have you always been true to me?" The nurse believes his supervisor has violated her professional ethics and should be counseled about this behavior; at the same time, he is afraid the supervisor will make life miserable for him if he reports the incident.

Researchers have attempted to develop models for explaining and measuring moral distress (Fry, Harvey, Hurley et al, 2002; Corley, Elswick, Gorman et al, 2001; Wilkinson, 1987). Use of these models has been limited because of the complexity of ethics and moral distress and the multiple variables that influence these phenomena. This is a promising area for nursing research and an emerging field within the study of nursing ethics.

To function effectively in today's complex health care arena, nurses need to study codes of ethics, ethical theories and principles, moral development, ethical dilemmas, and ethical decision-making models, all of which will be reviewed in this chapter. Such knowledge can serve to decrease their moral distress and increase their ability to participate in the resolution of ethical dilemmas. The accompanying Interview (p. 115) of respected ethicist Robert M. Veatch highlights some of the reasons why professional nurses need ethical decision-making skills.

NURSING CODES OF ETHICS

Having a **code of ethics** has long been a hallmark of disciplines considered to be professions. A code of ethics is an implied contract through which the profession informs society of the principles and rules by which it functions.

Ethical codes help with professional self-regulation, serving as guidelines to the members of the profession, who then can meet the societal

interview

with Robert M. Veatch, PhD,
Kennedy Institute of Ethics,
Georgetown University

Interviewer: Why do you think ethical decision making is important for nurses?

Veatch: All clinical decisions include an ethics component. Anyone with decision-making authority thus has the responsibility for making ethical choices. Since nurses are among the professional decision-makers in the health care arena, they will constantly be responsible for making ethical or moral choices. To do so is part of what it means to be a professional.

Interviewer: What do you believe are the most critical ethical challenges in the health care arena today and for the future?

Veatch: The single most critical ethical challenge in the health care area today is, in my view, the empowering of patients and agents for patients to become full, active partners in the clinical process. While health care professionals have special expertise in the science of health and special skills in delivering health care services, it is the patient (or patient-surrogate) who must make the critical choices in most cases. Empowering patients is the single most important thing a nurse can do. At the same time the nurse must assume full responsibility for his or her own conduct and must help keep other health professionals from assuming authority for areas that are rightly the patient's. Among the newer ethical questions that I consider to be critical are the allocation of scarce resources (how to set limits morally), how to respond to patients who make demands for services that violate the health professional's conscience, and how to show respect for philosophical and religious views of patients that reflect unusual or minority beliefs and values.

Interviewer: What, if any, role should the government play in deciding ethical cases?

Veatch: The government has a major role in deciding ethical cases. Most ethical disputes today involve matters about which reasonable people disagree. This means some neutral party must mediate such disputes and determine whose views should prevail. Hence, the government has a major role in determining whether consent is adequately informed and, if not, how patients can be protected from unwanted intrusion. On the other hand, patients may demand of health professionals services that the professional cannot in good conscience provide (such as abortion, euthanasia, or futile life support). The government must mediate these disputes and determine which, if any, services can be provided to patients who wish to refuse and which, if any services, the professional must provide against conscience. The government must also determine what the limits should be on professional codes of ethics.

Interviewer: In light of the Terri Schiavo case, has the cause for advance directives and living will been enhanced?

Veatch: The remarkable fact of the case of Terri Schiavo is that, in the end, the right course was followed. It is appropriate for the government to mediate disputes among concerned family members when they reach different conclusions about what an incompetent patient would have wanted or what would be in that person's best interest. After the most thorough review in the history of this country, the courts determined what most likely would have been her wishes and that course of action was followed. That is a strong endorsement of the advance directive and the related right of competent or formerly competent patients to express their wishes about terminal care and to have those wishes followed. I think it is very unlikely that dissenting family members and politicians will go this far in the future to attempt to circumvent the wishes of the patient as determined by the most neutral and fair procedures our society can establish.

need for trustworthy, qualified, and accountable caregivers. It is important to remember that codes are useful only if they are known and upheld by the members of the profession in their day-to-day practice.

American Nurses Association's *Code of Ethics for Nurses*

The *Code of Ethics for Nurses with Interpretive Statements* (American Nurses Association, 2001) is the nursing profession's expression of its ethical values and duties to the public. Beginning in 1896, nursing's *Code* has undergone no fewer than seven revisions, each clarifying meanings, defining terms, and making the *Code* more relevant to nursing practice at the time. *Codes* through the years have also reflected trends in social awareness issues, such as women's and patients' rights. The consequences of breaking the *Code* have become more specific with later versions.

The *Code of Ethics for Nurses with Interpretive Statements* (American Nurses Association, 2001) is the latest version of nursing's ethical code. The *Code of Ethics for Nurses* can be found on the inside back cover of this text. Interpretive statements can be found online (http://www.nursingworld.org/ethics/code/protected_nwcoe303.htm). A function of the American Nurses Association is the periodic review of the code to ensure that it reflects the dynamic nature of the profession, the health care environment in which nursing practice occurs, and the society in which we live.

The *Code* is backed by the American Nurses Association's *Nursing: Scope and Standards of Practice,* another very important document for professional nurses. It defines standards of practice and standards of professional performance. The current version of the *Scope and Standards of Practice* was published in 2004. Standard 12 of the *Scope* states, "the registered nurse integrates ethical provisions in all areas of practice" (American Nurses Association, 2004, p. 39). This standard attests to the importance of ethics in the profession and spells out eight measurement criteria to indicate achievement of the standard for the registered nurse. Examples of these criteria include "uses the *Code of Ethics for Nurses with Interpretive Statements* to guide practice" and "contributes to resolving ethical issues of patients, colleagues or systems as evidenced in such activities as participation on ethics committees" (American Nurses Association, 2004, p. 39). You may want to refer to Chapter 4 for more information on the *Scope and Standards of Practice.*

International Council of Nurses Code of Ethics for Nurses

The International Council of Nurses (ICN) also has published a code of ethics for the profession. This document discusses the rights and responsibilities of nurses related to people, practice, society, co-workers, and the profession. The ICN first adopted a code of ethics in 1953. Its last revision, adopted in 2000, represents agreement by more than 80 national nursing associations that participate in the international association. Inherent in the *International Council of Nurses Code for Nurses* is nursing's respect for the life, dignity, and rights of all people in a manner that is unmindful of nationality, race, creed, color, age, sex, political affiliation, or social status. The ICN's *Code for Nurses* can be viewed online (www.icn.ch/ethics.htm).

ETHICAL THEORIES

There is no single ethical theory recognized by all philosophers or ethicists or that can be applied universally in health care situations. Numerous theories have been developed, but few practicing nurses ascribe to the tenets of a single theory in their day-to-day delivery of care. In this section, selected ethical theories that nurse ethicists have identified as useful (deontology, utilitarianism, virtue ethics) are discussed in addition to the emerging theory of principalism.

Deontology

The term **deontology** has its origins from the Greek term *deon*, which means duty. Immanuel Kant (1724-1804) was the predominant proponent of deontology. He believed that an act was moral if it originated from good will. Ethical action consisted of doing one's duty or honoring one's obligations to human beings, inferring that to do one's duty was right; not to do one's duty was wrong. The outcomes or consequences of an action can be desired or deplored, but they are not relevant from an ethical perspective. In deontology, it is the intention of the action taken that is important from an ethical and moral perspective, not the consequences of the action, even if the consequence is negative.

Deontology can be further divided into act deontology and rule deontology. Act deontologists determine the right thing to do by gathering all the facts and then making a decision. Much time and energy are needed to judge each situation carefully in and of itself. Once a decision is made, there is commitment to universalizing it. In other words, if one makes a moral judgment in one situation, the same judgment will be made in any similar situation.

Rule deontologists, on the other hand, emphasize that principles guide our actions. Examples of rules might be "Always keep a promise" or "Never tell a lie." In all situations, the rule is to be followed. Deontologists are not concerned with the consequences of adhering to certain rules or actions. If the principle believed in is "Always keep a promise," the deontologist will keep promises, even if circumstances have changed. For example, if a father has promised that he will take his son to a baseball game and then a close family member becomes critically ill, the baseball game promise will be kept regardless of the changed circumstances.

In nursing, there are many rules and duties that nurses follow. One such rule is "Do no harm" (**beneficence**). Another justifiable rule is "The patient should be allowed to make his or her own decisions" (**autonomy**). Consider the situation of a severely depressed young man who wishes to end his life by committing suicide and asks for the nurse's assistance. Clearly, the rule about doing no harm conflicts with allowing the young man to make his own decisions. This is a clear

demonstration that dilemmas cannot always be resolved using theoretical approaches alone.

Utilitarianism

Utilitarianism is based on a fundamental belief that the moral rightness of an action is determined solely by its consequence. Utilitarianism theory was first described by David Hume (1711-1776) and was developed further by many notable philosophers, including Jeremy Benthal (1748-1832) and John Stuart Mill (1806-1873). Mill had a significant influence on utilitarian ethics as it is known today.

Those who subscribe to the tenets of utilitarian ethics believe that "what makes an action right or wrong is its utility, with useful actions bringing about the greatest good for the greatest number of people" (Guido, 2006, p. 4). In other words, it is right to maximize the greatest good for the benefit, happiness, or pleasure of the greatest number of people. The utilitarian approach to ethics assumes that it is possible to balance good and evil with a goal that most people experience good rather than evil. Utilitarian ethics calculates the effect of all alternative actions on the general welfare of present and future generations. Thus this position is also referred to as "calculus morality" (Davis, Aroskar, Liaschenko et al, 1997).

Professional health care providers employ utilitarian theory in many situations. The concept of triage, in which the sick or injured are classified by the severity of their condition to determine priority of treatment, is an example of utilitarianism. In triage, those who are so gravely ill or injured that they cannot possibly recover are not treated until all other patients have been treated. Although this seems cruel, when there are many more sick and wounded than available facilities to care for them, triage is accepted worldwide as an ethical basis for determining treatment.

Frequently, utilitarianism is the basis for deciding how health care dollars should be spent. For example, money is more likely to be spent on research for diseases that affect large numbers of people than for research on diseases that affect relatively few. Some health care systems, such as the National Health Service (NHS) in the United Kingdom, depend on utilitarian ethics as one determinant of who receives treatment. For example, inexpensive procedures that benefit large numbers of people, such as cataract surgeries, are easier to access than expensive ones, such as organ transplants, that benefit a few. A difficulty inherent in utilitarianism is that although the appeal is made to the happiness of the majority, the interest of the individual or minority, who also deserve help, may be overlooked.

Virtue Ethics

Virtue ethics was first noted in the works of Plato, Aristotle, and early Christians. According to Aristotle, virtues are tendencies to act, feel, and judge that develop through appropriate training but come from natural tendencies. This suggests that individuals' actions are built from a degree of inborn moral virtue (Burkhardt and Nathaniel, 2002).

Recently, bioethics literature has emphasized the character of the decision maker. Virtues refer to specific character traits, including but not limited to truth-telling, honesty, courage, kindness, respectfulness, compassion, fairness, and integrity. These virtues become obvious through one's behaviors and are expressions of specific ethical principles. Truthfulness, for example, embodies the principle of veracity. According to Butts and Rich (2005), when virtuous people are faced with ethical dilemmas they will automatically choose to do the right thing because they have developed character through life experiences.

Descriptions of character portray a way of being, rather than the process of decision making. From one's way of being flows a way of acting in both one's personal and one's professional life (Davis et al, 1997). A certain mental set does not guarantee right behavior, but it may predispose to right behavior. Despite the fact that a profession has a code of ethics, there is no guarantee that members of the profession will act in an ethical manner. The ability to respond to ethical dilemmas or situations in the health care arena is dependent upon the nurse's own integrity, honesty, courage, or other personal morals. Gallagher and

Wainwright (2005) suggest that "becoming an ethical practitioner requires commitment, personal investment and the intention and motivation to become a good nurse" (p. 24). It has been recognized that nurses' ways of being and acting are essential to the integrity of nursing practice and patient care. Nurses often practice in challenging circumstances in which they must rely on their own integrity to ensure that care is given conscientiously and consistently. Virtues may be what separates the competent nurse from the exemplary nurse. Table 5-1 summarizes the major points of the three primary ethical theories.

Principalism

Ethical principles have long been a means to analyze ethical problems in health care. The use of these principles as an emerging theory (**principalism**) is gaining popularity. This approach uses the key ethical principles of beneficence, nonmaleficence, autonomy, and justice in the resolution of ethical conflicts or dilemmas. In reality, most nurses are more knowledgeable of ethical principles than ethical theories and are more likely to use this approach when making ethical decisions. In addition to the four key principles described previously, other principles include fidelity and veracity. Further discussion of each principle follows.

ETHICAL PRINCIPLES

In order to practice in an ethical or moral way in nursing, the nurse ideally should demonstrate a general respect for humans. Inclusive in the concept of respect for persons is the notion of human dignity. The *Code of Ethics for Nurses* (American Nurses Association, 2001) states that "the nurse practices with compassion and respect for the inherent dignity, worth and uniqueness of every individual, unrestricted by considerations of social or economic status, personal attributes or the nature of health problems." Respect for persons requires that each person be respected as a unique individual equal to all others. This means valuing every aspect of a person's life, not just the parts that are easy to value because they

Table 5-1 PRIMARY ETHICAL THEORIES

Deontology	Moral rules are absolute and apply to all individuals.
	Concept of obligation overrides consequences of action.
	Duty must occur before value.
	Includes some religious traditions.
Utilitarianism	Moral rightness of actions is determined by their consequences.
	Basis found in the doctrine of psychological hedonism and the principle of utility that maximizes pleasure and minimizes pain.
	Interested in the greatest good for the greatest number.
Virtue Ethics	Introduces the character of the individual.
	Individual moral actions are based on innate moral virtue.
	Based on cardinal virtues (faith, hope, charity, wisdom).
	Focal virtues* as related to bioethics are compassion, discernment, trustworthiness, and integrity.

*Focal virtues identified by Beauchamp TL, Childress JF: *Principles of biomedical ethics*, ed 4, New York, 2001, Oxford University Press.

parallel our own value systems. Human dignity and respect for persons is the foundation of the six ethical principles discussed in this section: autonomy, beneficence, nonmaleficence, veracity, fidelity, and justice.

Autonomy

The principle of **autonomy** is based on the assertion that individuals have the right to determine their own actions and the freedom to make their own decisions. Respect for the individual is the cornerstone of this principle. Autonomy refers to the control individuals have over their own lives including determining their own course of action, in keeping with a plan they have chosen or helped develop. Autonomous decisions are based on (1) individuals' values, (2) adequate information, (3) freedom from coercion, and (4) reason and deliberation. Autonomous actions result from autonomous decisions. Examples of the use of autonomy by the patient include deciding to refuse treatment; giving consent for treatment or procedures; and obtaining information regarding results of diagnostic tests, diagnosis, and treatment options.

Disregard for autonomy, however, is glaringly evident in the health care system. Health care professionals often take actions that profoundly affect patients' lives without adequate consultation with the patients themselves. Many physicians and nurses operate, often unknowingly, within a paternalistic philosophy that implies that as health care providers with a vast knowledge base we are best equipped to make health care decisions for patients. Complicating the picture is the fact that some patients prefer to have decisions made for them, perhaps because of a lack of information or fears of making a poor choice.

Incorporating the principle of autonomy in all health care situations is difficult, if not impossible. Autonomy poses a problem for health care workers when the patient is incompetent to make decisions because of their physical condition, mental status, or developmental age. Examples of those unable to participate in decisions include infants or small children, mentally incompetent patients, and unconscious patients. Other patients may be unable to participate in decision making because of external constraints, such as financial limitations, lack of necessary information, or the norms of their culture. Nevertheless, the principle of autonomy is an increasingly important one in health care and nursing.

Beneficence

Beneficence is commonly defined as "the doing of good" and is often thought to be the most critical ethical principle in health care. In essence, one should always consider one's actions in the context of promoting good for others (i.e., the patient). While this sounds simple, health care providers are challenged daily when what is good for the patient may also cause harm to the patient or is in conflict with what the patient wants. For example, an elderly patient has become acutely confused and it has been determined that she is at high risk for falls, having fallen at home several times. The health care team decides that the patient is to be restrained at night; however, the patient becomes combative when restraints are applied. The patient is prevented from falling but has been psychologically harmed because of limitations on her independence and freedom of motion. (NOTE: Use of restraints is very controversial and is prohibited in some settings.)

Virtually everyone would agree that causing good and avoiding harm are important to all human beings—and certainly to health care professionals. It may seem surprising, therefore, how often conflicts center around this principle. Additional considerations may take precedence when there is conflict about the appropriate course of action. The application of the restraints in the above example causes some emotional harm to the patient but prevents more serious physical injury during the patient's acute confusion. In this sense, even though it inflicts harm in the short term, it is justified because of the long-term good that results.

In addition to consideration of both short-term and long-term benefits, the principle of beneficence may conflict with other ethical principles, most often autonomy. Even though a nurse or physician may understand that a particular treatment will do good for the patient, the patient may decide to forgo that treatment (autonomy) for a variety of reasons. In this instance, the health care provider should avoid acting paternalistically and recognize that the patient remains in a position of self-determination.

Nonmaleficence

Nonmaleficence is defined as the duty to do no harm. This principle is the foundation of the medical profession's Hippocratic Oath; it is like-

wise critical to the nursing profession. Inherent in the *Code of Ethics for Nurses* (American Nurses Association, 2001), the nurse must not knowingly act in a manner that would intentionally harm the patient. Although this point appears straightforward, the nature of health care dictates that some therapeutic interventions carry risks of harm for the patient, but the treatment will eventually produce great good for the patient. Classic examples of this are chemotherapy and bone marrow transplant procedures. Both interventions can make patients sicker and with both interventions the patient may acquire opportunistic infections, but the possibility of achieving a cure or remission of disease may justify the harm. The concept that justifies inflicting harm is referred to as the principle of **double effect.**

The principle of double effect considers the intended foreseen effects of actions by the professional nurse. The doctrine states that as moral agents we may not intentionally produce harm. It is ethically permissible, however, to do what may produce an evil or undesirable result if the intent is to produce an overall good effect (Beauchamp and Childress, 2001).

According to Guido (2006), four conditions must be present to justify the use of the double effect principle:

1. The action must be good or at least morally indifferent.
2. The health care provider must intend only the good effects.
3. The undesired effects cannot be a means to the end or good effect.
4. There is a favorable balance between desirable and undesirable effects (Guido, 2006, p. 6).

Veracity

Veracity is defined as "telling the truth." Truth telling has long been identified as fundamental to the development and continuance of trust among human beings. Telling the truth is expected. It is necessary to basic communication, and societal relationships are built on the individual's right to know the truth. Inherent in nurse-patient relationships is the understanding that nurses will be honest with their patients. However, in some instances nurses are constrained by a health care system that places limits on what a nurse can tell a patient. In these situations, the nurse participates in unintentional withholding of the truth. Intentional deception, however, is considered morally wrong.

Despite the well-established expectation of honesty, much intentional deception occurs between health professionals and people seeking health care. Persons seeking health care often are not completely truthful when giving their health histories. For example, they may not reveal the extent of their use of drugs or alcohol, may claim that they are adhering to a diabetic diet when they are not, or may lose weight just before a checkup and regain the weight as soon as the physical is completed.

At the same time, health care professionals are not always truthful in responding to patients' questions or inquiries for information relevant to their treatment or prognosis. They may avoid discussing certain topics or choose to answer only part of a patient's question, rather than giving all the known facts. Health care professionals are not responsible for false information given to them by their patients. They are responsible, however, for the information that they give to patients.

A number of reasons have been proposed to justify deception by health care professionals. For the most part, these justifications are related to the idea that patients would be better off not knowing certain information or that they are not capable of understanding the information. Based on these justifications, health care professionals often believe they have the right to decide what people should and should not know about their illnesses. Some justify not being truthful with a patient if they perceive that the patient may refuse medical treatment if they knew the complete truth. However, if both patient and health care provider are respectful of each other as individuals, it is difficult to accept that deception is ever justified. Based on findings from a literature review relevant to truth telling, Tuckett (2004) suggests that if a patient asks not to be told the truth the nurse can withhold the truth. He also posits that if a patient is mentally incompetent, autonomy and the capacity for self-determination have been forfeited, thereby justifying withholding of health care information.

Fidelity

The principle of **fidelity** refers to faithfulness or honoring one's commitments or promises to patients. The nurse is required to remain faithful in seriously considering all ethical mandates related to the practice of the profession. Through the process of licensure, nurses are granted the right to practice. The licensure process is intended to ensure that only a qualified nurse can practice nursing. When the nurse accepts licensure and becomes a part of the profession, it is mandated that he or she accept certain responsibilities as part of the contract with society. Burkhardt and Nathaniel (2002) state that nurses must be faithful in keeping their promises of respecting all individuals, upholding the *Code of Ethics for Nurses* (American Nurses Association, 2001), practicing within the scope of nursing practice, maintaining competence in nursing, abiding by the policies of the employing institution, and keeping promises to patients. Being faithful entails meeting reasonable expectations in all these areas.

When nurses receive patient assignments and accept reports on those patients, they are committed to provide care to those assigned to them. Failure to carry out the prescribed care is unethical and may constitute abandonment or neglect (Haynes, Boese, and Butcher, 2004).

Fidelity is the basis of the nurse-patient relationship. It suggests that one is faithful to the promises, agreements, and commitments made. This faithfulness creates the trust that is essential to any relationship. Most ethicists believe there is no absolute duty to keep promises, however. In every situation, the harmful consequences of the promised action must be weighed against the benefits of promise keeping (Burkhardt and Nathaniel, 2002).

Justice

The principle of **justice** states that equals should be treated the same and that unequals should be treated differently (Beauchamp and Childress, 2001). In other words, patients with the same diagnosis and health care needs should receive the same care. Those with greater or lesser needs should receive different care. Also at issue with justice is who receives health care and whether health care is a right or a privilege.

In health care, the most common concern about justice relates to allocation of resources. How much of our national resources should be appropriated to health care? What health care problems should receive the most financial resources? What patients should have access to health care services? According to the principle of justice, the answer to these questions is based on treating all individuals equally.

Numerous models have been developed for distributing health care resources. These models include the following:

1. To each equally
2. To each according to merit (this may include past or future contributions to society)
3. To each according to what can be acquired in the marketplace
4. To each according to need (Jameton, 1984)

All of these suggestions for distribution have merit and make it difficult to decide who should be treated and for what condition. Ideally, all patients would receive all available treatment and resources for their health needs. Unfortunately, this is not possible because of costs and limited supplies, such as transplantable organs. When the rich can buy the best health care available including lifesaving medical devices, or innovations, or organs, how does one apply the concept of justice? In addition, when disasters such as Hurricane Katrina strike and health care institutions are left with acutely ill patients and no electricity to operate medical devices that are treating patients, how does one decide what is just? A more disturbing issue in the discussion of justice has to do with disparities among ethnic minorities relevant to type of treatment and services offered. Research has demonstrated that allocation of resources in the health care system is not equitable among racial groups and that

"racial disparity exists in health care access, treatment options and outcomes" (Harrison and Falco, 2005, p. 252). This chapter's Cultural Considerations Challenge 5-1 describes health disparities in more detail.

Justice as a principle often leaves us with more questions than answers. It raises our consciousness about making ethical decisions but certainly does not determine what the answer should be, demonstrating once again that a more comprehensive method of resolving ethical dilemmas is necessary.

THEORIES OF MORAL DEVELOPMENT

In discussions regarding how one makes decisions about right and wrong or what ought to be done in ethical dilemmas, one must examine how a person develops morality. **Moral development** describes how a person learns to handle moral dilemmas from childhood through adulthood. Throughout the literature, particularly the nursing literature, the two most cited major theorists in moral development are Lawrence Kohlberg and Carol Gilligan. A brief discussion of each follows.

Kohlberg's Levels of Moral Development

Kohlberg (1976, 1986) proposed three levels of moral development, which he then subdivided into six stages. The levels are (1) preconventional, (2) conventional, and (3) postconventional. In the **preconventional** level, the individual is inattentive to the norms of society when responding to moral problems. Instead, the individual's perspective is self-centered. At this level, what the individual wants or needs takes precedence over right or wrong. A person in stage 1 of the preconventional level responds to punishment. In stage 2 the person responds to the prospect of personal reward. Kohlberg observed the preconventional level of moral development in children under 9 years of age as well as in some adolescents and adult criminal offenders.

The **conventional** level is characterized by making moral decisions that conform to the expectations of one's family, group, or society. The

Facts About Health Disparities

Health disparities include differences that occur by gender, race or ethnicity, education or income, disability, geographic location, or sexual orientation. Compelling evidence indicates that race and ethnicity correlate with persistent, and often increasing, health disparities among U.S. populations in all these categories.

The U.S. Department of Health and Human Services has selected six focus areas in which racial and ethnic minorities experience serious disparities in health access and outcomes:

1. Infant Mortality

African-American, American Indian, and Puerto Rican infants have higher death rates than white infants. In 2000 the African-American to white ratio in infant mortality was 2.5 (up from 2.4 in 1998). This widening disparity between African-American and white infants is a trend that has persisted over the last two decades.

2. Cancer Screening and Management

African-American women are more than twice as likely to die of cervical cancer than are white women and are more likely to die of breast cancer than are women of any other racial or ethnic group.

3. Cardiovascular Disease (CVD)

Heart disease and stroke are the leading causes of death for all racial and ethnic groups in the United States. In 2000 rates of death from diseases of the heart were 29 percent higher among African-American adults than among white adults, and death rates from stroke were 40 percent higher.

4. Diabetes

In 2000 American Indians and Alaska Natives were 2.6 times more likely to be diagnosed with diabetes compared with non-Hispanic whites, African-Americans were 2.0 times more likely, and Hispanics were 1.9 times more likely.

5. HIV Infection/AIDS

Although African-Americans and Hispanics represented only 26 percent of the U.S. population in 2001, they accounted for 66 percent of adult AIDS cases and 82 percent of pediatric AIDS cases reported in the first half of that year.

6. Immunizations

In 2001 Hispanics and African-Americans ages 65 and older were less likely than non-Hispanic whites to report having received influenza and pneumococcal vaccines.

From Office of Minority Health, Centers for Disease Control: Eliminating racial and ethnic health disparities, 2006 (website): http://www.cdc.gov/omh/AboutUs/disparities.htm.

person making moral choices based on what is pleasing to others characterizes stage 3 within this level. An individual in stage 4 of the conventional level makes moral choices based on some notion of what is desired by society. When confronted with a moral choice, people functioning at the conventional level follow family or cultural group norms. According to Kohlberg, most adolescents and adults generally function at this level.

The **postconventional** level consists of stage 5 and stage 6 and involves more independent modes of thinking than previous stages. The individual has developed the ability to define his or her own moral values. People at the postconventional level may ignore both self-interest and group norms in making moral choices. For example, they may sacrifice themselves on behalf of the group. Part of their moral reasoning and behavior is based on a socially agreed upon standard of human rights

(Haynes et al, 2004). In this highest level of moral development, people create their own morality, which may differ from society's norms. Kohlberg believed that only a minority of adults achieve this level.

Progression through Kohlberg's levels and their corresponding stages occurs over varying lengths of time for different individuals. The stages are sequential, they build upon each other, and each stage is characterized by a higher capacity for logical reasoning than the preceding stage.

Kohlberg (1976) suggested that certain conditions might stimulate higher levels of moral development. Intellectual development is one necessary characteristic. Individuals at higher levels intellectually are generally more advanced in moral development than those operating at lower levels of intellect.

An environment that offers people opportunities for group participation, shared decision-making processes, and responsibility for the consequences of their actions also promotes higher levels of moral reasoning. Further moral development is stimulated by the creation of conflict in settings in which the individual recognizes the limitations of present modes of thinking. For example, students have been stimulated to higher levels of moral reasoning through participating in courses on moral discussion and ethics (Kohlberg, 1973).

Gilligan's Levels of Moral Development

Gilligan (1982) was concerned that Kohlberg did not give adequate acknowledgment to the experiences of women in moral development. She recognized that Kohlberg's theories had largely been generated from research with men and boys, and believed that women's moral development was different from males'.

When women were tested using Kohlberg's levels of moral development, they scored lower than men. Gilligan believed that this was attributable not to inadequate moral development in women but to the fact that women's identities are largely dependent on relationships with others. Because of the basic difference in the way men

and women feel about relationships, which was not a part of Kohlberg's theory, Gilligan believed that Kohlberg's theory was inadequate to explain women's moral development.

She suggested that women view moral dilemmas in terms of conflicting responsibilities. The sequence she described included three levels and two transitions, with each level representing a more complex understanding of the relationship of self and others and each transition resulting in a crucial reevaluation of the conflict between selfishness and responsibility. Gilligan's levels of moral development are (1) orientation to individual survival, (2) a focus on goodness with recognition of self-sacrifice, and (3) the morality of caring and being responsible for others as well as self.

In Gilligan's view, the moral person is one who responds to need and demonstrates a consideration of care and responsibility in relationships. Gilligan described a moral development perspective focused on care. This perspective differed from the orientation toward justice described by Kohlberg (1973, 1976). As expected, women most often exhibited the care focus and men more often exhibited the justice focus.

Analysis of interviews with nurses suggests that nurses at times combine the care/justice perspective when forced to make ethical decisions (Chally, 1995). More recent work by Zickmund (2004) suggests that there has been a shift of nurses from the moral perspective of care to a justice orientation where universal rules and principles are used in moral decision making. One reason offered for this shift includes the notion that the nursing profession has begun to devalue caring as it becomes more scientific and technological. This chapter's Evidence-Based Practice Note (p. 125) explores how a preceptor can support ethical decision making by critical care nurses.

UNDERSTANDING ETHICAL DILEMMAS IN NURSING

Ethical dilemmas, as discussed in the Evidence-Based Practice Note, are a common occurrence in

☼ EVIDENCE-BASED PRACTICE

note

Critical care nurses are key care providers in critical care units, environments in which ethical dilemmas frequently occur. M.C. Hough, a doctoral student at Florida State University, wondered what factors might assist critical care nurses in ethical decision making. She designed a study to explore and describe ethical decision making in a critical care nursing practice.

A qualitative study design using ethnographic methods was used to accomplish this goal. Data triangulation was accomplished by using three techniques of data collection: (1) open-ended, in-depth semistructured interviews and probes; (2) participant observation; and (3) document analysis.

Fifteen critical care nurses with various experience and education levels were interviewed to ensure a representation similar to that found in typical clinical practices. Verbatim transcriptions of each tape-recorded interview were analyzed for content using The Ethnograph, a computer software program. Participant observation was conducted with a hospital ethics committee; the researcher attended monthly business meetings and requested copies of all ethics consultations for a 12-month period. Informal short interviews were used to clarify, explain, or describe relevant issues as the researcher attempted to learn what role the ethics committee played as a nontraditional form of education with critical care nurses in the area of ethical decision making.

Document analysis was also conducted. This consisted of examination of written records of ethics committee consultations over a 12-month period before beginning the research study.

The findings indicated that nurses who had the advantage of an experienced preceptor or coach, particularly during orientation, had the most focused reflection and the least difficulty with sound, systematic, ethical discourse and decision making. Nurses who did not have this coaching had the greatest difficulty identifying and resolving ethical dilemmas in clinical practice. While difficulty was more often seen with nurses with less than 5 years of experience, the lack of a coach or mentor caused even more senior nurses to experience difficulty with focused reflection.

Hough concluded that institutions could benefit from developing programs to educate critical care nurses about ethical decision making. Such programs would be enhanced by training preceptors to function as coaches during critical care orientation.

From Hough MC: *Walking the line: a qualitative study of critical care nursing and the importance of experiential learning in ethical decision making in clinical nursing practice*, PhD dissertation, Florida State University, 1998, Dissertation Abstracts.

nursing practice. Many ethical dilemmas arise in nursing because of conflicts between patients, their families, health care professionals, and institutions. The following section will explore the major issues involved in these conflicts: (1) personal value systems, (2) peers' and other professionals' behaviors, (3) patients' rights, (4) institutional and societal issues, (5) patient data access issues, and (6) global dilemmas.

Dilemmas Resulting From Personal Value Systems

Values are important preferences that influence the behavior of individuals. Value systems are learned beliefs that help people choose among difficult alternatives, even when there may not be a good choice.

Each person has a value system that has a beginning foundation in the beliefs, purposes, attitudes, qualities, and objects that are important to a child's early caregivers. In time, individuals develop their own value systems that are grounded in their culture and life experiences. A **personal value system** is a rank ordering of values with respect to their importance to the individual and to one another. Personal values are compatible with the lifestyle one chooses and are influential in the development of professional values.

Variations in value systems become highly significant when dealing with critical issues such as health and illness or life and death. Value systems enable people to resolve conflicts and decide on a course of action based on a priority of importance. In professional nursing it is not enough to recognize and act on one's personal values. In addition, one must determine whether the value system is ethical. Only after careful reflection can nurses take action based on their personal or professional values.

Identifying a personal value system and its influence on decision making helps one to understand behavior more clearly. In addition, it gives you clues as to why other people's choices are different from your own. The "Childhood Value Messages" exercise in Box 5-2 can help to identify values learned as a child that may still influence you today.

To see how value conflicts can affect health care delivery, consider the following patient-centered situation:

Mr. Glover was recently diagnosed with an inoperable glioblastoma (type of brain tumor). The physicians have offered radiation therapy as a palliative treatment to extend his life expectancy. Mr. Glover initially decided to follow through with the radiation, but before his first treatment, he opted to forgo treatment. The radiation oncologist called Mr. Glover's daughter and asked her to convince her father to receive the radiation treatments because the oncologist believed that both Mr. Glover's quality and quantity of life could be enhanced. Mr. Glover wanted only to live his last days enjoying his children, grandchildren, and fishing, not going to and from the radiation clinic.

What did the physician value? What did Mr. Glover value? How were these value systems in conflict? Is there an outcome that can satisfy everyone? What action should the nurse take to show sensitivity to Mr. Glover's personal value system?

Dilemmas Involving Peers' and Other Professionals' Behavior

All practicing nurses participate as members of the health care team. This involves cooperation and collaboration with other professionals. As is true in all situations involving human beings, conflicts can easily develop, particularly in stressful circumstances. These conflicts may be between two nurses, the nurse and physician, the nurse and agency policies, or the nurse and any other health care professional.

As discussed previously, conflicts can evolve because of differing value systems, cultures, education levels, or a variety of other factors. A nurse may believe that assisting with abortions is wrong, whereas the institution in which he or she is employed routinely performs abortions. This creates a conflict between the nurse's value system and the institution's practices. Conflicts relevant to human rights often center around one of the ethical principles discussed earlier: autonomy, beneficence, nonmaleficence, veracity, or justice.

A disturbing reality in health care is the presence of workers in all disciplines who are incompetent or who participate in actions that are considered unethical by other professionals. An incompetent worker may suffer from physical or mental impairment or may be ignorant of standards of care. Unethical actions result when health care workers break basic norms of conduct toward others, especially the patient, whatever the reason.

A serious issue today is the large number of nurses and other health care professionals impaired by drug dependence or other addictions. Deciding how and when to confront a suspected drug user may result in an ethical dilemma. This dilemma can be overwhelming. Nurses agonize over whether to report observed or suspected

Box **5-2** **Childhood Value Messages**

By the time we are about 10 years old, most of our values have already been "programmed." Values are taught to us by family members and friends, through the media, in churches and schools, and by watching other people. What are the value messages you learned as a child?

Recall as many values as you can remember hearing as a child and write them in the blanks provided below. Here are a few examples to get you thinking:

"Nothing worthwhile ever comes easy."

"Life is fatal—you're eternal."

"You can accomplish almost anything you want to if you persevere."

"Clean your plate; there are starving children in China!"

"You are your brother's keeper—reach out to others."

"Tell me the truth, and I won't punish you!"

"Get your work done first; then you can play."

Now it's your turn to write some of your childhood values. How many of these values still influence the way you think and act today? Which ones influence you professionally? If you want to further explore your values, you may do the following:

1. Next to each value on your list, write the person's name who taught or modeled that value.
2. Put a star next to those messages that are still your values today.
3. Put a check mark next to those messages that you need to alter.
4. How are some of these values still influencing you today? Is this a positive or negative influence?

    1. _____

    2. _____

    3. _____

    4. _____

    5. _____

    6. _____

    7. _____

    8. _____

Reprinted with permission of Uustal DB: *Clinical ethics and values: issues and insights in a changing healthcare environment*, East Greenwich, RI, 1993, Educational Resources in HealthCare.

instances of unethical conduct or incompetent care including impairment caused by alcohol or drugs. Fortunately, some employers and state nurses associations have developed plans to assist impaired nurses in getting the help they need and make provisions for them to return to the profession once they are far enough along in their recovery process. The board of nursing in each state as well as each state nurses association can provide information on specific programs for impaired nurses in the state. However, the process must begin with a co-worker who follows the ANA *standard of care* that obligates professional nurses to "report illegal, incompetent, or impaired"

colleagues (American Nurses Association, 2004, p. 39).

To understand the ethical dilemmas that can result from conflict between peers, consider the following nurse-centered situation:

Miss Corbin, RN, works on a surgical floor. She has just assisted in the transfer of Mr. Hudson to his room from the postanesthesia unit after surgery and noticed that he was resting comfortably. Miss Corbin sees a nurse colleague drawing up a pain medication. The nurse colleague returns to the medicine room 10 minutes later with an empty syringe. Miss Corbin asks, "Who needed pain medication?" The colleague replies, "Mr. Hudson.

He was in pain after surgery." Confused, Miss Corbin checks Mr. Hudson's room and learns from his wife that he has not asked for or received pain medication.

What should Miss Corbin do now? Is doing nothing and waiting to see if it happens again an option?

Dilemmas Regarding Patients' Rights

As health care has changed over the years so has the nature of relationships between providers and patients. Years ago, health professionals, particularly physicians, were considered "all-knowing" experts. Few patients questioned the physician, let alone demanded their basic human rights. Now consumers of health care are increasingly demanding to have a say in matters affecting their health care. A number of specialty groups have developed published lists of patient rights. Examples include *Declaration of the Rights of Mentally Retarded Persons, Dying Person's Bill of Rights, Pregnant Patient's Bill of Rights, Rights of Senior Citizens,* and the *United Nations Declaration of the Rights of the Child.* As consumers have become more aware of their rights, conflicts between patients, health care professionals, and institutions have developed. Many of the rights demanded by consumers are not only their moral rights but also their legal rights and have been upheld by the judicial system. In 1997 former President Bill Clinton created an Advisory Commission on Consumer Protection and Quality in the Health Care Industry with part of their responsibility to be the creation of a patient's bill of rights in health care. The American Hospital Association also supports a patient's bill of rights; this document, now called the Patient Care Partnership, outlines the rights of patients in regard to their treatment plan.

It is beyond the scope of this chapter to discuss all rights due patients. Some of the rights that have been identified in these documents are the right to privacy, the right to informed consent, the right to die, the right to confidentiality and respectful care, the right to care without discrimination, and the right to information concerning medical condition and treatment. In addition, patients have the right to be informed if any aspect of treatment is experimental. Based on that knowledge, patients have the right to refuse to participate in research studies.

The following case illustrates a conflict related to patients' rights to receive care that is culturally acceptable to them:

Mrs. Hamid recently immigrated to the United States from Iran with her husband, a college professor. It is important to her religious faith and cultural values that men not be present during labor and delivery or at any time when a woman's body is exposed. A female nurse-midwife is delivering Mrs. Hamid, but complications develop. Her baby's heart rate drops abruptly and a cesarean delivery is needed. The only obstetrical surgeon available for this emergency surgery is a man. What action should the nurse take to show sensitivity to Mrs. Hamid's personal value system and her culture?

Patient Self-Determination Act

A federal government–imposed safeguard for patients' rights, the Patient Self-Determination Act, gives patients the legal right to determine how vigorously they wish to be treated in life-or-death situations. This act forces individuals to think about the type of medical and nursing treatment they would want if they were to become critically injured or ill. At the time questions arise, the patient is often unconscious or too sick to make decisions or communicate personal wishes.

The Patient Self-Determination Act (PSDA), which went into effect in December 1991, calls for hospitals to abide by patients' advance directives. The PSDA specifies that any organization receiving Medicare or Medicaid funds must inform patients of state laws regarding directives, document the existence of directives in the patient's medical record, educate staff regarding directives, and educate the community about directives.

Advance directives are designed to ensure individuals the rights of autonomy, refusal of medical intervention, and death with dignity (Norman and Pinkham, 1994). Advance directives are legal documents that indicate the wishes of individuals in regard to end-of-life issues. Critically ill individuals can remain in charge of their own end-of-life decisions if their advance directives are carried out. Each time they access a health care institution patients should have in their possession their advance directives. In addition, copies should be given to significant others, primary care providers, and any legal counsel that may be involved with the patient. The best directive is one that has been notarized or developed in conjunction with a legal expert.

Families should talk about how each member wants critical situations to be handled. Individual preferences can then be understood. Ideally, family members, caregivers, and courts will not need to make decisions for the patient. Too often the first time a patient learns about advance directives is upon admission to a health care facility. The question then arises as to who is responsible for discussing this sensitive issue with the patient. The ideal time for patients to make difficult end-of-life decisions is well in advance of the need (Figure 5-1).

Advance directives have not been without controversy. One problem is that states have passed different legislations, and there is no guarantee that one state will honor another's advance directives. Another problem may arise when a person is designated as the proxy to decide about medical treatment if the patient cannot do so. In some situations, persons have been named as proxies without their knowledge. Some family members have vehemently disagreed with or refused to follow the directives of a parent or spouse. When family members are left to decide, conflict occurs if family members are not of one accord. This leaves health care providers with the quandary of what to do. Conflict also sometimes arises among caregivers who disagree about the correctness of honoring certain advance directives.

The following case illustrates a conflict among caregivers related to patients' rights:

A 28-year-old quadriplegic man is admitted to the hospital with pneumonia and severe pressure ulcers.

Figure 5-1
To avoid unwanted, life-prolonging interventions, patients must make end-of-life decisions early, discuss them with family members and caregivers, commit them to writing in advance directive documents, and periodically review and renew them. *(Courtesy Memorial Health Care System, Chattanooga, Tennessee.)*

He was injured 10 years ago in a motorcycle accident and has been in the care of his elderly grandmother for the past 4 years. The patient, who is of sound mind, asks not to be given antibiotics and to be allowed to die with dignity, receiving only comfort measures. At the insistence of the hospital administration, the physician orders intravenous antibiotics. What is the nurse's responsibility to this patient?

Dilemmas Created by Institutional and Societal Issues

There are many policies in health care institutions that govern both workers and patients. Nurses often experience ethical dilemmas when they disagree with the policies of their institution. The scope and complexity of nursing actions vary significantly from large multi-service medical centers to small clinics or offices. All organizations, however, that receive governmental funds are subject to public scrutiny and accountability. Ethical dilemmas between nurses and the organizations that employ them may develop over policies dictated by the organizations or mandated by governmental agencies. Some experts contend that nurses experience great difficulty when the correct course of action is known but they are unable to implement the ethically or morally correct action because of external constraints such as hospital policy (Austin, Lemermeyer, Goldberg et al, 2005). This chapter's Critical Thinking Challenge below summarizes a well-known family conflict over who decides when end-of-life decisions need to be made. It also describes the intense media interest that arose when the family conflict was complicated by a national debate over the right to die.

Controversial health care practices and policies at the institutional, local, state, or national level can also interfere with the nurse's ability to implement basic care safely and effectively. For example, grave concerns over health care have centered on its cost. The rising cost of health care over the past 35 years has prompted worry by individuals, groups, and communities as well as governmental officials. All health care agencies must stress cost-containment measures to survive. At times, cost-containment policies conflict with the value system of the nurse, whose goal is to provide high-quality, individualized patient care with sometimes limited resources. Mathes (2004) supports this notion and suggests that financial constraints and staffing limitations can add to the moral distress that nurses experience

---

<u>CRITICAL THINKING</u> *Challenge*

The life and death of Terri Schiavo is a family story—the story of a family divided by right to die issues (Dewan, 2003). In 1990 Terri Schiavo and her husband of 6 years, Michael, were living in St. Petersburg, Florida, hoping to have a family. On February 25 of that year, Terri suffered cardiac arrest and fell into a coma. In the following days, a feeding tube was inserted to provide hydration and nutrition to the young woman. In June 1990 her husband was appointed her legal guardian.

After nearly 3 years of therapy and rehabilitation efforts in various facilities, Michael Schiavo came to believe that medical experts who said his wife was in a persistent vegetative state were correct. Her parents, the Schindlers, disagreed and used every legal and emotional means at their disposal to prove otherwise. In the absence of written documentation as to her wishes, there was only her husband's report of a conversation they had to that effect, which her parents did not believe. In May 1998, over 8 years after her cardiac arrest, Michael Schiavo filed a petition to have the feeding tube removed, citing her alleged wish not to live on life support. A firestorm of legal activity ensued. What the courts were asked to decide was who has the more valid claim to make proxy life-or-death decisions—the family a person is born into or the spouse they choose to marry and know intimately during adulthood (Dewan, 2003).

The Schiavo case, with Michael Schiavo on one side and the Schindlers on the other, was argued in state courts for more than 7 years. Judges at all levels, the Florida legislature, Governor Jeb Bush, and both the Florida and the U.S. Supreme Courts were all involved in orders and counter-orders requiring repeated removals and reinsertions of the feeding tube. The case gained worldwide attention in 2005 when Congress and President George W. Bush tried an eleventh-hour move to override a Florida judge's order to remove Ms. Schiavo's feeding tube.

The days following the third and final removal of the feeding tube in March 2005 became a national death-watch, chronicled in every newspaper and television news show around the world. Thirteen days following the removal of the feeding tube, Terri Schiavo died. An autopsy confirmed the findings of persistent vegetative state, showing that much of her upper brain was destroyed and there was much damage to the lower brain (Wikipedia, 2006).

This tragic case is over but many questions remain: Who was right and who was wrong in this case? Was there any right choice? How might Terri Schiavo herself have felt about the attention focused on her case? What have we learned?

---

on the job, and these may make it difficult for nurses to provide the ideal level of care for patients.

Other institutional and societal concerns can result in ethical dilemmas for the nurse whose personal value system does not support the policies set forth by those in authority. Examples include policies concerning access to health care for the uninsured, elderly, children, and persons with acquired immunodeficiency syndrome (AIDS).

Ethics committees were created to assist with ethical dilemmas in institutional settings. These committees are multidisciplinary groups charged with the responsibility of providing consultation and emotional support in situations in which difficult ethical choices are necessary. Cases needing consideration are referred to the committee by those desiring help, usually clinical caregivers such as physicians and nurses.

The following vignette illustrates an ethical conflict between a nurse and the employing institution:

> Jennifer McLeod is a nurse working in a critical care unit. All beds in the unit are full. For the past 2 days, Ms. McLeod has been assigned to care for a 92-year-old woman who is critically ill with heart failure. The patient has no financial resources of her own, and no family member has seen her since she was admitted from a nursing home. She remains in very critical condition. Suddenly, orders come for the elderly woman to be transferred to a bed on a regular nursing unit. As she is being moved out of the critical care unit, word comes that a state senator's son with a non–life-threatening condition is to be admitted to the recently vacated bed. What action should the nurse take?

Dilemmas Created by Patient Data Access Issues

The advent of widespread computer use in health care institutions has created another area for ethical dilemmas. If institutional safeguards are not in place, nurses have easy and sometimes unrestricted access to confidential information regarding patients in the entire institution. With the typing of a password and a keystroke on the keyboard, information can be obtained from computers onsite as well as in distance sites. Those in positions to access health care information share a great responsibility to protect this information from unwarranted use by others, including themselves. Both access of confidential information by those not involved in the direct care of the patient and sharing of information that has been obtained through computer access with other people are unethical. The reality is, however, that health care workers, including nurses, sometimes access records of friends and family members out of curiosity.

Health care workers must examine how they use information technology in their work. Curtin (2005) noted that information technology, particularly the computerized electronic medical record, places great power in the hands of health care workers and exacerbates basic ethical problems that exist. She suggested that there should be a union of technology, ethics, and nursing to put in place safeguards to protect patient information. Computer ethics has been in existence since the 1970s, but in recent years there is renewed interest in scholarly inquiry in this field as the use of technology has permeated the health care institution. Professional nurses must take great care to protect patient information at all times. It is both an ethical and a legal responsibility.

The following example illustrates the type of ethical dilemma that can result from inappropriate information sharing:

> Susan, a first year nursing student, was observed by Beth, a more experienced student, as she read patient information on a third student known to both who was admitted to another service of the same facility. Neither Susan nor Beth was directly involved in the care of the third student. Considering Susan's inexperience, what steps should Beth take? If Susan was a senior, should Beth react any differently?

Dilemmas Created by Global Issues

Population migration has become an emotional topic in many of the wealthier nations, and the United States is no exception. There are a number of issues created by immigration, both legal and illegal, that affect health care in this nation. Issues range from overloaded emergency departments to inability to communicate with patients who do not speak English. Another issue to arise in recent years is the recruitment of nurses from other countries to work in this country.

As the nursing shortage intensifies and threatens to become worse as our population ages, some legislators have proposed changing American immigration laws to open the door wide to nurses from other countries (Dugger, 2006). The idea is heartily endorsed by the American Hospital Association, which reported in April 2006 that there were 118,000 vacancies for registered nurses nationwide. The federal government itself forecasted in 2002 an 800,000 shortfall of nurses by the year 2020. Removing the immigration cap for nurses would undoubtedly increase the flow of English-speaking foreign nurses, who could earn more in 1 month in the United States than they might in 6 months at home.

Countries expected to lose the most nurses under this scenario include the Philippines, which already loses several thousand nurses a year to this country, India, South Africa, and potentially China. Leaders in these countries decry the measure. A University of the Phillipines professor of medicine who headed that nation's National Institutes of Health stated, "I plead for justice. There has to be give and take, not just take, take, take by the United States" (Dugger, 2006).

The American Nurses Association is on record as opposing the measure, expressing disappointment that instead of increasing appropriations to expand nursing programs in this country, Congress is "outsourcing the education of nurses." This comes at a time when nearly 150,000 qualified applicants to American nursing schools were rejected because of inadequate numbers of faculty and facilities. The ANA was joined by Physicians for Human Rights in opposing the proposal. This could undermine our "multibillion-dollar effort to combat AIDS and malaria by potentially worsening the shortage of health workers in poor countries. We're pouring water in a bucket with a hole in it, and we drilled the hole" stated a physician with the advocacy group (Dugger, 2006).

The following example illustrates the type of ethical dilemma that can result from this particular global issue:

> A nurse becomes interested in an advertised position for recruiters for foreign nurses. She excitedly tells a friend about the benefits of this position: travel to exotic places and big bonuses for the number of nurses recruited. Her friend has some awareness of the professional and ethical issues surrounding recruitment of foreign nurses. What should she do?

ETHICAL DECISION MAKING

Nurses encounter situations daily that require them to make professional judgments and act on those judgments. The judgments or decisions are often made in conjunction with other persons involved in the situation: patients, families, and other health care professionals. Ethical decision making requires that the nurse make judgments or decisions when two or more of their values are incongruent. When an ethical decision is made, everyone must respect and value the perspectives held by others involved in the situation. Through respectful collaboration, the best decision can be reached in even the most difficult dilemma. Notice that it is suggested that "the best decision" will be made. In an ethical dilemma, there is not a right or wrong answer. Instead, we search for the best answer.

Ethical Decision-Making Model

Whether involved in a collective or individual decision, nurses need to be knowledgeable about suggested steps in **ethical decision making,** listed in Table 5-2. A variety of ethical decision-making models are available in published literature. Regardless of the author or professional discipline, the models share more similarities than differences. The steps are not always necessarily sequential nor are they intended to be rigid processes. Instead, ethical decision making is a process

Table 5-2 COMPARISON OF NURSING PROCESS WITH ETHICAL DECISION-MAKING MODEL

Nursing Process	Ethical Decision-Making Model
Assess	Clarify the ethical dilemma
	Gather additional data
Analyze	Identify options
Plan	Make a decision
Implement	Act
Evaluate	Evaluate

in which ideas are thoroughly examined to determine the best solution to a difficult situation.

The following steps can be used in ethical decision making:

1. Clarify the ethical dilemma.

   What is the specific issue in question? Who owns the problem and should actually make the decision? Who is affected by the dilemma? Determine the ethical principle or theory related to the dilemma. Are there value conflicts? What is the time frame for the decision?

2. Gather additional data.

   After clarifying the ethical dilemma, in most instances more information needs to be gathered. It is important to have as many facts as possible about the situation. Make sure you are up-to-date on any legal cases related to the situation because ethical and legal issues often overlap.

3. Identify options.

   Most ethical dilemmas have multiple solutions, some of which are more feasible than others. The more options that are identified, the more likely it is that an acceptable solution can be identified. Brainstorm with others and consider every possible alternative.

4. Make a decision.

   To make a decision, think through the options that are identified and determine each option's impact. Ethical principles and theories as well as universal basic human values may help determine the significance of each option. When confronted with an ethical dilemma, a decision should be made. Refusing to make a decision is not responsible professional behavior.

5. Act.

   Once a course of action has been determined, the decision must be carried out. Implementing the decision usually involves working collaboratively with others.

Case Study 5-1

Administration of Pain Medication

Mr. Joe Johnson is a 56-year-old white male admitted with the diagnosis of acute myocardial infarction (MI) and cardiogenic shock. He has a history of severe coronary artery disease (CAD) and has suffered several MIs over the past 3 years. The patient has an advance directive and a do-not-resuscitate (DNR) order on his chart. When the nurse assesses the patient, he is short of breath and diaphoretic with a blood pressure of 68/30 mm Hg and heart rate of 162 beats/min. His respirations are labored and rapid at 42 breaths/min. Mr. Johnson is mentally alert and states he is having crushing midsternal chest pain radiating into his jaw and down his left arm. He is crying and requesting that the nurse give him something for the pain. There is an order for IV morphine sulfate, 2-10 mg for pain every 1-2 hours as needed. The nurse on the departing shift refused to give the IV morphine because of the patient's compromised status and the fear of further depressing his respiratory and cardiac status. After receiving the report from his evening nurse, you enter the patient's room and find his wife and one of his sons. They are upset and demand you administer the IV pain medication immediately. What do you do?

6. Evaluate.

Unexpected outcomes are common in crisis situations that result in ethical dilemmas. It is important for decision makers to determine the impact an immediate decision may have on future ones. It is also important to consider whether a different course of action might have resulted in a better outcome. If the action accomplished its purpose, the ethical dilemma should be resolved. If the dilemma has not been resolved, engage in additional deliberation and reexamine alternative options.

Consider the six suggested ethical decision-making steps in the context of Case Study 5-1.

1. Clarify the ethical dilemma. The specific issue is the patient's right of autonomy versus the nurse's duty related to beneficence (to do good) and nonmaleficence (to do no harm). Mr. Johnson clearly owns the problem and appears alert enough to make a decision. Obviously, his wife and son are also affected by Mr. Johnson's pain, as is anyone who provides care for him. The dilemma needs to be resolved quickly because of the extent of the pain.

2. Gather additional data. A review of the medical record indicates that the patient has a do-not-resuscitate order. An experienced colleague tells the nurse about the double effect doctrine and the condition that must be met to justify its use. The nurse realizes that giving the medication to relieve the chest pain may further compromise the patient's already critical condition.

3. Identify options. Options include the following: (1) asking someone else to care for Mr. Johnson with the intention of avoiding the dilemma; (2) refusing to medicate Mr. Johnson and let him continue in pain; (3) medicating Mr. Johnson with 2 to 10 mg of morphine sulfate; and (4) asking for an order for a medication with fewer side effects.

4. Make a decision. The nurse determines that to allow the patient to be in severe pain is unacceptable. Morphine sulfate is without question the drug of choice. Thinking through the principle of double effect, the nurse realizes that the proposed action of administering the medication to relieve pain is intrinsically good. Only the good effect (relieving pain) is intended, but there is potential for the undesired and unintended effect (premature death) from giving the morphine sulfate. The situation is discussed with the patient and his family, indicating both positive and negative consequences of giving the pain medication. The nurse is honest enough to indicate that the morphine sulfate may cause him to stop breathing. Mr. Johnson, his family, and the nurse decide that it is appropriate to administer the medication.

5. Act. Proceed to administer the diluted IV morphine sulfate slowly over a 10-minute period, frequently checking Mr. Johnson's blood pressure. After a total of 6 mg of morphine is given, he states that the pain has been relieved.

6. Evaluate. It is important to determine whether the intended effect was achieved and also to identify any unintended effects. The patient's satisfaction and family's satisfaction with the decision are also important. (NOTE: This situation is based on a real-life case. The patient lived for another 5 hours free of pain. He and his family visited throughout these remaining hours of his life and reminisced about past family memories. The patient, his wife, and son all expressed much appreciation for the relief of pain. Read the nurse's verbatim account of this ethical dilemma in Box 5-3.)

Box 5-3 **Verbatim Account of Ethical Dilemma: Administration of Pain Medication**

This case clearly shows the struggle of the critical care nurse as she decided whether or not to medicate Mr. Johnson. The nurse decided to medicate this patient for his pain despite his unstable hemodynamic condition. She gave the following verbatim account:

When I came out of report, I can remember walking into that room. I walked up to the bed; I introduced myself. He was ice cold. He looked at me and said, "I know I'm dying; my family knows I'm dying. Please give me something for the pain. I just can't stand it." His heart rate was 162. His blood pressure was 68/30 and I'm thinking, "I'm going to have to give him something for the pain, and the real strong possibility here is the guy is going to die when I give him something for the pain."

When I was up to 3 mg of morphine, I remember his blood pressure dropped down to the mid-50s, and I'm sitting there thinking in the back of my mind that I have the training and the skills and I have the technology sitting just 5 feet away from the door, and I could just run out and grab some atropine. Instead I looked at him and said, "Joe are you still having chest pain?" He said, "Yes, please give me some more; I can't stand it." (Oddly enough, I remember thinking about the perspiration on my upper lip and the beads beginning to form on my forehead and thinking should I take time to wipe it off.) So I pushed another 0.25 mg of morphine, and I looked up at his monitor, and his heart rate was beginning to drop; his color was gray anyway. I sat there with him pushing the IV morphine slowly until I had given him about 6.5 mg. I remember checking his pressure, and it was about 46/20. We just sat there for about 4 or 5 minutes, and I asked him how he was feeling. He said that he was feeling a little bit better and the chest pain wasn't as bad. Gradually his pressure came up and about 10 minutes later his blood pressure was up to about 90/60 and he was pain free.

I can remember it was probably about three o'clock in the morning and I went in and was talking with him, and I asked him if he was having any pain. He said he wasn't having any pain. I put the blood pressure cuff on his arm. As it was coming down, I lost his pressure. I looked up at his monitor and his heart rate, which had gone back up to 130-140, was down to 90 and his blood pressure was about 70/50. I pumped it back up to recheck and his pressure was 65/30. I can remember looking at him, looking up at the monitor, and his heart rate was in the 60s. I looked up at the monitor, and then I looked down at Joe, and he had this look in his eyes. He just nodded his head to me. I reached over and touched his wife's hand. I just looked at her and said, "It's time!" I looked over at the son and said, "You had better get the rest of the family and bring them in." I checked Joe's blood pressure one last time. I think I heard it once in the mid-30s. His heart rate was below 40. I can remember stepping back and motioning for his son to come in. They started telling him how much they loved him, what a great father he was, and what a wonderful husband he was, just reminiscing. Actually, they had been reminiscing throughout the entire night, talking about baseball games and growing up, and family times.

By now I'm feeling kind of like an interloper, and I'm trying to back out of the room to give the family some privacy. Just when I was about to back out, Joe looked over and said, "Katie, come here," so I walked over to the bed. I had my stethoscope hanging from my neck. Joe reached up, he was very weak by this point, and grabbed my stethoscope and he pulled it and he pulled my head down and whispered in my ear, "Thank you for taking the time and sharing this with us. You don't know how much it means to all of us," and then he kissed my cheek. Needless to say, by now I'm crying, the entire family is crying, Joe is crying. I remember as I stood up Joe just looked at me and said, "Good-bye." Then each one of his children, his daughter-in-law, and his sister said good-bye to him and they all leaned down and kissed him. I remember he turned and looked at his wife and she said, "Joe, I love you so much," and he said, "Give me a kiss." She stood up, leaned over, and kissed him—and his heart stopped—he died.

Continued

The family had been glancing up at the monitor, and they saw the straight line and they all looked at me for confirmation. I nodded my head and said, "Yes, he's gone." The youngest son turned with tears streaming down his face … he walked over to me and put his arms around me and kissed me on the cheek and thanked me. Then every member of the family did the same thing.

It's been 9 years since this happened, but it seems like it was yesterday. It was one of those moments in your professional career that just touches your life so dramatically that I don't think I will ever forget it.

There is stress working in critical care, and a great many technical decisions and much expertise that you have to possess when you're making life-and-death decisions all the time. When something like this happens, it makes it all worthwhile. There are very few professions—in fact, I can't really think of any others—in which professionals have the privilege of sharing something like this with a family: being present when a human life ends.

I was placed in a situation where I had to make a decision. I had to weigh the possible ramifications that decision was going to have. Would I let this man continue to be in excruciating pain, having his life extended maybe 3 or 4 more hours and him die, and having that family remember his pain for the rest of their lives, or go ahead and give him the medication that was ordered with the chance that it might end his life? I can remember as I was walking over to the narcotic cabinet thinking that allowing the man to be in that much pain was certainly not ethical. I can remember when I finally made the decision to medicate him was when I was able to rationalize to myself that I wouldn't be giving him the medication to end his life, but I would be giving him the pain medication to end the pain, and that was an ethical decision!

This scenario had a positive outcome. Joe lived for about 5 more hours, but the last 5 hours he was pain free. His family was in and out; they reminisced about the past. They had good memories, not memories of pain and suffering.

Obviously, this type of situation does not occur every single shift when working in critical care, but it is a fairly common occurrence. It is these types of things that you have to deal with all the time. It can be very stressful, but it can also be very rewarding.

Catherine ("Katie") Hough, RN, PhD

Courtesy M. Catherine Hough.

SUMMARY OF *Key Points*

■ The terms *morals* and *ethics* are often used interchangeably. Technically, however, morals reflect what is done in a situation, whereas ethics are concerned with what should be done. Values are beliefs, ideals, and attitudes that one uses to guide behavior.

■ It is important that nurses are familiar with ethical theories and principles, moral development, and decision-making models to participate actively in resolving ethical dilemmas that

occur frequently in health care settings. Two major theorists in moral development are Kohlberg and Gilligan.

■ Codes of ethics, developed by the profession's members, are important to the development of the profession.

■ The ANA's *Code of Ethics for Nurses* serves as a guideline for nurses regarding ethical behavior.

■ The history of the *Code of Ethics for Nurses* is reflective of nursing's history as a profession.

- Ethical dilemmas occur in all areas of nursing practice.
- Respect for humans is the foundation for the six ethical principles of autonomy, beneficence, nonmaleficence, fidelity, veracity, and justice.
- Use of technology in health care institutions has compounded common ethical dilemmas and created new ones for health care workers.

- Dilemmas often occur because of conflicts between personal value systems, patients, families, health care professionals, institutions, and society.
- Ethical decision-making models are helpful in determining the best action to take when faced with an ethical dilemma.

CRITICAL THINKING QUESTIONS

1. Explain the differences among morals, values, and ethics. Give an example of each from your own value system.
2. How can the American Nurses Association's *Code of Ethics for Nurses* be used by the bedside nurse, by the home health nurse, and by student nurses?
3. Compare the American Nurses Association's *Code of Ethics for Nurses* with the International Council of Nurses *Code of Ethics for Nurses*. How are they similar, and how are they different?
4. Select an ethical theory or principle that is most congruent with your approach to ethical dilemmas. Use it as a basis for resolving the ethical dilemmas in this chapter. How well does it hold up under these test conditions?
5. Discuss your reactions to the following scenarios and questions in a small group:
   a. Mrs. Otto has recently undergone extensive surgery for gynecological cancer. The day after surgery, she asks for more pain medication than the physician has prescribed. You call for an order to increase the pain medication dosage, but she still complains every 2 hours that she cannot tolerate the pain. What should be done?
   b. Mrs. Loriz suffers from severe chronic pain, the cause of which has not been definitely diagnosed. Her husband has brought her into the emergency department for the fifth time this month asking for narcotic relief from the pain. In tears she states, "A shot of Demerol is the only thing that takes the edge off." She threatens suicide if she is sent

home without some help. The physician has ordered a placebo. What is the nurse's responsibility?
   c. Mr. Nelson, age 87, suffered a serious stroke. His wife of 65 years keeps a constant vigil at his bedside. After 4 weeks, he remains totally unresponsive and develops pneumonia. A tracheotomy is performed and a feeding tube inserted. Mrs. Nelson feels agreeing to a "do-not-resuscitate" order is letting her husband down but recognizes he has no quality of life. How should the nurse counsel Mrs. Nelson?
   d. Emily and Michael Mills are parents of a young child dying of Tay-Sachs disease. Emily recently found out she was pregnant and wants to know whether their second child is affected with the same disease. She undergoes genetic testing of the embryo, and to the parents' extreme dismay, they find that their second child also has Tay-Sachs disease. How can the nurse assist these parents in making a decision regarding the second pregnancy?
6. Answer the following questions, basing your answers on identified ethical principles:
   a. When is it acceptable to refuse an assignment?
   b. What is the nurse's duty when a patient confides that he wants to harm himself?
   c. Is health care a right?
   d. What should the nurse do when her personal values are in conflict with those of the patient?

REFERENCES

American Nurses Association: *Code of ethics for nurses with interpretive statements,* Washington, DC, 2001, American Nurses Publishing.

American Nurses Association: *Nursing: Scope and standards of practice,* Washington, DC, 2004, American Nurses Association.

Austin W, Lemermeyer G, Goldberg L et al: Moral distress in healthcare practice: the situation of nurses, *HEC Forum* 17(1):33-48, 2005.

Beauchamp TL, Childress JF: *Principles of biomedical ethics,* ed 4, New York, 2001, Oxford University Press.

Burkhardt MA, Nathaniel AK: *Ethics and issues in contemporary nursing,* ed 2, Albany, NY, 2002, Delmar.

Butts J, Rich K: *Nursing ethics: across the curriculum and into practice,* Sudbury, Mass, 2005, Jones and Bartlett.

Chally PS: Nursing research: moral decision making by nurses in intensive care, *Plast Surg Nurs* 15(2):120-124, 1995.

Corley MC, Elswick RK, Gorman M et al: Development and evaluation of a moral distress scale, *J Adv Nurs* 33(2):250-256, 2001.

Curtin LL: Ethics in informatics, *Nurs Admin Quart* 29(4):349-352, 2005.

Davis AJ, Aroskar MA, Liaschenko J et al: *Ethical dilemmas and nursing practice,* ed 4, Stamford, Conn, 1997, Appleton & Lange.

Dewan SK: It may be a family matter, but just try to define family, *The New York Times,* Oct 26, 2003, Section 4, p. 1.

Dugger CW: US plan to lure nurses may hurt poor nations, *The New York Times,* May 24, 2006.

Fry ST, Harvey RM, Hurley AC et al: Development of a model of moral distress in military nursing, *Nurs Ethics* 9(4):373-387, 2002.

Gallagher A, Wainwright P: The ethical divide, *Nurs Standard* 20(7):22-25, 2005.

Gilligan C: *In a different voice: psychological theory and women's development,* Cambridge, Mass, 1982, Harvard University Press.

Guido GW: *Legal & ethical issues in nursing,* ed 4, Upper Saddle River, NJ, 2006, Pearson Education.

Hardingham LB: Integrity and moral residue: nurses as participants in a moral community, *Nurs Philos* 5:127-134, 2004.

Harrison E, Falco SM: Health disparity and the nurse advocate: reaching out to alleviate suffering, *Adv Nurs Sci* 28(3):252-264, 2005.

Haynes L, Boese T, Butcher H: *Nursing in contemporary society: issues, trends and transition to practice,* Upper Saddle River, NJ, 2004, Pearson Prentice Hall.

Hough MC: *Walking the line: a qualitative study of critical care nursing and the importance of experiential learning in ethical decision making in clinical nursing practice,* PhD dissertation, Florida State University, 1998, Dissertation Abstracts.

International Council of Nurses: *International Council of Nurses code for nurses,* Geneva, Switzerland, 2000, International Council of Nurses.

Jameton A: *Nursing practice: the ethical issues,* Englewood Cliffs, NJ, 1984, Prentice-Hall.

Kohlberg L: Continuities and discontinuities in childhood and adult moral development revisited. In Kohlberg L, editor: *Collected papers on moral development and moral education,* Cambridge, Mass, 1973, Moral Education Research Foundation.

Kohlberg L: Moral stages and moralization: the cognitive developmental approach. In Lickona T, editor: *Moral development and behavior,* New York, 1976, Holt, Rinehart & Winston, pp 31-53.

Kohlberg L: A current statement on some theoretical issues. In Modgil S, Modgil C, editors: *Lawrence Kohlberg: consensus and controversy,* Philadelphia, 1986, Falmer, pp 485-546.

Mathes M: Ethical decision making and nursing, *MEDSURG* 13(6):429-431, 2004.

Nathaniel A: Moral distress among nurses, *Ethics Human Rights Issues Update* 1(3):3-6, 2002.

Norman EM, Pinkham DB: Advance directives: understanding their impact on care. In Strickland OL, Fishman DJ, editors: *Nursing issues in the 1990s,* Albany, NY, 1994, Delmar, pp 267-279.

Office of Minority Health, Centers for Disease Control: *Eliminating racial and ethnic health disparities,* 2006 (website):   http://www.cdc.gov/omh/AboutUs/disparities.htm.

Tuckett AG: Truth-telling in clinical practice and the arguments for and against: A review of the literature, *Nurs Ethics* 11(5):500-513, 2004.

Uustal DB: *Clinical ethics and values: issues and insights in a changing healthcare environment,* East Greenwich, RI, 1993, Educational Resources in HealthCare.

Wickipedia: *Terri Schiavo,* 2006 (website): http://en.wikipedia.org/wiki/Terri_Schiavo.

Wilkinson JM: Moral distress in nursing practice: experience and effects, *Nurs Forum* 23(1):16-29, 1987.

Zickmund SL: Care and justice: the impact of gender and profession on ethical decision making in the healthcare arena, *J Clin Ethics* 15(2):176-187, 2004.

6

Becoming a Nurse: Defining Nursing and Socialization into Professional Practice

Beth Perry Black and Kay Kittrell Chitty

Learning Outcomes

After studying this chapter, students will be able to:

- Describe the benefits of defining nursing and discuss how this is related to professional socialization.
- Compare early definitions of nursing with contemporary ones.
- Recognize the impact of historical, social, economic, and political events on evolving definitions of nursing.
- Identify commonalities in existing definitions of nursing.
- Develop personal definitions of nursing.
- Discuss how students' initial images of nursing are transformed through professional education and experiences.

- Differentiate between formal and informal socialization.
- Identify factors that influence an individual's professional socialization.
- Describe two developmental models of professional socialization and explain how they are used.
- Differentiate between the elements of professional socialization that are the responsibility of nursing programs and those that are the individual's responsibility.
- Describe strategies to ease the transition from student to professional nurse.

Definitions of nursing and nursing's scope of practice seek to describe who nurses are and what they do. They answer questions such as the following: "What is nursing?" "What is the role of the nurse?" "What is unique about nursing?" and "What are the boundaries of nursing practice?" Although the answers for these questions seem quite simple, agreement on a single definition of nursing has been elusive.

In this chapter we will first examine definitions of nursing and explore how they have evolved over time. Once you have a clearer idea of definitions of nursing, we will discuss how you will make the move from student to nursing student, and then from nursing student to professional nurse through the process of socialization. Defining nursing is an important first step in becoming a professional nurse in practice.

Having a clearer understanding of what nursing is, and, as Nightingale said, "what it is not," helps you move closer to incorporating the values of professional practice. This process of socialization takes time but is enhanced when you have a clear idea of what your end point is: safe, informed, and professional nursing practice.

DEFINING NURSING: HARDER THAN IT SEEMS

You may be surprised to learn that finding a universally acceptable definition of nursing has been difficult. Ask almost anyone on the street what nursing is and you will get answers that range from "they take care of people in the hospital" to "they help doctors." Few persons outside of the health care setting have a clear idea of what nurses are and what they do.

Even nurses themselves have been unable to agree on one definition. For more than 150 years, individuals, starting with Florence Nightingale, and organizations around the world such as the International Council of Nurses (ICN), the United Kingdom's Royal College of Nursing, and the American Nurses Association (ANA) have attempted to achieve a consensus on a definition of nursing. Some efforts have been more successful than others.

Most of the definitions reviewed in this chapter have some terms in common. Considering the variations in knowledge and technology during the different points in history when these definitions were written, the similarities are remarkable. All the definitions are rooted in history and were affected by significant political, economic, and social events that shaped the form of nursing as it is now known.

Why Define Nursing?

Why is it important to spend time trying to define nursing? Having an accepted definition of nursing is essential in a variety of ways and provides a framework for nursing practice. A definition establishes the parameters (or boundaries) of the profession and clarifies the purposes and functions of the work of nursing. In addition, a definition guides the educational preparation of aspiring practitioners and guides nursing research and theory development. Importantly, a clear definition makes the work of nursing visible and valuable to the public and to policy makers who determine when, where, and how nurses can practice. Norma Lang, an influential contemporary nursing leader, put it succinctly by stating, "If we cannot name it, we cannot control it, finance it, research it, teach it, or put it into public policy. It's just that blunt!" (Styles, 1991).

Definitions clarify purposes and functions

Nursing is a complex enterprise that is often confusing to its own practitioners, as well as to the public. Defining nursing assists people to grasp its nuances, many of which are not readily observable. Nursing benefits when people such as journalists, public policy makers, insurers, other health care professionals, and the public understand what it is that nurses do.

Definitions differentiate nursing from other health occupations

Over 200 different allied health occupations have been developed in the past several decades. Each new advance in technology bred a new "technician" who needed to be educated, hired, oriented, and paid with limited health care dollars, a trend that continues today. The resulting cost was a major factor leading to significant redesign of the health care system during the 1990s and required the redefining of roles within the system. In response to these changes, defining nursing became even more important in order to manage the overlap of nursing with other fields without losing the core identity of nursing.

Definitions influence health policy at local, state, and national levels

Policy makers, such as legislators and regulators, need to understand the role and scope of nursing. Without that understanding, they cannot institute good health care policy that maximizes use of nurses' particular skills to improve the health of the public.

A key reason to define nursing is that nursing practice is regulated at the state level. Nurse practice acts of each state need to reflect the increasing expertise and autonomy of nurses. When the roles of professional registered nurses, advanced practice nurses, licensed or vocational nurses, and nursing assistants are well defined, legislators can pass progressive laws regulating and expanding nursing practice. Otherwise, nurse practice acts may restrict nursing practice and inhibit professional growth.

Definitions aid in developing educational curricula and research agendas

When nursing faculty plan the curriculum of a school of nursing, one of the major determinants of the design is their definition of nursing. Without the foundation of a definition, what to include and how to prioritize the huge array of information today's nurses need to know would be extremely difficult and unwieldy. A definition of nursing provides a good starting point for curriculum development. In much the same way, nurse researchers cannot easily determine phenomena of interest for nursing unless they are clear about the boundaries and purposes of nursing actions that a definition of nursing sets in place.

Evolution of Definitions of Nursing

In the last century and a half as nursing was becoming progressively more formal as an area of study and practice, a number of attempts have been made to define nursing that reflect the profession's evolution over the years.

Nightingale defines nursing

Florence Nightingale was the first person to recognize the complex and multifaceted nature of nursing that led to difficulty in defining it. Considering how relatively undeveloped nursing was during her time, Nightingale's definitions contain surprisingly contemporary concepts. Remember that during Nightingale's day, formal schooling in nursing was just beginning. In *Notes on Nursing: What It Is and What It Is Not* (originally published in 1859), she became the first person to

attempt a written definition of nursing, stating, "And what nursing has to do . . . is put the patient in the best condition for nature to act upon him" (Nightingale, 1946, p. 75). She also wrote:

> I use the word *nursing* for want of a better. It has been limited to signify little more than the administration of medicines and the application of poultices. It ought to signify the proper use of fresh air, light, warmth, cleanliness, quiet, and the proper selection and administration of diet—all at the least expense of vital power to the patient (Nightingale, 1946, p. 6).

Although Nightingale lived in a time when little was known about disease processes and available treatments were extremely limited, these definitions foreshadowed contemporary nursing's focus on the therapeutic **milieu** (environment), as well as the modern emphasis on **health promotion** and **health maintenance.** She accurately observed that although simply possessing observational skills does not make someone a good nurse, without these skills a nurse is ineffective. Indeed, informed observation has always been an integral part of the process of nursing. Nightingale was also the first person to differentiate between nursing provided by a professional nurse using a unique body of knowledge and nursing care provided by a layperson such as a mother caring for a sick child.

Early twentieth-century definitions

Fifty years after Nightingale wrote *Notes on Nursing,* the search for a definition began in earnest. Following the English model, many schools of nursing had been established in the United States, and numbers of "trained nurses" were in practice. These nurses sought to develop a professional identity for their rapidly expanding discipline. Shaw's *Textbook of Nursing* (1907) defined nursing as an art: "It properly includes, as well as the execution of specific orders, the administration of food and medicine, the personal care of the patient" (pp. 1-2). Harmer's *Textbook of the Principles and Practice of Nursing* (1922) elaborated on Shaw's bare-bones definition: "The object of nursing is not only to cure the sick . . . but to bring health and ease, rest and comfort to mind and body. Its object is to prevent disease and to preserve health" (p. 3). The fourth edition of the Harmer text, which showed the influence of coauthor and nursing notable Virginia Henderson, redefined nursing: "Nursing may be defined as that service to an individual that helps him to attain or maintain a healthy state of mind or body" (Harmer and Henderson, 1939, p. 2). Henderson's perceptions represented the emergence of contemporary nursing and were so inclusive that they remained useful for many years. We will see her influence again in the next section.

Post–World War II definitions

World War II helped advance the technologies available to treat people, which, in turn, influenced nursing. The war also made nurses aware of the influential role emotions play in health, illness, and nursing care. Hildegard Peplau (1952), widely regarded as a pioneer among contemporary nursing theorists and herself a psychiatric nurse, defined nursing in interpersonal terms: "Nursing is a significant, therapeutic, interpersonal process. . . . Nursing is an **educative instrument** . . . that aims to promote forward movement of personality in the direction of creative, constructive, productive, personal and community living" (p. 16). Peplau reinforced the idea of the patient as an **active collaborator** in his or her own care.

During the late 1950s and early 1960s, the number of master's programs in nursing rapidly increased. As more nurses were educated at the graduate level and learned about the research process, they were eager to test new ideas about nursing. Nursing theory was born. (See Chapter 13 for an in-depth discussion of nursing theory.)

One of the theorists who began work during this early period of theory development was Dorothea Orem. Her 1959 definition captures the flavor of her later, more completely elaborated self-care theory of nursing: "Nursing is perhaps best described as the giving of direct assistance to a person, as required, because of the person's specific inabilities in **self-care** resulting from a situation of personal health" (Orem, 1959, p. 5). Orem's belief that nurses should do for a person only those things the person cannot do without assistance emphasized the patient's active role.

By 1960 Henderson's earlier definition had evolved into a statement that had such universal appeal that it was adopted by the International Council of Nurses:

> The unique function of the nurse is to assist the individual, sick or well, in the performance of those activities contributing to health or its recovery (or to a peaceful death) that he would perform unaided if he had the necessary strength, will or knowledge. And to do this in such a way as to help him gain independence as rapidly as possible (Henderson, 1960, p. 3).

Never before or since has one definition of nursing been so widely accepted both in the United States and throughout the world. Many believe it is still the most comprehensive and appropriate definition of nursing in existence.

Another pioneer nursing theorist, Martha Rogers, included the concept of the nursing process in her definition: "Nursing aims to assist people in achieving their **maximum health potential.** Maintenance and promotion of health, prevention of disease, nursing diagnosis, intervention, and rehabilitation encompass the scope of nursing's goals" (Rogers, 1961, p. 86).

Professional association definitions

Nursing organizations worldwide have also struggled with defining nursing. Definitions to be reviewed here include those of the American Nurses Association, the Royal College of Nursing, and the International Council of Nursing. As you read these definitions, notice that some new concepts and terms are introduced in the more recent American definitions. In the United States, nursing has defined itself as the health discipline that "cares," although recent discussion suggests that limiting nursing to "caring" only overlooks the significant role that nurses have in the curative processes of health care (Gordon, 2005).

American Nurses Association. The American Nurses Association (ANA) has published several definitions of nursing over the years. The second edition of *Nursing's Social Policy Statement* defined nursing comprehensively. This definition included six essential features of contemporary nursing practice (American Nurses Association, 2003, p. 5):

■ Provision of a caring relationship that facilitates health and healing

■ Attention to the range of human experiences and responses to health and illness within the physical and social environments

■ Integration of objective data with knowledge gained from an appreciation of the patient or group's subjective experience

■ Application of scientific knowledge to the processes of diagnosis and treatment through the use of judgment and critical thinking

■ Advancement of professional nursing knowledge through scholarly inquiry

■ Influence on social and public policy to promote social justice

A more succinct definition also put forth by the ANA is found in the preface to the *Code of Ethics for Nurses* (2001): "Nursing encompasses the prevention of illness, the alleviation of suffering, and the protection, promotion, and restoration of health in the care of individuals, families, groups, and communities" (p. 4).

Royal College of Nursing. The Royal College of Nursing (RCN) is the United Kingdom's voice of nursing and is the largest professional union of nurses in the world. This organization embarked upon an 18-month-long initiative to define nursing, culminating in the April 2003 publication of the document titled *Defining Nursing* (Royal College of Nursing, 2003).

The RCN definition of nursing has a core statement supported by six defining characteristics. The core statement is this:

> Nursing is the use of clinical judgment in the provision of care to enable people to improve, maintain, or recover health, to cope with health problems, and to achieve the best possible quality of life, whatever their disease or disability, until death.

The six defining characteristics are too lengthy to reprint here; however, the entire document is worthy of examination and reflection because of its comprehensiveness and thoughtfulness. You can locate it at www.rcn.org.uk/downloads/definingnursing/definingnursing-a5.pdf.

International Council of Nurses. The International Council of Nurses (ICN) is a federation of national nurses associations representing nurses in more than 120 countries. Although ICN's membership is diverse, their definition of nursing is quite similar to that of single-nation organizations such as the ANA and RCN. According to the ICN:

> Nursing encompasses autonomous and collaborative care of individuals of all ages, families, groups, and communities, sick or well, and in all settings. Nursing includes the promotion of health, prevention of illness, and the care of ill, disabled, and dying people. Advocacy, promotion of a safe environment, research, participation in shaping health policy and in patient and health systems management, and education are also key nursing roles (International Council of Nurses, 2003).

You can learn much more about the ICN online at www.icn.ch.

Definitions Developed by State Legislatures

One of the most significant definitions of nursing is contained in the nurse practice act of the state in which a nurse practices. Regardless of how restrictive or permissive it may be, this definition constitutes the legal definition of nursing in a particular state, and the professional nurse maintains familiarity with the latest version of the act. Ohio's **nurse practice act** contains wording typical of many states' acts (State of Ohio Board of Nursing, 2003):

> "Practice of nursing as a registered nurse" means providing to individuals and groups nursing care requiring specialized knowledge, judgment, and skill derived from the principles of biological, physical, behavioral, social, and nursing sciences. Such nursing care includes:

1. Identifying patterns of human responses to actual or potential health problems amenable to a nursing regimen;
2. Executing a nursing regimen through the selection, performance, management, and evaluation of nursing actions;
3. Assessing health status for the purpose of providing nursing care;
4. Providing health counseling and health teaching;
5. Administering medications, treatments, and executing regimens prescribed by licensed physicians, dentists, optometrists, and podiatrists; or until January 1, 2010, advanced practice nurses authorized to prescribe under section 4723.56 of the Revised Code;
6. Teaching, administering, supervising, delegating, and evaluating nursing practice.

It is no accident that the language in these nurse practice acts sounds like familiar nursing language. State nurses associations and boards of nursing are actively involved with legislators to assist them in drafting laws that accurately reflect the nature and scope of nursing. The current nurse practice act in each state can be obtained by calling or writing the state board of nursing. The addresses of the boards of nursing can be found on the Evolve website (www.evolve.elsevier.com/Chitty/professional/).

Before moving on to the next discussion on socialization, take time to look at the accompanying Critical Thinking Challenge 6-1. How would you define nursing?

BECOMING A NURSE: SHAPING YOUR PROFESSIONAL IDENTITY

Defining nursing means that you have determined the most salient elements of what it means to be a nurse: what a nurse is and what a nurse does. When you first decided to become a nurse, you had certain preconceived notions about what nursing was and how you saw yourself as a nurse. Your desire to be a nurse may have been shaped by an illness experience of your own or a family member. Becoming a nurse may simply be something that you have always wanted to do without a

---

CRITICAL THINKING *Challenge 6-1*

Nursing is . . .

Instructions: Using your thoughts, as well as elements of others' definitions, write your own definition of nursing. Explain it to a classmate, giving your rationale for what you included and excluded. Keep it among your professional papers to refer to in later years. See how it evolves over time.

---

specific event that spurred this desire. Or you may be pragmatic in your career choice by selecting a profession in which demand is high and the risk of unemployment is low. Whatever the reason you elected to pursue a career in nursing, your image of nursing and what it entails is almost certainly going to be changed while in nursing school. Your thinking about nursing should change, develop, and mature over the course of your education.

While many students enter the profession of nursing with the worthy goal of "taking care of people," how this goal is translated into practice remains something of a mystery until you begin your studies as a nursing student. Being a student of nursing is the first of many steps in socializing you into professional practice: the goal of **socialization** is the development of **professionalism.** The goal of your nursing education is not simply teaching you the tasks of nursing, although they are important elements of your practice. The overriding goal of your education is to teach you to think like a nurse, to see the world of health care through the lens of nursing, and to respond to the effects of both educational and clinical experiences by developing professionalism.

This process requires that students **internalize,** or take in, new knowledge, skills, attitudes, behaviors, values, and ethical standards and make these a part of their own professional identity. For the RN returning to school for a BSN, a modification of an already-formed professional identity occurs. This process of internalization and development or modification of an occupational identity is known as professional socialization; it begins during the period students are in formal nursing programs and continues as they practice in "the real world."

EDUCATION AND PROFESSIONAL SOCIALIZATION

Nursing faculty are concerned with creating educational experiences that encourage and facilitate the transition from student to professional nurse. How does a student make the transition from a novice struggling to understand what is going on to a person who thinks and feels like a nurse? Learning any new role is derived from a mixture of formal and informal socialization. We have all been socialized into a variety of roles over the course of our lives. One that is so familiar to you now is the role of student in a generic sense. You learned in kindergarten that there are particular ways to behave in class, times to sit quietly and times to play, ways to get the teacher's attention, and, definitely, ways that you did not want to get the teacher's attention! You learned the "rules" of being a student and, unless you were particularly incorrigible, you learned your role as a student early and well.

In nursing, **formal socialization** includes classroom lectures, assignments, and lab experiences taught by faculty, such as planning nursing care, writing a paper on professional ethics, learning steps of a physical examination on a healthy child, starting an IV, or practicing communication with a psychiatric patient (Figure 6-1). Formal socialization proceeds in an orderly, building-block fashion, such that new information is based on previous information. For that reason, advanced nursing students are often encouraged to manage a larger number of patients than they did as novice students when their skills were fewer and less tested.

Informal socialization includes lessons that occur incidentally, such as the unplanned observation of a nurse teaching a young mother how to care for her premature infant, participating in a student nurse association, or hearing nurses discuss patient care in the nurses' lounge. Part of professional socialization is simply absorbing the culture of nursing, that is, the rites, rituals, and valued behaviors of the profession. This requires that students spend enough time with nurses in work settings for adequate exposure to the nursing culture to occur. Most nurses agree that informal socialization experiences were often more powerful and memorable than formal socialization in their own development.

Figure 6-1
During formal socialization, students internalize the knowledge, skills, and beliefs of nursing in planned educational experiences and interactions with faculty and other nurses. *(Courtesy Emory University/Nell Hodgson Woodruff School of Nursing.)*

Learning a new vocabulary is also part of professional socialization. Each profession has its own **jargon** that is generally not well understood by outsiders. Professional students in any field usually enjoy acquiring the new vocabulary and practicing it among themselves. While the vocabulary of any profession can be confusing and complex, the student quickly becomes fluent as a function of both formal and informal socialization. The student should be aware, however, that certain informal vocabulary overheard on nursing units is not always appropriate in professional settings and may actually be denigrating to patients or their families. A wise student will decide early to forgo these sorts of negative characterizations.

Learning any new role creates some degree of anxiety. Many of us remember the distress we felt when going to school for the first time as a young child. Some new students may find themselves particularly anxious as clinical experiences begin; the uncertainty of the situation, the unfamiliar language, the presence of patients with serious medical diagnoses, and a keen sense of the importance of the work of nursing can all contribute to this anxiety. This is not uncommon and may conjure up memories of our early days of formal education.

Once the initial nerves and excitement of entering nursing school have worn off, students may find themselves dealing with disappointment and frustration when their learning expectations come into conflict with educational realities. Students' ideas of what they need to learn, when they need to learn it, and what might be the best way to learn it may differ from how their education actually unfolds. Students sometimes become disillusioned when they observe nurses behaving in ways that conflict with their ideas and ideals about how nurses should behave. Knowing in advance that these things may happen can help students accurately assess the sources of their anxiety and manage it more effectively.

Factors Influencing Socialization

As students progress through nursing programs, a variety of factors challenge their customary ways of thinking. These include personal feelings and beliefs, some of which may conflict with professional values. For example, if students have strong religious beliefs, they may be uncomfortable working with patients who have no such belief or whose beliefs are different from their own. Yet the very first statement in the *Code of Ethics for Nurses* (American Nurses Association, 2001) requires that nurses work with all patients regardless of their beliefs. However, if you have a strong moral objection to a particular belief system of a patient or a negative reaction to a patient based on some characteristic of the patient, you should seek out your clinical faculty or other professional mentor to discuss your reaction and determine how to handle your conflicted feelings in an appropriate and professional way. This is not an uncommon response in nursing students as their sphere of contact with others different from themselves grows.

When children are growing up, they are first influenced by the values, beliefs, and behaviors of the significant adults around them. Later, peers become a significant influence. These influences also shape ideas about health, health care, and nursing. A common issue in nursing practice revolves around negative health behaviors of patients. If a nurse's family valued fitness, for example, it may be difficult for that nurse to empathize with an obese patient with heart disease who refuses to exercise even though there are clear health benefits. In this example, a family value (fitness) comes into conflict with a professional value (nonjudgmental acceptance of patients). Other patient issues that sometimes challenge students' values are substance abuse; self-destructive behaviors; abortion; issues related to sexuality, such as sexual identity, infertility, genetic manipulation; and end-of-life issues.

All people have **biases;** however, unexamined biases are more likely to influence behavior than examined ones. Nurses need to be aware of their biases and discuss them with peers, instructors, and professional role models. Failure to do so may adversely affect the nursing care provided to certain patients. Professional nurses make every effort to avoid imposing their personal beliefs on others (see Chapter 9 for further discussion of self-awareness and nonjudgmental acceptance as necessary attributes of professional nurses). Becoming a professional nurse requires learning how to deal with values conflicts such as these while respecting patients' differing viewpoints. This cannot be taught but is the responsibility of each aspiring professional. The key point here is that you should begin to identify those "hot button" issues that seem to affect you negatively, so that you can understand your own responses and how to set them aside while still providing excellent care of your patients.

As seen from this brief overview, socialization is much more than the transmission of knowledge and skills. Socialization serves to develop a common nursing consciousness and is the key to keeping the profession vital and dynamic while preserving its fundamental focus on human responses in health and illness.

A New Factor Influencing Socialization—Distance Learning

Distance learning in nursing is a fast-growing phenomenon. More nursing schools are utilizing technology to deliver education to nurses who do not have access to traditional on-campus programs. Initially, single courses or continuing education short courses were offered by distance education. Today, entire nursing curricula are offered by distance learning and the amount of on-campus time may be very limited. Many programs today routinely use highly technological resources such as video teleconferencing and online courses. This trend is expected to increase as demand and technological developments continue. Even within traditional nursing curricula, some content is taught online with infrequent classroom sessions.

Questions about whether students could achieve educational outcomes through distance learning have been answered: they can and do pass their courses, some with distinction, using these methodologies (Anderson, 2004; Hurst, 2005). Questions then arose about whether professional

attitudes and values—in other words, professional socialization—could be effectively achieved through distance education. Although more study is needed, initial indicators have been positive (Cragg, Plotnikoff, Hugo et al, 2001; Nesler, Hanner, Melburg et al, 2001).

MODELS OF PROFESSIONAL SOCIALIZATION

The transition from student to professional is a topic of importance to nurse researchers interested in creating effective means of professional socialization. During the 1970s and 1980s, a number of models of professional socialization of basic and RN students were developed. Cohen (1981) and Hinshaw (1976) described developmental models appropriate for beginning nursing students. Bandura (1977) described a type of socialization he called *modeling*, which is useful when learning any new behavior. Benner (1984) identified five stages nurses pass through in the transition from "novice to expert." Two of these models, Cohen's and Benner's, are presented in more detail below. Although these models were developed in the early 1980s, they serve to describe processes of transition and socialization that many faculty have come to recognize as almost universal among nursing students.

Cohen's Model of Basic Student Socialization

Cohen (1981) proposed a model of professional socialization consisting of four stages. Basing her work on developmental theories and studies of beginning students' attitudes toward nursing, she asserted, "Students must experience each stage in sequence to feel comfortable in the professional role" (p. 16). She believed that a positive outcome in all four stages is necessary for satisfactory socialization to occur. Readers may wish to compare themselves and nursing classmates against these four stages. A reminder, however: although it is interesting and potentially useful, this model has not been subjected to rigorous testing or scientific validation. However, this model does appear to fit the behaviors that experienced faculty note in the development of students' socialization into professional practice.

Cohen identified the first stage in her model, stage I, as unilateral dependence. Because they are inexperienced and lack knowledge, students at this stage rely on external limits and controls established by authority figures such as teachers. During stage I, students are unlikely to question or analyze critically the concepts teachers present because they lack the necessary background to do so. An example of a student operating in a unilateral dependent stage would be the student who agrees to a clinical assignment without questioning the clinical faculty's thinking about the appropriateness of the assignment or what the student may gain from the assignment. The student "soaks in" the faculty's direction and discussion about the patient without yet making linkages of his or her own in thinking about the patient's condition. Fundamentally, students at this stage do as they are told because they lack the experience and knowledge to question.

In stage II—negativity/independence—students' critical thinking abilities and knowledge bases expand. They begin to question authority figures. Cohen called this occurrence cognitive rebellion. Much as young children learn that they can say no, students at this level begin to free themselves from external controls and to rely more on their own judgment. They think critically about what they are being taught. This is a stage when students begin to question, "Why do I have to learn about this? This isn't nursing!" or complain, "I will never learn to give an injection to a patient if I have to sit here reading about the nursing process!" This can be stage where a student's fledgling independence may cause some lack of judgment in the clinical setting, much as a toddler may overestimate his or her own powers of mobility or dexterity. In addition, students at this stage may begin to demand "more difficult" patient situations to manage and resist faculty's (more informed) judgment that the student is not yet ready for complex patients.

Stage III—dependence/mutuality—is characterized by what Cohen described as students'

more reasoned evaluation of others' ideas. They develop an increasingly realistic appraisal process and learn to test concepts, facts, ideas, and models objectively. Students at this stage are more impartial; they accept some ideas and reject others. This is a time when students begin to appreciate the usefulness of the nursing process in organizing care and begin to use more sophisticated critical thinking skills.

In stage IV—interdependence—students' needs for both independence and mutuality (sharing jointly with others) come together. Students develop the capacity to make decisions in collaboration with others. The successfully socialized student completes stage IV with a self-concept that includes a professional role identity that is personally and professionally acceptable and compatible with other life roles. Faculty appreciates the maturity and trustworthiness that students exhibit when they reach this stage in their professional development. These students are often highly self-directed, seeking out learning experiences in order to maximize their knowledge before the completion of their formal education. Table 6-1 summarizes the key behaviors associated with each of Cohen's stages.

Benner's Stages of Nursing Proficiency (Basic Student Socialization)

Patricia Benner, a nurse, was curious about how nurses made the transition from inexpert beginners to highly expert practitioners. She described a process consisting of five stages of nursing practice, on which she based her 1984 book, *From Novice to Expert*. The stages Benner described are "novice," "advanced beginner," "competent practitioner," "proficient practitioner," and "expert practitioner." Advancing from stage to stage occurs gradually as nurses gain more experience in patient care. Clinical judgment is stimulated when the nurse's "preconceived notions and expectations" (p. 3) collide with, or are confirmed by, the realities of everyday practice.

In 2000, many years after she generated this model, Benner's work was one of several theories presented to a group attempting to demonstrate

Table 6-1   Cohen's Model of Basic Student Socialization

Stage	Key Behaviors
I: Unilateral dependence	Reliant on external authority; limited questioning or critical analysis
II: Negativity/independence	Cognitive rebellion; diminished reliance on external authority
III: Dependence/mutuality	Reasoned appraisal; begins integration of facts and opinions following objective testing
IV: Interdependence	Collaborative decision making; commitment to professional role; self-concept now includes professional role identity

Data from Cohen HA: *The nurse's quest for professional identity*, Menlo Park, Calif, 1981, Addison-Wesley.

how learning theories apply to adult skill acquisition. They tested and confirmed that Benner's model was valid, and they suggested that her stages apply to any adult learning situation (Hom, 2003).

Benner's novice stage, or stage I, begins with students entering nursing school. Because they generally have little background on which to base their clinical behavior, they must depend rather rigidly on rules and expectations established for them. Their practical skills are limited. For example, a novice nurse is faced with the request of a mother to let her 2-year-old child take "just a peek" at his newborn sister, even though it is against hospital protocol to allow children to visit when the newborn is in the room with the mother. The novice is very uncomfortable with the request because it is against the rules. The novice denies the request, citing the hospital rules.

By the time learners enter the advanced beginner period, or stage II, they have discerned that a particular order exists in clinical settings (Benner, Tanner, and Chesla, 1996). Their performance is marginally competent. They can base their actions on both theory and principles but tend to experience difficulty formulating priorities, viewing many nursing actions as equally important. When faced with the same situation as the novice nurse and the mother of a 2-year-old, the advanced beginner is still likely to deny the mother's request, but the nurse also has an understanding of the needs of the mother to see her 2-year-old in addition to spending time with the new infant. The advanced beginner suggests

that the mother send the infant to the nursery and then have an uninterrupted visit with her older child.

Competent practitioners, or stage III learners, usually have 2 to 3 years' experience in a setting. As a result, they feel competent, organized, and efficient most of the time. These feelings of mastery are a result of planning and goal-setting skills and the ability to think abstractly and analytically. These learners can coordinate several complex demands simultaneously. For example, the competent nurse spends a few moments at the start of his or her shift, examining the needs of each patient and planning fundamental care. At this stage, the competent nurse understands that situations change quickly and that planning is the best way to ensure that care gets implemented even when emergencies or unexpected events arise. This nurse may or may not allow the 2-year-old child to visit with his new sister; however, the nurse will examine the needs of everyone carefully and many of the exigencies involved before making a final decision about allowing the toddler "a peek" at his baby sister.

Proficient practitioners (stage IV) have typically been in practice 3 to 5 years. These nurses are able to see patient situations holistically rather than in parts, to recognize and interpret subtleties of meaning, and to easily recognize priorities for care. They can focus on long-term goals and desired outcomes. These experienced nurses are likely to be leaders on their units, having a wealth of experience and commitment to nursing.

Concerned with patient outcomes rather than institutional rules, the proficient nurse would likely understand in a holistic way the needs of the mother and her 2-year-old son and their desire to incorporate the new infant into their family. This nurse is likely to allow the "rules" to be broken in deference to the needs of the family.

Expert practitioner, or stage V, status is reached only after extensive practice experience. These nurses perform intuitively, without conscious thought, automatically grasping the significance of the patient's complete experience. They move fluidly through nursing interventions, acting on the basis of their feeling of "rightness" of nursing action. They may find it difficult to express verbally why they selected certain actions, so integrated are their responses. Both to themselves and to observers, their expertise seems to "come naturally." Expert nurses on occasion have difficulty deconstructing their work, that is, being able to describe what they experience clinically, because it comes so naturally to them. The expert nurse might even initiate a suggestion to the newborn's mother that the 2-year-old "take a peek" at his baby sister because this nurse recognizes the complexities of incorporating a new member into the family.

Table 6-2 summarizes Benner's stages from novice to expert. Box 6-1 contains a nurse's experience as a student that demonstrated the clear difference between novice and expert nursing.

Actively Participating in One's Own Professional Socialization

Many schools of nursing have programs for registered nurses with associate degrees or diplomas to return for completion of their bachelor of science in nursing (BSN) degree. These students have special socialization needs as they return to the classroom, sometimes after many years of practice. Davidhizar, Gigen, and Reed (1993) recommended some strategies for RNs to decrease the stress they experience upon returning to school. Although written for returning students, these strategies could apply to all students:

■ Actively involve yourself in the learning process.
■ Keep your eye on the prize. You are temporarily uncomfortable but will ultimately get something you want (such as certification, promotion, sense of self-confidence, personal growth, or graduate school).
■ Keep your perspective. You are in school by choice. No one is doing this to you.
■ Set aside preconceived ideas, prejudices, and habits. Give yourself and the school experience a chance.
■ Open up your creative side, your abstract thinking, and your willingness to engage in

---

Table 6-2   BENNER'S STAGES OF NURSING PROFICIENCY (BASIC STUDENT SOCIALIZATION)

Stage	Nurse Behaviors
I: Novice	Has little background and limited practical skills; relies on rules and expectations of others for direction
II: Advanced beginner	Has marginally competent skills; uses theory and principles much of the time; experiences difficulty establishing priorities
III: Competent practitioner	Feels competent, organized; plans and sets goals; thinks abstractly and analytically; coordinates several tasks simultaneously
IV: Proficient practitioner	Views patients holistically; recognizes subtle changes; sets priorities with ease; focuses on long-term goals
V: Expert practitioner	Performs fluidly; grasps patient needs automatically; responses are integrated; expertise comes naturally

Data from Benner P: *From novice to expert: excellence and power in clinical nursing practice*, Menlo Park, Calif, 1984, Addison-Wesley.

Box 6-1 **From Novice to Expert: "How Did You Know That?"**

The difference between a novice and an expert nurse was demonstrated to me in a very stark way when I was in my first semester of nursing school. I was assigned to a surgical unit with other junior students. Our clinical instructor, Janie, had 8 years of surgical intensive care unit experience as an RN, and had been a faculty member for several years. The fact that she was 7 months pregnant never deterred her or slowed her down in any way. Janie just always seemed to know when we needed her, even when we didn't know we needed her.

I had finished my patient's morning care, a kind elderly man who was going to be transferred to a long-term care facility later that morning. Because I was not busy, I asked one of the other students on the unit if she needed any help. Her patient was fairly complex, having been transferred from the surgical ICU the night before. He had a deep sacral decubitus ulcer that needed to be assessed, in addition to gangrene in his lower extremities. She asked me to help turn him so she could assess his sacral area. Using our best communication skills, we told the patient exactly what we were going to do, that we were going to turn him on his side and assured him that we were not going to hurt him.

Being the two novices that we were, we were fascinated by the size and depth of the ulcer and spent what seemed like several minutes staring at it. The patient never complained about the position we were holding him in. We continued to try to figure out what to do with regard to his pressure sore. I finally took a look at his face and began to reassure him that we were almost done. Then I realized that he was not responding. My novice assessment: "He looks funny" ("funny" in an odd way, not in a humorous way).

Thank goodness Janie, the expert nurse and clinical faculty, was walking past the patient's door. She heard my novice assessment and immediately understood the severity of "looking funny" to a new student. In my memory she became airborne as she dashed into the room; in reality she simply walked in, made an immediate and correct assessment of the patient and called a code. He was in a full cardiac arrest. My novice classmate and I stood cowering in the corner as the room was quickly filled with persons responding to the emergency. I wondered how Janie knew what to do with so little effort and so much intuition. I envied her calmness and leadership in the resuscitation effort, the placement of a pacemaker in the patient, and coordination of his transfer back to the ICU.

My novice assessment: "He looks funny." Her expert assessment: "New students, can't describe patient. Complex patient. Risk for variety of complications due to prolonged bed rest and post-op infection, unresponsive, cyanotic, eyes open, not breathing, no heart rate. Call code, lower head of bed, start CPR, make sure IV is patent, make sure oxygen is available, etc, etc . . ."

To her credit, Janie took my classmate and me to lunch that day, encouraging us to discuss what had happened and reassuring us that nothing we did caused him to have an arrest. She allowed us to work through our own considerable distress. And I knew that I wanted to be "just like her" when I became an RN. Twenty-seven years later, I am still grateful for her example of compassionate expert nursing.

Beth Black, PhD, RN
UNC at Chapel Hill School of Nursing

hypothetical thinking. Everything need not be immediately applicable in the work setting to be of value.

- Be receptive to feedback, even if it is critical. If you were perfect, you would not need to be here.
- Develop your time management skills. Learn to use bits of time, such as listening to tapes while driving.
- Get a mentor for emotional support—another nurse, older friend, relative, or faculty member.

- Use faculty members as resources. They want to be helpful but cannot read your mind or discern what you need.

For other ideas about how to become an active participant in your own socialization process, use the checklist in Box 6-2.

SOCIALIZATION TO THE WORK SETTING

When nurses graduate, professional socialization is not over. In fact, the intensity of their socialization

---

Box 6-2 A Do-It-Yourself Guide to Professional Socialization

Listed below are 20 possible behaviors demonstrated by students who take responsibility for their own professional socialization. Place a check next to the behaviors you regularly exhibit. Be honest with yourself.

1. I interact with other students in and out of class.
2. I participate in class by asking intelligent questions and initiating discussion occasionally.
3. I have formed or joined a study group.
4. I use the library, labs, and teachers as resources.
5. I organize my work so that I can meet deadlines.
6. If I have a conflict with another student or a teacher, I take the initiative to resolve it.
7. I do not let minor personality problems distract me from my goals.
8. I seek out new learning experiences and sometimes volunteer to demonstrate new skills to others.
9. I have chosen professional role models.
10. I am realistic about my performance.
11. I try to accept constructive criticism without becoming defensive.
12. I recognize that trying to do good work is not the same as doing good work.
13. I recognize that each teacher has different expectations, and it is my responsibility to learn what is expected by each.
14. I demonstrate respect for my teachers' time by making appointments whenever possible.
15. I demonstrate respect for my classmates, patients, and teachers by never coming to class or clinical unprepared.
16. I recognize my responsibility to help create a dynamic learning environment and am not satisfied to be merely an academic spectator.
17. I participate in the student nurse association and encourage others to do the same.
18. I represent my school with pride.
19. I project a professional appearance.
20. One of my goals is to become a self-directed, lifelong learner.

Scoring: 1-10 checks—You need to examine your behavior and think about taking more responsibility for your own socialization; 11-15 checks—you are active in your own behalf; try to begin using some of the remaining behaviors on the list or come up with your own; more than 15 checks—you are a role model of positive action in your own professional socialization process.

is likely to increase as their exposure to nursing and the culture of nursing increases. Most experts believe that socialization, similar to learning, is a lifelong activity. The transition from student to professional nurse is another of life's challenges and, similar to most challenges, is one that helps people grow.

It can seem that just as students become well socialized to the culture of the educational setting, they graduate and must become **resocialized** to a work setting. Most new nursing graduates feel somewhat unprepared and overwhelmed with the responsibilities of their first positions. Although agencies that employ new graduates realize that the orientation period will take time, graduates may have unrealistic expectations of themselves and others.

During the early days of practice, most graduate nurses quickly realize that the ideals taught in school are not always possible to achieve in everyday practice. This is largely a result of time constraints and produces feelings of conflict and even guilt. In school, students are taught to spend time with patients and to consider their emotional as well as physical needs. In practice, the emphasis may seem to be on finishing tasks or completing checklists and flow sheets. Talking with patients, engaging in patient teaching, or counseling family members may be viewed as an unproductive use of time. In the early days of professional practice, having time to do comprehensive, individualized nursing care planning, a staple of life for nursing students, may seem like an unrealistic luxury. Box 6-3 describes the feelings of a new graduate following her first 9 months of practice.

Speed of functioning is another area in which new nurses vary widely. By the end of a well-planned orientation, new graduates should be able to manage an average patient load without too much difficulty. Time management is a skill that is closely related to speed of functioning. Managing your time well means managing yourself well and requires self-discipline. The ability to organize and prioritize nursing care for a group of patients is the key to good time management.

(It is also an asset to students!) Box 6-4 and Figure 6-2 provide guidance on how to keep poor time management from becoming a problem while you are a student. Once you have established good time management skills, they will carry over to the work setting.

New nurses also must adapt to collaborating with other nursing care personnel, such as nursing assistants, patient care technicians, and other unlicensed assistive personnel who help them in caring for patients. This is a difficult adjustment for some nurses who are unaccustomed to delegating, are unsure of the abilities of others, or believe only they can provide quality care.

An overlooked aspect of stress in new graduates is the sheer physical fatigue caused by 8- to 12-hour shifts accompanied by the standing, walking, lifting, bending, and stooping that patient care requires. Many new graduates have never spent an entire shift on a unit during schooling. When physical fatigue combines with

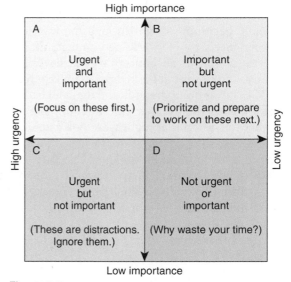

Figure 6-2
Setting priorities is an important aspect of time management. Use this grid to determine whether a task should go to the top, middle, or bottom of your daily "to do" list or whether it is a time-waster and should be ignored.

Box **6-3** **Letters from a New Graduate**

It's hard for me to find words where I should begin. I love the nursing profession and am so glad I have chosen this career path for myself, though this has undoubtedly been the most difficult 8 months of my life. It is exhausting and overwhelming at times. I am finally beginning to feel more comfortable in my role as a nurse, though it often depends on the day and the challenges each shift brings.

I work on an infant unit at [a large midwestern children's hospital], which is a wonderful place to start my career. I am also still working 12-hour nights, which has been a tough adjustment. I'm afraid I'm not a "true nightshifter," however, and at some point in the next few months may need to transition to a different shift.

My head spins when I reflect back on how much I've already learned and how much more there still is for me to learn! There really is no way I could have mentally prepared myself for what this first year of nursing has brought to me thus far, but I do know now that this is what I was meant to do.

I look forward to the day when I begin to be more confident of my abilities on a daily basis, when the transition from "novice" to a bit more experienced actually happens. I am sure that time will come soon, but in the meantime I am just taking things day by day.

I have seen many of my friends from nursing school go through these transitions as well as myself. It helps to hear the voice of an experienced and wise nurse. It gives me hope that things will eventually get better and the courage to keep at it—that there is a light at the end of this long tunnel.

Sincerely,

Liza Davis, B.S.N.

One month later:

It's interesting to think back to the first time I wrote to you just a few short weeks ago. I feel as if I am finally beginning to go through the transition I have long awaited. I had my first very difficult experience a couple weeks ago on the unit. It was a new admit of a 2-year-old in severe respiratory distress, who in all honesty should never have come to my floor, an acute care unit. I spent 4 consecutive hours at his bedside as we kept him stabilized, then finally was able to transfer him to the PICU. It was quite stressful, and though I had no idea how to handle the situation initially, I somehow had it all figured out as time went on. The doctors involved in his case were fantastic, as were the other nurses on that night who took care of my other patients for me. I never realized how well it went until the next day at work when I told my story to my co-workers. Their first question was, "Did he code on you?" and when I said "No," they replied with, "Well then you did your job well." Since my experience that night, I have felt much more confident and at ease with what I am doing, that I might actually be becoming a "good nurse." I really feel as if that experience was a turning point for me.

I still take each day for what it brings as I know how quickly things can turn bad with a patient. I do know that each day seems to get a bit easier, however, and hope I will continue on this path. It certainly has been a trying journey, but I know I am a better person because of it.

Liza

| Box 6-4 | Time Management Self-Assessment |

Effective time management is a skill that can be developed. Listed are principles reflecting good time management. For each of statements A through J, circle the answer that most closely characterizes how you manage your time.

A. I spend some time each day planning how to accomplish school and other responsibilities.
   0. Rarely
   1. Sometimes
   2. Frequently
B. I set specific goals and dates for accomplishing tasks.
   0. Rarely
   1. Sometimes
   2. Frequently
C. Each day I make a "to do" list and prioritize it. I complete the most important tasks first.
   0. Rarely
   1. Sometimes
   2. Frequently
D. I plan time in my schedule for unexpected problems and unanticipated delays.
   0. Rarely
   1. Sometimes
   2. Frequently
E. I ask others for help when possible.
   0. Rarely
   1. Sometimes
   2. Frequently
F. I take advantage of short but regular breaks to refresh myself and stay alert.
   0. Rarely
   1. Sometimes
   2. Frequently
G. When I really need to concentrate, I work in a specific area that is free from distractions and interruptions.
   0. Rarely
   1. Sometimes
   2. Frequently
H. When working, I turn down other people's requests that interfere with completing my priority tasks.
   0. Rarely
   1. Sometimes
   2. Frequently
I. I avoid unproductive and prolonged socializing with fellow students or employees during my workday.
   0. Rarely
   1. Sometimes
   2. Frequently
J. I keep a calendar of important meetings, dates, and deadlines and carry it with me.
   0. Rarely
   1. Sometimes
   2. Frequently

Scoring: Give yourself 2 points for each "Frequently," 1 point for each "Sometimes," and 0 points for each "Rarely." If your score is 0-10, you need to improve your time management skills; 11-15, you are doing fine but can still improve; 16-18, you have very good time management skills; and 19-20, your time management skills are superior!

the mental and emotional stress of decision making, efforts to become integrated into a peer group, uncertainty about policies or procedures, and lack of role clarity, sensory overload is almost certain to occur.

This chapter's Cultural Considerations Challenge 6-1 contains the description of one nurse's early adjustment to nursing practice. Still in practice after 25 years, this man entered and remained in nursing at a time when few men considered nursing as a profession.

"Reality Shock": When Ideals and Reality Collide

A reality of nursing today is the shortage of nurses to provide care in a complex health care system with an aging population and more persons living with chronic illness. Working conditions are

Cultural Considerations Challenge   6-1

A Look Back at a Man's Career in Nursing in a Small Rural Setting

I "fell into" the nursing profession by chance, not planning to become a nurse at first. At the time I made my decision to become a nurse, I was working in construction and took a part-time job as a nursing assistant at the small 40-bed community hospital in my home town. The male assistants were called "orderlies" back then. I think we were called "orderlies" because we were expected to keep order when patients became "unruly," which they sometimes did. The biggest change for me when I became a licensed professional was assuming responsibility for my actions. In working as an orderly/assistant, I had someone else take responsibility. That was fun. I could leave my worries at work. When I became an RN, I realized that "the buck stops here," so to speak. As an RN, it became MY responsibility to make a decision. I looked forward to my work every evening, because every day it was always something new and interesting. Twenty-five years later, it still is.

I selected my BSN program because I felt that it was the best program in the state. I still think that. The nursing program was tough but I don't recall feeling out of place, even though I was one of very few males in my class, maybe 3 or 4 of more than 100 students. I had good friends in school and we supported each other through clinicals, exams, and complaints about all those things nursing students complain about. After graduation, I had to decide whether to go back to the small community hospital where I had worked as an orderly or stay at the large university teaching hospital where I had trained. I find myself occasionally wondering how my life would have been different had I stayed at the teaching hospital. But now, I don't think I'd trade my experiences in a small community hospital with fewer than 100 beds.

In this beautiful setting near the mountains, I grew to know a lot of people in the small community. I knew their histories, their families, and many of their individual idiosyncrasies. I still see some of these patients in the community from time to time, and they remember that I was their nurse. Working in a small community hospital gave me experiences like these that I wouldn't have had in a large referral hospital. I look back on my early days in nursing rather fondly at times. From a "male" perspective, it did seem that I was called on quite a bit to do a lot of the heavy labor of the unit! I recall only one other male RN in the little community hospital. He worked in the ER and I didn't have a lot of contact with him, other than taking report on a patient from time to time.

I left the small hospital 11 years ago to work in a larger hospital, forcing me to grow professionally because the patients are more acutely ill in the cardiac care unit where I now work. Another substantial difference is that there are a lot of men who are RNs. Occasionally, I'll even work a shift where all of the nurses are men. I have always felt like I fit in as a nurse because my values are the same as other nurses that I know, males and females.

Twenty-five years after graduation, I am still glad I made the decision to become a nurse. I have many interests outside of nursing which keep me busy. But the challenges of nursing never grow old. As a nurse, no two days are alike. I think that's what holds me in this position in spite of the stress of working in a cardiac care unit. That's what I liked about it in the beginning, and that's what I still like about it today.

Kim Elder, BSN, RN
UNC at Chapel Hill School of Nursing, '81

sometimes very difficult, especially when acuity (severity of illness) of the patients is high and staffing is low. Despite the rewards of a career spent in nursing, nursing can be difficult at times. A current challenge in nursing is retention: keeping nurses in nursing. Replacing nurses who leave is extremely expensive for hospitals (Atencio, Cohen, and Gorenberg, 2003). Many of the difficulties faced by nurses now are not very different from other times of shortage when the needs of the health care system were greater than the profession could provide. This section is intended to leave you in a more powerful position to understand some of the negative feelings you may experience as you make the transition into professional nursing. Because as the saying goes, "forewarned is forearmed," we are including some discussion of not only how to recognize these feelings but also how to manage them so that you will remain an involved, well-prepared, and productive professional nurse.

"**Reality shock**" (Kramer, 1974) was a term used to describe the feelings of powerlessness and ineffectiveness experienced by new graduates, a term that is still relevant more than 30 years later. Psychological stresses generated by reality shock decrease the ability of individuals to cope effectively with the demands of the new role. Causes of reality shock include the following:

- Absence of positive reinforcement (such as coaching) and frequent communication
- Lack of support, such as faculty availability
- The gap between the ideals taught in school and the actual work setting
- The inability to implement desired nursing care because of circumstances such as a heavy case load or time constraints

Unfortunately, some new nurses "drop out" at this point, rather than taking steps to resolve reality shock. Kramer identified several ways nurses may drop out:

- Disengaging mentally and emotionally
- Driving oneself and others to the breaking point by trying to do it all
- "Job hopping"—looking for the perfect, non-stressful job that is completely compatible with professional values

- Prematurely returning to school
- Burning out—a condition of unresolved reality shock with subsequent emotional exhaustion
- Leaving the nursing profession entirely, which neither nursing nor society can afford

Much can be done to reduce reality shock in the transition from student to professional. Students must recognize that schools cannot provide enough clinical experience to make graduates comfortable on their first day as new nurses. They can take responsibility for obtaining as much practical experience as possible outside of school. Working in a health care setting during summers, on school breaks, and on weekends may be helpful. They should avoid work during the school week, if at all possible, or keep it to an absolute minimum because academic responsibilities take priority during that time, and exhausted students make poor learners.

Some schools offer programs in which students are paired with practicing nurses (**preceptors**) and work closely with them to experience life as a registered nurse. If your school offers such a program, take advantage of it. If not, seek out information about similar programs at area hospitals. Many agencies, including hospitals and the military, are now providing excellent opportunities for students nearing graduation to function in expanded roles.

Talking with other new graduates about your feelings is one of the best ways to combat reality shock. Take the initiative to form a group for mutual support—others need it too! Another interpersonal strategy is to seek a professional mentor. A **mentor** is an experienced nurse who is committed to nursing and to sharing knowledge with less experienced nurses to help advance their careers. A mentor can be a great source of all types of knowledge, as well as another source of support. Having a mentor is different from having a preceptor. Mentoring involves the formation of a long-term relationship through which ideas, experiences, and successful behavior patterns are shared.

Ask a nurse whose work you admire to be your mentor and identify what he or she can offer. Some inexperienced nurses are fearful of approaching potential mentors with this request. They should remember that this process is not a one-way street; it has benefits to both parties because it complements and validates the mentor's knowledge and self-esteem, as well as provides important information and support to the nurse being mentored. To get the most from a mentoring relationship, first understand your professional and personal needs and select a mentor who seems to share your values and beliefs. Set up specific times to meet and be willing to communicate openly with your mentor (Hagenow and McCrea, 1994). A mentoring relationship is a powerful tool by which a new nurse can benefit from the experience, wisdom, and feedback from someone who has "been there"—who understands your experience because he or she has experienced the same thing.

The Internet provides opportunities for nursing students to learn more about the profession of nursing and to assist with socialization into practice. One excellent website for student nurses is www.nursingnet.org. This website was created and is maintained by practicing nurses who seek to improve professionalization in nursing.

Care of self is an important activity as you begin your career in the care of others. Have you ever noticed that when you are traveling on an airline, the flight attendants instruct you, in the case of an emergency, to put on your own oxygen mask first? Then you are prepared to help those around you. The same principle applies here. You will provide better care to others if you care for yourself first, such as eating nutritiously, exercising regularly, avoiding tobacco and excessive alcohol use, seeking spiritual support if that is important to you, and having friends outside of work—all of those things that you know are "good for you." The stronger and healthier you are physically, psychologically, and spiritually, the better prepared you are to face the demands of your transition into the important work of nursing.

In the final analysis, you—and only you—are responsible for your own lifelong professional socialization. Those nurses who maintain a good balance between their work and personal lives and who have reasonable expectations of the work of nursing without sacrificing their own values and ideals have great potential to be effective nurses over a long career.

SUMMARY OF *Key Points*

- Although attempts to define nursing have been under way since the days of Nightingale, efforts have generally fallen short of capturing the diversity and richness that constitutes nursing.
- Definitions reviewed in this chapter have more commonalities than differences.
- Definitions change over time as society and nursing change and as each individual's perceptions about, and experiences in, nursing change.
- The dynamic nature of the nursing profession, society, and health care will likely prevent us from ever developing one eternal, universally accepted definition of nursing.
- Professional socialization is a critical process that turns novices into fully functioning professionals.
- Two major components of socialization to professional nursing are socialization through education and socialization in the workplace.
- Conceptual models of professional socialization that identify stages in the process and key behaviors occurring at each stage are applicable to nursing.
- Individuals have responsibility for actively participating in their own professional socialization. They should identify needed learning experiences and seek opportunities that provide these experiences.
- Reality shock is a stressful period that new nurses may experience when entering nursing practice. Understanding the stages of reality shock and how to resolve them can assist new graduates through this transition.
- Mentors can be valuable resources in enhancing and enriching the professional socialization experience.

CRITICAL THINKING QUESTIONS

1. Obtain your school's definition of nursing. How is it similar to or different from definitions in this chapter?
2. From the definitions of nursing presented in this chapter, select the one you most prefer and explain your choice.
3. How might new technologies, economic factors, social trends, and new practice options for nurses affect future definitions of nursing? How might these factors affect the scope of nursing?
4. If you are already a practicing nurse, how has your personal definition of nursing changed over time? How have you seen the scope of nursing change since you entered practice?
5. Obtain a copy of the nurse practice act for your state. Find the legal definition of nursing and compare it with other definitions found in this chapter. How are they alike and how are they different? How does your state define the scope of nursing practice?
6. Describe how both formal and informal socialization experiences in school are modifying your image of nursing.
7. Examine one of the two models of socialization discussed in this chapter and place yourself in one of the stages. Give your rationale for that placement. If none of the models or stages fits your experience, create your own model (or stage) and share it with the class.
8. List five things you can do to take active responsibility for your own professional socialization.
9. Interview a new nurse and discuss his or her experience with reality shock. How is this individual handling the transition from student to practicing nurse? What can you learn from his or her experience?
10. Identify several personal and professional areas in which a mentor might be helpful to you. Select a potential mentor and talk with him or her about your needs.

REFERENCES

American Nurses Association: *Code of ethics for nurses,* Washington, DC, 2001, American Nurses Publishing.

American Nurses Association: *Nursing's social policy statement,* ed 2, Washington, DC, 2003 (website): nursebooks.org.

Anderson ET: Impact of community health content on nurse practitioner practice: a comparison of classroom and web-based teaching, *Nurs Ed Perspect* 25(4):171-175, 2004.

Atencio BL, Cohen J, Gorenberg B: Nurse retention: is it worth it? *Nurs Economic$* 21(6):262-268, 299, 2003.

Bandura A: *Social learning theory,* Englewood Cliffs, NJ, 1977, Prentice-Hall.

Benner P: *From novice to expert: excellence and power in clinical nursing practice,* Menlo Park, Calif, 1984, Addison-Wesley.

Benner P, Tanner CA, Chesla CA: *Expertise in nursing practice: caring, clinical judgment, and ethics,* New York, 1996, Springer.

Cohen HA: *The nurse's quest for professional identity,* Menlo Park, Calif, 1981, Addison-Wesley.

Cragg CE, Plotnikoff RC, Hugo K et al: Perspective transformation in RN-to-BSN distance education, *J Nurs Ed* 40(7):317-322, 2001.

Davidhizar R, Gigen JN, Reed C: RN to BSN: avoiding the pitfalls, *Health Care Supervisor* 12(1):48-56, 1993.

Gordon S: *Nursing against the odds: how health care cost cuts, media stereotypes and medical hubris undermine nurses and patient care,* Ithaca, NY, 2005, Cornell University Press.

Hagenow NR, McCrea MA: A mentoring relationship: two viewpoints, *Nurs Manag* 25(12):42-43, 1994.

Harmer B: *Textbook of the principles and practice of nursing,* New York, 1922, Macmillan.

Harmer B, Henderson V: *Textbook of the principles and practice of nursing,* ed 4, New York, 1939, Macmillan.

Henderson V: *Basic principles of nursing care,* London, 1960, International Council of Nurses.

Hinshaw AS: *Socialization and resocialization of nurses for professional nursing practice,* New York, 1976, National League for Nursing.

Hom EM: Coaching and mentoring new graduates entering perinatal nursing practice, *J Perinat/Neonat Nurs* 17(1):35-49, 2003.

Hurst J: *EDTNA/ERCA J Renal Care* 31(3):160-163, 2005.

Kramer M: *Reality shock: why nurses leave nursing,* St Louis, 1974, Mosby.

International Council for Nurses: *The ICN definition of nursing,* 2003 (website): www.icn.ch/definition.htm.

Nesler MS, Hanner MB, Melburg V et al: Professional socialization of baccalaureate nursing students: can students in distance nursing programs become socialized? *J Nurs Ed* 40(7):293-302, 2001.

Nightingale F: *Notes on nursing: what it is and what it is not,* Philadelphia, 1946, JB Lippincott, Reprint (originally published in 1859).

Orem D: *Guidelines for developing curricula for the education of practical nurses,* Washington, DC, 1959, Government Printing Office.

Peplau H: *Interpersonal relations in nursing: a conceptual frame of reference for psychodynamic nursing,* New York, 1952, GP Putnam's Sons.

Rogers M: *Educational revolution in nursing,* New York, 1961, Macmillan.

Royal College of Nursing: *Defining nursing,* 2003 (website): www.rcn.org.uk/downloads/definingnursing/definingnursing-a5.pdf.

Shaw CW: *Textbook of nursing,* ed 3, New York, 1907, Appleton.

State of Ohio Board of Nursing: *Law and rule information,* 2003 (website): www5.state.oh.us/nur/Law_and_Rule.htm.

Styles MM: Bridging the gap between competence and excellence, *ANNA J* 18(4):353-366, 1991.

Educational Patterns in Nursing

Kay Kittrell Chitty

Learning Outcomes

After studying this chapter, students will be able to:

- Trace the development of basic and graduate education in nursing.
- Discuss the influence of early nursing studies on nursing education.
- Describe traditional and alternative ways of becoming a registered nurse.
- Discuss program options for registered nurses and students with nonnursing baccalaureate degrees.
- Differentiate between licensed practical/vocational nurses and registered nurses.

- Explain the difference between licensure and certification.
- Define accreditation and analyze its influence on the quality and effectiveness of nursing education programs.
- Discuss recommendations of the Institute of Medicine (IOM) and major nursing organizations regarding transforming nursing education.
- Identify current and future challenges in nursing education.

Diversity is the major characteristic of nursing education today. Influenced by a variety of factors—societal changes, periodic shortages, historical factors, public expectations, professional standards, legislation, national studies, and constant changes in the health care system— many different types of nursing education programs currently exist.

In 2006 there were 1,547 state approved programs preparing registered nurses (RNs) in the United States (Figure 7-1). Of these, 58.8 percent were associate degree programs, 37.2 percent were baccalaureate programs, and 4 percent were diploma programs (National League for Nursing, 2006). In addition to the basic registered nurse programs, there were also 417 master's programs and 109 doctoral programs (Fang, Wilsey-Wisniewski, and Bednash, 2006). Also included in the educational system of nursing are a large number of practical nursing programs (LPN/LVN programs), continuing education programs, and advanced practice certification programs.

---

*Educational terms and definitions used in this chapter are congruent with those used by the American Association of Colleges of Nursing, as defined in *2005-2006 Enrollment and Graduations in Baccalaureate and Graduate Programs in Nursing,* (Fang, Wilsey-Wisniewski, and Bednash, 2006).

This chapter provides an orientation to the multiple and sometimes confusing nursing educational pathways in existence today. This coverage includes the history behind educational programs, descriptions of the various programs, and trends and future issues.

DEVELOPMENT OF NURSING EDUCATION IN THE UNITED STATES

Florence Nightingale is credited with founding modern nursing and creating the first educational system for nurses. After hospitals came into existence in Western Europe, and before the influence of Florence Nightingale, nurses had no formal preparation in giving care, because there were no organized programs to educate nurses until the late 1800s. Before this time, nursing care was administered either by the patient's relatives or by self-trained persons who were often held in low regard by society.

Nightingale revolutionized and professionalized nursing by stressing that nursing was not a domestic, charitable service but a respected occupation requiring advanced education. In 1860 she opened a school of nursing at St. Thomas's

Figure 7-1
In 2006 there were 1547 programs preparing registered nurses in the United States and its territories. Students entering nursing today are diverse in terms of age, sociocultural background, and gender.

Hospital in London and established the following principles, which were considered highly innovative at the time:

1. The nurse should be trained in an educational institution supported by public funds and associated with a medical school.
2. The nursing school should be affiliated with a teaching hospital but also independent of it.
3. The curriculum should include both theory and practical experience.
4. Professional nurses should be in charge of administration and instruction and should be paid for their instruction.
5. Students should be carefully selected and should reside in "nurses' houses" that form discipline and character.
6. Students should be required to attend lectures, take quizzes, write papers, and keep diaries. Student records should be maintained (Notter and Spalding, 1976).

Nightingale also believed that nursing schools should be financially and administratively separate from the hospitals in which the students trained. This was not the case, however, when nursing schools were first established in the United States.

The first training schools for nurses in the United States were established in 1872. Located at Bellevue Hospital in New York, the New England Hospital for Women and Children in New Haven, Connecticut, and Massachusetts General Hospital in Boston, the course of study was 1 year in length. These schools became known as the "famous trio" of nursing schools. In October 1873, Melinda Anne (Linda) Richards became the first "trained nurse" educated in the United States. By 1879 there were 11 U.S. nursing training schools. Other schools rapidly developed, and by 1900 there were 432 hospital-owned and hospital-operated programs in the United States (Donahue, 1985). These early training programs differed in length from 6 months to 2 years, and each school set its own standards and requirements. Upon graduation from these programs, students were awarded a diploma. The term **diploma program** was, and still is, used to identify hospital-based nursing education programs. The primary reason for the schools' existence was to staff the hospitals that operated them. The education of student nurses was not always the primary concern.

Early Studies of the Quality of Nursing Education

Nursing leaders of the early 1900s were concerned about the poor quality of many of the recently-formed nurse training programs. They initiated studies about nursing and nursing education to prompt changes. October 1899 marked the culmination of some 4 years of work by the American Society of Superintendents of Training Schools for Nurses. Isabel Hampton Robb chaired a Society-selected committee to investigate a means to prepare nurses better for leadership in schools of nursing. Teachers College, which had opened in New York 10 years earlier for the training of teachers, seemed the logical location for the leadership training of nurses. A program, originally designed to prepare administrators of nursing service and nursing education, began as an 8-month course in hospital economics (Donahue, 1985).

Mary Adelaide Nutting came to Teachers College in 1907 as the first nursing professor the world had ever known. Under her direction, the department progressed and became a pioneer in nursing education. The school became known as the "Mother House" of collegiate education because it fostered the initial movements toward undergraduate and graduate degrees for nurses (Donahue, 1985). In 1912 Nutting conducted a nationwide investigation of nursing education, *The Educational Status of Nursing,* that focused on the living conditions of students, the material being taught, and the teaching methods being used (Christy, 1969).

Another major study of nursing education was published in 1923. Titled *The Study of Nursing and Nursing Education in the United States* and referred to as the **Goldmark Report,** the study focused on the clinical learning experiences of students, hospital control of the schools, the desirability of establishing university schools of nursing, the lack of funds specifically for nursing

education, and the lack of prepared teachers (Kalisch and Kalisch, 1995).

The year 1924 marked another first in nursing education, when the Yale School of Nursing was opened as the first nursing school to be established as a separate university department with an independent budget and its own dean, Annie W. Goodrich. The school demonstrated its effectiveness so well that in 1929 the Rockefeller Foundation ensured the permanency of the school by awarding it an endowment of $1 million (Kalisch and Kalisch, 1995).

In 1934 a study entitled *Nursing Schools Today and Tomorrow* reported the number of schools in existence, gave detailed descriptions of the schools, described their curricula, and made recommendations for professional collegiate education (National League of Nursing Education, 1934). In 1937 *A Curriculum Guide for Schools of Nursing* was published, outlining a 3-year curriculum and influencing the structure of diploma schools for decades after its publication (National League of Nursing Education, 1937).

Although published over a 30-year period and undertaken by different groups, these early studies consistently made five similar recommendations:
1. Nursing education programs should be established within the system of higher education.
2. Nurses should be highly educated.
3. Students should not be used to staff hospitals.
4. Standards should be established for nursing practice.
5. All students should meet certain minimum qualifications upon graduation.

These studies set the stage for the development of the educational programs that exist today.

EDUCATIONAL PATHWAYS TO BECOMING A REGISTERED NURSE

Today, preparation for a career as a registered nurse usually begins in one of three ways: in a hospital-based diploma program, a baccalaureate degree program, or an associate degree program. These basic programs vary in the courses offered, length of study, and cost. Following the completion of a basic program for registered nurses, graduates are eligible to take the National Council Licensing Examination for Registered Nurses (NCLEX-RN). Upon successful completion of the licensing examination, graduates may legally practice as registered nurses and use the credential RN. Employment and career advancement vary depending on the type of basic program attended (Figure 7-2).

Having three different educational routes to achieve RN licensure is confusing to the public—and even to many nurses themselves. In the following sections, each type of basic program is described, along with its history, unique characteristics, and special issues. These basic programs are discussed in the chronological order in which they were developed.

Diploma Programs

The hospital-based diploma program was the earliest form of nursing education in the United States. At the peak of diploma education in the 1920s and 1930s, approximately 2000 programs existed, with numerous programs in almost every state. Since their numbers peaked in the first third of the twentieth century, the number of

diploma programs has decreased, with a dramatic decline since the mid-1960s when nursing education moved rapidly into collegiate settings. In 1960 there were approximately 800 diploma programs in the United States. Today there are only 62 (National League for Nursing, 2006). This decline in the number of diploma programs is attributable to several factors: the growth of associate degree and baccalaureate degree programs in nursing, which moved the education of nurses into the mainstream of higher education; the inability of hospitals to continue to finance nursing education; accreditation standards that have made it difficult for diploma programs to attract qualified faculty; and the increasing complexity of health care, which has required nurses to have greater academic preparation.

Despite the significant decrease in the number of diploma programs, many outstanding nurses practicing today received their basic nursing education in these programs. In the early days of formal nurses' "training" in this country—that is, during the late 1800s and early 1900s—diploma programs provided one of the few avenues for women to obtain formal education and jobs. Most of the early programs followed a modified

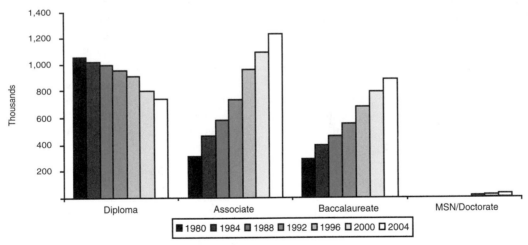

Figure 7-2
Distribution of the RN population according to basic nursing education, 1980-2004. *(From U.S. Department of Health and Human Services:* The registered nurse population, March 2004: preliminary findings from the national sample survey of registered nurses, *Washington, DC, 2006, Government Printing Office, p 2.)*

apprenticeship model. Lectures were given by physicians, and clinical training was supervised by head nurses and nursing directors. Nursing courses paralleled medical areas and included surgery, obstetrics, pediatrics, operating room experience, and, somewhat later, psychiatry. Students were sometimes sent to affiliated institutions where they could obtain experiences that were not available at the home hospital.

The schedule was demanding, with classes being held after patient care assignments were completed. Critics charged that students were used as inexpensive labor to staff the hospitals and that education was given a lower priority. The truth of those charges varied, depending on which hospital was scrutinized, but there is no question that early nursing students virtually ran the hospitals. Programs lasted 3 years, and at graduation, students were awarded diplomas in nursing. Today, most diploma programs are about 24 months in duration.

A problem that many diploma program graduates faced was that hospitals were not part of the higher education system in the United States. Therefore most colleges and universities did not recognize the nursing diploma as an academic credential and often refused to give college credit for courses taken in diploma programs, regardless of the quality of the courses, students, and faculty. Most diploma programs today have established agreements with colleges and universities that allow students to earn college credit in courses such as English, psychology, and the sciences, thereby enabling them to attain advanced standing in a baccalaureate program upon completion of the diploma program.

Baccalaureate Programs

Armed with the early studies of nursing education, nursing leaders continued to push for nursing education to move into the mainstream of higher education, that is, into colleges and universities where other professionals were educated. They believed that nurses needed a baccalaureate degree, the Bachelor of Science in Nursing (BSN), to qualify nursing as a recognized profession and to provide leadership in administration, teaching, and public health.

By the time the first baccalaureate nursing program was established in 1909 at the University of Minnesota, diploma programs were numerous and firmly entrenched as the system for educating nurses. This first baccalaureate program was part of the University's School of Medicine and followed the 3-year diploma program structure. Despite its many limitations, it was the start of the movement to bring nursing education into the recognized system of higher education.

Seven other baccalaureate programs in nursing were established by 1919 (Conley, 1973). Most of the early baccalaureate programs were 5 years in duration. This structure provided for 3 years of nursing education and 2 years of liberal arts. The growth in the numbers of these programs was slow both because of the reluctance of universities to accept nursing as an academic discipline and because of the power of the hospital-based diploma programs. The theoretical, scientific orientation of the baccalaureate program was in sharp contrast to the "hands on" skill and service orientation that was the hallmark of hospital-based diploma education.

Influences on the growth of baccalaureate education

National studies of nursing and nursing education stated and restated the need for nursing education and practice to be based on knowledge from the sciences and humanities. Chief among these studies was Esther Lucille Brown's report *Nursing for the Future,* more commonly known as the **Brown Report** (Brown, 1948). Published in 1948, the Brown Report recommended that basic schools of nursing be placed in universities and colleges, with effort made to recruit men and minorities into nursing education programs. This report, sponsored by the Carnegie Foundation, was widely reviewed, discussed, and debated.

In 1965 the American Nurses Association (ANA) published a **position paper** entitled *Educational Preparation for Nurse Practitioners* *and Assistants to Nurses.* Although not all nursing historians agree, this paper, which subsequently created conflict and division within nursing, had a significant influence on the growth of baccalaureate education in nursing. In preparing the position paper, the ANA studied nursing education, nursing practice, and trends in health care. It concluded that baccalaureate education should become the basic foundation for professional practice. The ANA position paper made four major recommendations:

1. Education for all those who are licensed to practice nursing should take place in institutions of higher learning.
2. Minimum preparation for beginning professional nursing practice should be the baccalaureate degree in nursing.
3. Minimum preparation for beginning technical nursing practice should be the associate degree in nursing.
4. Education for assistants in the health service occupations should consist of short, intensive preservice programs in vocational education institutions rather than on-the-job training programs (American Nurses Association, 1965).

Despite tremendous opposition from proponents of diploma and associate degree programs, in 1979 the ANA further strengthened its resolve by proposing three additional positions:

1. By 1985 the minimum preparation for entry into professional nursing practice should be the baccalaureate degree in nursing.
2. Two levels of nursing practice should be identified (professional and technical) and a mechanism to devise competencies for the two categories established by 1980.
3. There should be increased accessibility to high-quality career mobility programs that use flexible approaches for individuals seeking academic degrees in nursing (American Nurses Association, 1979).

The controversy created by the initial ANA position paper and the additional 1979 resolutions continued for many years. Practicing nurses across the United States, who were mainly diploma program graduates, as well as hospitals that supported diploma programs vehemently protested the recommendations.

In 1970 the National Commission for the Study of Nursing and Nursing Education published a report entitled *An Abstract for Action* (Lysaught, 1970). Also known as the **Lysaught Report,** it made recommendations concerning the supply and demand for nurses, nursing roles and functions, and nursing education. Among the priorities identified by this study were (1) the need for increased research into both the practice and education of nurses and (2) enhanced educational systems and curricula (Lysaught, 1970).

In the early 1980s the National Commission on Nursing published two reports suggesting that the major block to the advancement of nursing was the ongoing conflict within the profession about educational preparation for nurses. These studies recommended establishing a clear system of nursing education, including pathways for educational mobility and development of additional graduate education programs.

Another major national nursing group supporting the baccalaureate as the entry credential was the **National League for Nursing (NLN).** The organization's membership consists of nurses, faculty members, health care agencies, all types of nursing programs, and nonnursing citizens who are supportive of nursing. After much debate, in 1982 the NLN board of directors approved the *Position Statement on Nursing Roles: Scope and Preparation,* which affirmed the nursing baccalaureate degree as the minimum educational level for professional nursing practice and the associate degree or diploma as the preparation for technical nursing practice (National League for Nursing, 1982).

In 1996 the American Association of Colleges of Nursing (AACN) board approved a position statement *The Baccalaureate Degree in Nursing as Minimal Preparation for Professional Practice.* This document supports, among other things, articulated programs, which enable associate degree nurses to attain the baccalaureate degree. This document was updated in 2000. It can be found online (http://www.aacn.nche.edu/Publi-cations/positions/baccmin.htm).

Baccalaureate programs today

Today, baccalaureate programs provide education for both basic students who are preparing for licensure and registered nurses returning to school to obtain a baccalaureate degree in nursing. This section focuses on the program characteristics of prelicensure baccalaureate education, also known as **basic programs.** Baccalaureate programs for registered nurses are discussed later in this chapter.

Basic baccalaureate programs combine nursing courses with general education courses in a 4- or 5-year curriculum in a senior college or univer-sity. Students may be admitted to the nursing program as entering freshmen or after com-pleting certain liberal arts and science courses. Students meet the same admission requirements to the university as other students and often must meet even more stringent requirements to be admitted to the nursing major.

Courses in the nursing major focus on nursing science, communication, decision making, leader-ship, and care to persons of all ages in a wide variety of settings (Figure 7-3). Baccalaureate education takes place in 4-year colleges and uni-versities where nursing students interact with the larger student population. This promotes diverse thinking, cultural awareness, and broad social-ization.

Faculty qualifications in baccalaureate pro-grams are usually higher than in other basic nursing programs. A minimum of a master's degree or, increasingly, a doctorate in nursing or a related field is required. The requirement of a doctorate ensures that nursing faculty members are able to meet the teaching, research, and service requirements expected of faculty in universities.

Baccalaureate graduates are prepared to take the **National Council Licensing Examination for Registered Nurses** and, after licensure, assume beginning practice and ultimately leadership positions in any health care setting, including hospitals, community agencies, schools, clinics,

Figure 7-3
Clinical experience is a vitally important aspect of every basic nursing program.

and homes (National League for Nursing, 1997). Graduates with baccalaureate degrees are also prepared to move into graduate programs in nursing and advanced practice certification programs. Programs granting a baccalaureate are the most costly of the basic programs in terms of time and money, but such an investment results in long-term professional advancement. Today, there is great demand for baccalaureate gra-duates, and they enjoy the greatest career mobil-ity of all basic program graduates in nursing.

According to the American Association of Colleges of Nursing's 1998 *The Essentials of Bac-calaureate Education for Professional Nursing Practice,* "Nurses who graduate from bachelor's degree programs should possess the skills to 'communicate, collaborate, and negotiate' in delivering high quality care to patients and fami-lies" (AACN, 1998, p. 1). The AACN document also stressed that baccalaureate-prepared nurses are providers, designers, and managers of care in a dramatically changing health care system and their education should include an increased emphasis on economics, epidemiology, genetics. gerontology, global perspectives, and telecommunications (AACN, 1998).

Associate Degree Programs (ADN)

Associate degree in nursing (ADN) education is the newest form of basic preparation for registered nurse practice. Begun in 1952 as a result of a post World War II nursing shortage, based upon a model developed by **Dr. Mildred Montag,** and fueled by the community college movement of the 1950s, associate degree programs are now the most common type of basic nursing education program in the United States and graduate the most registered nurse candidates of all the basic programs.

The popularity of ADN programs is attributable to several features: accessibility of community colleges, low tuition costs, part-time and evening study opportunities, shorter duration of programs, and graduates' eligibility to take the licensure examination for registered nurses.

When first envisioned by Dr. Montag as part of her doctoral dissertation, associate degree programs were proposed as a solution to a nursing shortage. She suggested a shorter program designed to prepare nurse technicians who would function under the supervision of professional nurses. Associate degree nurses were to work at the bedside, performing routine nursing skills for patients in acute and long term care settings. The original associate degree program, as outlined by Montag (1951), offered general education courses in the first year and nursing courses in the second year. Montag originally viewed the associate degree as a final, end-point degree, not a stepping stone to the baccalaureate degree in nursing.

In practice, Montag's original conceptions of associate degree programs have been greatly modified. Associate degree curricula now offer more nursing credits than she suggested. They also include content on leadership and clinical decision making, abilities that Montag did not foresee in technical nurses. Because of additions to the curriculum, it is now virtually impossible for students to complete an associate degree in only 2 years. Associate degree graduates are employed in a wide variety of settings and usually function autonomously alongside baccalaureate and diploma graduates. In the educational system of nursing today, the associate degree can be a step in the progression to the baccalaureate degree or master's degree.

In 1990 the NLN Council of Associate Degree Programs prepared a document entitled *Educational Outcomes of Associate Degree Nursing Programs: Roles and Competencies.* This document was written in response to a national effort to differentiate the competencies of the associate degree nurse from those of the baccalaureate nurse. The document identified associate degree competencies in three roles: provider of care, manager of care, and member within the discipline of nursing. In response to a changing health care delivery system, the document was revised in 2000. Entitled *Educational Competencies for Graduates of Associate Degree Nursing Programs,* the revised document emphasizes "diversity in health care, clinical decision making, assessment, patient education, continuity of care, collaboration, and leadership" (NLN, 2000, viii) as additional aspects of ADN education. Box 7-1 reviews landmarks in the history of nursing education.

External Degree Programs

External degree programs in nursing are different from traditional basic nursing education in that students attend no classes. Learning is independent and is assessed through highly standardized and validated competency-based outcomes assessments, leading to the description, "virtual university." Students are responsible for arranging their own clinical experiences in accordance with established standards.

Excelsior College, formerly known as the New York Regents External Degree Nursing Program, is the most well-recognized external degree model. Beginning in 1970 with an associate degree program, Excelsior College now offers associate

Box 7-1 Landmarks in the History of Nursing Education

1860—Florence Nightingale founded the first organized program to educate nurses at St. Thomas's Hospital in London.

1872—The "famous trio," the first year-long training schools for nurses, was established in the United States, founded at Bellevue Hospital, the New England Hospital for Women and Children, and Massachusetts General Hospital.

1873—Melinda Anne (Linda) Richards became the first "trained nurse" to graduate in the United States.

1899—Teachers College, Columbia University, offered the first postgraduate course in hospital economics for nurses.

1907—Mary Adelaide Nutting became the first nursing professor at Teachers College, Columbia University.

1909—The first baccalaureate program in nursing was established at the University of Minnesota.

1923—The Goldmark Report was published, the first such report focusing on hospital control of schools of nursing and lack of proper teacher preparation.

1924—Yale University established the first nursing school as a separate university department with its own dean, Annie W. Goodrich.

1932—The first doctoral degree in nursing education (EdD) was granted by Teachers College.

1934—The first PhD program in nursing was initiated by New York University.

1948—Esther Lucille Brown's report *Nursing for the Future* was published, recommending that basic nursing programs be situated in colleges and universities rather than in hospitals.

1952—The first Associate Degree in Nursing program, based on Dr. Mildred Montag's model, was established to prepare nurse technicians.

degree, baccalaureate, and master's degrees in nursing. All the nursing programs are accredited by the National League for Nursing Accreditation Commission (NLNAC).

Since 1981 the California State University Consortium has offered a statewide external degree baccalaureate program in nursing. The California program is for registered nurses already holding current licenses to practice in the state.

There are numerous external degree programs in existence today, many of which are marketed online and by direct mail. Prospective students must exercise caution to choose only bona fide accredited programs that are affiliated with recognized colleges and universities.

Articulated Programs

In response to the demand for educational mobility, **articulation** (movement) between programs has become much more common in today's nursing education system. The purpose of articulation is to facilitate opportunities for nurses to move up the educational ladder. An example of a fully articulated system is the licensed practical nurse/associate degree in nursing/bachelor of science in nursing/master of science in nursing (LPN/ADN/BSN/MSN) program in which students spend the first year preparing to be an LPN and the second year completing the associate degree. If desired or necessary, students can "stop out" of the program at the end of the first year, take the licensure examination for practical nursing, and return to the associate degree program at a later time. On the other hand, they may continue study in the program after the initial 2 years to earn a baccalaureate degree and even continue for a master's or doctoral degree.

Multiple-entry, multiple-exit programs are difficult to develop. A tremendous amount of joint institutional planning is needed to work out equivalent courses and to keep the programs congruent with one another. A change in one curriculum dictates changes in all the others. These challenges explain why fully articulated programs have been slow to develop. In increasing numbers, however, articulation agreements between baccalaureate and ADN programs and between ADN and LPN programs are being established that facilitate student movement between programs and accept transfer credit between institutions. These requirements often result in acceleration or advanced placement within the higher-degree school.

In spite of the difficulties in developing them, several state legislatures have mandated their public institutions to create articulation programs to facilitate upward educational mobility for nurses. Other states have statewide voluntary articulation plans, while still others have individual school-to-school agreements in place. Table 7-1 lists the types of articulation agreements for all 50 states and the District of Columbia.

ALTERNATIVE EDUCATIONAL PROGRAMS IN NURSING

In addition to the basic programs leading to entry-level nursing practice, several **alternative educational programs** exist.

Baccalaureate Programs for Registered Nurses

After nursing organizations of the 1960s and 1970s publicly advocated for the baccalaureate degree to be the minimum education level for professional practice, the demand for the nursing bachelor's degree increased. Employers of nurses recognized that broadly educated nurses matched well with the complexities of health care. As a result, many supported the baccalaureate as a requirement for career mobility. Diploma and associate degree graduates returned to school in increasing numbers. Today, many students enter ADN programs with plans to earn a baccalaureate degree ultimately. Baccalaureate programs for RNs allow them, as well as diploma nurses, to accomplish this goal.

Registered nurses with diplomas and associate degrees were not always welcomed into baccalaureate programs. In the early years of baccalaureate education for RNs, many schools required these students to take courses in areas the students believed they had already mastered. For a number of years, there were barriers for these nurses in completing their baccalaureate degrees. Now, however, the majority of baccalaureate programs have recognized the legitimacy and importance of **RN-to-baccalaureate in nursing** education and have developed alternative tracks

Table 7-1   NURSING EDUCATION PROGRAM ARTICULATION AGREEMENTS BY TYPE AND STATE

State	Statewide Agreement	Individual Agreement	Mandated Agreement
	X		
Alaska	X		
Arizona	X		
Arkansas	X		
California		X	
Colorado	X		
Connecticut			X
Delaware	X		
District of Columbia	X		
Florida			X

Table 7-1   Nursing Education Program Articulation Agreements by Type and State—cont'd

State	Statewide Agreement	Individual Agreement	Mandated Agreement
Georgia	X		
Hawaii		X	
Idaho	X		
Illinois	X		
Indiana		X	
Iowa	X		
Kansas	X		
Kentucky		X	
Louisiana	X		
Maine		X	
Maryland			X
Massachusetts		X	
Michigan		X	
Mississippi	X		
Missouri	X		
Montana		X	
Nebraska		X	
Nevada		X	
New Hampshire	X		
New Jersey	X		
New Mexico		X	
New York		X	
North Carolina			X
North Dakota	X		
Ohio	X		
Oklahoma	X		
Oregon		X	
Pennsylvania	X		
Rhode Island		X	
South Carolina			X
South Dakota	X		
Tennessee	X		
Texas			X
Utah		X	
Vermont		X	
Virginia		X	
Washington			X
West Virginia		X	
Wisconsin	X		
Wyoming	X		

Key to articulation agreement types: Statewide: Articulation plans and models are in place for public and sometimes private institutions; often these agreements apply to all programs in a state's university and community college system; 24 states and the District of Columbia. Individual: Arrangements are made on a school-to-school basis; a blanket agreement does not exist; 18 states. Mandated: State laws exist regulating the transfer of credit between public institutions; 8 states.
Source: American Association of Colleges of Nursing: Fact sheet: *Articulation agreements among nursing education programs*, Washington, DC, 2006, AACN.

to accommodate the unique learning needs of the registered nurse student.

Baccalaureate programs for registered nurses are most often offered by universities that also offer basic nursing education in baccalaureate programs. The registered nurse students may be integrated with the basic students, or they may be enrolled in a separate or partially separate sequence. Some baccalaureate programs for registered nurses are free-standing; that is, they are offered by colleges that do not have a basic baccalaureate nursing program or in single-purpose institutions.

Most 4-year colleges and universities allow the transfer of general education credits from associate degree nursing programs. With increasing frequency, transfer credit is given for nursing courses as well, or there is the option of receiving credit for previous nursing courses through a variety of advanced placement methods such as examinations, demonstrations, and portfolios.

For diploma graduates, transfer credit is usually given for previous college courses, such as English, if they were included as part of the diploma program and taught by college faculty. Options for advanced placement of diploma graduates into baccalaureate programs are extremely variable, and prospective registered nurse students should seek detailed information to select a program that fits individual needs and goals.

The demand for the baccalaureate degree by large numbers of associate degree and diploma graduates continues to be strong. More nurses are returning to school to prepare for the wider opportunities offered by the baccalaureate degree. With broad preparation in clinical, scientific, community health, and patient education skills, the baccalaureate nurse is well positioned to move across community-based settings such as home health care, outpatient centers, and neighborhood clinics, where opportunities are fast expanding.

Programs for Second Degree Students

A noteworthy trend is the significant increase in the number of students with baccalaureate degrees in other fields making a career change to nursing. The educational system in nursing has responded to this group of students by offering options to the traditional basic baccalaureate education. Increasingly, baccalaureate programs offer these students an accelerated or fast track sequence, awarding either a second baccalaureate degree or, in some cases, a master's degree in nursing. Accelerated master's degree programs in nursing for individuals with bachelor's degrees in another field are known as **generic master's degree** programs. They usually require about three years to complete, depending on the number of prerequisite courses. Graduates take the registered nurse licensure examination (NCLEX-RN) after completing the generic master's program.

Another educational track for students with baccalaureate degrees in other fields was the **generic nursing doctorate (ND).** This degree is discussed later in this chapter (see History of Doctoral Education in Nursing).

PRACTICAL NURSING PROGRAMS (LPN OR LVN)

Nursing education includes a large number of programs preparing practical nurses. **Practical nurses (LPNs/LVNs)** are differentiated from registered nurses by education and licensure and have a limited scope of practice. Licensed practical nurses (LPNs) or licensed vocational nurses (LVNs) are considered technical workers in nursing.

Practical nursing programs became a significant component of the nursing field during World War II. These programs were created to satisfy the demand for nurses and programs that could produce nurses quickly. The first planned curriculum for practical nursing was developed in 1942. Although national accreditation is available for practical nursing programs, the majority of LPN/LVN programs have state approval rather than national accreditation.

Practical nursing education typically lasts 12 months and takes place in a variety of settings: vocational/technical schools, community colleges, and high schools. Many LPN/LVN programs now offer credit for prior learning to health care workers such as hospital aides, orderlies, paramedics, emergency medical technicians, and military corps personnel. These individuals often enter nursing through practical nursing programs.

Graduates of practical nursing programs must pass the **National Council Licensing Examination for Practical Nursing (NCLEX-PN)** to become licensed. The scope of their practice focuses on meeting basic patient needs in hospitals, long term care facilities, and homes. They must practice under the supervision of a physician or registered nurse and are not a substitute for RNs.

Many newly licensed practical nurses plan to become registered nurses, with the majority of these individuals either taking courses or planning to begin registered nurse courses in 1 to 2 years. National statistics from 2001, the last year for which figures are available, show that 9.5 percent of all licensed RNs have practiced previously as LPNs or LVNs, indicating that many are achieving their goal of becoming registered nurses (U.S. Department of Health and Human Services, 2001).

ACCREDITATION OF EDUCATIONAL PROGRAMS

The concept of accreditation of educational programs in nursing is important. Although all nursing programs must be approved by their respective state boards of nursing for graduates to take the licensure examination, nursing programs may also seek accreditation, which goes beyond minimum state approval. **Accreditation** refers to a voluntary review process of educational programs by a professional organization. The organization, called an accrediting agency, compares the educational quality of the program with established standards and criteria. Accrediting agencies derive their authority from the U.S. Department of Education. Two agencies are responsible for accrediting nursing educational programs today, as described below.

Prospective nursing students should inquire about the accreditation status of any nursing program they are considering. Qualifying for certain scholarships, loans, and military service usually depends on being enrolled in an accredited program. Acceptance into graduate programs in nursing may also depend on graduation from an accredited baccalaureate program. Employers of nurses are usually interested in hiring nurses who are graduates of accredited programs.

From 1952 through 1996, the National League for Nursing was the only official professional accrediting organization for master's, baccalaureate, associate degree, diploma, and practical nursing programs in the United States. In 1997, as a result of a mandate from the U.S. Department of Education, a separate division of the NLN was created. The new division, the **National League for Nursing Accreditation Commission (NLNAC),** assumed responsibility for all NLN national program accreditation activity. Accreditation is conducted through four NLNAC councils: the Council of Associate Degree Programs, the Council of Diploma Programs, the Council of Baccalaureate and Higher Degree Programs, and the Council of Practical Nursing Programs. Each council develops its own accreditation program and criteria and revises them periodically.

Accreditation of nursing schools grew out of concerns repeatedly expressed in reports and by leaders of the profession about the lack of quality and standards for nursing education. An accredited program voluntarily adheres to standards that protect the quality of education, public safety, and the profession itself. Accreditation provides both a mechanism and a stimulus for programs to initiate periodic self-examination and self-improvement. It assures students that their educational program is accountable for offering quality education.

Accrediting bodies establish standards by which a program's effectiveness is measured. Programs under review prepare reports, known as self-studies, that show how the school meets each standard. The self-study is reviewed by a volunteer team composed of nursing educators from the type of program being reviewed, and an on-site program review is conducted by the same team. Following the site visit, the visitors' report and the program's self-study are reviewed by the appropriate NLNAC council, and a decision is made about the accreditation status of each nursing program.

Once accredited and in good standing, continuing accreditation reviews take place every 8 to 10 years. Programs that do not meet standards may be placed on warning and given a specific time period to correct deficiencies. Accreditation can be withdrawn if deficiencies are not corrected within the specified time.

In 1996 the **American Association of Colleges of Nursing (AACN)** organized the **Commission on Collegiate Nursing Education (CCNE)** and began the process of acquiring recognition from the U.S. Department of Education as the national accrediting body for baccalaureate and higher degree nursing programs. CCNE began operation in 1998 and has subsequently established an organizational structure, policies and procedures, and accreditation standards and criteria. In December 1999 CCNE received a recommendation from the National Advisory Committee on Institutional Quality and Integrity, a panel of the U.S. Department of Education, that the Secretary of Education grant initial recognition of CCNE as a national agency for the accreditation of baccalaureate and graduate nursing education programs. This status was renewed in 2002. The establishment of a second national accrediting body for nursing education represented a significant development in the evolution of the nursing profession. Schools and colleges of nursing have a choice of which accrediting body they wish to use.

GRADUATE EDUCATION IN NURSING

A variety of economic, educational, and professional trends are fueling the demand for registered nurses with **advanced degrees** (master's or doctorates). The rapidly changing health care system requires nurses to possess increasing knowledge, clinical competency, greater independence, and autonomy in clinical judgments. Trends in community-based nursing centers, case management, complexity of home care, sophisticated technologies, and society's orientation to health and self-care are rapidly causing the educational needs of nurses to expand, thereby requiring graduate education.

Nurses who have advanced education can become researchers, nurse practitioners, clinical specialists, educators, and administrators. Some open their own clinics, where they provide direct care and serve as consultants to businesses and health care agencies. Chapter 1 describes some of the opportunities open to nurses with advanced degrees. Certainly, having a workforce of highly educated nurses will further strengthen the profession.

Master's Education

The purpose of master's education is to prepare persons with advanced nursing knowledge and clinical practice skills in a specialized area of practice. Teachers College, Columbia University, is credited with initiating graduate education in nursing. Beginning in 1899, the college offered a postgraduate course in hospital economics, which prepared nurses for positions in teaching and hospital administration. From this limited beginning, there has been consistent growth in the number of master's nursing programs in the United States.

Over the last 30 years, the growth in numbers of master's programs in nursing has been dramatic. In 1970 there were 70 programs. In 2005 there were 378. Enrollment in master's nursing degree programs grew from 19,958 in 1986 to 42,646 in 2005. A majority of these students were attending school part-time (Berlin, Wilsey, and Bednash, 2005; Fang, Wilsey-Wisniewski, and Bednash, 2006).

Most nurses in the 1950s and 1960s viewed the master's degree in nursing as a terminal (final) degree. The master's degree was considered the highest degree nurses would ever need. Early master's programs were longer and more demanding than master's programs in other disciplines. Master's programs in the 1950s and 1960s prepared students for careers in nursing administration and nursing education.

With the rapid development of doctoral programs for nurses during the 1970s, however, the master's degree could no longer be considered a terminal degree. Programs were shortened from as long as 2 years to the approximate 1-year length of master's study in most other disciplines. Advanced practice through clinical specialization became the emphasis. Master's programs in nursing are most often found in senior colleges and universities that have basic baccalaureate programs in nursing. These programs may also seek voluntary accreditation from the NLNAC Council of Baccalaureate and Higher Degree Programs or from the CCNE.

Entrance requirements to master's programs in nursing usually include the following: a baccalaureate degree from an accredited program in nursing, licensure as a registered nurse, completion of the Graduate Record Examination (GRE) or other standard aptitude test, a minimum undergraduate grade point average (GPA) of 3.0, recent work experience as a registered nurse in an area related to the desired area of specialization, and specific goals for graduate study.

The average traditional program length is 18 to 24 months of full-time study, although part-time study and fast track curricula are far more common today than in the past. The curriculum includes theory, research, clinical practice, and courses in other disciplines. Master's students generally select both an area of clinical specialization, such as adult health or gerontology, and an area of role preparation, such as informatics, administration, or teaching. Students may be required to write a comprehensive examination and/or to complete a thesis or research project.

Major areas of role preparation include administration, case management, informatics, health policy/health care systems, teacher education, clinical nurse specialist, nurse practitioner, nurse-midwifery, nurse anesthesia, and other clinical and nonclinical areas of study.

As illustrated in Figure 7-4, all other role preparation fields trailed nurse practitioner preparation in popularity. Nearly 52 percent of all master's level students enrolled in 2004 were pursuing the nurse practitioner credential. Other role preparation majors included 8.6 percent preparing for clinical specialist roles, 6.7 percent for administration/management, 6.9 percent for nurse anesthesia, and 7.4 percent for teaching. The remaining master's students were specializing in various other majors or were undeclared (Fang et al, 2006). Clinical specialization choices for NP graduates included (in descending order of popularity) family NP, adult NP, pediatric NP, gerontological NP, women's health NP, neonatal NP, adult acute care NP, pediatric acute care NP, adult psychiatric/mental health NP, family psychiatric/mental health NP, and dual or combined tracks (Fang et al, 2006).

With the increasing demand for nurse practitioners, master's programs have expanded their practitioner tracks. Master's programs offering nurse practitioner options increased from 108 in 1992 to 306 in 2004 (Berlin et al, 2005; Fang et al, 2006).

The master of science (MS) and the master of science in nursing (MSN) are the two most common graduate degrees offered. A recent option in master's education is the RN/MSN track, which allows registered nurses who are prepared at the associate degree or diploma level and who meet graduate admission requirements to enter a program leading to a master's degree rather than a baccalaureate degree. Other recent graduate program options are combined degrees such as the master of science in nursing/master of business administration (MSN/MBA) for nurse administrators or the master of science in nursing/juris doctor (MSN/JD) for nurse attorneys. Clearly, diversity in nursing education extends to the graduate as well as the basic level.

Doctoral Education

Doctoral programs in nursing prepare nurses to become faculty members in universities, administrators in schools of nursing or large medical centers, researchers, theorists, and advanced practitioners. Doctoral programs in nursing offer

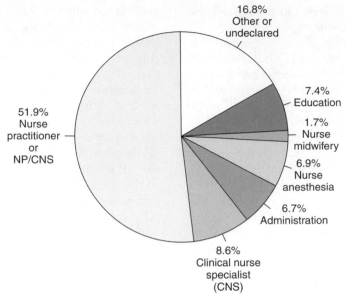

Figure 7-4

By a large margin, master's graduates in 2004-2005 selected role preparation as nurse practitioners. The much smaller number of students choosing teacher education is cause for concern about the future supply of nursing faculty. *(Data from Fang D, Wilsey-Wisniewski SJ, and Bednash GD:* 2005-2006 Enrollment and graduations in baccalaureate and graduate programs in nursing, *Washington, DC, American Association of Colleges of Nursing.)*

several degree titles, including the doctor of nursing science (DNSc), the doctor of philosophy (PhD), and the doctor of nursing practice (DNP).

History of doctoral education in nursing

Formal doctoral education for nurses began at Columbia University's Teachers College in 1910 with the creation of the Department of Nursing and Health. The first student completed her work for the doctor of education (EdD) with a major in nursing education and was awarded her doctorate in 1932. Seventy years later in 2002, Teachers College was still granting an EdD in nursing education.

In 1934 New York University initiated the first PhD program for nurses. The programs at Teachers College and New York University provided many of the profession's early leaders, who worked over the years for improvement in nursing education (Parietti, 1990).

From 1934 through 1953, no new nursing doctoral programs were opened. In 1954 the University of Pittsburgh opened the first PhD program in clinical nursing and clinical research in the United States. As the 1950s drew to a close, a total of only 36 doctoral degrees had been awarded in nursing (Parietti, 1990).

Because of the limited number of nursing doctoral programs, most nurses in the 1950s and 1960s earned doctorates in nonnursing fields, such as education, sociology, and physiology. Doctoral education for nurses moved into a new phase when the federal government initiated nurse scientist programs in 1962. These programs were created to increase the research skills of nurses and provide faculty for the development of doctoral programs in nursing. The nurse scientist programs were discontinued in 1975 after more universities began offering doctoral programs in nursing.

A program offering the nursing doctorate (ND) to students as their first nursing degree was begun at Case Western Reserve University in 1979. The ND program was designed for students with baccalaureate degrees in fields other than nursing. The program, which has been phased out, was based on that school's philosophy that professional nursing education should begin at the postbaccalaureate level. Following completion of 900 clinical hours, ND graduates were eligible to take the registered nurse licensure examination before continuing to the postlicensure portion of the program. Graduates were prepared for leadership positions in practice, business, management, research, and education. All programs currently offering the Doctor of Nursing (ND) are transitioning to the Doctor of Nursing Practice (DNP) discussed below (AACN, 2004).

The 1970s saw a major increase in the number of doctoral programs in nursing. In that decade alone, 15 new doctoral programs were established. Between 1970 and 1980, the number of programs increased to 22, and between 1980 and 1990, the number more than doubled, from 22 to 48 (Parietti, 1990). In 1996 the number of doctoral programs stood at 66 (National League for Nursing, 1997). By 2005 that number had risen to 97 (Fang et al, 2006).

Current status of doctoral education in nursing

Doctoral degrees for students with prior degrees in nursing include the Doctor of Nursing Science (DNSc) and the Doctor of Philosophy (PhD). Both of these degrees build on master's preparation in nursing. The DNSc is viewed as a professional practice degree. Conceived as an advanced practice degree with an emphasis on clinical research, the DNSc is intended to bridge the gap between practice and research (Allen, 1990). In contrast, the PhD is considered an academic degree and prepares scholars for research and the development of theory.

In October 2004, the members of the American Association of Colleges of Nursing debated and passed a resolution calling for a new doctoral degree, the Doctor of Nursing Practice (DNP). Designed to replace the master's degree, nurses who wish to practice in advanced roles, such as nurse practitioner or nurse-midwife, would be required to complete the DNP. Proponents of this change suggest that it would put nursing on an even footing with other health care disciplines, several of which are moving in the same direction. Conversely, the proposed change could increase confusion within and outside of the profession about the qualifications of nurses prepared at the doctoral level. It could also discourage nurses from seeking the PhD in nursing and thereby further deepen the shortage of nurse faculty prepared in the manner of other professors on campus (Dracup and Bryan-Brown, 2005). The debate over this proposal is ongoing.

Enrollment trends indicate that there is continued demand for doctoral education in nursing. During the 1990s, the number of programs as well as the number of requests for admission to these programs greatly increased. This trend has partially stemmed from the requirement of a doctorate for academic advancement and tenure for university nursing faculty. A doctorate is required to become a competent researcher who can compete for grants and develop nursing science. This advances the profession as a whole. Doctoral programs that prepare nurses predominantly for research and teaching reported 3466 students enrolled in 2005. Far fewer students complete their doctoral programs, however, with most students enrolled only part-time. For example, in 2005 only 417 students (12 percent) actually completed research-focused doctorates in 97 reporting doctoral programs (Fang et al, 2006). This low completion rate further aggravates the nursing faculty shortage, discussed later in this chapter. It is projected that large numbers of nurses with doctoral degrees will be needed in the future as positions requiring this degree expand in universities and throughout the health care system.

CERTIFICATION PROGRAMS

Licensure and certification are both forms of credentialing of nurses. **Licensure** refers to state regulation of the practice of nursing and is required of individuals at the entry point to practice. It assures public safety by assessing basic competence. **Certification** goes beyond licensure by validating a high level of knowledge and proficiency in a particular practice area. It is voluntarily pursued by individual nurses and is therefore a credential that has professional but not legal status.

Certification means that a certificate is awarded by a certifying body as validation of specific qualifications demonstrated by a registered nurse in a defined area of practice. A comprehensive examination is required to become certified, as well as documentation of experience, letters of reference, and other documents. Currently, more than 45 organizations offer advanced practice certification (Yoder-Wise, 2006). Box 7-2 lists examples of the professional associations that currently grant certification.

Certified nurses may have greater earning potential, wider employment opportunities, a broader scope of practice, status, and prestige than noncertified nurses. Increasingly, they are eligible for insurance reimbursement for their services. Requirements for admission to certification programs vary, with some requiring only registered nurse licensure and others requiring either a baccalaureate or a master's degree.

The **American Nurses Credentialing Center (ANCC),** a subunit of the ANA, provides 39 different certification programs for registered nurses at the associate degree, baccalaureate, and advanced practice levels. **Advanced practice nurses (APNs)** certified by the ANCC must have master's degrees and demonstrate successful completion of a certification examination based on nationally recognized standards of nursing practice and designed to test their special knowledge and skills. For certain specialties, candidates also must show evidence of specified clinical practice experience. Once granted, certification is effective for 3 to 5 years, whereupon the individual

---

Box **7-2** **A Sample of Certifying Organizations in Nursing***
■ AACN Certifying Corporation (Critical Care)   ■ American Association of Diabetes Educators   ■ American Association of Spinal Cord Injury Nurses   ■ American Board for Occupational Health Nurses, Inc.   ■ American College of Nurse Midwives   ■ American Nurses Credentialing Center (40 areas of certification)   ■ American Organization of Nurse Executives   ■ American Psychiatric Nurses' Association   ■ Board of Certification for Emergency Nursing   ■ Council on Recertification of Nurse Anesthetists   ■ National Association of Neonatal Nurses   ■ National Association of Nurse Practitioners   ■ National Certification Corporation for Obstetric, Gynecologic, and Neonatal Specialties   ■ National Board for Certification of School Nurses   ■ Pediatric Nursing Certification Board   ■ Rehabilitation Nursing Certification Board

*A complete list of certifying boards can be obtained by writing to the *Journal of Continuing Education in Nursing*, Slack, Inc., 6900 Grove Drive, Thorofare, NJ 08086. Ask for the Annual Continuing Education Survey. Also available online (http://www.jcenonline.com/survey.asp).

must apply for recertification based either on retesting or by demonstrating continuing education credits and evidence of ongoing clinical practice.

In response to the need to create uniformity in the numerous certification programs, the ANCC and more than a dozen other certification boards formed the American Board of Nursing Specialties (ABNS) in 1991. Membership is open to certifying bodies that have met the standards and principles of ABNS. The organization's stated aims are to promote standards of excellence in nursing certification and to increase public awareness of the value of certification.

Nurses holding certification at the associate degree/diploma level use the initials RN, C (Registered Nurse, Certified) after their names. Certified baccalaureate nurses are entitled to use RN, BC (Registered Nurse, Board Certified). Those certified as clinical specialists use APRN, BC (Advanced Practice Registered Nurse, Board Certified). Box 7-3 lists the areas in which the ANCC offers certification.

Although certification is a desirable concept, several challenges must be overcome in regard to the current methods of certification. With so many different organizations offering certification, the lack of uniformity of programs, testing, and practice requirements must be examined. How the profession can ensure certification standards and who should be responsible for certification of nurses are continuing concerns.

Many in the nursing profession believe that nurses should be certified in a standardized manner by one nationally recognized certifying board. The American Association of Colleges of Nursing has been particularly vocal in this regard and issued position statements in 1994 and 1998 emphasizing standardization goals (American Association of Colleges of Nursing, 1998). Judging from the proliferation of certifying bodies, this is a goal the profession has yet to attain.

CONTINUING EDUCATION

Continuing education (CE) is a term used to describe non–degree-seeking ways in which nurses maintain expertise during their professional careers. It differs from staff development, which refers to how an agency or institution assists its employees in maintaining competence. Continuing education opportunities are those sought by individual nurses themselves. Continuing education for nurses takes place in a variety of settings: colleges, universities, hospitals, community agencies, professional organizations, and professional meetings. Continuing education is available in many formats, such as workshops, institutes, conferences, short courses, evening courses, telecourses, and instructional modules offered in professional journals and by professional organizations online.

The American Nurses Credentialing Center (ANCC) is responsible for standards of continuing education, accreditation of programs offering continuing education, transferability of CE credit from state to state, and development of guidelines for recognition systems within states.

Box **7-3** **Areas of Certification Offered by the American Nurses Credentialing Center (ANCC) in 2006 and Their Corresponding Credentials**

Advanced Practice Exams—APRN, BC (Advanced Practice Registered Nurse, Board Certified)

- Acute Care Nurse Practitioner
- Adult Nurse Practitioner
- Family Nurse Practitioner
- Gerontological Nurse Practitioner
- Pediatric Nurse Practitioner

Continued

- Adult Psychiatric and Mental Health Nurse Practitioner
- Family Psychiatric and Mental Health Nurse Practitioner
- Clinical Nurse Specialist in Gerontological Nursing
- Clinical Nurse Specialist in Adult Health Nursing
- Clinical Nurse Specialist in Pediatric Nursing
- Clinical Nurse Specialist in Adult Psychiatric and Mental Health Nursing
- Clinical Nurse Specialist in Child and Adolescent Psychiatric and Mental Health Nursing
- Clinical Nurse Specialist in Public/Community Health Nursing
- Clinical Nurse Specialist in Home Health Nursing
- Advanced Diabetes Management—Clinical Nurse Specialist
- Advanced Diabetes Management—Nurse Practitioner
- Advanced Diabetes Management—Registered Dietitian
- Advanced Diabetes Management—Registered Pharmacist
- Nursing Administration, Advanced (RN, CNAA-BC)

Specialty Nursing Exams—RN–BC (Registered Nurse–Board Certified)
- Cardiac/Vascular Nurse
- Gerontological Nurse
- Informatics Nurse: Baccalaureate degree in nursing
- Informatics Nurse: Baccalaureate degree in other relevant field of study
- Medical-Surgical Nurse
- Nursing Professional Development
- Pediatric Nurse
- Perinatal Nurse
- Psychiatric and Mental Health Nurse
- Nursing Administration (RN, CNA-BC)
- Ambulatory Care Nursing
- Nursing Case Management
- Pain Management

From American Nurses Credentialing Center: Accessed June 13, 2006, from http://nursingworld.org/ancc/cert/index.html.

The **contact hour** is the measure of continuing education credit. Generally, nurses receive 1 contact hour of CE credit for each 50 or 60 minutes they spend in a continuing education course.

A major nationwide trend is **mandatory continuing education.** Before renewing their licenses in states and territories with mandatory continuing education, nurses must provide evidence that they have met contact hour requirements. The requirement for mandatory continuing education is a government's way of ensuring that nurses remain up to date in their profession. In 2005 mandatory continuing education credit as a prerequisite for license renewal was required in 27 states and U.S. territories. The number of CE hours required ranged from a low of 10 hours in 2 years in Rhode Island to a high of 50 hours every 2 years (or national certification) in New Mexico (Yoder-Wise, 2006). Box 7-4 lists mandatory continuing education states and territories.

Continuing Education Through Distance Learning (DL)

Now that the technology is available to create virtual universities, nursing education has recognized the value of distance learning as a means to help nurses continue learning. **Distance learning (DL)** is an umbrella term used to describe courses offered by electronic means, such as on television or online. Distance learning offerings span the gamut from stand-alone continuing education modules to entire degrees offered online. DL offers several major positive features (AACN, 1999):

- It increases access to nursing education for adults in midcareer, who represent a growing proportion of the undergraduate nursing population.
- It increases access to nursing education in rural areas underserved by higher education.
- It increases the efficiency of the shrinking number of nursing faculty members by allowing them to reach larger audiences than in traditional nursing classes on campuses.
- It allows practicing nurses to obtain continuing education credits without leaving home.

Box 7-4	States and Territories Requiring Continuing Education for License Renewal*

- Alabama
- Alaska
- Arkansas
- California
- Delaware
- Florida
- Iowa
- Kansas
- Kentucky
- Louisiana
- Massachusetts
- Michigan
- Minnesota
- Nebraska
- Nevada
- New Hampshire
- New Mexico
- North Mariana Islands
- Ohio
- Puerto Rico
- Rhode Island
- South Carolina
- Texas
- U.S. Virgin Islands
- Utah
- West Virginia
- Wyoming

*A current list of states and territories requiring continuing education for license renewal can be obtained by writing to the *Journal of Continuing Education in Nursing*, Slack, Inc., 6900 Grove Drive, Thorofare, NJ 08086. Ask for a reprint of their Annual Continuing Education Survey. Also available online (http://www.jcenonline.com/survey.asp).

As more colleges of nursing offer coursework and entire degrees through distance learning, the issue of adequate and properly supervised clinical experience arises. Technology may again provide at least a partial answer to this dilemma through the use of virtual reality. Virtual reality "employs computers and other multimedia peripherals to produce a simulated (i.e., virtual) environment that users perceive as comparable to real-world objects and events" (Simpson, 2003). DL students validate their clinical competence in a number of traditional ways, including preceptorships, clinical examinations, demonstrations, and clinical portfolios. Preliminary research findings on the outcomes of these courses indicate when properly structured, well monitored, and offered to carefully selected students, achievement levels of DL students are comparable to those of traditional students (Zucker and Asselin, 2003).

When technology is used carefully and courses offered through DL are constructed properly, there is no reason to limit these offerings. This is particularly true in an era when the numbers of nurses, faculty, and researchers fall well below national projections of need.

CHALLENGES IN NURSING EDUCATION

A number of challenges face nursing education. Two major challenges are discussed in this section: the inability of nursing programs to produce enough nurses to meet the need because of faculty and other resource shortages; the need to transform nursing education to meet the complex health care needs of the nation for the future.

Faculty and Other Resource Shortages Threaten Nation's Supply of Nurses

Despite the fact that enrollments and graduations in associate and baccalaureate degree programs across the nation have increased over the past 5 years, the number of employed nurses still falls short of current needs and will fall further behind as the population ages. As the general population ages, so does the nurse faculty population. Nationally, the mean age for faculty members was 49.7 years in 1993. By 2002 this average had risen to 51.1 years and by 2006, almost two thirds of all full-time nursing faculty members were 45-60 years old (National League for Nursing, 2006). This trend will result in increasing numbers of faculty retirements in the next decade. The faculty shortage, already affecting some areas of the country, is predicted to become severe in the majority of the nation's schools of nursing by the year 2010 (AACN, 2003). Data from the 2005-2006 academic year show that over 37,000 qualified applicants were not accepted in basic baccalaureate problems alone because of insufficient faculty, insufficient clinical sites, or other insufficient resources (Fang et al , 2006).

Recognizing that the shortage of faculty was reaching critical proportions, in April 2003 the AACN issued an official report, known as a white paper, outlining the problem (AACN, 2003). Among their findings were the following:

- A 2000 national sample of schools reported 7.4 percent faculty vacancies, with only 20 of 220 schools reporting no vacancies. Although this may not seem like a large vacancy rate, it has a considerable impact because of teacher/student ratios mandated by nursing accreditation bodies. Accredited schools are required to limit the size of a faculty member's clinical supervision responsibilities to 10 students at any one time.
- Reasons for faculty shortages include the following: age and retirement time lines; an inadequate pool of younger faculty for replacement; resignations for nonacademic jobs; decrease in the overall number of graduates from both master's and doctoral programs; average age of doctoral graduates (46.2 years) as compared with graduates of all professions (33.7 years), meaning that the number of productive work years for these older faculty members is curtailed; plans of new doctoral graduates to work outside education; average academic salaries lower than those in clinical areas and continuing budgetary constraints within most higher education systems, making salary increases unlikely; and expanding expectations of the faculty role. Furthermore, faculty members are challenged more and more by nontraditional students who demand more individual attention—at the same time as they are increasingly required to do research, service, and publishing.

The AACN (2003) white paper suggested numerous additional strategies for dealing with the faculty shortage (see the entire 2003 report at www.aacn.nche.edu/publications/whitepapers/facultyshortages.htm). Faculty shortages are severe and seriously affect the nation's supply of registered nurses. Interest in nursing careers is strong, but access to professional nursing programs is increasingly difficult and is expected to become even more so for the foreseeable future.

Need to Transform Nursing Education

As the twentieth century came to a close, nursing organizations turned their attention to the future. A number of organizations issued reports identifying changes needed in nursing education to prepare nurses for practice in the twenty-first century. The reports included the NLN's *A Vision for Nursing Education* (1993; see also National League for Nursing, 1995), the AACN's *Nursing Education's Agenda for the 21st Century* (AACN, 1993, 1999), and the report from the Pew Health Professions Commission entitled *Health Professions Education for the Future: Schools in Service to the Nation* (O'Neil, 1993). Although the three organizations advocated somewhat different approaches and strategies, several common themes emerged in their reports. Common emphases included the following eight points:

1. Schools should recruit diverse students and faculties that reflect the multicultural nature of society.
2. Curricula and learning activities should develop students' critical thinking skills.
3. Curricula should emphasize students' abilities to communicate, form interpersonal relationships, and make decisions collaboratively with patients, their families, and interdisciplinary colleagues.
4. The number of advanced practice nurses should be increased, and curricula should emphasize health promotion and health maintenance skills for all nurses.
5. Emphasis should be placed on community-based care, increased accountability, state-of-

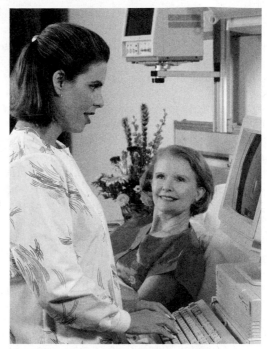

Figure 7-5
Information management is more important than ever in nursing. This nursing student is developing information technology skills to manage multiple sources of patient information successfully.

the-art clinical skills, and increased information management skills (Figure 7-5).
6. Cost-effectiveness of care should be a focus in nursing curricula.
7. Faculty should develop programs that facilitate program articulation and career mobility.
8. Continuing faculty development activities should support excellence in practice, teaching, and research.

These eight areas of emphasis remain as relevant today as they were when first identified in the 1990s.

Others also recognized the need to reshape nursing education to meet the challenges of future patient care through improved nursing practice. In 1999 the National League for Nursing launched a 5-year project entitled *Transforming the Landscape for Nursing Education*. The purpose of this project was to begin a national dialogue on skills and competencies, types of programs and curricula, academic and community partnerships, standards for future program types, and research initiatives for nursing education. Plans for this transformation included discovering the core knowledge needed to bridge education and practice; differentiating between knowledge and outcome competencies for a continuum of practice; identifying research on curricula, methods, and instructional strategies for core curricula common to basic preparation for health professions; developing seamless program articulation along the continuum of nursing education; and creating infrastructures that provide for ongoing communication among leaders in education and practice (National League for Nursing, 1999).

In April 2002 the ANA issued a document entitled *Nursing's Agenda for the Future: The Future Vision for Nursing*. The vision for nursing education articulated in this paper included the valuing of nursing education by the public; education programs that are accessible, affordable, and flexible; adequate faculty with high qualifications who engage in innovative teaching, clinical practice, and research; learning environments conducive to the creativity of faculty and students; evidence-based education; safe, quality care; and partnerships to enhance clinical experiences, meet the needs of special populations, and promote professional involvement. The following five strategies were outlined for achieving the vision: (1) establish congruence between the educational enterprise and societal needs; (2) enrich the high caliber of nursing faculty; (3) attain clarity in education about nursing roles and scopes of practice; (4) work for universal excellence in nursing education; and (5) promote the value of nursing education to the profession and the public (see the entire ANA 2002 report at www.nursingworld.org/naf/).

Some experts believe that education of all health professions is in need of systemic change. A notable example is the 2003 Institute of Medicine's report *Health Professions Education: A Bridge to Quality*. This report built upon the 2001 IOM report *Crossing the Quality Chasm: A New Health System for the 21st Century*, which recommended a complete restructuring of clinical education across all health professions. As a follow-up to the initial report, a multidisciplinary summit of health profession leaders met in 2002; this high-level panel composed of 150 participants recommended the goal of "an outcome-based education system that better prepares clinicians to meet both the needs of patients and the requirements of a changing health system" (IOM, 2003). Five major problems were identified in all health professions' education. They were the following (Institute of Medicine, 2003):

1. Students are not being educated to care for the increasingly diverse, elderly, and chronically ill patient populations.
2. Students are not being prepared to work in teams, but once in practice, they are usually expected to work in interdisciplinary teams.
3. Students are not consistently educated in how to find, evaluate, and use the rapidly expanding scientific evidence upon which practice should be based.
4. There is little opportunity to learn how to identify, analyze, and eliminate the root causes of errors and other quality problems in health care delivery systems.
5. Students often are not provided basic informatics training to enable them to access information and use computerized order entry systems.

They recommended that all the health professions develop and share a set of core competencies that would result in better educational quality and relevance. This exhaustive report can be read in its entirety online (http://darwin.nap.edu/books/0309087236/html).

The important thing for students of nursing to recognize about these reports is that nursing organizations and leaders are constantly analyzing the changes in the health care system and working to set standards by which high-quality educational programs can be designed, implemented, and evaluated. The complexity of health care delivery systems and the dynamic nature of the patient populations served, the shortage of faculty, and the lack of human and financial resources make this a challenging task. However, there is no question that the transformation of nursing education over the next 2 decades will be significant.

Other Challenges

In addition to the two major challenges discussed above, nursing education must address a variety of other issues, including job market fluctuations; increasing competition for clinical learning sites by all health profession schools; diminishing resources in institutions of higher education and the high cost of operating nursing education programs; and the inability of some nursing programs to meet accreditation standards.

SUMMARY OF *Key Points*

- The development of nursing education has been influenced by a number of factors, leading to a diverse array of program offerings.
- First provided in hospitals, entry-level nursing education has evolved into three major types of basic programs: diploma, baccalaureate, and associate degree, each of which has a range of features.
- Alternatives such as baccalaureate degree programs for registered nurses, external degree programs, accelerated options for postbaccalaureate students, and online programs contribute to a rich, yet complex educational picture for registered nurses.
- Voluntary accreditation is designed to ensure the quality of nursing education programs.
- Schools have found it necessary to restrict enrollments because of faculty shortages, lack of clinical sites, and budget constraints.
- Life-long learning through continuing education is considered essential for all professionals, particularly in practice-based disciplines such

as nursing. Continuing education is now mandated as a prerequisite for relicensure in 27 states and U.S. territories, and this number is expected to increase.
- The problem of reduced resources in nursing education may soon reach crisis proportions, and weaker schools may close. This is a result of underfunding of higher education in general and, in particular, diminishing sources of federal and state funding for schools of nursing.
- Graduate programs in nursing are not preparing adequate numbers of nursing educators to meet current and future needs. Faculty shortages are already developing, and a severe faculty shortage is expected nationwide by 2010.
- In response to changes in higher education and the health care system, national organizations have suggested initiatives to revise educational requirements and program emphases for the twenty-first century that will enable future registered nurses at all levels to meet the changing health care needs of society.

CRITICAL THINKING QUESTIONS

1. What factors did you use to determine the type of basic nursing program you entered? Knowing what you know now, what changes, if any, would you make in your choice?
2. How would you advise a high school student interested in nursing to select a program?
3. Should nursing have only one basic program type that leads to entry into the profession? Discuss the pros and cons of a single program. In what part of the higher education system should this basic program be located? What academic credential should be awarded at the completion of the program? In what ways would the unification of nursing education strengthen the profession?
4. What content areas and skills should be included in basic nursing programs to prepare graduates for contemporary nursing practice? What should be eliminated to make room for this content?

5. Offering complete articulation of all types of nursing education from practical nursing through doctoral study seems like a logical course of action. Should all states mandate program articulation? Why or why not?
6. Discuss the merits and drawbacks of mandatory continuing education from viewpoints of both nurses and consumers of nursing care.
7. What unique contributions to nursing are possible by nurses with master's-level education? With doctoral-level degrees?
8. Find out which of the national accrediting bodies, NLNAC or CCNE, accredits your school or college. Research their standards online (visit Evolve for WebLinks related to the content of this chapter: http://evolve.elsevier.com/Chitty/professional/) and analyze how your school meets those standards.

REFERENCES

Allen J, editor: *Consumer's guide to doctoral degree programs in nursing,* New York, 1990, National League for Nursing.

American Association of Colleges of Nursing: *Nursing education's agenda for the 21st century,* Position statement, Washington, DC, 1993, revised 1999, American Association of Colleges of Nursing.

American Association of Colleges of Nursing: *Certification and regulation of advanced practice nurses,* Position statement, Washington, DC, 1994, revised 1998, American Association of Colleges of Nursing.

American Association of Colleges of Nursing: *The baccalaureate degree in nursing as minimal preparation for professional practice,* Position statement, Washington, DC, 1996, American Association of Colleges of Nursing.

American Association of Colleges of Nursing: *The essentials of baccalaureate education for professional nursing practice,* Washington, DC, 1998, American Association of Colleges of Nursing.

American Association of Colleges of Nursing: *Distance technology in nursing education: a white paper,* Washington, DC, 1999 (website): http://www.aacn.nche.edu/Publications/WhitePapers/whitepaper.htm.

American Association of Colleges of Nursing: *Faculty shortages in baccalaureate and graduate nursing programs: scope of the problem and strategies for expanding the supply,* Washington, DC, 2003, American Association of Colleges of Nursing.

American Association of Colleges of Nursing: *The practice doctorate in nursing: a position statement,* Washington, DC, 2004, American Association of Colleges of Nursing.

American Association of Colleges of Nursing: *Fact sheet: articulation agreements among nursing education programs,* Washington, DC, 2006, American Association of Colleges of Nursing.

American Nurses Association: *Educational preparation for nurse practitioners and assistants to nurses,* Position paper, Kansas City, Mo, 1965, American Nurses Association.

American Nurses Association: *A case for baccalaureate preparation in nursing,* Kansas City, Mo, 1979, American Nurses Association.

American Nurses Association: *Nursing's agenda for the future: the future vision for nursing,* Washington, DC, 2002, American Nurses Association.

American Nurses Credentialing Center: Accessed June 13, 2006, from http://nursingworld.org/ancc/cert/index.html.

Berlin LE, Wilsey SJ, Bednash GD: *2004-2005 enrollment and graduations in baccalaureate and graduate programs in nursing,* Washington, DC, 2005, American Association of Colleges of Nursing.

Brown EL: *Nursing for the future,* New York, 1948, Russell Sage Foundation.

Christy T: Portrait of a leader: M. Adelaide Nutting, *Nurs Outlook* 17(1):20-24, 1969.

Conley V: *Curriculum and instruction in nursing,* Boston, 1973, Little, Brown.

Donahue MP: *Nursing: the finest art: an illustrated history,* St Louis, 1985, Mosby.

Dracup K, Bryan-Brown CW: Doctor of nursing practice: MRI or total body scan, *Am J Crit Care* 14(4):278-281, 2005.

Fang D, Wilsey-Wisniewski SJ, Bednash GD: *2005-2006 Enrollment and graduations in baccalaureate and graduate programs in nursing,* Washington, DC, 2006, American Association of Colleges of Nursing.

Institute of Medicine: *Crossing the quality chasm: a new health system for the 21st century,* Washington, DC, 2001, National Academies Press.

Institute of Medicine: *Health professions education: a bridge to quality,* Washington, DC, 2003, National Academies Press.

Kalisch P, Kalisch B: *The advance of American nursing,* ed 3, Boston, 1995, Little, Brown.

Lysaught J: *An abstract for action,* New York, 1970, McGraw-Hill.

Montag M: *The education of nursing technicians,* New York, 1951, Putnam.

National League for Nursing: *Position statement on nursing roles: scope and preparation,* New York, 1982, National League for Nursing.

National League for Nursing, Council of Associate Degree Programs: *Educational outcomes of associate degree nursing programs: roles and competencies,* New York, 1990, National League for Nursing.

National League for Nursing: *A vision for nursing education,* New York, 1993, National League for Nursing.

National League for Nursing: *Emerging environment for nursing education and practice examined during two-year vision campaign: news from the National League for Nursing,* New York, 1995, National League for Nursing.

National League for Nursing, Center for Research in Nursing Education and Community Health: *NLN guide to undergraduate RN education,* ed 5, Sudbury, Mass, 1997, NLN Press and Jones and Bartlett.

National League for Nursing: *Transforming the landscape: executive summary,* Biennial Convention, June 5, 1999, Miami Beach, Fla.

National League for Nursing: *Educational competencies for graduates of associate degree nursing programs,* New York, 2000, National League for Nursing.

National League for Nursing: *A guide to state approved schools of nursing 2006 RN, 58th edition,* New York, 2006, National League for Nursing.

National League for Nursing: *Nurse educators 2006,* New York, 2006, National League for Nursing.

National League of Nursing Education: *Nursing schools today and tomorrow,* New York, 1934, National League of Nursing Education.

National League of Nursing Education: *A curriculum guide for schools of nursing,* New York, 1937, National League of Nursing Education.

Notter L, Spalding E: *Professional nursing, foundations, perspectives and relationships,* ed 9, Philadelphia, 1976, JB Lippincott.

O'Neil EH: *Health professions education for the future: schools in service to the nation,* San Francisco, 1993, Pew Health Professions Commission.

Parietti E: The development of doctoral education in nursing: a historical overview. In Allen J, editor: *Consumer's guide to doctoral degree programs in nursing,* New York, 1990, National League for Nursing, p 1532.

Simpson R: Welcome to the virtual classroom, *Nurs Admin Quart* 27(1):83-86, 2003.

U.S. Department of Health and Human Services: *The registered nurse population, March 2000: findings from the national sample survey of registered nurses,* Washington, DC, 2001, Government Printing Office.

U.S. Department of Health and Human Services: *The registered nurse population, March 2004: preliminary findings from the national sample survey of registered nurses,* Washington, DC, 2006, Government Printing Office.

Yoder-Wise PS: Annual CE survey: state certifying board/associations: CE and competency requirements, *J Contin Educ Nurs* 37(1):5-13, 2006.

Zucker DM, Asselin M: Migrating to the web: the transformation of a traditional RN to BS program, *J Contin Educ Nurs* 34(2):86-89, 2003.

Critical Thinking, the Nursing Process, and Clinical Judgment

Beth Perry Black and Kay Kittrell Chitty

Learning Outcomes

After studying this chapter, students will be able to:

- Define critical thinking in nursing.
- Contrast the characteristics of "novice thinking" with those of "expert thinking."
- Explain the purpose and phases of the nursing process.
- Differentiate between nursing orders and medical orders.
- Explain the differences between independent, interdependent, and dependent nursing actions.

- Describe evaluation and its importance in the nursing process.
- Define clinical judgment in nursing practice and explain how it is developed.
- Devise a personal plan to use in developing sound clinical judgment.

Almost every nurse-patient encounter is an opportunity for the nurse to assist the patient in moving to a higher level of wellness. Whether or not this actually happens depends in large measure on the nurse's ability to think critically about the patient's particular needs and how best to meet them. It also depends on the nurse's ability to use a reliable problem-solving approach that leads to sound clinical decisions about the patient's priority nursing needs. Underlying this admittedly simplistic description is the assumption that patients are not passive recipients of nursing care but are active participants in care to the extent of their ability.

This chapter explores several important and interdependent aspects of thinking and decision making in nursing: critical thinking, the nursing process, and clinical judgment.

DEFINING CRITICAL THINKING

Defining critical thinking is a complex task that requires an understanding of how people think through problems. Educators and philosophers struggled with definitions of critical thinking for several decades. In 1990 the American Philosophical Association's Committee on Pre-College Philosophy published an expert consensus statement (Box 8-1) describing critical thinking and the ideal critical thinker (American Philosophical Association, 1990). This expert statement was the culmination of 3 years of work by Facione and others who synthesized the work of numerous persons who had defined critical thinking. In his 2006 update of his essay *Critical Thinking: What It Is and Why It Counts,* Facione (2006) suggested that giving a definition of critical thinking that can be memorized by the learner is actually antithetical to critical thinking! This means that the very definition of critical thinking does not lend itself to simplistic thinking and memorization. Paul and Elder's (2005) definition of critical thinking is similar: "Critical thinking is a process by which the thinker improves the quality of his or her thinking by skillfully taking charge of the structures inherent in thinking and imposing intellectual standards upon them." They go on to describe a "well-cultivated critical thinker" as one who:

- Raises questions and problems, and formulates them clearly and precisely
- Gathers and assesses relevant information, using abstract ideas for interpretation
- Arrives at conclusions and solutions that are well-reasoned and tests them against relevant standards

- Is open-minded and recognizes alternative ways of seeing problems, and has the ability to assess the assumptions, implications, and consequences of alternative views of problems
- Communicates effectively with others as solutions to complex problems are formulated

The similarities are evident between Facione's and Paul and Elder's definitions: critical thinking is a process that requires disciplined engagement of the intellect to solve problems most effectively.

You may be asking, "What does this have to do with nursing?" The answer is very simple. Making good clinical judgments requires excellent critical thinking skills. As a practitioner of professional nursing responsible and accountable for your own decisions, the development of critical thinking skills is crucial as you provide nursing care for patients with increasingly complex conditions. Critical thinking skills provide the nurse with a powerful means of determining patient needs, interpreting physician orders, and intervening appropriately. Box 8-2 presents an example of the importance of critical thinking in the provision of safe care.

Box **8-1** | **Expert Consensus Statement Regarding Critical Thinking and the Ideal Critical Thinker**

We understand critical thinking (CT) to be purposeful, self-regulatory judgment that results in interpretation, analysis, evaluation, and inference, as well as explanation of the evidential, conceptual, methodological, criteriological, or contextual considerations upon which that judgment is based. CT is essential as a tool of inquiry. As such, CT is a liberating force in education and a powerful resource in one's personal and civic life. While not synonymous with good thinking, CT is a pervasive and self-rectifying human phenomenon. The ideal critical thinker is habitually inquisitive, well-informed, trustful of reason, open-minded, flexible, fair-minded in evaluation, honest in facing personal biases, prudent in making judgments, willing to reconsider, clear about issues, orderly in complex matters, diligent in seeking relevant information, reasonable in the selection of criteria, focused in inquiry, and persistent in seeking results that are as precise as the subject and the circumstances of inquiry permit. Thus educating good critical thinkers means working toward this ideal. It combines developing CT skills with nurturing those dispositions that consistently yield useful insights and that are the basis of a rational and democratic society.

From American Philosophical Association: Critical thinking: a statement of expert consensus for purposes of educational assessment and instruction, *The Delphi report: research findings and recommendations prepared for the committee on pre-college philosophy,* 1990, ERIC Document Reproduction Services, pp 315-423.

CRITICAL THINKING IN NURSING

You may be wondering at this point, "How am I ever going to learn how to make connections among all of the data I have about a patient?" This is a common response for a nursing student who is just learning some of the most basic psychomotor skills in preparation for practice. You need to understand that, just like learning to give injections safely and maintaining a sterile field properly, you can learn to think critically. This involves paying attention to how one thinks and making thinking itself a focus of concern. A nurse who is exercising critical thinking asks the following questions: "What assumptions have I made about this patient?" "How do I know my assumptions are accurate?" "Do I need any additional information?" and "How might I look at this situation differently?"

Nurses just beginning to pay attention to their thinking processes may ask these questions after nurse-patient interactions have ended. This is known as **reflective thinking.** Reflective thinking is an active process valuable in learning and changing behaviors, perspectives, or practices. Nurses can also learn to examine their thinking processes during an interaction as they learn to "think on their feet." This is a characteristic of expert nurses. As you move from novice to expert, your ability to think critically will improve with practice. In Chapter 6 you read about Dr. Patricia Benner (1984, 1996), who studied the differences in expertise of nurses at different stages in their careers, from novice to expert. So it is with critical thinking; novices think differently than experts. Box 8-3 summarizes the differences in novice and expert thinking.

Critical thinking in nursing, however, involves more than good problem-solving strategies. It is a complex, purposeful, disciplined process that has specific characteristics that make it different from run-of-the-mill problem solving. Consciously developed to improve patient outcomes, critical thinking by the nurse is driven by the needs of the patient and family. Critical thinking in nursing is

---

Box **8-2** Using Critical Thinking Skills to Improve a Patient's Care

Mr. Smith is a 77-year-old man admitted to your general medicine unit with several problems, including dehydration secondary to severe nausea and vomiting and a urinary tract infection. His medication orders include hydrochlorothiazide 50 mg q AM for mild hypertension, ampicillin 2 g q 6 hours. His IV order is D_5LR at 125 ml/hour. His lab values show a serum potassium level of 2.6 mEq/L. You recognize that this is low. Mr. Smith seems weak and lethargic; his urine output has been 35 ml/hour for the past 2 hours. You are concerned about him and his condition.

A nurse using good critical thinking skills will note the following: the source of his dehydration, his antibiotic order for his UTI, his low potassium level, his IV rate, his low urinary output, and his daily use of a diuretic known to be associated with potassium loss. His lethargy and weakness could be a product of his age and general condition, but you also know that they are signs of hypokalemia. Critical thinking does not stop at noting these issues, however. Critical thinking requires making a judgment about what to do with your concerns. A nurse not using critical thinking may simply follow physician orders with the expectation that Mr. Smith will feel better once his dehydration is reversed and his UTI is adequately treated. Using your good critical thinking skills, however, you come to the conclusion that Mr. Smith may be better supported with a different approach to his care. You call his physician to discuss your concerns, describing in detail the "big picture." The specific, detailed information that you communicate clearly allows the physician to reconsider Mr. Smith's medical regimen and proceed from a more informed position. The next day you are pleased to see Mr. Smith walking in the hall when you come onto the unit at the beginning of your shift. He says that he feels "like a new person."

Box **8-3** Novice Thinking Compared With Expert Thinking

Novice Nurses

- Tend to organize knowledge as separate facts. Must rely heavily on resources (e.g., texts, notes, preceptors). Lack knowledge gained from actually doing (e.g., listening to breath sounds).
- Focus so much on actions that they tend to forget to assess before acting.
- Need clear-cut rules.
- Are often hampered by unawareness of resources.
- Are often hindered by anxiety and lack of self-confidence.
- Must be able to rely on step-by-step procedures. Tend to focus more on procedures than on the patient response to the procedure.
- Become uncomfortable if patient needs preclude performing procedures exactly as they were learned.
- Have limited knowledge of suspected problems; therefore they question and collect data more superficially.
- Tend to follow standards and policies by rote.
- Learn more readily when matched with a supportive, knowledgeable preceptor or mentor.

Expert Nurses

- Tend to store knowledge in a highly organized and structured manner, making recall of information easier. Have a large storehouse of experiential knowledge (e.g., what abnormal breath sounds sound like, what subtle changes look like).
- Assess and think things through before acting.
- Know when to bend the rules.
- Are aware of resources and how to use them.
- Are usually more self-confident, less anxious, and therefore more focused.
- Know when it is safe to skip steps or do two steps together. Are able to focus on both the parts (the procedures) and the whole (the patient response).
- Comfortable with rethinking a procedure if patient needs require modification of the procedure.
- Have a better idea of suspected problems, allowing them to question more deeply and collect more relevant and in-depth data.
- Analyze standards and policies, looking for ways to improve them.
- Are challenged by novices' questions, clarifying their own thinking when teaching novices.

From Alfaro-LeFevre R: *Critical thinking in nursing: a practical approach*, ed 2, Philadelphia, 1999, WB Saunders. Reprinted with permission.

undergirded by the standards and ethics of the profession. Nurses who think critically seek to build on patients' strengths while honoring patients' values and beliefs (Alfaro-LeFevre, 1999). They are engaged in a process of constant evaluation, redirection, improvement, and increased efficiency. Be aware that critical thinking involves far more than stating your opinion. You must be able to describe how you came to a conclusion and support your conclusions with explicit rationales.

This is a different way of thinking for most people and requires practice. Dimensions of critical thinking include both cognitive skills and "habits of the mind" (Scheffer and Rubenfeld, 2000). Box 8-4 summarizes these characteristics and offers an opportunity for you to evaluate your progress as a critical thinker.

An excellent continuing education self-study module designed to improve your ability to think critically can be found online (www.nursing-

Box **8-4** Self-Assessment: Critical Thinking

Directions: Listed below are 15 characteristics of critical thinkers. Mark a plus sign (+) next to those you now possess, mark IP (in progress) next to those you have partially mastered, and mark a zero (0) next to those you have not yet mastered. When you are finished, make a plan for developing the areas that need improvement. Share it with at least one person and report on progress weekly.

Characteristics of Critical Thinkers: How Do You Measure Up?

_____ Inquisitive/curious/seeks truth

_____ Self-informed/finds own answers

_____ Analytical/confident in own reasoning skills

_____ Open-minded

_____ Flexible

_____ Fair-minded

_____ Honest about personal biases/self-aware

_____ Prudent/exercises sound judgment

_____ Willing to revise judgment when new evidence warrants

_____ Clear about issues

_____ Orderly in complex matters/organized approach to problems

_____ Diligent in seeking information

_____ Persistent

_____ Reasonable

_____ Focused on inquiry

Modified from Facione PA: Critical thinking: a statement of expert consensus for purposes of educational assessment and instruction, "The Delphi Report," Milbrae, California: The California Academic Press, 1990.

spectrum.com; at the Continuing Education link, request course number CE168d). You can also begin to learn about the many facets of critical thinking by participating with classmates in the Critical Thinking Challenge, Six Caps, on p. 193. This exercise will allow you to practice thinking through the various questions that need to be asked in response to very complex patient and family issues.

THE NURSING PROCESS AS AN INTELLECTUAL STANDARD

Critical thinking requires systematic and disciplined use of universal intellectual standards (Paul and Elder, 2005). In the practice of nursing, the **nursing process** represents a universal intellectual standard by which problems are addressed and solved. The nursing process is a method of critical thinking focused on solving patient problems in professional practice. The nursing process is "a designated series of actions intended to fulfill the purposes of nursing—to maintain the patient's wellness—and, if this state changes, to provide the amount and quality of nursing care the situation demands to direct the patient back to wellness" (Yura and Walsh, 1983). Similar to Henderson's definition of nursing, Yura and Walsh stated that "if wellness cannot be achieved, then [the purpose of the nursing process is] to contribute to the patient's quality of life, maximizing his resources as long as life is a reality" (p. 71).

A simple example of using a process approach to problem solving is illustrated by examining a daily decision that you and most other people face: how to dress for the day. Before putting on your clothes, there are several factors you need to

CRITICAL THINKING *Challenge 8-1*

Six Caps

This is an hour-long group activity designed to clarify the various types of thinking that constitute critical thinking. For every six participants, you will need six pieces of colored paper (one white, one red, one black, one yellow, one green, and one blue). You will also need six straight pins. Divide the group into smaller groups of six and give each group member a pin and piece of colored paper. Each person draws a cap on the paper and pins it to his or her shirt in plain view. These represent the six "thinking caps," that is, the various types of thinking to be explored:

White cap—Information. Asks the questions, "What information do we have, what is needed, and how can we get it?"

Red cap—Feelings, intuition, and emotion. Asks the questions, "What are we, the patient, and the family feeling, and how do we know?"

Black cap—Policies, codes, standards, protocols, laws. Asks the questions, "What are the standards we should consider, and what are the risks?"

Yellow cap—Optimism. Asks the questions, "What are the benefits, who benefits, and what are the values being expressed?"

Green cap—Growth. Asks the questions, "Why don't we try it this way?" and "What are some different alternatives?"

Blue cap—Focuses on thinking. Asks the questions, "How are we going to proceed in thinking through this situation?" and "What have we achieved and what do we want to achieve?"

Read the case study below (or one prepared by your teacher) and discuss it from the viewpoint of each "cap." Identify issues for reflection. Then switch "thinking caps." Discuss the case study again. How easy or difficult was it to change your type of thinking? Do some types of thinking come more naturally to you than others? Which ones will you have to work to develop? Do you see value in each type of thinking? When the group reconvenes, summarize what you have learned on a flip chart.

Case Study for Six Caps

Marianne is a 79-year-old woman who was admitted to the emergency department yesterday with a severe headache. Shortly after admission, she became unresponsive; a brain scan revealed she had suffered a hemorrhagic stroke. Marianne's pupils are dilated and do not respond to light; she is breathing with the assistance of a respirator. Her elderly husband and three adult children are all assembled. The physician has recommended surgery to remove the blood clot but cannot offer much assurance that she will recover function. She has no advanced directives, but her husband wants to "try everything." The children believe that she would not want to undergo this surgery only to be kept alive with poor quality of life, which they agree is the likely outcome. The ethics committee is assembled to assist the family in making the decision. Before meeting with the family, the committee meets to discuss the situation.

Modified from De Bono E: Edward de Bono's mind pack, London, 1995, Dorling-Kindersley; Kenney LJ: Using Edward de Bono's six hats game to aid critical thinking and reflection in palliative care, *Int J Palliat Nurs* 9(3):105-112, 2003.

consider. What is the expected temperature? Will it be clear, raining, or snowing? How much time will be spent outdoors? Are there any activities planned that require special dress? Next, you probably look at the possible clothing choices. Some clothes may be out of season, and others need repairs, are too dressy or casual, or do not fit quite right. After considering the environmental factors, the day's activities, and your mood, you select the day's clothing. After dressing, you may look in a mirror to evaluate how you look. You may then modify your outfit based on your image in the mirror. At this point, you have solved the problem of clothing yourself. You have identified a problem, considered various factors related to the problem, identified possible actions, selected the best alternative, evaluated the success of the alternative selected, and made adjustments to the solution based on the evaluation. This is the same general process nurses use in solving patient problems through the nursing process.

For individuals outside the profession, nursing is commonly and simplistically defined in terms of tasks nurses perform (e.g., give injections). Many students get frustrated with activities and courses in nursing school that are not focused on these tasks, believing themselves that the tasks of nursing are nursing. Even within the profession, the intellectual basis of nursing practice was not articulated until the 1960s, when nursing educators and leaders began to identify and name the components of nursing's intellectual processes. This marked the beginning of the nursing process.

During the 1970s and 1980s, debate about the use of the term diagnosis began. Up until that time, diagnosis was considered to be within the scope of practice of physicians only. Nurses were not supposed to diagnose conditions in patients. This began to change in 1973 when the National Group for the Classification of Nursing Diagnosis, now called **NANDA International (NANDA),** published its first list of nursing diagnoses. The purpose of this group was (and is) to identify terminology and definitions that may be used and tested as nursing diagnoses.

Nursing diagnosis is the identification of those problems amenable to nursing intervention and that may be managed independently by nurses. In 2006 NANDA published its sixth edition of *Nursing Diagnoses: Definitions and Classifications* that included 167 NANDA approved diagnoses, 5 new diagnoses, and 3 revised diagnoses. Newly approved nursing diagnoses include "impaired religiosity," "readiness for enhanced religiosity," "risk for dysfunctional grieving," "risk for impaired religiosity," "and sedentary lifestyle." Revised diagnoses include "dysfunctional grieving," "disturbed energy field," and "risk for spiritual distress."

Here is a simple example of how one of the newly approved nursing diagnoses may be used:

> A pregnant woman at 40 weeks of gestation who is in labor with a fetus that has been identified as having a serious, life-threatening condition may have a medical diagnosis of "term labor." After careful nursing assessment and the application of critical thinking skills, the vigilant nurse may describe a nursing diagnosis of "risk for dysfunctional grieving" based on NANDA's (2006) taxonomy that describes perinatal risk factors associated with this diagnosis that apply to this patient.

A more detailed discussion of nursing diagnosis is located in the next section of this chapter.

The nursing process as a method of clinical problem solving is taught in nursing curricula across the United States, and many states refer to it in their nurse practice acts. The nursing process has sometimes been the subject of criticism among nurses. In recent years some nursing leaders have questioned the use of the nursing process, describing it as linear, rigid, and mechanistic. They believe that the nursing process contributes to linear thinking and stymies critical thinking. They are concerned that the nursing process format, and rigid faculty adherence to it, encourages students to copy from published sources when writing care plans, thus inhibiting the development of a holistic, creative approach to patient care (Mueller, Johnston, and Bligh, 2002). Certainly the nursing process can be taught, learned, and used in a rigid, mechanistic, and linear manner. Ideally, the nursing process is used as a creative approach to thinking and decision making in nursing. Because the nursing process is an integral aspect of nursing education, practice, standards, and law nationwide, learning to use it as a mechanism for critical thinking and as a dynamic and creative approach to patient care is a worthwhile endeavor. Despite reservations among some nurses about its use, the nursing process remains the cornerstone of nursing standards, legal definitions, and practice and, as such, should be well understood by every nurse.

PHASES OF THE NURSING PROCESS

Like many frameworks for thinking through problems, the nursing process is a series of organized steps, the purpose of which is to impose some discipline and critical thinking on the provision of excellent care. Identifying specific steps makes the process clear and concrete but can cause nurses to use them rigidly. Keep in mind that this is a process, that progression through the process may not be linear, and that it is a tool to use, not a road map to follow rigidly. More creative use of the nursing process may occur by expert nurses who have a greater repertoire of interventions from which to select. For example, if a newly hospitalized patient is experiencing a great deal of pain, a novice nurse might proceed by asking family members to leave so he or she can provide a quiet environment in which the patient may rest. An expert nurse would realize that the family may be a source of distraction from the pain or may be a source of comfort in ways that the nurse may not be able to provide. The expert nurse, in addition to assessing the patient, is willing to consider alternative explanations and interventions, enhancing the possibility that the patient's pain will be relieved.

Phase 1: Assessment

Assessment is the initial phase or operation in the nursing process. During this phase, information or data about the individual patient, family, or community are gathered. Data may include physiological, psychological, sociocultural, developmental, spiritual, and environmental information. The patient's available financial or material resources also need to be assessed and recorded in a standard format; each institution usually has a slightly different method of recording assessment data.

Types of data

Nurses obtain two types of data about and from patients: subjective and objective. **Subjective data** are obtained from patients as they describe their needs, feelings, strengths, and perceptions of the problem. Subjective data are frequently referred to as *symptoms*. Examples of subjective data are statements such as, "I am in pain" and "I don't have much energy." The only source for these data is the patient. Subjective data should include physical, psychosocial, and spiritual information. Subjective data can be very private. Nurses must be sensitive to the patient's need for confidence in the nurse's trustworthiness.

Objective data are the other types of data that the nurse will collect thråough observation, examination, or consultation with other health care providers. These data are measurable, such as pulse rate and blood pressure, and include observable patient behaviors. Objective data are frequently called *signs*. An example of objective data that a nurse might gather includes the observation that the patient, who is lying in bed, is diaphoretic, pale, and tachypneic, clutching his hands to his chest.

Objective data and subjective data usually are congruent; that is, they usually are in agreement. In the situation just mentioned, if the patient told the nurse, "I feel like a rock is crushing my chest," the subjective data would substantiate the nurse's observations (objective data) that the patient is having chest pain. Occasionally subjective and objective data are in conflict. A stark example of incongruent subjective and objective data well-known to labor and delivery nurses is when a pregnant woman in labor describes ongoing fetal activity (subjective data); however, there are no fetal heart tones (objective data) and the infant is stillborn. Incongruent objective and subjective data require further careful assessment to ascertain the patient's situation more completely and accurately. Sometimes incongruent data reveal something about the patient's concerns and fears. In order to get a clearer picture of the patient's situation, the nurse should use the best communication skills he or she possesses in order to increase the patient's trust, which will result in more openness.

Sources of patient data

Patient data can be obtained from many sources (Figure 8-1). The patient is considered the only

primary source. Sources of data such as the nurse's own observations or reports of family and friends of the patient are considered **secondary sources. Tertiary sources** of data include medical records and information gathered from other health care providers such as physical therapists, physicians, or dietitians.

Methods of collecting patient data

A number of methods are used when collecting patient data. The patient interview is a primary means of obtaining both subjective and objective data. The interview typically involves a face-to-face interaction with the patient that requires the nurse to use the skills of interviewing, observation, and listening. Many factors influence the quality of the interview, including the physical environment in which the interaction occurs. If the patient is not in a private room, the open exchange of information may not occur easily. Sometimes the presence of family members constrains the flow of information from a patient, especially when dealing with sensitive or private issues. Similarly, if an interview takes place in a cold, noisy, or public place, the type of data obtained may be affected by environmental distractions. Internal factors related to the patient's condition can influence the amount and the type of data obtained. For example, when interviewing a patient who is having difficulty breathing, the verbal data obtained by the interview may be limited, but careful observation and attentive listening can yield much information about the patient's condition.

Physical examination is the second method for obtaining data. Nurses use physical assessment techniques of inspection, auscultation, percussion, and palpation to obtain these data (Figure 8-2). A third method of obtaining data is through consultation. Consultation is discussing patient needs with health care workers and others who are directly involved in the care of the patient. Nurses

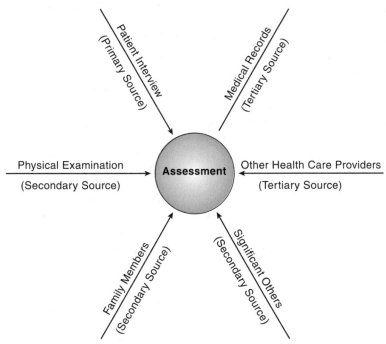

Figure 8-1
Patient data originate from primary, secondary, and tertiary sources.

also consult with patients' families to obtain background information and their perceptions about the patients' needs.

Organizing patient data

Once patient data have been collected, they must be sorted or organized. A number of methods have been developed to assist nurses in organizing patient data. Abdellah's 21 nursing problems, Henderson's 14 nursing problems, Yura and Walsh's human needs approach, and Gordon's 11 functional health patterns are commonly used frameworks for collecting and organizing patient data. Contemporary nursing theorists continue to develop other organizing frameworks, including those of Madeleine Leininger, Sister Callista Roy, Dorothy Orem, and others you will read about in Chapter 13. Nurses choose different methods of organizing patient data depending on personal

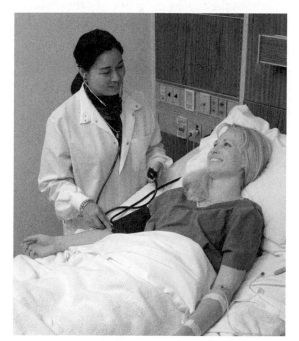

Figure 8-2
Physical examination is a secondary source of objective assessment data. (*Photo courtesy Hamilton Medical Center, Dalton, Georgia.*)

preference and the method used in the agencies where they are employed.

Confidentiality of patient data

A word of caution is needed in regard to patient data. Earlier, it was mentioned that patients confide personal information to nurses only if they believe the nurse is trustworthy. Patients need to know and trust that nurses share such information only with the other treatment team members. Nurses must respect patients' privacy rights and should never discuss patient information with anyone who does not have a work-related need to know. This is not only an ethical issue, but it is also a legal issue. Patients' privacy is now protected by Federal law (see Health Insurance Portability and Accountability Act [HIPAA] on page 99).

A complicating factor in ensuring patients' privacy in the age of information technology is that vast amounts of patient data may be stored and retrieved relatively easily. Although the issues of confidentiality and access to electronically stored data have yet to be fully resolved, each nurse should be entrusted to never violate a patient's privacy by revealing patient information except to other members of that patient's treatment team.

Phase 2: Analysis and Diagnosis

During the data-gathering phase of the nursing process, nurses obtain a great deal of information about their patients. These data must first be validated, and then compared with norms to sort out data that might indicate a problem or identify a pattern. Next, the data must be clustered or grouped so that problems can be identified and their cause discerned. This process is known as data analysis and results in the identification of one or more nursing diagnoses. Knowledge from the biological sciences, social sciences, and nursing enables nurses to analyze relationships among various pieces of patient data.

Nursing diagnosis

Nursing diagnosis was defined by Gordon (1976) as "actual or potential health problems which nurses, by virtue of their education and experience, are capable and licensed to treat" (p. 1299). In 1990 NANDA defined nursing diagnosis as "a clinical judgment about individual, family, or community responses to actual or potential health problems/life processes (which) provide the basis for selection of nursing interventions to achieve outcomes for which the nurse is accountable" (North American Nursing Diagnosis Association, 1990).

NANDA diagnoses.   For 3 decades NANDA has worked to develop a comprehensive list of nursing diagnoses. The composition of NANDA originally included nursing educators, theorists, and practitioners from the United States and Canada who first met in 1973 at the National Conference Group to develop standard terminology, content, and format for nursing diagnoses. The group became NANDA in 1982 and has continued to meet every 2 years to revise the original list of approved diagnoses. After each revision, new diagnoses are tested by nurses in practice settings to evaluate their appropriateness and usefulness. This is a continuing process. Membership in NANDA is now open worldwide to nurses and nursing groups interested in advancing nursing diagnosis. A list of the 2005-2006 NANDA-approved nursing diagnoses can be found on the Evolve website (**www. evolve.elsevier.com/Chitty/professional/**).

NANDA-approved nursing diagnoses consist of five components (NANDA, 2003, pp. 263-264):

1. Label—Concise term or phrase that names the diagnosis
2. Definition—Term or phrase that clearly delineates meaning and helps differentiate from similar diagnoses
3. Defining characteristics—Clusters of observable cues or inferences
4. Risk factors—Factors that increase vulnerability to an unhealthful event
5. Related factors—Factors that precede, are associated with, or relate to the diagnosis

All nursing diagnoses must be supported by data, which NANDA refers to as defining characteristics, also known as signs and symptoms.

Remember that a sign is observable and is objective, whereas a symptom is reported by the patient and is subjective. An easy way to understand the difference is to remember the difference between the words in the commonly used phrase "nausea and vomiting." Nausea is a subjective report of a specific feeling by a patient but is not directly observable by the nurse. Vomiting, on the other hand, is objective, verifiable, and quantifiable. It is a clear sign that the patient's report of nausea (a symptom) was correct.

WRITING NANDA NURSING DIAGNOSES. Accurate diagnosis of human responses is very important. All nursing actions flow from the diagnosis, and inaccurate diagnoses can lead to lost time and wasted resources and may endanger the patient. Accuracy of diagnosis is a professional behavior, one of nursing's accountabilities (Lunney, 2001).

A format used to write the diagnostic statement, called the PES format (Box 8-5), was developed by Gordon (1987). In this format, the P stands for the concise description of the problem, using the NANDA diagnostic label, for example, "ineffective breathing pattern."

The E part of the statement stands for etiology, or cause, and begins with the words "related to." These related factors are conditions or circumstances that can cause or contribute to the development of the problem. To extend the previous example, "ineffective breathing pattern related to anxiety," explains the cause of the ineffective breathing pattern as the patient's high anxiety level. The etiology part of the statement is important, because if the cause were decreased energy or fatigue rather than anxiety, the nurse would

---

Box **8-5** Writing Nursing Diagnoses
P = Problem (NANDA diagnostic label)   E = Etiology (causal factors)   S = Signs and symptoms (defining   characteristics)

need to select different nursing actions to solve the problem. A diagnosis may be technically correct but if the etiology is incorrect, interventions are likely to be ineffective.

The last part of the diagnostic statement is S, which stands for signs and symptoms, or as NANDA calls them, "defining characteristics." Thus the complete diagnostic statement for our sample diagnosis might be "ineffective breathing patterns related to anxiety as manifested by dyspnea, nasal flaring, use of accessory muscles to breathe, and respiratory rate of 24/minute." Some nurses use the phrase "as evidenced by" or "AEB" to preface to the list of defining characteristics.

Prioritizing nursing diagnoses. After diagnoses are identified, the nurse must put them in order of priority. Two common frameworks are used to establish priorities. One of these considers the relative danger to the patient. Using this framework, diagnoses that are life threatening are the nurse's first priority. Next are those that have the potential to cause harm or injury. Last in priority are those diagnoses that are related to the overall general health of the patient. Thus a diagnosis of "ineffective airway clearance" would be dealt with before "sleep pattern disturbance," and "sleep pattern disturbance" could have priority over "knowledge deficit."

Another framework used to prioritize diagnoses is Maslow's (1970) hierarchy of needs (refer to Chapter 12, Figure 12-2). When this framework is used, there is an inverse relationship between high-priority nursing diagnoses and high-level needs. In other words, highest priority is given to diagnoses related to basic physiological needs. Diagnoses related to higher-level needs such as love and belonging or self-esteem, although important, have priority only after basic physiological needs are met.

Except in life-threatening situations, nurses should take care to involve patients in identifying priority diagnoses. Because varied sociocultural factors have a great impact on the manner in which patients prioritize problems, nurses must be aware of these factors and take them into consideration when planning patient care. The nurse's own cultural perspective must not take priority over that of the patient in determining priorities. For example, many maternity nurses are very strong proponents of breastfeeding and consider it one of their priorities in assisting new mothers to establish effective breastfeeding patterns. However, for some women, breastfeeding is not a cultural norm or a desirable outcome of new motherhood. While it may be difficult to understand for the maternity nurse who has expertise in the benefits of breastfeeding, imposing the nurse's cultural and professional perspective on the patient is unacceptable and can lead to diminished effectiveness of nursing care in other domains in which the new mother needs assistance.

Medical diagnosis and nursing diagnosis

Nursing diagnosis is different from medical diagnosis and was never intended to be a substitute for it. Rather than focusing on what is wrong with the patient in terms of a disease process, a nursing diagnosis identifies the problems the patient is experiencing as a result of the disease process, that is, the **human responses** to the illness, injury, or threat.

An important difference between nursing diagnosis and medical diagnosis is that nursing diagnoses address patient problems that nurses can treat legally and within their scope of practice. It would do little good for nursing diagnoses to include "appendicitis" because appendicitis is a medical diagnosis requiring surgery, and nurses may not perform surgery. An appropriate nursing diagnosis for a patient after an appendectomy might be "ineffective airway clearance related to incisional pain." Because it is legal in all states for nurses to provide comfort measures and to assist patients to cough and deep breathe, this would be both an appropriate and a legal nursing diagnosis that is remedied by nursing interventions. The medical diagnosis becomes a platform from which nursing diagnoses are developed: a patient with a new medical diagnosis of diabetes will have some very specific nursing diagnoses and interventions based on the requirements of the medical condition (diabetes) that caused the patient to seek care. Medical and nursing diagnoses are not competing issues; they are related and should lead to both medical and nursing interventions that are complementary and effective.

Phase 3: Planning

Planning is the third phase in the nursing process. Planning begins with identification of patient goals and determination of ways to reach those goals. Goals are used by the patient and the nurse to guide the selection of interventions and to evaluate patient progress. Bloom's taxonomy (as described by Clark, 2001) (Box 8-6) provides a simple description of domains of learning that drive the development of patient goals: psychomotor, cognitive, and affective goals. This taxonomy identified domains of educational activities that are well suited to nursing.

Just as nursing diagnoses are written in collaboration with the patient, goals should also be agreed on by both nurse and patient unless collaboration is impossible, such as when the patient has an altered mental status, is a young child, or is incapacitated in some way. In that event, family members or significant others can collaborate with the nurse. Goals give the patient, family, significant others, and nurse direction and make them active partners.

Writing patient goals and outcomes

The terms goal and objective are frequently used interchangeably. Note that the word "objective" is used differently here than its earlier use as an adjective describing observable and measurable data. In terms of outcomes, the word "objective" is a noun and means a goal or specific aim of intervention. Goals or objectives are statements of what is to be accomplished and are derived from the diagnoses. Because the problem or diagnosis is written as a patient problem, the goal should also be stated in terms of what the patient will do rather than what the nurse will do. The goal begins with the words "the patient will" or "the patient will be able to." The goal sets a general direction, includes an action verb, and should be both attainable and realistic for the patient.

Outcome criteria are specific and make the goal measurable. Outcome criteria define the terms under which the goal is said to be met, partially met, or unmet. Each diagnosis has at least one patient goal, and each patient goal may have several outcome criteria. Effective outcome criteria state under what conditions, to what extent, and in what time frame the patient is to

---

| Box **8-6** | Bloom's Taxonomy |

A taxonomy is a classification system. Bloom, an educator, described types of learning in terms of domains of educational activities. This taxonomy is helpful for nursing:

■ **Psychomotor Domain:** Involves physical movement and increasingly complex activities in the motor-skill arena. Learning in this domain can be assessed by measures such as distance, time, and speed.
Nursing goal: Patient will move from bed to chair 3 times today without assistance.

■ **Cognitive Domain:** Involves knowledge and intellectual skills. Cognitive skills range from simple recall to complex tasks such as synthesis and evaluation.
Nursing goal: Patient will list five signs of illness in her newborn infant by the date of hospital discharge.

■ **Affective Domain:** Involves the emotions, such as feelings, values, and attitudes.
Nursing goal: Patient will describe feeling more accepting of new colostomy within 1 week of providing ostomy self-care.

Setting nursing goals using Bloom's taxonomy is a simple way to address three important domains of the patient's needs. A single patient is likely to have goals in each of these domains.

act. For the postoperative patient who had an abdominal procedure, a sample patient goal with outcome criteria might be, "The patient will have effective bowel elimination as evidenced by having one soft, formed stool every other day without the use of laxatives or enemas within 2 weeks." It is easy to see that this goal is written in terms of what the patient will do (have a bowel movement at least every other day), is measurable (one soft, formed stool), gives conditions (without the use of laxatives or enemas), and has a specified time frame for accomplishment (2 weeks).

Establishing a time frame for patient goals to be met is important. **Short-term goals** may be attainable within hours or days. They are usually specific and are small steps leading to the achievement of broader, long-term goals. For example, "The patient will lose 2 pounds" is a short-term goal, and the time limit for accomplishment can be brief, perhaps a week or 10 days. **Long-term goals,** however, usually represent major changes or rehabilitation. A goal such as "The patient will lose 75 pounds" may take months or perhaps even years to accomplish, and the time frame should be set accordingly. Setting realistic goals in terms of both outcomes and time is extremely important. Frustration and discouragement can occur when goals are unrealistic in outcomes or time.

The nurse can be a good resource for helping patients in determining accessible goals. For example, assume that your patient is a young man with a severely injured thigh and knee from a single-car automobile accident. The injury will require several orthopedic surgeries. To complicate matters, he has a nosocomial (hospital-acquired) infection in his surgical site. One day, he mentions to you that his goal is to run a marathon within a year. Running a marathon is a worthy goal and is reachable eventually for this young man. However, as his nurse, you recognize the importance of setting some short-term goals right now that will improve his health and better the chances of achieving his goal of running a marathon. Your care plan should reflect the short-term, attainable goals (such as walking with a walker the length of the hallway twice a day) that he needs to reach in the meantime that will move him towards his long-term, personal goal.

Cultural congruency is an important consideration in setting patient goals and selecting interventions. A culturally congruent intervention is one that is developed within the broad social, cultural, and demographic context of the patient's life. The patient is more likely to benefit from an intervention that is tailored to his or her specific sociocultural needs and interests. While cultural congruency is an important element to effective intervention, the nurse must take care not to stereotype patients or assume that "all _____" (fill in the blank) like the same things, will react the same way, or respond to the same intervention. The Cultural Consideration Challenge on p. 202 describes three published accounts of nursing situations with specific cultural implications for intervention.

Selecting interventions and writing nursing orders

After short-term and long-term goals are identified through collaboration between nurse and patient, the nurse writes **nursing orders.** Nursing orders are actions designed to assist the patient in achieving a stated goal. Every goal has specific nursing orders, which may be carried out by a registered nurse (RN) or delegated to other members of the nursing staff.

Nursing orders and medical orders differ. Nursing orders refer to interventions that are designed to treat the patient's response to an illness or medical treatment, whereas medical orders are designed to treat the actual illness or disease. An example of a nursing order is "Teach turning, coughing, and deep-breathing exercises prior to surgery." These activities are designed to prevent postoperative respiratory problems caused by immobility. They are appropriate nursing orders because prevention of complications due to immobility is a nursing responsibility. Nursing orders may include instructions about consultation with other health care providers, such as the dietitian, physical therapist, or pharmacist.

Cultural Considerations *Challenge*

Impact of Culture on Nursing Interventions

These articles (one clinical issue and two research papers) demonstrate the recognition of the impact of culture on three different groups of patients in planning interventions.

- Jewish patients and their families had a wider view of the Jewish community as part of a cohesive family during end-of-life care than hospice professionals did in a qualitative study of 11 professional hospice caregivers and 5 Jewish family members who had used hospice services. The professional staff considered only the patient and family members as a group and did not include the community. The authors found that professional caregivers needed to restructure their care "to preserve and accommodate those values and beliefs that strengthen the meaning of life and death for individuals and families." Leininger's cultural care theory was the theoretical framework used to guide this study (Bonura, Fender, and Roesler, 2003).

- Using a social support framework, researchers examined the feasibility of the use of a pregnancy support website for low-income African-American women. Basing their work on the issue of health disparity in which African-American women have a disproportionate number of low–birth-weight infants, these researchers developed a culturally congruent website that provided information on pregnancy-related health behaviors and other pregnancy issues. They found that the women used the website and that the discussion board was the most effective way of delivering informative social support. The "ask-a-nurse" page was also popular. The researchers found that younger women, who may be more comfortable with computers, were the heaviest users of this novel intervention (Herman, Mock, Blackwell et al, 2005).

- With the increase in the numbers of Mexican immigrants to the United States, nurses need to be aware of the challenges related to social support for childbearing women who may not understand English well. These Mexican women may have few, if any, close relatives and may be unaware of American childbirth customs. The authors suggested that the primary short-term goal for the woman is to be able to trust her health care provider. Nurses who have knowledge of the social support needs of their Mexican patients can help the patient prevent emotional distress by identifying resources for social support. Educational interventions such as childbirth classes offered in Spanish are particularly useful. The authors suggest that inclusion of interventions in prenatal care that enhance a woman's social support may increase the likelihood of good adjustment to motherhood (Martinez-Schallmoser, MacMullen, and Telleen, 2005).

Adapted from Bonura D, Fender M, Roesler M: Culturally congruent end-of-life care for Jewish patients and their families. In Neville K, editor: *The research connection: the psychosocial and nursing advisory board to the New Jersey Commission on Cancer Research*, Vol 1, Trenton, NJ, 2003, State of New Jersey Commission on Cancer Research; Herman J, Mock K, Blackwell D et al: Use of a pregnancy support web site by low-income African American women, *JOGNN* 34(6):713-720, 2005; Martinez-Schallmoser L, MacMullen NJ, Telleen S: Social support in Mexican American childbearing women, *JOGNN* 34(6):755-760, 2005.

Types of nursing interventions.   Nursing interventions are of three basic types: independent, dependent, or interdependent. **Independent interventions** are those for which the nurse's intervention requires no supervision or direction by others. Nurses are expected to possess the knowledge and skills to carry out independent actions safely. An example of an independent nursing intervention is teaching a patient how to examine her breasts for lumps. The nurse practice act of each state usually specifies general types of independent nursing actions.

Dependent interventions do require instructions, written orders, or supervision of another health professional, usually a physician. These actions require knowledge and skills on the part of the nurse but may not be done without explicit directions. An example of a dependent nursing intervention is the administration of medications. Although a physician or advanced practice nurse must order medications in in-patient settings, it is the responsibility of the nurse to know how to administer them safely and to monitor their effectiveness. The nurse also must question orders that he or she feels are incongruent with safe care or are not within accepted standards of care.

The third type, **interdependent interventions,** includes actions in which the nurse must collaborate or consult with another health professional before carrying out the action. One example of this type of action is the nurse implementing orders that have been written by a physician in a protocol. **Protocols** define under what conditions and circumstances a nurse is allowed to treat the patient, as well as what treatments are permissible. They are used in situations in which nurses need to take immediate action without consulting with a physician, such as in an emergency department, a critical care unit, or a home setting.

Writing the plan of care

Once interventions are selected, a written plan of care is devised. Some health care agencies use individually developed plans of care for their patients. The nurse creates and develops a plan for each patient. Others use standardized plans of care that are based on common and recurring problems. The nurse then individualizes these standard plans of care. An advantage of using standardized plans is that they can decrease the time spent in generating a completely new plan each time a patient is seen. These plans are easily computer-generated, with the nurse making selections from menus to individualize the plan to the particular patient. The amount of time needed to update and document these plans is then vastly decreased. Computer use also facilitates data collection for research.

Because of the decreasing average length of stay for patients in health care facilities, the increasing focus on achieving timely patient outcomes in the specific time frame permitted by reimbursement systems, and the emphasis by accrediting bodies on multidisciplinary care, many agencies adopted the use of multidisciplinary plans of care known as **critical paths,** care tracks, or care maps. A critical path for congestive heart failure can be found on the Evolve website (**www.evolve.elsevier.com/Chitty/professional**). Critical paths have been replaced with other types of multidisciplinary care plans in some settings. Whatever the type in use in a given setting, multidisciplinary care plans are written in collaboration with physicians and other health care providers and establish a sequence of short-term daily outcomes that are easily measured. This type of care planning facilitates communication and collaboration among all members of the health care team. It also permits comparisons of outcomes between treatment plans as well as among health care facilities. As with the nursing process, unyielding adherence to the critical path without taking a patient's idiosyncratic responses into consideration can negatively affect patient outcomes and is a detriment to successful nursing care.

The development of appropriate plans of care depends on the nurse's ability to employ critical thinking. Nurses must be able to analyze information and arguments, make reasoned decisions, recognize many viewpoints, and question and seek answers continuously. At the same time, nurses must be logical, flexible, and creative and take initiative while considering the holistic nature of each patient.

Phase 4: Implementation of Planned Interventions

Implementation, the fourth phase or operation of the nursing process, occurs when nursing orders are actually carried out. Most people think of nursing as "doing something" for or to a patient. Notice, however, that in using the nursing process, nurses do a great deal of thinking, analyzing, and planning before the first actual nursing action takes place.

Professional nurses understand the crucial nature of the first three phases of the nursing process in ensuring that safe and appropriate care occurs. Nurses who forgo these essential phases and move immediately into action are not providing care in a responsible, professional manner. Patients feel a greater sense of trust in nurses who are providing care when dependent, independent, and interdependent orders are planned and carried out in an orderly, competent manner. Common nursing interventions include such actions as managing pain, preventing postoperative complications, educating patients, and performing procedures (such as wound care and catheter insertion) that are ordered by other health care providers. As the nurse carries out planned interventions, he or she is continually assessing the patient, noting responses to nursing interventions and modifying the care plan or adding nursing diagnoses as needed. Documentation of nursing actions is an integral part of the implementation phase.

Phase 5: Evaluation

Evaluation is the final phase of the nursing process. In this phase, the nurse examines the patient's progress in relation to the goals and outcome criteria to determine whether a problem is resolved, is in the process of being resolved, or is unresolved. In other words, the outcome criteria are the basis for evaluation of the goal. Evaluation

may reveal that data, diagnosis, goals, and nursing interventions were all on target and that the problem is resolved.

Evaluation may also indicate a need for a change in the plan of care. Perhaps inadequate patient data were the basis for the plan, and further assessment has uncovered additional needs. The nursing diagnoses may have been incorrect or placed in the wrong order of priority. Patient goals may have been inappropriate or unattainable within the designated time frame. It is possible that nursing actions were incorrectly implemented.

Evaluation is a critical phase in the nursing process and one that is often slighted. The best nursing care plan is one that is evaluated frequently and changed in response to the patient's condition. Sometimes a care plan will reflect all of the most common nursing interventions used to treat specific diagnoses; it is not enough, however, to continue to do the "right things" if the patient is not improving in the expected manner. If, on evaluation, the problem is not resolving in a timely way or will not resolve at all, the nursing care plan must be revised to reflect the necessary changes.

In addition to evaluating the individual plan of care, nurses are responsible for evaluating the quality of care that all patients receive. Several terms are currently used for this process, including total quality management (TQM), continuous quality improvement (CQI), and quality improvement (QI). Regardless of the terminology, the goal is the same: to improve health care and the way in which it is delivered.

DYNAMIC NATURE OF THE NURSING PROCESS

Although the phases in the nursing process are discussed separately here, in practice they are not so clearly delineated nor do they always proceed from one to another in a linear fashion. As seen in Figure 8-3, the nursing process is dynamic, meaning that nurses are continuously moving from one phase to another and then beginning the process again. Often a nurse performs two or more

Assessment

Analysis of
data/formulation
of nursing
diagnosis

Evaluation

Nursing care
planning/
outcomes
identification

Implementation
of care plan

Figure 8-3
The nursing process is a dynamic, nonlinear tool for
critical thinking about human responses.

phases at the same time, for instance, observing a
wound for signs of infection (assessment) while
changing the dressing on the wound (intervention)
and asking the patient the extent to which pain has
been relieved by comfort measures (evaluation).

Now that you have read about the phases of
the nursing process, we will look back at the
opening scenario. The problem that was identified was the necessity to wear appropriate
clothing. Data, both objective (the temperature
outdoors) and subjective (the mood one is in),
were gathered. Selection was made and implemented, and an evaluation of the implementation was carried out by looking in the mirror.
This comparison reveals that problem solving is
something each person does every day. The use of
the nursing process simply provides professional
nurses with a patient-oriented framework with
which to solve clinical problems.

An example of using the nursing process in a
high-priority clinical situation is described in
Box 8-7. This case study demonstrates how using
the nursing process becomes so natural that
experienced nurses go through the phases fluidly
and automatically. While no responsible nurse
would take the time to write out this care plan in
advance of acting on a diagnosis of "ineffective
airway clearance," you should understand that the
nursing process is exactly the same for those high-

priority nursing situations that require immediate action and those that will evolve over time.

DEVELOPING CLINICAL JUDGMENT IN NURSING

Becoming an effective nurse involves more than
critical thinking and the ability to use the nursing
process. It depends heavily on developing excellent **clinical judgment.** Clinical judgment consists of informed opinions and decisions based
on empirical knowledge and experience. Nurses
develop clinical judgment gradually as they gain
a broader, deeper knowledge base and clinical
experience. Extensive direct patient contact is the
best means of developing clinical judgment.

Critical thinking and clinical reasoning used
in the nursing process are both important aspects
of clinical judgment. A nurse who has developed
sound clinical judgment knows what to look for
(e.g., elevation of temperature in a surgical
patient), draws valid conclusions about possible
alternative meanings of signs and symptoms (e.g.,
postoperative infection, atelectasis, dehydration),
and knows what to do about it (e.g., listen to
breath sounds, assess for dehydration, check
incision for redness and drainage, seek another
opinion, notify the physician). Developing sound
clinical judgment requires recalling facts, recognizing patterns in patient behaviors, putting facts
and observations together to form a meaningful
whole, and acting on the resulting information in
an appropriate way.

Knowing the limitations of your expertise is
an important aspect of clinical judgment. Most
nurses have an instinctive awareness of when
they are approaching the limits of their expertise
and will seek consultation with other professionals as needed. Your state's nurse practice act,
health agency policies, school policies, and the
professions' standards of practice all provide
guidance in making the decision about nursing
actions within your scope of practice. Nursing
students, whether new to nursing or registered
nurses in baccalaureate programs, must consider
policies and standards in determining their scope
of practice in any given nursing situation.

Box **8-7** Nursing Process Case Study of a High-Priority Diagnosis

You have just received a report from the day shift about Mr. Burkes. You were told that he had been admitted with a diagnosis of cancer of the tongue and that he had a radical neck dissection yesterday. He has a tracheostomy and requires frequent suctioning of his secretions. He is alert and responds by nodding his head or writing short notes.

When you enter his room, you note that he is apprehensive and tachypneic, and is gesturing for you to come into the room. You auscultate his lungs and note coarse crackles and expiratory wheezes. You can see thick secretions bubbling out of his tracheostomy. He has poor cough effort.

Based on these data, you realize that a priority nursing diagnosis is ineffective airway clearance. You immediately prepare to perform tracheal suctioning. As you are suctioning, you watch the patient's nonverbal responses and note that he is less apprehensive when the suctioning is completed. You also auscultate the lungs and note that there are decreased crackles and that the expiratory wheezes are no longer present. Mr. Burkes writes "I can breathe now" on his note pad.

  I. Assessment
   A. Subjective data
      1. None because of inability to speak
   B. Objective data
      1. Tracheostomy with copious, thick secretions
      2. Tachypnea
      3. Gesturing for help
      4. Coarse crackles and expiratory wheezes
      5. Poor cough effort
 II. Analysis
   A. Ineffective airway clearance related to copious, thick secretions
III. Plan
   A. Short-term goal: Patient will maintain patent airway as evidenced by absence of expiratory wheezes and crackles, decreased signs of anxiety and air hunger.
   B. Long-term goal: Patient will have patent airway as evidenced by his ability to clear the airway without the use of suctioning by the time of discharge.
IV. Implementation
   A. Assess lung sounds every hour for crackles and wheezes.
   B. Suction airway as needed.
   C. Elevate head of bed to 45 degrees.
   D. Teach patient abdominal breathing techniques.
   E. Encourage patient to cough out secretions.
 V. Evaluation
   A. Short-term goal: Achieved as evidenced by decreased crackles and absent wheezes when auscultating the lungs; patient appears less anxious, indicated by writing that he "can breathe now."
   B. Long-term goal: Will be evaluated before discharge.

Box **8-8** Clinical Judgment: Nine Key Questions

1. **What major outcomes (observable beneficial results) do we expect to see in this particular person, family, or group when the plan of care is terminated?** Example: The person will be discharged without complications, able to care for himself, 3 days after surgery. Outcomes may be addressed on a standard plan, or you may have to develop these outcomes yourself. Make sure any predetermined outcomes in standard plans are appropriate to your patient's specific situation.

2. **What problems or issues must be addressed to achieve the major outcomes? Answering this question will help you prioritize.** You may have a long list of actual or potential health problems needing to be structured in order to set your priorities.

3. **What are the circumstances?** Who is involved (e.g., child, adult, group)? How urgent are the problems (e.g., life-threatening, chronic)? What are the factors influencing their presentation (e.g., when, where, and how did the problems develop)? What are the patient's values, beliefs, and cultural influences?

4. **What knowledge is required?** You must know problem-specific facts (e.g., how problems usually present, how they are diagnosed, what their common causes and risk factors are, what common complications occur, and how these complications are prevented and managed); nursing process and related knowledge and skills (e.g., ethics, research, health assessment, communication, priority setting); related sciences (e.g., anatomy, physiology, pathophysiology, pharmacology, chemistry, physics, psychology, sociology). You must also be clearly aware of the circumstances, as addressed in question 3 above.

5. **How much room is there for error?** In the clinical setting, there is usually minimal room for error. However, it depends on the health of the individual and the risks of interventions. A healthy, young postoperative patient with no chronic illnesses may tolerate early mobility after surgery better than an elderly person with a history of multiple chronic problems requiring numerous medications. While their orders for postoperative ambulation may be identical and your commitment to their safe care exactly the same for these two patients, excellent clinical judgment based on your assessments allows you to conclude that the young patient is safe walking in the hallway with a family member, while the elderly patient needs your assistance and guidance during early ambulation.

6. **How much time do I have?** Time frame for decision making depends on (1) the urgency of the problems (e.g., there is little time in life-threatening situations, such as cardiac arrest) and (2) the planned length of contact (e.g., if your patient will be hospitalized only for 2 days, you have to be realistic about what can be accomplished, and key decisions need to be made early).

7. **What resources can help me?** Human resources include clinical nurse educators, nursing faculty, preceptors, experienced nurses, advanced practice nurses, peers, librarians, and other health care professionals (such as pharmacists, nutritionists, physical therapists, physicians). The patient and family are also valuable resources (usually they know their own problems best). Other resources include texts, articles, other references, computer databases, decision-making support, national practice guidelines, and facility documents (e.g., guidelines, policies, procedures, assessment forms).

8. **Whose perspectives must be considered?** The most significant perspective to consider is the patient's point of view. Other important perspectives include those of the family and significant others, caregivers, and relevant third parties (e.g., insurers).

9. **What is influencing my thinking?** Identify your personal biases and any other factors influencing your critical thinking and therefore your clinical judgment.

From Alfaro-LeFevre R: *Critical thinking in nursing: a practical approach*, ed 2, Philadelphia, 1999, WB Saunders. Reprinted with permission.

Box 8-9 **Self-Assessment: Developing Sound Clinical Judgment**

Answer the following questions honestly. When finished, make a list of the items you need to work on in your quest to develop sound clinical judgment. Keep the list with you and review it frequently. Seek opportunities to practice needed activities.

1. Use References
   - Do I look up new terms when I encounter them to make them part of my vocabulary?
   - Do I familiarize myself with normal findings so that I can recognize those outside the norm?
   - Do I use research findings and base my practice on scientific evidence?
   - Do I learn the signs and symptoms of various conditions, what causes them, and how they are managed?
2. Use the Nursing Process
   - Do I always assess before acting, stay focused on outcomes, and make changes as needed?
   - Do I always base my judgments on fact, not emotion or hearsay?
3. Assess Systematically
   - Do I have a systematic approach to assessing patients to decrease the likelihood that I will overlook important data?
4. Set Priorities Systematically
   - Do I evaluate both the problem and the probable cause before acting?
   - Am I willing to obtain assistance from a more knowledgeable source when indicated?
5. Refuse to Act Without Knowledge
   - Do I refuse to perform an action when I do not know the indication, why it works, and what risks there are for harm to this particular patient?
6. Use Resources Wisely
   - Do I look for opportunities to learn from others, such as teachers, other experts, or even my peers?
   - Do I seek help when needed, being mindful of patient privacy issues?
7. Know Standards of Care
   - Do I read facility policies, professional standards, school policies, and state board of nursing rules and regulations to determine my scope of practice?
   - Do I know the clinical agency's policies and procedures affecting my particular patients?
   - Do I attempt to understand the rationales behind policies and procedures?
   - Do I follow policies and procedures carefully, recognizing that they are designed to help me use good judgment?
8. Know Technology and Equipment
   - Do I routinely learn how to use patient technology such as IV pumps, patient monitors, computers?
   - Do I learn how to check equipment for proper functioning and safety?
9. Give Patient-Centered Care
   - Do I always remember the needs and feelings of the patient, family, and significant others?
   - Do I value knowing my patients' health beliefs and values within their own cultural contexts?
   - Do I "go the extra mile" for patients?
   - Do I demonstrate the belief that every patient deserves my very best efforts?

Adapted from Alfaro-LeFevre R: *Critical thinking in nursing: a practical approach*, ed 2, Philadelphia, 1999, WB Saunders, pp 88-92. Used with permission.

Communication and Collaboration in Nursing

Kay Kittrell Chitty

Learning Outcomes

After studying this chapter, students will be able to:

- Describe therapeutic use of self.
- Identify and describe the phases of the traditional nurse-patient relationship.
- Explore the role self-awareness plays in the ability to use nonjudgmental acceptance as a helping technique.
- Identify their own communication strengths and challenges.
- Discuss factors creating successful or unsuccessful communication.

- Explain the concept of professional boundaries.
- Differentiate between therapeutic and social relationships.
- Evaluate helpful and unhelpful communication.
- Demonstrate components of active listening.
- Identify key prerequisites of collaboration.
- Explain the impact of gender and cultural diversity on nurse-patient and other professional relationships.

Interpersonal skills are very important to professional nurses. Regardless of the settings in which they work and the roles they assume within those settings, most nurses interact with many people every day. The way in which they relate to patients, families, colleagues, and other professionals and nonprofessionals determines the level of comfort and trust others feel and, ultimately, the success of their interactions. All the clinical skills in the world cannot overcome poor interpersonal relationships. This chapter includes information that can enhance the development of self-awareness, nonjudgmental acceptance of others, communication skills, and collaboration skills, all of which are essential components of effective interpersonal relationships in nursing.

THERAPEUTIC USE OF SELF

Hildegard Peplau, a pioneer in nursing theory development, first focused on the importance of the nurse-patient relationship in her 1952 book *Interpersonal Relations in Nursing*. She called using one's personality and communication skills to help patients improve their health status "therapeutic use of self" (Peplau, 1952).

The ability to use oneself therapeutically can be developed. Nurses develop this ability by acquiring certain knowledge, attitudes, and skills that assist them in relating effectively to patients, patients' families, co-workers, and other health care professionals.

The Traditional Nurse-Patient Relationship

The nursing process can begin only after the nurse and patient establish their initial therapeutic **nurse-patient relationship.** Awareness of the three identifiable phases of the nurse-patient relationship helps nurses to be realistic in their expectations of this important relationship. Each of three phases—orientation, working, and termination—is sequential and builds on previous phases.

The orientation phase

The **orientation phase,** or introductory phase, is the period often described as "getting to know you" in social settings. Relationships between nurses and their patients have much in common with other types of relationships. The chief similarity is that there must be trust between the two parties for the relationship to develop. Nurses cannot expect patients to trust them automatically and to reveal their innermost thoughts and feelings immediately.

During the orientation phase, nurse and patient assess one another. Early impressions made by the nurse are important. Some people have difficulty accepting help of any kind, including nursing care. Putting the patient at ease with a pleasant, unhurried approach is important during the early part of any nurse-patient relationship.

During the orientation phase, the patient has a right to expect to learn the nurse's name, credentials, and extent of responsibility. The use of simple orienting statements is one way to begin: "Good morning, Mr. Davis. I am Jennifer Carter, and I am your nurse until noon today. I am responsible for your total care while I am here."

Developing trust. The orientation phase includes the beginning development of trust. Notice the use of the term "beginning develop-

ment." Full development of trust is slow and may take months of regular contact. A fact of contemporary nursing practice is that patient interactions may be brief, sometimes lasting only minutes. However, even in the most abbreviated contacts, nurses must orient patients and help them feel comfortable and as trusting as possible.

Certain behaviors help patients develop trust in the nurse. A straightforward, nondefensive manner is important. Answering all questions as fully as possible and admitting to the limits of your knowledge also facilitate trust. Promise to find out the answers to all questions and report the information to the patient as soon as possible. Meet with patients at the designated times or make arrangements to let them know of a change in plans. Use active listening behaviors and accept the patient's thoughts and feelings without judgment.

Congruence between verbal and nonverbal communication is a key factor in the development of trust. Communicating in a congruent manner requires that nurses be aware of their own thoughts and feelings and be able to share those with others in a nonthreatening manner. The self-assessment of communication patterns in Box 9-1 is the type of activity that can help improve self-awareness.

Developing an initial understanding of the patient's problem or needs also starts in the orientation phase. Because patients themselves often do not clearly understand their problems or may be reluctant to discuss them, nurses must use their communication skills to elicit the information needed in order to make a nursing diagnosis. Communication skills useful in nurse-patient interactions are discussed later in this chapter.

Tasks of the orientation phase. By the end of a successful orientation phase, regardless of its length, several things will have happened. First, the patient will have developed enough trust in the nurse to continue to participate in the relationship. Second, the patient and nurse will see each other as individuals, unique from all others and worthy of one another's respect. Third, the patient's perception of major problems and needs will have been identified. And fourth, the

Box 9-1 **Communication Patterns Self-Assessment**

Directions: Answer the following true-or-false questions as honestly as possible; then review your answers and draw at least two conclusions about your habitual communication patterns. Check your conclusions for accuracy with a friend who knows your style of communicating well.

1. I usually listen about as much as I talk.
2. I rarely interrupt others.
3. I pay close attention to what others say.
4. I usually make eye contact with the person I am talking with.
5. I can usually tell if someone is angry or upset.
6. I would hesitate to interrupt someone to ask for clarification.
7. People often tell me personal things about themselves.
8. I find it is best to change the subject if someone gets too emotional.
9. If I can't "make things better" for a friend with a problem, I feel uncomfortable.
10. I am comfortable talking with people much older or much younger than I am.
11. When there is conflict, I tend to:
    a. avoid.
    b. verbally attack.
    c. give in.
    d. become autocratic.

approximate length of the relationship will have been estimated, and the nurse and patient will have agreed to work together on some aspect of the identified problems. This agreement, whether formalized in writing or informally agreed upon, is sometimes called a "contract." An example of a contract that might emerge from the orientation phase of the relationship with a patient newly diagnosed with diabetes is an agreement to work together on his ability to calculate and inject his daily insulin requirement.

The working phase

The second phase of the nurse-patient relationship is called the **working phase,** because it is during this time that the nurse and patient tackle tasks outlined in the previous phase. Because the participants now know each other to some extent, there may be a sense of interpersonal comfort in the relationship that did not exist earlier.

Nurses should recognize that in the working phase patients may exhibit alternating periods of intense effort and periods of resistance to change. Continuing the example of the patient with dia-

betes, the nurse can anticipate that he will experience some degree of difficulty in accepting the life changes the illness causes. He may show progress in learning to give himself insulin one week but not be able to demonstrate injection technique the next week. Nurses who become frustrated when a patient's progress toward self-care is not smooth and sustained must realize that regression is an ego defense mechanism that occurs as a reaction to stress and that regression often precedes periods of positive behavioral change.

It is difficult to make and sustain change. Patience, self-awareness, and maturity are required of nurses during the working phase. Continued building of trust, use of active listening, and other helpful communication responses facilitate the patient's expression of needs and feelings during the working phase.

The termination phase

The **termination phase** includes those activities that enable the patient and the nurse to end the relationship in a therapeutic manner. The process of terminating the nurse-patient relationship begins in the orientation phase when participants estimate the length of time it will take to accomplish the desired outcomes. This is part of the informal contract.

As in any relationship, positive and negative feelings often accompany termination. The patient and nurse feel good about the gains the patient has made in accomplishing goals. They may feel sadness about ending a relationship that has been open and trusting. People tend to respond to the end of relationships in much the same way they have responded to other losses in life. Feelings of anger and fear may surface, in addition to sadness.

Feelings evoked by termination should be discussed and accepted. Summarizing the gains the patient has made is an important activity during this phase. The importance of the relationship to both patient and nurse can be shared in a caring manner.

The giving and receiving of gifts at termination has different meanings for different people. The meaning of such behavior should be explored in a sensitive manner, and the agency's policies on gifts should be consulted.

Because termination is often painful, participants are sometimes tempted to continue the relationship on a social basis, and requests for addresses, phone numbers, and e-mail addresses are not uncommon. The nurse must realize that professional relationships are different from social relationships. It is not helpful to stay in touch with patients following termination of a professional nurse-patient relationship. Other differences between social and professional relationships are outlined in Box 9-2.

During the course of a professional career, every nurse will experience countless nurse-patient relationships, each with its own meaning and duration. If nurses can view each new relationship both as an opportunity to assist another human being to grow and change in a positive, healthful way and as a challenge to grow and change themselves, the rewards of nursing will be rich indeed.

Developing Self-Awareness

Awareness of oneself, called self-awareness, is basic to effective interpersonal relationships, especially the nurse-patient relationship. Robert

---

Box 9-2 **Differences in Social and Professional Relationships**

Social Relationships

- Evolve spontaneously
- Not time-limited
- Not necessarily goal-directed; broad purpose is pleasure, companionship, sharing
- Centered on meeting both parties' needs
- Problem solving is rarely/occasionally a focus
- May or may not include nonjudgmental acceptance
- Outcome is pleasure for both parties

Professional Relationships

- Evolve through recognized phases; use planned and purposeful interactions
- Limited in time with termination date often predetermined
- Goal-directed; systematic exploration of identified problem areas
- Centered on meeting patient's needs; does not address nurse's needs
- Problem solving is a primary focus
- Includes nonjudgmental acceptance
- Outcome is improved health status of patient

Burns, the eighteenth-century Scottish poet, described the rarity of true self-awareness in his poem "To a Louse": "Oh wad some Power the giftie gie us/To see oursels as ithers see us!" (Barke, 1955).

As Burns knew, few people have the innate capacity to recognize their own emotional needs, biases, and blind spots, as well as their impact on others. With practice, however, most can become more effective in doing so, thus improving self-awareness.

An important guideline in professional nursing is this: nurses should get their own emotional needs met outside of the nurse-patient relationship. When nurses' strong unmet needs for acceptance, approval, friendship, or even love enter into their relationships with patients, professionalism is lost, and relationships become social in nature. Becoming aware of one's needs and making conscious efforts to meet those needs in private life make professional, therapeutic relationships with patients possible. As discussed earlier and summarized in Box 9-2, there are important differences in social and professional relationships.

The subject of professional boundaries was explored in a brochure published by the National Council of State Boards of Nursing (1996). It defined **professional boundaries** as "the spaces between the nurse's power and the client's vulnerability. The power of the nurse comes from the professional position and the access to private knowledge about the client" (p. 1). Boundary violations occur when "there is confusion between the needs of the nurse and those of the client" (p. 2).

According to the NCSBN brochure, nurse-patient relationships can be plotted on a continuum of professional behavior that ranges from underinvolvement (such as distancing, disinterest, neglect) through a zone of helpfulness to over-involvement (such as excessive personal disclosure by the nurse, secrecy, role reversal, or sexual misconduct). Both underinvolvement and over-involvement can be detrimental to patient and nurse (p. 3). Box 9-3 describes a case in which a nurse was disciplined by his state board of nursing for failing to honor the professional boundaries between a nurse and patient.

Box 9-4 contains seven "guiding principles to determining professional boundaries and the continuum of professional behavior" (p. 4) from the NCSBN brochure. The brochure was so often requested that the NCSBN has now developed an entire continuing educational module about professional boundaries. It is offered online for continuing education (CE) credit (http://www.learningext.com/products/generalce/boundaries/boundariesabout.asp).

Nurses care for a diverse array of patients whose values, beliefs, and lifestyles may challenge the nurses' own. Patients sometimes are attractive or repellant to nurses. Sometimes nurses find themselves meeting their own needs to be liked or needed through relationships with patients. Nurses who have emotional reactions to patients, positive or negative, sometimes feel disturbed or guilty about these feelings. Part of self-awareness is recognizing one's feelings and understanding that although feelings cannot be controlled, behaviors can. Effective nurses control their behavior to prevent their own prejudices, beliefs, and needs from intruding into nurse-patient relationships.

Avoiding Stereotypes

Stereotypes are prejudices and attitudes developed through interactions with family, friends, and others in each individual's social and cultural system. It is not uncommon for even well-educated professionals to have stereotypical expectations of groups of people different from themselves. These stereotypes are established through childhood experiences and affect relationships with people in the stereotyped group. Because stereotypes and prejudices tend to persist despite contrary experiences, they are irrational, or illogical, beliefs.

The subtle intrusion of stereotyped expectations into the nurse-patient relationship can cause disturbed patterns of relating. For example, the expectation that elderly people are irritable

Box 9-3 **Legal Note: Nurse's Relationship With Patient Results in Disciplinary Action**

Tapp v. Board of Registered Nursing, 2002 WL 31820206 P.2d -CA

This case involved a California registered nurse at a psychiatric facility in Fresno who was accused of having sexual relations with his former patient following her discharge. The patient was hospitalized for emotional problems related to sex. She was hospitalized on a unit where the nurse worked the night shift. They became friendly; he brought her small gifts, gave her his telephone number, and called her during his off-work hours. After she was discharged, they spoke often by telephone and he began to visit her at her apartment. On one occasion, the nurse gave her a tablet of a controlled substance.

One week following her discharge, they began a sexual relationship that lasted for 2 weeks. Shortly after the relationship ended, the patient was readmitted, "suffering adverse effects from the affair" (p. 4). The California Board of Registered Nursing initiated disciplinary proceedings for "acts of unprofessional conduct." An administrative law judge heard testimony, made a determination of misconduct, and recommended that the nurse's license be revoked, but stayed the revocation and recommended that the nurse be placed on probation for 5 years on multiple conditions. The California Board of Registered Nursing disagreed and ordered the revocation of his license. There were subsequent appeals, dismissals, and further appeals.

Nurses must realize that there can be no socialization between themselves and patients, particularly sexual in nature. Not only was this nurse's behavior with this patient during her hospitalization "highly improper, but his socialization with the patient after her discharge from the hospital, not to mention the fact that he provided the patient with a controlled substance, was ample reason to impose strict disciplinary action" (p. 5).

Abstracted from Nurse's Relationship with Patient Results in Disciplinary Action: *Nursing Law's Regan Report* 43(8):4-5, 2003.

Box 9-4 **Principles for Determining Professional Boundaries**

1. The nurse, not the patient, is responsible for delineating and maintaining boundaries.
2. The nurse should work within the "zone of helpfulness," which is neither aloof or too intense/emotionally involved.
3. The nurse should examine any boundary crossing, be aware of its potential implications, and avoid repeated crossings.
4. Variables such as the care setting, community influences, client needs, and the nature of therapy affect the delineation of boundaries.
5. Actions that overstep established boundaries to meet the needs of the nurse are boundary violations.
6. The nurse should avoid dual relationships in which the nurse has a personal or business relationship, as well as the professional one.
7. Post-termination relationships are complex because the client may need additional services, and it may be difficult to determine when the nurse-client relationship is truly terminated.

Adapted from National Council of State Boards of Nursing: *Professional boundaries: a nurse's guide to the importance of appropriate professional boundaries*, Chicago, 1996, NCSBN.

and demanding may cause the nurse to avoid elderly patients or to treat their complaints as unimportant: "just another grumpy old person."

Professional nurses deliver high-quality care to all patients regardless of ethnicity, age, gender, religion, lifestyle, or diagnosis. The *Code of Ethics for Nurses* (see inside back cover of this text) calls upon nurses to do this. Nurses are not without stereotypes and prejudices, however, and must strive to be aware of their own irrational feelings toward patients. Every professional nurse's goal is to accept all patients as individuals of dignity and worth who deserve the best nursing care possible.

Becoming Nonjudgmental

Acceptance is not always easy, because prejudices are strong and are often outside our awareness. This means that judging others as "good" or "bad" may occur automatically, usually unconsciously. It is important to remember that acceptance conveys neither approval nor disapproval of patients and their personal beliefs, habits, expressions of feelings, or chosen lifestyles. **Nonjudgmental acceptance** means that nurses acknowledge all patients' rights to be different and to express their "differentness."

Therapeutic use of self begins with the ability to convey acceptance to patients and requires self-awareness and nonjudgmental attitudes on the part of nurses. Ongoing examination of attitudes toward others is both a lifelong process and an essential part of self-awareness and interpersonal growth.

Reconceptualizing the Nurse-Patient Relationship: Theory of Human Relatedness

The type of nurse-patient relationship (NPR) discussed in the previous section is the traditional model taught and practiced since the middle of the twentieth century. It is based on several assumptions that no longer hold true in many settings where nurses practice in today's fast-paced health care system. These assumptions are as follows (Hagerty and Patusky, 2003):

■ The NPR is linear and proceeds through several phases, each building on the preceding one.

■ Building trust is essential during early phases of the NPR.

■ Time and repeated contacts are required to establish an effective NPR.

■ Patients desire relationships with nurses, wish to receive services from them, and will cooperate and comply with those nurses.

Although the traditional, time-honored NPR is still appropriate in many settings, the assumptions on which it is based are being challenged by today's health care realities. The reality is that patients today are more acutely ill, nurses' workloads have increased, and the time nurses spend with patients may be quite limited, sometimes to only one or two contacts. Are these more limited NP contacts therefore doomed, or can we rethink the NPR and find ways to modify it to suit today's streamlined caregiving contexts?

Hagerty and Patusky (2003) proposed reconceptualizing the NPR using the theory of human relatedness as a framework. They recommended approaching each nurse-patient contact as an opportunity for connection and goal achievement rather than as one step in a lengthy relationship-building process. They also recommended that nurses approach their patients with a sense of the patient's autonomy, choice, and participation (p. 147), putting the relationship on a more equitable basis than the traditional nurse-patient relationship, which gives much of the power to the nurse. Research into these concepts continues.

These ideas can form the basis for classroom discussion and provide "new insights and opportunities for assessment, intervention, and research toward positive, hopeful, and efficacious nursing care" (Hagerty and Patusky, 2003, p. 149).

COMMUNICATION THEORY

Communication is the exchange of thoughts, ideas, or information and is at the heart of all relationships. Communication is a dynamic process that is the primary instrument through which change occurs in nursing situations. Nurses use their communication skills in all phases of the nursing process. These skills are vital to effective nursing care and to effective interaction with others in health care.

Jurgen Ruesch (1972, p. 16), a pioneer communications theorist, defined communication as "all the modes of behavior that one individual employs, conscious or unconscious, to affect another: not only the spoken and written word, but also gestures, body movements, somatic signals, and symbolism in the arts."

Communication begins the moment two people become aware of each other's presence. It is impossible not to communicate when in the presence of another person, even if no words are spoken. Even when alone, people routinely engage in "self-talk," which is an internal form of communication.

Levels of Communication

Communication exists simultaneously on at least two levels: verbal and nonverbal. **Verbal communication** consists of all speech and represents part of communication. Much communication is **nonverbal communication,** which consists of grooming, clothing, gestures, posture, facial expressions, tone and volume of voice, and actions, among other things (Figure 9-1). Words can be used to hide feelings, but individuals tend to exercise less conscious control over nonverbal communication than verbal communication. Therefore the nonverbal component is considered a more reliable expression of feeling. Certainly nurses must pay as much attention to nonverbal messages as they do to verbal ones.

Consider this example: a nurse who is preparing a patient for a breast biopsy notices that the patient keeps her head turned away and will not look at the nurse. When the nurse says, "Is there anything you want to talk about or ask?" the patient responds, "No, I'm fine." The wise nurse would pay more attention to her nonverbal communication than to the spoken word. If the nurse pays attention only to the patient's words, her underlying feelings would be ignored. The nurse's job in evaluating this patient's needs is made more difficult by the incongruence between her verbal and nonverbal messages.

Figure 9-1

Nonverbal communication consists of grooming, clothing, gestures, posture, facial expressions, tone and volume of voice, and actions. Nonverbal communication is particularly important to patients whose ability to speak is impaired. (*Courtesy Medical University of South Carolina.*)

When **congruent** communication occurs, the verbal and nonverbal aspects match and reinforce each other. In **incongruent** communication, the words and nonverbal communication do not match. Incongruent communication creates confusion in receivers, who are unsure to which level of communication they should respond. Nurses should be alert to incongruent communication for clues to patients' unexpressed feelings.

Elements of the Communication Process

Ruesch identified five major elements that must be present for communication to take place: a sender, a message, a receiver, feedback, and context. The **sender** is the person sending the message, the **message** is what is actually said plus accompanying nonverbal communication, and the **receiver** is the person receiving the message. A response to a message is termed **feedback.** The setting in which an interaction occurs—including the mood, relationship between sender and receiver, and other factors—is known as the **context.** All of these elements are necessary for communication to occur.

Consider the classroom situation. During a lecture, the professor is the sender, the lecture is the message, and students are the receivers. The professor (sender) receives feedback from the students (receivers) through their facial expressions, alertness, posture, attentiveness, and comments. The atmosphere in the classroom is the context. If the atmosphere is a relaxed one of give-and-take between students and professor, the feedback is quite different from feedback in a more formal context. Figure 9-2 shows the relationships among the five elements of communication.

Operations in the Communication Process

In addition to the five elements of communication, Ruesch also identified three major operations in communication: perception, evaluation, and transmission.

Perception

Perception is the selection, organization, and interpretation of incoming signals into meaningful messages. In the classroom situation just described, students select, organize, and interpret various pieces of the professor's message or lecture. Each student perceives the information differently, based on factors such as personal experience, previous knowledge, alertness, sensitivity to subtleties of meaning, and sociocultural background. This is sometime referred to as an individual's perceptual screen, through which all incoming messages are filtered.

Evaluation

Evaluation is the analysis of information received. Is the content of the professor's lecture useful? Is it important or relevant to the students' needs? Is it likely to be on the next test? Each student evaluates the message in a different manner.

Transmission

Transmission refers to the expression of information, verbal or nonverbal. While the professor is transmitting his verbal message to the students, his or her nonverbal behavior of excitement, uncertainty, confusion, or boredom with the subject matter also transmits a message to the class.

Factors influencing perception, evaluation, and transmission

Perception, evaluation, and transmission are influenced by many factors. The gender and culture of the sender and receiver; the interest and mood of both parties; the value, clarity, and length of the message; the presence or absence of feedback; and the atmosphere of the context all are powerful influences. Also involved are individuals' needs, values, self-concepts, sensory and intellectual

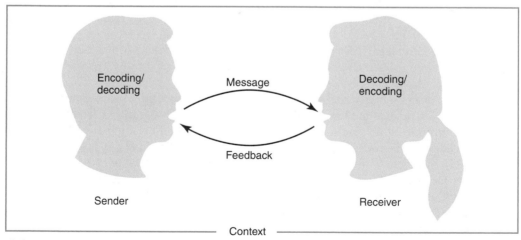

Figure 9-2
Elements of the communication process.

abilities or deficits, and sociocultural conditioning. Given the variety of factors involved, it is clear that communication is a complex human activity worthy of nurses' attention.

HOW COMMUNICATION DEVELOPS

Humans learn to communicate through a certain developmental sequence, which begins in infancy. Infants use somatic language to signal their needs to caretakers. **Somatic language** consists of crying; reddening of the skin; fast, shallow breathing; facial expressions; and jerking of the limbs. The sequence progresses to action language in older infants. **Action language** consists of reaching out, pointing, crawling toward a desired object, or closing the lips and turning the head when an undesired food is offered. Last to develop is verbal language, beginning with repetitive noises and sounds and progressing to words, phrases, and complete sentences.

If a child's development is normal, any one or combination of these forms of communication can be used. Somatic language usually decreases with maturity, but because it is not under conscious control, some somatic language may persist past childhood. A familiar example is facial blushing when embarrassed or angry. The development of communication is determined by inborn and environmental factors. The amount of verbal stimulation an infant receives can enhance or retard the development of language skills. The extent of a caretaker's vocabulary and verbal ability is therefore influential. Some families engage in lengthy discussions on a variety of issues, thereby providing intense verbal stimulation, whereas others are quieter and less verbal.

Nonverbal communication development is similarly influenced by environment. Some families communicate through nonverbal gestures such as touch or facial expressions, which children learn to "read" at young ages. Other families ascribe to the adage "Children should be seen and not heard," thus discouraging verbal expression and increasing dependence on nonverbal cues for communicating. The ability to communicate effectively is dependent on a number of factors.

Primary among these are the quantity and quality of verbal and nonverbal stimulation received during early developmental periods.

CRITERIA FOR SUCCESSFUL COMMUNICATION

Everyone has had the experience of being the sender or receiver of unsuccessful communication. A simple example is arriving for an appointment with a friend at the wrong time or wrong place because of a communication mix-up. Unsuccessful communication creates little harm when done under social circumstances. In nursing situations, however, accurate, complete communication is vitally important. Nurses can achieve successful communication on most occasions if they plan their communication to meet four major criteria: feedback, appropriateness, efficiency, and flexibility.

Feedback

When a receiver relays to a sender the effect of the sender's message, **feedback** has occurred. Feedback was identified as one of Ruesch's five elements necessary for communication (see Figure 9-2). It is also a criterion for successful communication. In making the social appointment mentioned previously, if the receiver of the message had said, "Let's make sure I understand you. We'll meet at 12:30 on Tuesday at Cafe Al Fresco," that feedback could have led to successful communication.

In a nurse-patient interaction, a nurse can give feedback to a patient by saying, "If I understand you correctly, you have pain in your lower abdomen every time you stand up." The patient can then either agree or correct what the nurse has said: "No, the pain is there only when I arise in the morning." Effective nurses do not assume that they fully understand what their patients are telling them until they feed the statement back to the patient and receive confirmation.

Appropriateness

When a reply fits the circumstances and matches the message, and the amount is neither too great nor too little, **appropriateness** has been achieved.

In day-to-day conversation among acquaintances passing on the street, most people recognize the question "How are you?" as a social nicety, not a genuine question. The individual who launches into a lengthy, detailed description of how his morning has gone has communicated inappropriately. The reply does not fit the circumstances, and the quantity is too great. An appropriate response is, "Fine, and how are you?"

If a patient asks, "When is my lunch coming?" just after having eaten lunch, the nurse will be alert to other inappropriate messages by this patient that may signal a variety of problems. In this instance, the inappropriate message does not match the context.

Efficiency

Efficiency means using simple, clear words that are timed at a pace suitable to participants. Explaining to an adult that she will have "an angioplasty" tomorrow morning may not result in successful communication. Telling her she will have "an angioplasty, a procedure in which a small balloon is threaded into an artery and inflated to open up the vessel so more blood can flow through," will more likely ensure her understanding. This message would not be an efficient one for a small child, however. Messages must be adapted to each patient's age, verbal level, and level of understanding.

Some examples of patients who require special assistance in evaluating and responding to messages are young children, the mentally ill, some people with neurological deficits, the developmentally disabled, and those recovering from anesthesia or on pain medication. For efficient communication to occur, nurses must recognize patients' needs and adjust messages accordingly.

Flexibility

The fourth criterion for successful communication is **flexibility.** The flexible communicator bases messages on the immediate situation rather than preconceived expectations. When a student nurse who plans to teach a patient about diabetic diets enters the patient's room and finds the patient crying, the student must be flexible enough to change gears and deal with the feelings the patient is expressing. Pressing on with the lesson plan in the face of the patient's distress shows a lack of compassion as well as inflexibility in communicating.

Nurses can learn to use these four measures of successful communication to enhance their effectiveness with patients. The continuing absence or malfunction of any of these four criteria can create disturbed communication and hamper the implementation of the nursing process.

BECOMING A BETTER COMMUNICATOR

People are not born as good communicators. Communication skills can be developed if you are willing to put forth a moderate amount of time and energy. Becoming a better listener, learning a few basic helpful responding styles, and avoiding common causes of communication breakdown can put you on the path to becoming a better communicator.

Listening

A requirement of successful verbal communication in any setting is listening, but too often we hear without listening. **Active listening** is a method of communicating interest and attention. Fostering an unrushed manner and using such signals as good eye contact, nodding, and "mumbles" ("mm-hmm") and encouraging the speaker ("Go on" or "Tell me more about this") help to communicate interest. Facing the speaker squarely with an inviting facial expression and using an **open posture** (relaxed; arms uncrossed) also communicate interest. Sit, bend, or stoop to place your eye level at that of the patient and repeat (reflect) what you hear, including feelings, checking to be sure you heard correctly. These indications of interest and active listening will help you focus on patients and tune into the meanings behind their words (listening with the "third ear").

Having someone listen to concerns, even if no problem solving takes place, may be therapeutic.

Ventilation is the term used to describe the verbal "letting off steam" that occurs when talking about concerns or frustrations. The experience of feeling "listened to" is becoming so rare in contemporary American society that a columnist for *The Christian Science Monitor* was prompted to write about it (Gardner, 1990; see News Note below).

Nurses may have difficulty listening for a variety of reasons. They may be intent on accomplishing a task and be frustrated by the time it takes to be a good listener. They may be planning their own next response and not hear what the patient is saying. They may be distracted by a vibrating pager or cell phone. Similar to other people, nurses have their own personal and professional problems that sometimes preoccupy them and interfere with effective listening. Nurses must remember that no verbal message can be received if the receiver (the nurse) is not listening.

Three common listening faults include interrupting, finishing sentences for others, and lack of interest. It is important for nurses to remember that what the patient is saying is just as important as what the nurse wishes to say.

Being listened to meets the patient's emotional need to be respected and valued by the nurse. Listening can help avert problems by letting people ventilate about the pressures they feel. Hospitalized patients particularly may feel that their lives are out of control and that they are isolated or invisible. They may need to discuss those feelings with someone who will listen without becoming defensive (Figure 9-3).

Nurses at all levels find listening a useful and rewarding skill. Nurse managers often use listening as a tool for dealing with staff members' problems and concerns and find that no other intervention is required. Listening is a talent that can be developed; properly used, it can be an

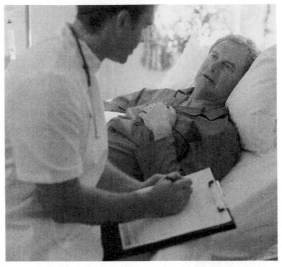

Figure 9-3
Being an active listener is an important part of communication. *(Courtesy Hamilton Medical Center, Dalton, Georgia.)*

*news*note *Where Did All the Listeners Go?*

When everybody learned how to tune out their machines—blabbing-off radio and television ads, hanging up on computer phone calls, and so on—they also learned how to tune out other people.

During the talkiest era ever, nobody listens. Or so it is assumed. In his new novel, *A Tenured Professor*, Harvard economist John Kenneth Galbraith puts it nicely: "By long custom, social discourse in Cambridge is intended to impart and only rarely to obtain information. People talk; it is not expected that anyone will listen. A respectful show of attention is all that is required until the listener takes over in his or her turn."

But wait. Just as it seems that the glazed-over eye and the numbed ear typify the Age of the Non-Listener, there is heartening news.

In Milwaukee, the Roman Catholic Archdiocese is sponsoring six "listening sessions" to give Catholic women a chance to express their feelings about abortion.

The first session, held last month in a college gymnasium in Fond du Lac, Wisconsin, drew 100 women. While participants gathered in small groups to discuss the volatile issue, Archbishop Rembert Weakland, who organized the event, moved from table to table, listening and reportedly saying little.

Archbishop Weakland, considered one of the more liberal Catholic leaders, has been criticized within his church for his gesture. But as he explained to a reporter, "The polarization about this issue has become so great that I had to admit we needed dialogue about it within the Catholic community."

It is one thing for equals to listen to equals, or for subordinates to listen to those in authority. But it is a high tribute when individuals in power listen to those below them.

Once upon a time, being a "good listener" was considered a social grace. At least 51 percent of the world were "good listeners." They were also called women. A young woman learned by example that her gender role was to listen to what others—especially men—were saying. Her mouth was primarily for smiling at what she heard, with an occasional rhythmic "uh-huh."

Today that "uh-huh" is increasingly likely to come from a stranger. Lending an ear has become a paid profession. As if to signify a national hunger for "listening sessions," an entire industry has sprung up.

Eight-year-olds phone latchkey hotlines for after-school comfort and conversation while Mom—the original "good listener"—is off at work. Bereaved dog and cat owners call on pet grief counselors for animal-loving shoulders to cry on. Even technology offers an ear, this one electronic, as answering machines and voice mailboxes do more and more of the listening.

Then of course there is the biggest listening post of all, the talk show. What does it say about the desperate yearning for an audience, any audience, that guests are willing to bare their souls and share their most intimate secrets not with close friends but with Oprah, Phil, Geraldo—and millions of TV viewers?

Is this what it takes to get a word in edgewise in the late 20th century?

Outside the TV studio, other cameras reveal that finding a "good listener"—or any listener at all—can be a tricky business in classrooms as well, especially for women.

Catherine Krupnick, a researcher at the Harvard Graduate School of Education, videotaped thousands of hours of college classes. She discovered that even when male students made up just one tenth of a class, the men would do one quarter of the talking. Other studies over the past two decades confirm Ms. Krupnick's findings, showing that professors are more likely to call on men.

The philosopher Mortimer Adler has called listening "the untaught skill." Those like Archbishop Weakland may be thought of as pioneers in retraining. But the changeover from mouth to ear won't come easily. The thing about listening is that it takes more time and, in fact, more thought than merely talking.

When a reporter, after one of the "listening sessions" in Wisconsin, asked the Archbishop what he thought, he gave the right answer: "I'm still listening."

—*Marilyn Gardner*

essential part of a nurse's communication repertoire.

Using Helpful Responding Techniques

There are many helpful responding techniques nurses can use to demonstrate respect and encourage patients to communicate openly. Helpful responses that have already been discussed in this chapter include being nonjudgmental, observing body language, and using active listening. Other useful responses include demonstrating empathy, asking open-ended questions, giving information, using reflection, and being silent. Each will be explained.

Empathy

Empathy consists of awareness of, sensitivity to, and identification with the feelings of another person. Nurses can empathize with patients even if they have not experienced an event in their own lives exactly like the one the patient is experiencing. If nurses have had a similar or parallel experience, empathy is possible. For example, the feeling of loss is familiar to most nurses, even though they may not personally have lost a close family member.

Empathy is different from sympathy in that the sympathetic nurse enters into the feeling with the patient, whereas the empathic nurse appreciates the patient's feelings but is not swept along with the feelings. "You seem upset about the upcoming procedure" is an example of a nursing statement that demonstrates empathy.

Open-ended questions

An **open-ended question** is one that causes the patient to answer fully, giving more than a "Yes" or "No" answer. Open-ended questions are very useful in data gathering and in the opening stages of any nurse-patient interaction. For example, asking a patient, "Are you in pain?" may elicit only a confirming "Yes." Saying to him, "Tell me about your pain" is more likely to elicit information about the site, type, intensity, and duration of the pain, therefore making the nurse-patient interaction more useful.

Giving information

An essential part of nursing is providing information to patients and their significant others. Giving information includes sharing knowledge that the recipients are not expected to know. Nurses provide information when they tell patients what to expect during diagnostic procedures, inform them of their rights as patients, and teach them about their conditions, diets, or medications.

An important distinction every nurse needs to make is the difference between providing information and giving opinions. While providing information is a helpful aspect of the nursing role, giving opinions is considered unhelpful. Instead, nurses should encourage patients to consider their own values and opinions as primary in importance. The nurse's opinion is not relevant.

Reflection

The nurse using reflection is serving as a mirror for the patient. **Reflection** is a method of encouraging patients to think through problems for themselves by directing patient questions back to the patient. Reflection implies respect because the nurse believes the patient has adequate resources to solve the problem without outside assistance. In response to the patient's question, "Do you think I should go through with this surgery?" the nurse can reflect the question: "Your thinking on this question is most important. Do you think you should have the surgery?"

Silence

Although silent periods in social conversations often feel uncomfortable, using silence in nurse-patient relationships can be a helpful response. Using silence means allowing periods of reflection during an interaction without feeling pressure to "fill the gap" with conversation or activity. For example, when a patient has just been given upsetting news, sitting quietly without making any demands for conversation may be the most therapeutic response a nurse can make at that time. "Being with" patients is often just as valuable as "doing for" them. Professional nurses learn to use both of these tools and find time in their busy schedules to be with patients.

There are many more helpful responding styles nurses can use in their interactions with patients. The five discussed here, once practiced and mastered, can be a foundation upon which to build.

Culturally Sensitive Communication

Because communication is the means by which people connect, nurses must take cultural differences into consideration when planning and implementing care. No hard and fast rules can be given because communication practices are unique for each individual and vary widely for people from the same cultural backgrounds. Various elements to assess include dialect, style, volume, use of touch, emotional tone, gestures, stance, space needs, and eye contact (Davidhizar, Dowd, and Giger, 1998).

Culturally sensitive nurses recognize that even when individuals speak the same language, sender and receiver may perceive different meanings because of unique life experiences. Patients may be unwilling to share certain information with nurses because of cultural taboos. Nurses may inadvertently offend patients or family members by violating cultural norms concerning touch, space, and eye contact.

Later in this chapter, Box 9-5 provides strategies for communicating effectively with coworkers of different cultural backgrounds. It is easily adapted for use with patients and provides guidelines for promoting cross-cultural communication.

Avoiding Common Causes of Communication Breakdown

Just as there are many factors influencing successful communication, unsuccessful communication can occur for many reasons. A sender may send an incomplete or confusing message. A message may not be received, or it may be misunderstood or distorted by the receiver. Incongruent messages may cause confusion in the receiver. In nursing situations, there are several common causes of communication breakdown. These

include failing to see each individual as unique, failing to recognize levels of meaning, using value statements, using false reassurance, and failing to clarify unclear messages.

Failing to see the uniqueness of the individual

Failing to see the uniqueness of each individual is a frequent cause of communication breakdown. This failure is caused by preconceived ideas, prejudices, and stereotypes, illustrated by the following interchange between a patient and a nurse:

Patient: "My back is really hurting today. I can hardly turn over in bed."

Nurse: "I guess we have to expect these little problems when we get older."

This nurse has pigeonholed the patient in a specific group, "old people," and therefore does not react to the patient as an individual. The nurse could have promoted continued communication by responding to the patient as an individual:

Nurse: "Tell me exactly how your back hurts, Mrs. Jameson."

Failing to recognize levels of meaning

When nurses recognize no level of meaning other than superficial ones, communication breakdown can occur. Patients often give verbal cues to meanings that lie under the surface content of their verbalizations:

Patient: "It's getting awfully warm in here."

Nurse: (Responding only to surface meaning) "I'll adjust the air conditioning for you."

This response does not help the patient express himself fully. A different type of response focuses on the symbolic level of meaning:

Nurse: "Perhaps the questions I am asking are making you uncomfortable."

Although it takes a lot of experience to know when and how to respond to symbolic communication, nurses should be aware of its existence.

Using value statements and clichés

Using value statements and clichés is another communication problem. The use of clichés, which are trite, stereotyped expressions, is common in social conversation. Consider the prevalence of the cliché "Have a good day." This statement has come to have little real meaning. This common error can cut off communication by showing the patient that the nurse does not understand the patient's true feelings.

Patient: "My mother is coming to see me today."

Nurse: "How nice. Do you want to put on a fresh gown?"

This nurse has failed to verify whether the patient actually wishes to see her mother. In fact, the patient and her mother may have a difficult relationship, and the patient may dread the impending visit. By assuming otherwise, the nurse has contributed to communication breakdown. This patient probably will not attempt to discuss her relationship with her mother any further with this nurse. A more helpful response would be:

Nurse: "How do you feel about her visit?"

This allows the patient to ventilate her feelings about her mother's visit, whether positive or negative. The nurse has conveyed a genuine interest in the patient's true feelings.

Giving false reassurance

Using **false reassurance** is another communication pitfall. It may help the nurse feel better but does not facilitate communication and help the patient.

Patient: "I'm so afraid the biopsy will be cancer."

Nurse: "Don't worry. You have the best doctor in town. Besides, cancer treatment is really good these days."

For a fearful patient, this type of glib reassurance does not help. This nurse has no way of knowing that the patient's concerns are not legitimate. She may indeed have cancer. A more sensitive response would be:

Nurse: "Why don't we talk about it?"

This kind of response keeps the lines of communication open between patient and nurse.

Failing to clarify

Failing to clarify the patient's unclear statements is a fifth common communication pitfall.

Patient: "I've got to get out of the hospital. They have found out I'm here and may come after me."

Nurse: "No one will harm you here."

This nurse has responded as if the patient's meaning was clear. A clarifying response might be:

Nurse: "Who are 'they,' Mrs. Johnson?"

Confused patients or those with psychiatric illnesses often communicate in ways that are difficult to understand. It is reassuring to patients to know that nurses are trying to understand them, even if they are not always successful. Communication is facilitated by **clarification** responses.

Practicing Helpful Responses

Nurses can practice using helpful responses and avoiding common communication pitfalls with family members, friends, and co-workers, as well as in patient contacts. Being a good communicator takes practice and usually feels unnatural at first. Any new behavior takes time to integrate into habitual patterns. By continuing to practice, nurses soon find themselves feeling more natural. They find that these newly acquired skills are beneficial both professionally and personally. The accompanying Critical Thinking Challenge compares different responses in a nurse-patient interaction.

Caring Through Holistic Communication

Holistic communication is "the art of sharing emotional and factual information. It involves letting go of judgments and appreciating the patient's point of view" (Klagsbrun, 2001, p. 116). Think about those words; how reassuring would it be to you right now to have someone who, without judgment, appreciated your point of view? Virtually all nurses begin their professional lives wanting to give patients that kind of attention. But the reality of too many patients and too little time often reduces communication to its barest essentials. Proponents of the holistic view of communication believe that it speeds the healing process, whereas functional communication, which consists of instructions and quick responses, inhibits it.

CRITICAL THINKING *Challenge*

Helpful and Unhelpful Responding Techniques

Directions: Critique both interactions, identifying the helpful and unhelpful responses used by the nurse. Describe how you imagine the patient might feel at the close of each interaction. Identify what the nurse has accomplished in each instance.

Mr. Goodman has been admitted to the hospital for coronary bypass surgery. During the admission process, the following interactions might take place.

Interaction One

Nurse: Mr. Goodman, I am Mrs. Scott. Can I get some information about you now?

Patient: Okay.

Nurse: You're here for bypass surgery?

Patient: Yes, that's what they tell me.

Nurse: (Taking blood pressure) Do you have any allergies to foods or medications?

Patient: Not that I know of. I've never been in a hospital before.

Nurse: Well, your blood pressure looks good. (Silence while patient has thermometer in mouth.) This is a really nice room—just remodeled. I know you'll be comfortable here. Will your wife be coming to see you tonight? (Removes thermometer)

Patient: My wife is sick. She hasn't been able to leave home for 2 years. I don't know what will happen to her while I am here.

Nurse: Gosh, I'm so sorry to hear that. I guess having you back home healthy is what she wants though, isn't it? And you've got a great surgeon. Well, I've got to run now. Check on you later.

Interaction Two

Nurse: Good afternoon, Mr. Goodman. I'm Mrs. Scott, and I'll be your nurse this evening. If this is a good time, I'd like to ask you some questions and complete your admission process.

Patient: Okay.

Nurse: First, I'll get your temperature and blood pressure, and then we'll talk. (Silence while nurse takes vital signs.) Everything looks good. Do you have any allergies to foods or medications?

Patient: Not that I know of. I've never been in a hospital before.

Nurse: Hospitals can be a little overwhelming, especially when you've never been a patient before. Now, would you please tell me in your own words why you are here?

Patient: Well, the doc tells me I have a clogged artery, and I need a bypass. I guess they'll open up my heart.

Nurse: What exactly do you know about the surgery?

Patient: Not too much, really. He told me yesterday that I need it right away—and here I am.

Nurse: It sounds like you need some more information about what will happen. Later this evening I will come back, and we'll talk some more. Are you expecting to have visitors tonight?

Patient: No, my wife can't leave home. I don't know what she will do without me while I'm here. This came up so suddenly.

Nurse: I can see that this is a serious concern for you. We can explore some possibilities when I come back this evening. I'll plan to come around 7:15, if that suits you.

Patient: Sure, I can use all the help I can get.

Some nurses fear that holistic communication will take too much time. But when patients are listened to in this way, their anxiety decreases and they complain less, call for attention less often, feel more understood and valued, and "are more likely to comply with their treatment plan" (Klagsbrun, 2001, p. 116).

Holistic communicators actively attend to their patients through such intentional gestures as using an accepting facial expression or warm eye contact, turning toward the patient with open posture, and encouraging expression of concerns. They show a willingness to listen to whatever issues the patient needs to share by asking simple, open-ended questions such as, "How are you right now?"

Holistic communicators use the principles of active listening—that is, listening to the whole person and paying "gentle, compassionate attention to what has been said or implied" (Klagsbrun, 2001, p. 116). This kind of being present with patients means avoiding analyzing, judging, or problem solving. It means avoiding defensiveness, even when the patient is critical of you or your co-workers. In addition, it has a beneficial effect on the well-being of nurses and patients.

COMMUNICATION WITH PROFESSIONAL COLLEAGUES

This chapter has focused on nurse-patient communication as the core of the nursing process and foundation of the therapeutic use of self. In addition to patients and their families, however, nurses must also communicate effectively with an ever-increasing array of professional and unlicensed personnel including physicians, lab, pharmacy, and medical records personnel, other nurses, and allied health personnel, to name a few. Socialization into health care professions tends to be discipline specific. It typically does not emphasize the strengths of other disciplines and what they can offer as patient care teammates (Lindeke and Block, 2001). This tunnel vision tends to create territoriality in which each discipline defends its own turf rather than promoting collegiality and collaboration. Health care delivery suffers when the members of the health care team fail to use the talents of all or experience communication breakdown.

As a general rule, nurses can use with colleagues the same communication skills that have been discussed as part of nurse-patient communication. Sensitivity to cultural differences where they exist and thoughtful use of electronic communication devices are both essential in today's increasingly diverse and technology-driven workplace. The value of face-to-face communi-

cation cannot be overemphasized. The attitude of respect for others, regardless of position, is essential. Active listening, acceptance, and being nonjudgmental are key elements, as are the conscious use of feedback, appropriateness, efficiency, and flexibility.

Effective Use of Electronic Communication Devices

The past decade has brought an unprecedented proliferation of electronic communication devices such as cell phones, PDAs, e-mail, voice mail, and faxes. It is not uncommon to see nurses with "ear buds" in place talking (presumably) with other staff members even as they care for patients. This is insensitive and sends a very clear message to patients that they and their needs are secondary. The use of e-mail presents another set of problems and can lead to misunderstanding because the facial expression, tone of voice, and other contextual cues are not visible to message recipients and are therefore subject to misinterpretation. A few common-sense guidelines are useful to prevent the use of technological communication devices from creating a barrier to nurse-patient or nurse-colleague communication:

- Give your full attention to the person you are with. Avoid checking your cell phone or PDA for messages while conversing with others.
- Adapt a courteous tone in e-mail and voice mail messages regardless of how rushed you are; remember the recipient cannot see your nonverbal communication.
- Avoid the use of jargon in verbal and written communication; use acronyms only when you are confident of their universal understanding.
- Keep messages short; include only necessary useful details without being abrupt or curt.
- When receiving a message, read, listen, and evaluate the entire message before reacting.

Communication in Today's Multicultural Workplace

Sensitivity to cultural differences in communication is essential in today's culturally diverse workplace. The composition of the health care workforce is being rapidly transformed by the

Box 9-5 **Strategies to Promote Effective Communication in the Multicultural Workplace**

- Pronounce names correctly; when in doubt, ask for the correct pronunciation.
- Use proper titles of respect (e.g., doctor, reverend, mister). Be sure to ask for the person's permission to use his or her first name or wait until you are given permission to do so.
- Be aware of gender sensitivities. If uncertain about the marital status of a woman or her preferred title, it is best to refer to her as "Ms." (pronounced miz) initially; then at the first opportunity, ask her what she prefers to be called.
- Be aware of subtle linguistic messages that may convey bias or inequality, for example, referring to a white male as "Mr." while addressing an African-American female by her first name.
- Refrain from Anglicizing or shortening a person's given name without his or her permission, for example, calling a Russian American "Mike" instead of Mikhael, or shortening the name of Italian American Maria Rosaria to Maria. The same principle applies to the surname.
- Call people by their proper name. Avoid slang such as "girl," "boy," "honey," "dear," "guy," "fella," "babe," "chief," "mama," "sweetheart," or similar terms. When in doubt, ask whether a particular term is offensive.
- Refrain from using slang, pejorative, or derogatory terms when referring to persons from particular ethnic, racial, or religious groups.
- Identify people by race, color, ethnic origin, religion, or physical handicap/disability only when necessary and appropriate.
- Avoid using words and phrases that may be offensive to others. For example, "culturally deprived" or "culturally disadvantaged" implies inferiority, and "nonwhite" implies that white is the normative standard.
- Avoid clichés and platitudes, such as, "Some of my best friends are Mexicans" or "I went to school with African-Americans."
- In communications, use language that includes all staff.
- Do not expect a staff member to know all the other employees of his or her background or to speak for them. They share ethnicity, not necessarily the same experiences, friendships, or beliefs.
- Refrain from telling stories or jokes demeaning to certain ethnic, racial, age, or religious groups. Also avoid those pertaining to gender-related issues or to persons with physical or mental disabilities.
- Avoid remarks that suggest to staff from diverse backgrounds that they should consider themselves fortunate to be in the organization. Do not compare their employment opportunities and conditions to people in their country of origin.
- Remember that communication problems multiply in telephone communications because important nonverbal cues are lost and accents may be difficult to interpret.

Adapted with permission from Andrews MM: Transcultural perspectives in nursing administration, *JONA* 28(11):34, 1998.

population demographics of the nation. Diversity in age, race, gender, ethnicity, country of origin, sexual orientation, and disability is present, creating opportunities for nurses to develop skill in transcultural communication.

Culture is the lens through which all other aspects of life are viewed. Culture determines an individual's health beliefs and practices. It also affects profoundly the meaning individuals attribute to work. Different cultures view caring for the sick in widely varying ways, such as a divine calling, a religious vocation, or an occupation for the lower classes.

The meaning of work in a given culture also affects how people of that culture communicate. Andrews (1998) pointed out that verbal or nonverbal communication issues are often at the root of conflict in the multicultural health care setting. According to Andrews, the decision to speak directly with someone, send a memorandum, make a phone call or e-mail, or not to communicate at all should be made only after taking the receiving staff member's cultural preferences into consideration. Strategies for promoting effective cross-cultural communication in the workplace are found in Box 9-5.

Wise nurses do not leave their communication skills at the patient's bedside but use them throughout their personal and professional lives. Using clear, simple messages and clarifying the intent of others constitute a positive goal in all personal and professional communication. As with patients, trust must exist before communication with co-workers can be effective.

COLLABORATION SKILLS: THE KEY TO EFFECTIVE TEAMWORK

Collaboration is a complex process that builds on communication. Collaboration in health care settings is far more than simply cooperation, negotiation, or compromise. It implies working jointly with other professionals, all of whom are respected for their unique knowledge and abilities, to improve a patient's health status or to solve an organizational problem. It involves sharing knowledge and authority and is nonhierarchical (Henneman, Lee, and Cohen, 1995).

Collaboration may occur as an outgrowth of a long-standing relationship or it can be in a fleeting encounter. It can even occur electronically. Making the most of all collaboration opportunities enhances positive patient outcomes. As mentioned earlier, schools rarely use a collaborative model of education. Once out of school, however, professionals must collaborate when a complex problem that is beyond one individual's ability to solve arises (Gerardi and Morrison, 2005).

In spite of the fact that nurses are educated as individuals, most of the time they work in teams. To work effectively on teams, collaboration skills are essential. For collaboration to occur, a variety of human and organizational factors must be in place.

Human Factors in Collaboration

Although it may seem to state the obvious, all collaborating parties must be willing to work together if the collaboration is to be successful. They must have attained a level of readiness to collaborate through education, maturity, and prior experience (Henneman et al, 1995). They must know what knowledge and expertise they bring to the table and have confidence in the worth of their contributions. They must understand their own limits and their discipline's boundaries while respecting what other professions and professionals can contribute. Above all, they must communicate effectively, trust one another, and be committed to working together (Kramer and Schmalenberg, 2003). Box 9-6 contains a checklist to help you determine if you are ready to collaborate.

Organizational Factors in Collaboration

Just as the people involved must have certain attributes that facilitate collaboration, the organization in which the collaboration takes place also must be supportive. According to Henneman and col-

---

Box **9-6** **Are You Ready to Collaborate? Key Components of Effective Collaboration**

Respect for the other parties involved
Emotional maturity
Confidence in own knowledge
Willingness to learn
Cooperative spirit
Belief in a common purpose
Value unique perspectives of other disciplines
Willingness to negotiate
Know own limits
Communicate
Self-knowledge
Self-awareness (e.g., biases, values, goals)
Positive regard for opinions that differ
Not threatened by conflict

leagues (1995), factors supporting collaboration include a flat, as opposed to a multi-tiered, organizational structure; encouragement and support of individuals to act autonomously; recognition of team accomplishments, as opposed to individual accomplishments; cooperation, as opposed to competition; and valuing of knowledge and expertise, rather than titles or roles. Collaborative organizations have values that support equality and interdependence rather than status and pecking orders. Creativity and shared vision are also valued (Kramer and Schmalenberg, 2003).

The collaborative process (Gardner, 2005) entails a number of steps if it is to be successful. They include the following:

- Identification of the stakeholders (who has a stake in the outcome?)
- Identification of the problem(s) to be solved
- Identification of barriers or roadblocks on the road to solution
- Clarification of the desired outcomes (agree upon criteria for success)
- Clarification of the process (how will we approach the task?)
- Identification of who will be responsible for each step in the task
- Evaluation (have we met our criteria for success?)

Outcomes of Collaboration

Collaboration is a positive process that benefits the people involved, as individuals and as a group; the organization in which they work; and health care consumers. Increased feelings of self-worth, a sense of accomplishment, esprit de corps, enhanced collegiality and respect, and increased productivity, retention, and employee satisfaction are positive benefits of collaboration (LeTourneau, 2004). Collaboration among health care professionals also holds great promise for enhancing positive patient outcomes (Kramer and Schmalenberg, 2003).

Nurse-Physician Collaboration

Among the most problematic relationships that nurses encounter during practice are those with physicians. Educational, status, and gender differences must be overcome. Despite rising male enrollments in nursing schools and even more dramatic female enrollments in medical schools, practicing physicians are predominantly male and practicing nurses overwhelmingly female. This leads to differences in styles of communicating and behaving that can cause challenges in collaborative relationships.

During female-dominated nursing school experiences, most nurses are encouraged to view physicians as teammates and to collaborate with them whenever possible. Male-dominated medical schools, however, tend to instill in their graduates a hierarchical model of teamwork with the physician at the top of the hierarchy. These two divergent cultures, when combined with gender differences in communication and teamwork patterns, further complicate the relationship between the two professions. Too often, gender differences are interpreted as professional differences, leading to further misunderstanding.

People realize that there are differences in communication styles and behavior among individuals of different cultures. What too few people recognize is that gender is a type of culture, because men and women grow up learning different lessons about what is appropriate adult behavior. From birth, boy babies and girl babies are dressed differently, given different toys, praised for different types of behavior, and socialized to gender-specific behavior in dozens of more subtle ways. Teachers treat boys and girls differently; authors of children's books and television scripts depict men and women differently (Heim, 1995). Is it any wonder that as adults, men and women may have differing expectations of professional relationships?

Women tend to treat other people as equal, regardless of their position in the organizational hierarchy. They spend time chatting with others, building and maintaining relationships, and frequently make friends at work. Even when in management roles, they tend to tell people what to do indirectly. In general, they come to meetings expecting to discuss the issues and make decisions depending on the outcome of the discussion. They value the process aspects of decision making as much as the outcome and tend to seek consensus in decision making (Heim, 1995). This can cause them to seem tentative or unsure to task-oriented people.

Men tend to see other workers as above, below, or parallel to them in the organizational structure and to treat them accordingly. They tend to be task-oriented, chat less, are friendly but tend not to become friends with co-workers, and are likely to tell subordinates what to do directly. In general, they come to meetings already having discussed the issues, made decisions beforehand, and lined up the votes they need to get their decisions approved. They are more goal-oriented and pay less attention to process than to outcome (Heim, 1995). They tend to focus on justice issues and rule out alternatives. This can cause them to seem headstrong to more consensus-oriented people.

Beyond gender differences, medicine and nursing have differing cultures. This is sometimes termed the care-cure conflict. Differences of opinion are inevitable when the basic approach to problems is different, as they are with nursing and medicine. Conflict can be either destructive or constructive. When participants have conflict negotiation skills, conflict can lead to creative solutions and an atmosphere where diverse ideas are welcome.

In collaborative relationships, conflict can be categorized as emotionally-based or task-based. Emotionally-based conflicts are attributable to relationships while task-based conflicts are a result of differences of opinion over how to approach a task or achieve a mutual goal.

Constructive conflict negotiation skills can be developed (Gerardi and Morrison, 2005). Examples of these skills include the following:

- Acknowledge the conflict.
- Recognize and affirm that positives can result from conflict.
- Facilitate debate over task issues while redirecting concerns away from the personal level.
- Promote expression of varying perspectives.
- Monitor tone of voice, eye contact, defensive nonverbal posture.

- Avoid locking into a fixed position; explore alternatives and opportunities to synthesize several ideas to create a new one.
- Share power; elicit everyone's opinions and look for win-win situations.
- Stay focused on the desired outcome.

Successful collaboration requires a focus on both relationships and the task at hand. Differences in gender culture create challenges in all aspects of personal and professional life if they are not understood. Understanding the differences in communication styles between nurses and physicians serves to increase self-awareness and minimize assumptions and erroneous interpretations. For insight into how gender culture may affect your working relationships, take the gender culture self-assessment in the Cultural Considerations Challenge on p. 233 and discuss it in a small group composed of both genders.

Collaboration With Assistive Personnel

Relationships between registered nurses and unlicensed assistive personnel, formerly known as nurse's aides or nursing assistants, affect quality of care and patient outcomes. All too often, mutual respect and cooperation are missing in these important relationships, and both groups feel frustrated and unappreciated. Because nursing is not as ethnically diverse as the total population, ethnic and cultural differences can complicate the relationship between nurses and unlicensed personnel. Language is often a barrier as are nonverbal and other culturally determined behaviors, such as the value placed on punctuality. Differences in beliefs, values, perceptions, and priorities create conflict, result in poor teamwork, reduce job satisfaction, and ultimately have a negative impact on patient care (Grossman and Taylor, 1995).

Hayes (1994) reported on team building sessions with registered nurses and unlicensed personnel on three general hospital units. The purpose was to identify and align the needs of work-related relationships in both groups with the needs of the nursing unit. This is a key step in team building, which was the model chosen to encourage collaboration between the two groups.

Cultural Considerations *Challenge*

Gender Culture Self-Assessment

Directions: For each of the paired statements, select the one that most accurately expresses your experiences or feelings.

Column One	Column Two
I prefer to compete to win.	I prefer to find win-win solutions.
I like to work where I know the hierarchy so that I know what is expected of me.	I like to work in situations where power is equally shared.
When I lead a meeting, I prefer to sit in front of the group or at the head of the table.	When I lead a meeting, I prefer to sit with the group or in a circle.
In arriving at a decision, I study the options, select one, and move ahead with it.	In arriving at a decision, I usually ask several other people for their opinions.
I define a "team player" as someone who follows orders, supports the leader unquestioningly, and does what is needed no matter how he or she feels.	I define a "team player" as someone who shares ideas, listens even when they disagree, and works collaboratively.
I can disagree or even argue with my friends and not allow it to affect the friendship.	I expect my friends to side with me in disagreements and tend to take it personally if they do not.
In the workplace, competent people do not worry about being nice.	In the workplace it is possible to be both competent and nice.
I spend little time in getting to know my co-workers personally.	It is worthwhile to spend time getting to know my co-workers on a personal level.

Scoring instructions: If most of your checks were in Column One, you have a traditionally male gender style. When you work with women, you can anticipate some challenges because of differences in behavior and conversational styles. These challenges can be overcome. If most of your checks were in Column Two, you have a traditionally female gender style. When you work with men, you can anticipate some challenges because of differences in behavior and conversational styles. These challenges can be overcome. If your checks were about equally balanced between Column One and Column Two, you have a combination of male and female gender styles. You should be able to work easily with both men and women.

Teams were defined as groups of workers with a fairly stable composition. They worked interdependently and "shared a common purpose" (Hayes, 1994, p. 52). To emphasize that the nurses and unlicensed personnel needed to work cooperatively, researchers asked each group questions, such as the following: "What do you need from each other to make your day go better?" "What is important for you to have in the way of working relationships on this nursing unit?" "What do you need from the registered nurses?" "What do you need from the nursing assistants?" (Hayes, 1994, p. 52).

Unlicensed personnel reported needing to feel welcome, appreciated, and respected but instead reported feeling unwelcome, unrecognized, and unappreciated. They did not realize that registered nurses were expected to plan, supervise, and evaluate the work of unlicensed personnel. The registered nurses expressed the need to feel competent as managers and to have unlicensed personnel comply with requests and give feedback about assigned activities. Some registered nurses reported that they preferred to complete work themselves rather than experience embarrassment when unlicensed personnel failed to comply with their requests.

Team-building sessions centered around identifying problematic feelings and misperceptions and correcting them. For example, in response to the unlicensed personnel's belief that their contributions to patient welfare were unappreciated, the registered nurses replied, "We could not run the unit without you" and "What you do makes the difference in how comfortable the patients feel" (Hayes, 1994, p. 53).

During team building with these groups, Hayes reported that misperceptions were aired and discussed and expectations were clarified. Registered nurses' legitimate authority and legal responsibility for unlicensed personnel were clarified. The result was an increase in mutual respect and understanding.

To stress the importance of positive working relationships, Diann B. Uustal, clinical ethicist and consultant, adapted the familiar poem "Children Learn What They Live" to apply to colleagues (Box 9-7). It reminds us that professional co-workers, as much as patients, deserve respectful concern.

Box **9-7** **Colleagues Learn What They Live**

If a colleague lives with hostility, s/he learns to fight.
If a colleague lives with ridicule, s/he learns to be shy.
If a colleague lives with shame, s/he learns to feel guilty.
If a colleague lives with tolerance, s/he learns to be patient.
If a colleague lives with encouragement, s/he learns confidence.
If a colleague lives with praise, s/he learns to appreciate.
If a colleague lives with fairness, s/he learns justice.
If a colleague lives with security, s/he learns to have faith.
If a colleague lives with approval, s/he learns to like her/himself.
If a colleague lives with acceptance and friendship, s/he learns to find satisfaction in professional nursing.

Adapted with permission of Uustal DB: *Values and ethics in nursing: from theory to practice*, East Greenwich, RI, 1985, Educational Resources in Nursing and Wholistic Health.

SUMMARY OF *Key Points*

- The "therapeutic use of self" means using one's personality and communication skills effectively while implementing the nursing process to help patients improve their health status.
- Phases in the traditional nurse-patient relationship include the orientation phase, the working phase, and the termination phase. Short-term patient contacts in today's streamlined care delivery system also present opportunities for connection and goal achievement.
- In long-term nurse-patient relationships, each phase has specific tasks that should be accomplished before progressing to subsequent phases.
- Acceptance of others' values, beliefs, and lifestyles is important in nursing.
- Developing awareness of biases can help nurses to prevent the intrusion of these biases into nurse-patient relationships.
- Communication is the core of all relationships and is the primary instrument through which desired change is effected in others.
- Communication is both verbal and nonverbal and consists of a sender, a receiver, a message, feedback, and context.

- Perception, evaluation, and transmission are the three major operations in communication.
- Communication develops sequentially, beginning with somatic language and progressing to action language and then to verbal language.
- Communication may be successful or unsuccessful. Successful communication meets four major criteria: feedback, appropriateness, efficiency, and flexibility.
- Active listening is a key factor in holistic communication.
- Unsuccessful communication is caused by a variety of factors that can be identified and eliminated.
- In addition to communicating well with patients, nurses use communication skills to collaborate effectively with physicians, other nurses, unlicensed personnel, and other members of the health care delivery team.
- Professional nurses must be sensitive to sociocultural factors such as ethnicity and gender that can affect communication and collaboration.

CRITICAL THINKING QUESTIONS

1. Explain what is meant by the term "therapeutic use of self."
2. List the phases of the traditional nurse-patient relationship and describe the tasks of each.
3. Identify ways nurses can quickly "connect" with patients and help them move toward wellness during short-term opportunities.
4. Explain why nonverbal communication may be more revealing than verbal communication.
5. List as many factors as you can that influence the communication process.
6. Identify a recent interaction you have had in which communication was incongruent. Analyze the effect of the incongruence on the communication. When are people most likely to use incongruent communication?
7. Some experts suggest that the traditional nurse-patient relationship should be reconceptual-

ized to fit today's fast paced health care settings. Others believe that nurses should challenge the direction of health care and advocate for a return to more traditional, patient-centered health care. Write a paragraph supporting one of these two divergent views. Share your paragraph with a small group of classmates.
8. Think of a person with whom you have experienced difficult communication. Identify which of the barriers to successful communication are functioning in that person's communication with you and analyze your responses to that person.
9. Describe a collaborative experience you have had with another health care professional. What factors differentiated it from cooperation or compromise?

REFERENCES

Andrews MM: Transcultural perspectives in nursing administration, *JONA* 28(11):30-38, 1998.

Barke J, editor: *Burns' poems and songs,* London, 1955, Collins.

Davidhizar R, Dowd S, Giger JN: Recognizing abuse in culturally diverse clients, *Health Care Supervisor* 17(2):10-20, 1998.

Gardner DB: Ten lessons in collaboration, *Online J Issues Nurs* 10(1):1-6, Jan 31, 2005, available online: http://www.nursingworld.org/ojin/topic26/tpc26_1.htm.

Gardner M: Where did all the listeners go? *Christian Science Monitor,* April 27, 1990, p 14.

Gerardi DS, Morrison F: Managing conflict creatively, *Criti Care Nurs/Suppl,* February 2005.

Grossman D, Taylor R: Cultural diversity on the unit, *Am J Nurs* 95(2):64-66, 1995.

Hagerty BM, Patusky KL: Reconceptualizing the nurse-patient relationship, *Image: J Nurs Scholar* 35(2):145-150, 2003.

Hayes PM: Team building: bringing RNs and NAs together, *Nurs Manag* 25(5):52-55, 1994.

Heim P: Getting beyond "she said, he said," *Nurs Admin Quart* 19(2):6-18, 1995.

Henneman EA, Lee JL, Cohen JI: Collaboration: a concept analysis, *J Adv Nurs* 21(1):103-109, 1995.

Klagsbrun J: Listening and focusing: holistic health care tools for nurses, *Nurs Clin N Am* 36(1):115-130, 2001.

Kramer M, Schmalenberg C: Securing "good" nurse/physician relationships, *Nurs Manag* 34(7):34-38, 2003.

LeTourneau B: Physicians and nurses: friends or foes? *J Healthcare Manag* 49(1):12-14, 2004.

Lindeke L, Block D: Interdisciplinary collaboration in the 21st century, *Minnesota Med* 8(6):42-45, 2001.

National Council of State Boards of Nursing: Professional boundaries: a nurse's guide to the importance of appropriate professional boundaries, Chicago, 1996, NCSBN, available online: www.ncsbn.org/public/resources/res/expectnurse.pdf.

Nurse's Relationship with Patient Results in Disciplinary Action: *Nursing Law's Regan Report* 43(8):4-5, 2003.

Peplau H: *Interpersonal relations in nursing,* New York, 1952, GP Putnam's Sons.

Ruesch J: *Disturbed communication: the clinical assessment of normal and pathological communicative behavior,* New York, 1972, WW Norton.

Uustal DB: *Values and ethics in nursing: from theory to practice,* East Greenwich, RI, 1985, Educational Resources in Nursing and Wholistic Health.

10

Illness, Culture, and Caring: Impact on Patients, Families, and Nurses

Kay Kittrell Chitty

Learning Outcomes

After studying this chapter, students will be able to:

- Differentiate between acute and chronic illness.
- Describe the stages of illness.
- Explain behavioral responses to illness.
- Distinguish between internal and external influences on illness behaviors.
- Discuss the influence of culture on illness behaviors.
- Describe the characteristics of the culturally competent* nurse.

- Explain the concept of spiritual nursing care.
- Identify spiritual nursing interventions.
- Explain the physical, emotional, and cognitive effects of stress.
- Discuss how family functioning is altered during illness.
- Explain the necessity of and strategies for self-care by nurses.

Although prevention and health maintenance activities are primary functions of nurses, many nurse-patient interactions center on the management of illness. A unique characteristic of nursing is the emphasis on viewing patients holistically. Nurses recognize that human beings are complex organisms with physical, mental, emotional, spiritual, social, and cultural components—all of which affect how a person responds when ill. The effective nurse takes each of these dimensions into consideration when planning nursing care.

This chapter explores the stages of illness, illness behaviors, cultural factors that influence how people behave during illness, and the impact of illness and culture on patients, families, and nurses. It also explores briefly the reasons why nurses need to develop balance in their lives and engage in self-care.

ILLNESS

Illness is a highly personal experience. It is differentiated from disease in that **disease** is an alteration at the tissue or organ level causing reduced capacities or reduction of the normal life span. Illness is usually considered a subjective

---

*The term "culturally sensitive" may also be used; it is believed by some to be a more realistic goal.

state. One may feel ill in the absence of a disease. Conversely, health care professionals may define a state of illness, such as hypertension, even in the absence of subjective symptoms in the ill person.

People's perceptions of change in body image or loss of function or body part play a major role in whether or not they see themselves as ill. People with mild arthritic changes who have no decrease in their activities and who need to use only over-the-counter analgesics such as aspirin may not consider themselves ill. To a radiologist looking at an x-ray, however, arthritic changes indicating a disease process may be evident.

Whether the presence of illness is determined by the individual or by a health care provider, illness is experienced differently by individuals and their families. Culture plays a powerful role in health beliefs and behaviors; it also determines how individuals and families react to illness. The nurse's responses to patients must be defined in terms of these unique reactions.

Acute Illness

Illnesses can be classified as either acute or chronic. **Acute illness** is characterized by severe symptoms that are relatively short-lived. Symptoms tend to appear suddenly, progress steadily, and subside quickly. Depending on the illness, the patient may or may not require medical attention. The common cold is an example of an acute illness that does not usually require a health care provider's attention. Others, such as acute appendicitis, may be fatal without rapid medical intervention. Unless complications arise, people suffering from acute illness usually return to their previous level of wellness. Some acute illnesses, such as acute myocardial infarction, may lead to chronic conditions, such as congestive heart failure.

Individuals with sudden, catastrophic injuries, such as a spinal cord injury, experience dramatic and extensive change. They face physical limitations, significant modifications in daily living, and changes in social roles. Daily, they must bear challenges that most people consider unbearable. Evidence-Based Practice Note on p. 239 describes a study of how individuals with catastrophic ill-

nesses and injuries cope with their disabilities (Dewar and Lee, 2000).

Chronic Illness

A **chronic illness** usually develops gradually, requires ongoing medical attention, and may continue for the duration of the person's life. Hypertension, diabetes, and Parkinson's disease are examples of chronic illnesses; they can be treated but not cured.

It is increasingly important for nurses to understand chronic illnesses and their impact, because they are one of the fastest-growing health problems in the United States. It is estimated that one third to one half of the U.S. population has one or more chronic illnesses. Factors such as sedentary lifestyles, obesity, and the aging of the population are expected to contribute to a continued increase in the number of chronically ill Americans for the foreseeable future.

Chronic illnesses are caused by permanent changes that leave residual disability. They vary in severity and outcomes, but there is generally not an end point at which normal health is regained. Some chronic illnesses are progressively debilitating and result in premature death, whereas others are associated with a normal life span, even though functioning is impaired. Some chronic illnesses go through periods of **remission,** when symptoms subside, and **exacerbation,** when symptoms reappear or worsen.

Chronic illnesses are pervasive and life-altering. They lead to altered individual functioning and disruption of family life. Long-term medical management of chronic illness can create financial hardship as well. Patients with chronic illness need to make lifestyle changes, often many changes simultaneously. They must begin doing things they are not accustomed to doing and stop doing things they normally do. Patients with diabetes, for example, must begin monitoring their blood glucose levels and change their eating habits. Box 10-1 presents the similarities and differences between acute and chronic illnesses.

Being diagnosed with an acute or chronic illness can be a major life crisis. The emotional reactions of the patient and family sometimes

EVIDENCE-BASED PRACTICE

note

Canadian nurse researchers Anne Dewar and Elizabeth Lee wondered how individuals with catastrophic illness and injury faced challenges that others considered unbearable and that tested the limits of human endurance. They conducted individual interviews with 28 men and women from 18 to 75 years of age. These interviewees had endured chronic conditions, such as spinal cord injuries, multiple sclerosis, or major burns, for time periods ranging from 3 to 25 years. The researchers analyzed subjects' responses using grounded theory methods, a qualitative research methodology. The theoretical framework selected by the researchers was symbolic interactionism, which seeks to determine the relationship between the individual and the social world in which he or she lives.

They found that these individuals experienced three phases in bearing their difficulties. The researchers termed these phases *finding out*, *facing reality*, and *managing reality*. They discovered that the individuals in their study did not progress through stages, as others have suggested, but instead the phases flowed together and were reexperienced continuously. These individuals used three enduring strategies in all phases, which the researchers termed *protecting*, *modifying*, and *boosting*. Protecting involved insulating oneself from further emotional pain by limiting requests for assistance and not sharing emotional distress with significant others. Modifying meant learning to manage the physical, emotional, and social aspects of a condition by learning new skills and diffusing their emotions to preserve their social support, that is, not "whining." Boosting meant efforts to enhance self-esteem, such as comparing themselves with others who were in worse condition.

Dewar and Lee concluded that "the burdens of chronic illness and injuries [are] exceedingly complex, as individuals are forced to rebuild an image of themselves, manage their daily lives, and preserve relationships with others. Social support is important but forces the sufferer to make modifications to meet the needs of others as well as his or her own" (p. 924). They recommended that nurses and other health care professionals "accept and support the individual's need to express emotions such as anger, sorrow, and despair in all phases of the illness" (p. 922).

Abstracted from Dewar AL, Lee EA: Bearing illness and injury, *West J Nurs Res* 22(8):912-926, 2000.

present a greater challenge than dealing with the physical aspects of the disease. Most medical and nursing attention, however, is focused on physical symptoms and the disease process rather than emotions (Cassidy, 1999). Box 10-2 describes how one patient experiences a chronic illness, lupus erythematosus, and describes its impact on her feelings, family responsibilities, and relationships.

STAGES OF ILLNESS

Adjustment to illness is a process. Although the behaviors are different for each person, people who are ill tend to progress through certain recognizable stages. Ellis and Nowlis (1994) have identified five stages: disbelief and denial, irritability and anger, attempting to gain control, depression and despair, and acceptance and participation. Nurses encounter patients in each stage, so it is important to have some understanding of the types of behaviors associated with each. Remember that a person's culture affects how he or she responds to illness and that the studies by Ellis and Nowlis were done with people of individualistic, Western cultures. Also remember that stage theories are convenient ways

Box **10-1** Types of Illness

Acute	Chronic
• Sudden onset of symptoms	• Gradual onset of symptoms
• Symptoms progress quickly from mild to severe	• Symptoms may be mild or vague; once illness is resolved may have remissions and exacerbations
• Patient usually returns to former level of functioning	• Illness continues through the life span
• Changes often not permanent but may progress to chronic illness	• Changes are permanent and progressive
• Does not usually require long-term behavioral change/treatment	• Requires long-term behavioral change/treatment
• May represent a life crisis	• Often represents a life crisis

Box **10-2** **Comments of a Patient With a Chronic Disease: Lupus Erythematosus**

If there is one thing I want to say to nurses who work with patients with chronic disease, it is "Be patient and understand our problems and feelings." When I go to the doctor's office or to the hospital, I usually leave feeling guilty because I have been impatient with everyone I saw. Guilt and anger are the two feelings I seem to have had since I was diagnosed with this disease. I alternate between being angry that I got lupus and feeling that I should be grateful for the fact that I have something I can at least live with when others are not so fortunate.

I guess the thing that bothers me most is that the nurses keep telling me what changes I need to make to take better care of myself. They never seem to understand that I am doing the best I can do. I can't possibly get the amount of rest they seem to think I need, and I can't avoid as much stress as they seem to think I should avoid. Both my husband and I work hard at our jobs, and I hate asking him and my sons to take over my responsibilities at home when I am sick, so I wind up compromising. I ask them to help some and I do more than I should. When I get the lecture from the nurses on how I should take better care of myself, I usually just nod and say that I will, even when I know that I probably won't be able to.

—**Anonymous**

of conceptualizing and learning, but often human beings do not fit neatly into the identified stages.

Stage I: Disbelief and Denial

According to Ellis and Nowlis (1994), the first stage results from difficulty in believing that the signs and symptoms being experienced are caused by illness. Often, there is a belief that the symptoms will go away. Fear of illness often leads to the hope that the symptoms will subside without treatment.

Denial is a defense mechanism that people sometimes use to avoid the anxiety associated with illness. People who pride themselves on their vigor and health may downplay the significance of symptoms. If this occurs, they may avoid treatment or attempt inappropriate self-treatment. Extended denial can have serious results, because some illnesses, left untreated, may become too advanced for effective treatment.

Stage II: Irritability and Anger

As the ability to function is altered by illness, irritability results. Anger is directed toward the body because it is not performing as it should. With the current emphasis on wellness and prevention, anger may be directed inward, and guilt feelings may occur for failing to prevent the illness. Anger may also be directed toward others—spouse, family members, co-workers, or health care providers.

Stage III: Attempting to Gain Control

In this stage, people may consult their health care provider or use over-the-counter medications, folk practices, or home remedies. They are aware that they are ill and usually experience some concern or even fear about the outcome. These fears usually stimulate treatment-seeking behavior as a way of gaining control over the illness, but fears may also lead to further denial and avoidance. Family members may become involved, encouraging the person to seek treatment or follow medical advice.

Stage IV: Depression and Despair

Depression is perhaps the most common mood that occurs with illness. The ability to work is altered, daily activities must be modified, and the sense of well-being and freedom from pain are lost. Illness results in many types of loss, and depression is a normal response. The severity of the depression varies according to the severity and length of the illness, as well as the individual's personality characteristics and coping abilities. Individuals with chronic illnesses often undergo cycles of depression as remissions and exacerbations occur.

Stage V: Acceptance and Participation

By the time this stage occurs, the patient has acknowledged the reality of illness and is ready to participate in decisions about treatment. Active involvement and the hope attached to pursuing treatment usually lead to increased feelings of mastery and serve to decrease depression.

Not all individuals go through every stage, and they do not necessarily go through them at the same rate or in the same order. Those with acute illnesses may progress through stages in a different way than those with chronic illnesses. As mentioned, culture plays a major role in how people respond to illness. Box 10-3 summarizes the stages of illness.

THE SICK ROLE

Although illness is highly subjective and is experienced differently by each individual, a number of factors influence how a particular person will respond. One important factor is the cultural expectation about how people should behave when ill. Children learn the part they are expected to play as an ill person through **parental modeling**—that is, by observing how their parents respond to major and minor illnesses. Do their significant adult figures avoid work and other activities when ill, or do they forge ahead stoically, ignoring minor illness or pain?

Each culture generally requires that certain criteria be met before people can qualify as "sick." Talcott Parsons (1964), a renowned sociologist, identified five attributes and expectations of the **sick role** that guided the view of illness in Anglo-American society for decades. According to Parsons, the sick Anglo-American:

1. Is exempt from social responsibilities.
2. Cannot be expected to care for himself or herself.
3. Should want to get well.

Box **10-3** Stages of Illness

Stage I: Disbelief and Denial
Stage II: Irritability and Anger
Stage III: Attempts to Gain Control
Stage IV: Depression and Despair
Stage V: Acceptance and Participation

From Ellis J, Nowlis E: *Nursing: a human needs approach*, ed 5, Philadelphia, 1994, JB Lippincott.

4. Should seek medical advice.

5. Should cooperate with the medical experts.

In other words, Parsons' definition of the sick role includes behavior that is dependent, passive, and submissive. For decades, Parsons' sick role expectations were taught in medical and nursing schools and guided the way health care providers viewed patients' reactions to pain and illness for many years. In our multicultural society, however, this view is no longer adequate, because different cultures have differing sick role expectations.

The cultural composition of the nation and the world is changing. By 2010 whites will be the smallest ethnic minority in the world. Nurses, regardless of their own cultural backgrounds, must strive to provide culturally competent care to patients of many diverse cultures. With more than 66 different categories of race listed in the 2000 U.S. Census, this can seem like an overwhelming task. In fact, it is probably impossible for nurses to master the subtleties of every culture they encounter. Nurses can learn about their patients' culturally determined health care and illness beliefs, values, and practices, however, by consistently performing cultural assessments. These instruments will be discussed later in this chapter.

The current Anglo-American expectation is that people should accept responsibility for their own care rather than completely submit to health care providers; this is the consumer-oriented approach to health care. There is a presumption that ill people should want to get well and should behave in a way that leads to wellness.

This expectation that ill persons should want to get well and return to their normal activities as quickly as possible means that patients should cooperate in the treatment process and, to a great extent, become submissive and compliant, placing themselves in the hands of the caretakers. Persons who refuse to take medications as ordered or who refuse to perform prescribed activities, such as adhering to an exercise program or therapeutic diet, are viewed in a negative light. Their friends and family members may become irritated at their lack of participation in getting well again. Their caregivers call them "noncompliant." Often what is missing is an understanding of the patient's perception of the illness. Shifting from a focus of caring for patients to partnering with them is helpful in overcoming negative attitudes.

In caring for patients with acute and chronic illnesses, it is important for nurses to refrain from making judgments about patients' lifestyle choices. Emphasis should be placed on encouraging and reinforcing healthy behaviors. Education and support are important role functions for the nurse, especially in the management of patients with chronic disorders.

Working with patients with chronic illnesses can be particularly challenging for nurses. The inability of modern medicine to cure disease sometimes leads caregivers to feel hopeless and powerless. They may also feel overwhelmed and inadequate at times. Self-aware nurses recognize these feelings and do not allow them to interfere with the nurse-patient relationship.

Illness Behaviors

Although some behaviors are expected of sick people, there is also a wide variation in responses. Each person who is newly diagnosed with hypertension, for example, behaves somewhat differently from other people with the same condition. Both internal and external variables affect how an individual acts when ill (see Box 10-4). An ill individual's personality has a great deal of influence on the response to illness. Past experiences with illness and cultural background also influence illness behaviors.

Internal influences on illness behaviors

Personality structure is an internal variable that determines, to a large extent, how one manages illness. Personality characteristics the nurse should consider when assessing the ill person are dependence/independence, coping ability, hardiness, learned resourcefulness, resilience, and spirituality.

Box 10-4 Internal and External Influences on Illness Behavior	
Internal Influences	**External Influences**

• Dependence/independence needs
• Coping ability
• Hardiness
• Learned resourcefulness
• Resilience
• Spirituality
	• Past experiences
	• Culture
	  • Communication patterns
	  • Personal space norms
	  • Role expectations
	  • Values
	  • Ethnocentrism

Dependence and independence. Patients' needs for dependence are unrelated to the severity of their illnesses. Some patients adopt a passive attitude and rely completely on others to take care of them. Others deny they are ill or have problems with being dependent and try to continue living as independently as they did before becoming sick.

We have all encountered sick people who have expressed views such as, "I don't ask any questions—I know that my doctor and nurses know what is best for me, and I do what they tell me." Perhaps you also know someone who reacted to illness by saying, "They don't know what they are talking about. I don't need to be in bed, and I don't need to take that medicine." These two sentiments are at the opposite ends of the **dependency** continuum.

People who perceive themselves as helpless may be more willing to submit to health care personnel and do what they are told. Those who are used to being in charge and see themselves as independent may resent the enforced dependency of hospitalization and illness. These two different attitudes are illustrated in Case Study 10-1.

Both overly dependent and overly independent behavior can be frustrating to nurses, who sometimes become angry with patients who request help with activities they are capable of doing themselves. The patient who is too dependent requires assistance to assume gradually more responsibility. The patient who needs to be "in charge" may have problems turning control over to caregivers and is often too independent. This patient needs assist-

Case Study 10-1

EXAMPLE 1: Dependence

Mrs. Johnson has been in the hospital for several days following major abdominal surgery. Even after she progressed to the point at which she could feed herself, turn over in bed, and go to the bathroom unaided, she continued to call for assistance when she needed to turn over in bed or to get out of bed. She now calls the nurse every few minutes, making some small request that she is quite capable of performing for herself. She is communicating to the nurse that she needs a great deal of assistance and is demonstrating overly dependent behavior.

EXAMPLE 2: Independence

One hour ago Mr. Thomas returned to his room after surgery. The nurse found him trying to get out of bed by himself. He did not call to ask for assistance, although he is still groggy from anesthesia. He says that he is used to doing things for himself and feels uncomfortable asking the nurses for help. Mr. Thomas is demonstrating behavior that is too independent for his current physical status.

ance in recognizing limitations and using available resources to meet his or her needs.

Because nurses most often focus on promoting patient independence, they may react negatively to patients who are exhibiting dependent behavior. It is important for the nurse to be aware of personal feelings about dependent behaviors and to keep in mind that these behaviors may be the patient's way of signaling an increased need for security or support. Sometimes independence may not be the desired outcome. For patients with chronic illnesses who must rely on others for assistance in meeting their needs, too much independence may actually be dysfunctional (Whiting, 1994) as well as dangerous.

Coping ability. An individual copes with disease or illness in a variety of ways. **Coping** is a term that described the methods a person uses to assess and manage demands. With an acute illness, coping is generally short-term and leads to a return to the pre-illness state. With chronic disorders, coping behaviors must be used continuously.

Sick people use coping methods to deal with the negative consequences of the disorder, such as pain or physical limitations. Each individual has a unique coping repertoire that is called into play to achieve a sense of control. With chronic health problems, there is a continuous need for adjustments to maintain well-being and prevent the feelings of despair that can result from high stress conditions (Bowsher and Keep, 1995).

Hardiness and learned resourcefulness. Hardiness and learned resourcefulness are two concepts that have received attention as personal characteristics related to coping. **Hardiness** is viewed as a function of resistance to stressful life events (Bowsher and Keep, 1995). The interrelated dimensions of hardiness include the tendency to believe that one can influence the course of events, to view change as a challenge, and to feel commitment to values or goals.

The person with high levels of hardiness is believed to be better able to manage the changes associated with illness and to have less physical illness resulting from stress. Hardy people are likely to perceive themselves as having some control over a situation, even when ill. This feeling can affect a person's sense of well-being and adaptation to acute and chronic health problems.

Zauszniewski (1995) described the concept of **learned resourcefulness** as a characteristic useful in promoting adaptive, healthy lifestyles. Throughout life, individuals acquire a number of skills that enable them to cope effectively with stressful situations. The resulting attitude of self-control can be particularly helpful in reducing the feelings of depression and helplessness that often accompany the numerous stressors of chronic illness.

The nurse can enhance both hardiness and resourcefulness by teaching new coping skills. Stress inoculation and skills in self-regulation, problem solving, conflict resolution, and emotion control are examples of the types of educational interventions the nurse may implement.

Resilience. Scholars studying human behavior have often noted that some children did well in spite of difficult circumstances that defeated others. They attributed the differing reactions as a function of the phenomenon of resilience. **Resilience** is an aspect of coping that can be defined as "a pattern of successful adaptation despite challenging or threatening circumstances" (Humphreys, 2001). Resilient responses are thought to be a result of three factors:

- Disposition (i.e., temperament, personality, overall health and appearance, and cognitive style)
- Family factors such as warmth, support, and organization
- Outside support factors, such as a supportive network and success in school or work

Resilience can be thought of as both a process and an outcome. It can develop over a person's lifetime and can be taught, modeled, and learned (Wolin, 1993).

The study of resilience has broadened to include adolescents and adults who face difficult, traumatic, or adverse circumstances. It has also been applied to adults with critical illness, battered women, survivors of sexual abuse, and others. You can expect to see much more about resilience as this phenomenon continues to be studied and better understood. A useful website to help you begin understanding the concept of resilience can be found online (www.projectresilience.com).

Spirituality. The concept of spirituality is receiving increased interest in society as a whole, as well as in nursing. Spirituality is defined as "inner strength related to belief in and sense of connectedness with a higher power" (Chilton, 1998). The degree of spiritual awareness varies from individual to individual. This awareness can be dormant or suppressed, or it may be expressed through religious worship and prayer, although it is not necessarily manifested in overt religious practices (Cavendish et al., 2000). Religion is a specific way of organizing rituals and beliefs to create meaning. Spirituality is a larger umbrella concept under which religion resides. Spirituality is less differentiated than religion and can include concepts and beliefs from many religions and philosophies.

Spiritual growth occurs over the life span and is a very internal process. Spiritual growth consists of increasing awareness of meaning, connectedness, purpose, and values in life (Cavendish et al., 2000).

The role of spiritual beliefs in health and illness has only recently been formally investigated. A growing number of scholars and health professionals think that spiritual beliefs have psychological, medical, and financial benefits that can be proved scientifically. Questions about the effects of intercessory prayer (prayer by others on behalf of a sick person) have been debated. Since 2000, $2.3 million of public funds have been expended on the study of prayer's effects. A scientifically rigorous, privately funded study of more than 1800 heart surgery patients was conducted over nearly a decade. To the disappointment of many, it found that intercessory prayer had no effect on recovery (Carey, 2006). The debate will undoubtedly continue.

One of the leading proponents of the spirituality and healing movement in American medicine is Dr. Herbert Benson, a Harvard Medical School cardiologist and founder of the Mind/Body Institute. He originated the "relaxation-response" therapy to reduce stress in patients with hypertension, chronic pain, and other stress-related illnesses. According to Benson, many people use prayer as part of the relaxation response (Benson and Stark, 1996). The Mind/Body Medical Institute of Pathway Health Network in Boston has studied the effects of the relaxation response and asserts the following benefits (Larson, 1996):

- A 36 percent reduction in physician visits by chronic pain patients
- Significantly fewer postoperative complications in open heart surgery patients
- Lowered blood pressure and decreased use of medications in 80 percent of hypertensive patients
- A 50 percent reduction in health maintenance organization (HMO) visits by relaxation-response users

Another indication of the priority of meeting patients' spiritual needs in health care settings is the increase in chaplain presence in some inpatient and outpatient settings. More than 90 percent of the patients surveyed believed that having a chaplain available was helpful, and 60 percent were more likely to return to a hospital with a pastoral presence in an otherwise frightening and confusing environment (Larson, 1996).

The Joint Commission on Accreditation of Healthcare Organizations, the International Council of Nursing, the American Association of Colleges of Nursing, and the National Council of State Boards of Nursing all acknowledge that **spiritual nursing care** is a responsibility that goes beyond calling the chaplain. Yet many nurses experience barriers to rendering spiritual nursing care. These barriers range from feelings of inadequacy, lack of knowledge, embarrassment, their own spiritual uncertainty, lack of preparation, lack of privacy, lack of time, or failure to see it as a nursing role (McEwen, 2005).

Nurses are encouraged to view spirituality as one aspect of the whole human person and to assess patients for spiritual distress. They should recognize the individuality and value of each patient's spiritual beliefs and encourage their use in coping with illness. Spiritual distress is a

NANDA (2003) diagnosis meaning "a disturbance in the belief or value system that provides strength, hope, and meaning to life." Patients who question the meaning of suffering and the meaning of life, who express anger at God, or who view illness as punishment from God are experiencing spiritual distress.

Experts (Cavendish et al, 2000; McEwen, 2005) have identified a number of ways nurses can help patients engage their spirituality:

- Assess human responses in the spiritual domain.
- Be present for patients; listen actively.
- Allow patients to discuss beliefs in a higher power or the hereafter without introducing your own religious beliefs.
- Help patients explore what is meaningful and important in their lives.
- Value patients' inner strengths and motivations.
- Encourage patients to trust messages from an inner voice or divine providence.
- Pray with patients or read scripture, if you are comfortable doing so.
- Understand that how nurses connect with patients affects patient outcomes.
- Go beyond caring for physical needs and respect and facilitate religious practices.
- Obtain assistance of spiritual care experts.

Nurses are participating in the use of spirituality in healing. St. Francis Hospital's Congregational Nurse Program in Evanston, Illinois, for example, is reaching 15,000 local families in an interfaith health project. Following training as congregational nurses, nurses spend approximately 20 hours weekly at churches and other places of worship providing classes, counseling, and referrals. They dovetail their efforts with the spiritual beliefs and customs of each congregation. As you learned in Chapter 1, the faith community nurse concept is being implemented in numerous communities around the United States. By respecting and treating the whole person, these practitioners are affirming that a key dimension of health and healing is the spiritual dimension.

External Influences on illness behaviors

External factors that bear on illness behaviors include past experiences and cultural group membership. Both directly influence how an individual perceives and responds to illness. The values that guide feelings about illness and steer a person toward particular methods of treatment are acquired primarily in the family of origin and in the culture.

Past experiences. Adults who were pampered during childhood illnesses may accept being ill fairly easily. Relying on others for care may not bother them, and they may settle into the sick role easily. Adults who received childhood messages such as "It is weak to be ill" or "One must keep going even when not feeling well" may have difficulty accepting illness and the restrictions that accompany it. Still other adults who experienced traumatic hospitalizations as children or who were threatened with injections for misbehaving may see hospitals and nurses as threatening. Clearly, these adults behave differently when ill.

Nurses should determine the patient's past experiences with illness and the health care system during a careful admission assessment. They can then use these findings to individualize care.

Culture. Culture is a pattern of learned behavior and values that are reinforced through social interactions, shared by members of a particular group, and transmitted from one generation to the next. Culture exerts considerable influence over most of an individual's life experiences. Meanings attached to health, illness, and perceptions of treatment are affected to a large degree by a person's culture. Culture determines when one seeks help and the type of practitioner consulted. It also prescribes customs of responding to the sick. Culture defines whether illness is seen as a punishment for misdeeds or as the result of inadequate personal health practices. It influences whether one goes to an acupuncturist, an herbalist, a folk healer, or a traditional physician.

Beginning in the early 1970s, schools of nursing began including cultural concepts in their curricula. Increasing numbers of universities and colleges offered graduate programs in transcultural nursing. The Transcultural Nursing Society was legally incorporated in 1981, and in 1988 it began certifying nurses in transcultural nursing. Through oral and written examinations and evaluation of educational background and working experiences, a qualified nurse can become a certified transcultural nurse (CTN) (Andrews, 1992).

The Transcultural Nursing Society began publishing the *Journal of Transcultural Nursing* in 1989. By 1993 a resolution was adopted by the American Nurses Association's House of Delegates to identify and determine strategies to promote diverse and multicultural nursing in the workforce (Kirkpatrick and Deloughery, 1995).

Changes in the nursing workforce are needed in order to deal more effectively with commonalities and differences in patients. Significant disparities exist between the health status of whites and nonwhites in the United States. For example, the death rate for heart disease is more than 40 percent higher in African-Americans than in the white population. Similarly discouraging disparities exist in death rates for cancer and HIV/AIDS, among other diseases. Although these disparities may be due in part to education, poverty, and lifestyle factors, there is a growing unease among health professionals that racism may play a role. As a result, professional associations such as the American Nurses Association, the Joint Commission for the Accreditation of Healthcare Organizations, and the federal government have all endorsed standards for culturally appropriate health care services. The profession of nursing is largely white, which underscores the need for culturally competent nurses. Clearly, transcultural nursing is an important field of study, practice, and research and an essential one in today's increasingly diverse society.

THE CULTURALLY COMPETENT NURSE. Knowledge of a patient's culture directs the nurse in understanding behaviors and planning appropriate approaches to patient problems. Because culture may guide the patient's response to health care providers, and their interventions, it is necessary for the nurse to be knowledgeable about cultural influences. This is known as **cultural competence.** Understanding a patient's cultural background can facilitate communication and support establishing an effective nurse-patient relationship. Conversely, lack of understanding can create barriers that impede nursing care.

The shared values and beliefs in a culture enable its members to predict each other's actions. They also affect how members react to each other's behavior. When nurses work with patients from cultures about which little is known, they lack these familiar guidelines for predicting behavior. This can cause anxiety and feelings of distrust in both patient and nurse. Some of the issues that can arise when nurses care for patients from other cultures include stereotyping, communication difficulties, misperceptions about personal space, differing values and role expectations, and ethnocentrism.

STEREOTYPING. In an effort to predict behavior, nurses may stereotype or "pigeon-hole" patients from different cultures. It is important that nurses refrain from **stereotyping** members of cultures or ethnic groups that are different from their own. When providing nursing care, one size does not fit all. **Cultural conditioning** is a term that means people are culture-bound. They are unconscious of their own innate values and beliefs and assume that all people are basically alike, that is, that all people share their values and beliefs.

It is important to recognize that the health care professions create cultural conditioning in their practitioners during school. Nursing is no exception. Nurses tend to hold their knowledge and beliefs about health in high regard and may devalue people who do not possess similar knowledge and beliefs. Individualized planning is always the best basis for care, whatever the patient's culture or ethnic group. Failure to individualize care often results in noncompliance, dissatisfaction with care, and poor outcomes (Taylor, 2005).

COMMUNICATION. The nurse should keep in mind that patterns of communication are strongly influenced by culture. The Asian patient who smiles and nods may be communicating politeness and respect rather then agreeing or indicating understanding. Anglo-Americans tend to value a direct approach to problems, but in other cultures, subtlety and indirectness may be valued. Although Western culture values direct eye contact, some cultures view this as impolite, particularly direct eye contact between men and women.

PERSONAL SPACE AND STRUCTURE. The amount of **personal space** needed is another factor that varies depending on cultural experience. Some cultures use touch as a major form of communication; in others, touching between persons who are not considered family is disrespectful. Culture also has a primary influence on the type of stress its members experience at various points in their lives. Every society places stress on its members at one or more stages of development. For instance, Anglo-American adolescents are typically under great stress as they struggle with independence. Amish adolescents tend to experience less stress, because their behavior during this period of development is more rigidly prescribed by their culture.

VALUES. Values held by the nurse may conflict with patients' cultural values. In the Navajo culture, for example, great value is placed on keeping pain and discomfort to oneself. Letting others know how you feel is seen as weak. The nurse who expects patients to ask for medication when in pain may assume that the Navajo patient is comfortable when the opposite is actually the case. On the other hand, a nurse who values suffering in silence may underrate the discomfort of a patient who comes from a culture that promotes dramatic expression of discomfort.

ROLE EXPECTATIONS. The role expectations of nurses also vary from culture to culture. A common Anglo-American view of nurses is that they treat people as equals, are passive, and take direction from physicians. These patients feel free to ask questions of their nurses. Asians, however, may expect nurses to be authoritative, to provide directives, and to be expert practitioners who take charge. Out of respect for authority, they may not speak until spoken to and may verbally agree with anything nurses propose. Case Study 10-2 illustrates a cultural difference between patient and nurse in expressing pain.

ETHNOCENTRISM. Nurses respond to sick people based not only on their formal education but also on their own socialization and culture. All too often people are unaware of their own biases and tend to be ethnocentric. **Ethnocentrism** is the inclination to view one's own cultural group as superior to others and to view differences negatively. For example, some nurses are intolerant of patients who do not speak English and either avoid them or spend little time with them (Kulwicki, Miller, and Schim, 2000).

The nurse who identifies how personal beliefs and expectations can influence care is better able to recognize and deal with any prejudices that may impede patient care. Cultural assessment, therefore, begins with self-assessment. To begin a cultural self-assessment, examine your own values. What behaviors do you expect from people who are ill? Toward what groups do you have prejudices or biases? The nurse who is frustrated by the difficulty of caring for a patient from a different culture may benefit from taking a few

Case Study 10-2

Cultural Expression of Pain

Mrs. L, a 42-year-old Asian woman, became ill and required surgery while visiting her daughter in the United States. Following surgery, she was placed on a patient-controlled analgesia (PCA) pump. The nurse explained to Mrs. L how to self-administer medication when she felt pain. Mrs. L smiled and nodded her head when asked whether she understood the instructions. Much later the nurse noticed that this patient appeared to be in great pain. After talking with Mrs. L's daughter, the nurse realized that Mrs. L had not understood how to use the equipment but was unwilling to ask for additional instructions or complain of pain.

minutes to imagine what it would be like to be hospitalized in a foreign country. Candidly answering the questions in the Cultural Consideration Challenge below will help you begin the important process of self-assessment.

Cultural assessment. An important step in meeting the challenge of providing nursing care to diverse patients is the **cultural assessment.** Cultural assessments are used to identify beliefs, values, and health practices that may help or hinder nursing interventions. Dr. Madeleine Leininger, nurse anthropologist, nurse theorist, and founder of transcultural nursing, advocated that nurses routinely perform cultural assessments to determine patients' culturally specific needs (Leininger, 1999). To demystify the process, it may be helpful to think of cultural assessment as "merely asking people their preferences, what they think, who we should talk to in making a decision" (Villaire, 1994, p. 138). There are numerous cultural assessment instruments available. Some of these instruments require in-depth interviews and comprehensive data gathering, which may require more time than is available in today's health care settings.

You can continue the process of becoming a culturally competent nurse by using the "Cultural Assessment Checklist" in the Cultural Considerations Challenge on p. 250. It was designed for use by home health nurses but is easily adapted for use in other settings. Its concise yet comprehensive nature takes into account the limited amount of time nurses may have to get to know new patients—but also recognizes the necessity of developing a culturally congruent plan of care if desired outcomes are to be achieved.

Culturally competent nurses take cultural differences into consideration, usually interpret patient behavior accurately, and recognize problems that need to be managed. They realize that cultural norms must be included in the plan of care to prevent conflicts between nursing goals and patient/family goals. They recognize that planning culturally congruent care is the most time-effective

---

✦ *Cultural Considerations Challenge*

Sociocultural Self-Assessment

Directions: Use your answers to these questions to better understand your own social and cultural beliefs and expectations.

1. To what groups do I belong? What is my cultural heritage? My socioeconomic status? My age-group? My religious affiliation?
2. How do I describe myself? What parts of the description come from the groups to which I belong?
3. What kinds of contact have I had with persons from different groups? Do I assume that others have the same values and beliefs that I have?
4. What makes me feel proud about my group affiliations? Am I ethnocentric in my attitudes and behavior? What would I change about my group affiliations if I could? Why?
5. Have I ever experienced the feeling of being rejected by another group? Did this experience heighten my sensitivity to other cultures or cause me to denigrate others different from myself?
6. When I was growing up, what messages did I get from parents and friends about people from groups different from mine? Do these attitudes cause me any difficulty today?
7. What are the major stereotypes I hold about people from different groups? Do these biases help or hinder me in developing cultural sensitivity?
8. To work effectively with people from different cultural groups, what do I need to change about myself?

Cultural Considerations *Challenge*

Cultural Assessment Checklist

Patient-identified cultural/ethnic group

_____

Religion _____

Etiquette and Social Customs

- Typical greeting. Form of address: Handshake appropriate? Shoes worn in home?
- Social customs before "business." Social exchanges? Refreshment?
- Direct or indirect communication patterns?

Nonverbal Patterns of Communication

- Eye contact. Is eye contact considered polite or rude?
- Tone of voice. What does a soft voice or a loud voice mean in this culture?
- Personal space. Is personal space wider or narrower than in the American culture?
- Facial expressions, gestures. What do smiles, nods, and hand gestures mean?
- Touch. When, where, and by whom can a patient be touched?

Client's Explanation of Problem

- Diagnosis. What do you call this illness? How would you describe this problem?
- Cause. What caused the problem? What might other people think is wrong with you?

- Course. How does the illness work? What does it do to you? What do you fear most about this problem?
- Treatment. How have you treated the illness? What treatment should you receive? Who in your family or community can help?
- Prognosis. How long will the problem last? Is it serious?
- Expectations. What are you hoping the nurses will do for you?

Nutrition Assessment

- Pattern of meals. What is eaten? When are meals eaten?
- Sick [comfort] foods.
- Food intolerance and taboos.

Pain Assessment

- Cultural responses to pain.
- Patient's perception of pain response.

Medication Assessment

- Patient's perception of "Western" medications.
- Possible pharmacogenetic variations.

Psychosocial Assessment

- Decision maker.
- Sick role.
- Language barriers, translators.
- Cultural/ethnic community resources.

Reprinted with permission of Narayan MC: Cultural assessment in home healthcare, *Home Healthcare Nurse* 15(10):663-672, 1997.

way to achieve the desired goals (Figure 10-1). In addition, being knowledgeable about other cultures promotes feelings of respect and enhances understanding of attitudes, behaviors, and the impact of illness. The accompanying Interview with Dr. Madeleine Leininger provides insights into her vast experience and strongly held beliefs about cultural competence in nursing. For further study in cultural competence, several websites containing valuable resources and links are

http://www.transculturalcare.net, http://www.culturediversity.org, and http://www.tcns.org.

IMPACT OF ILLNESS ON PATIENTS AND FAMILIES

Regardless of culture, illness results in a number of changes for both patients and families. Common experiences include behavioral and emotional changes, changes in roles, and disturbed family dynamics. Illness creates stress and other emotional responses. Factors affecting responses to illness include personality before illness; suddenness, extent, and duration of required lifestyle changes; individual and family resources for dealing with the stress of illness; the life-cycle stage of the patient and family; previous experiences with illness or crisis; and social support (Lewis, 1998). Religious faith also plays a role in responses to illness.

Severe illnesses that profoundly affect physical appearance and functioning are more likely to result in high levels of anxiety and extensive behavioral changes than are short-term, non–life-threatening illnesses. The impact of a chronic illness is significant and continues for the lifetime of the patient. When planning holistic nursing

inter**view** *with Dr. Madeleine Leininger, Founder of Transcultural Nursing*

Interviewer: Dr. Leininger, please tell us what you mean by the term "culturally competent."

Dr. Leininger: **Culturally competent** care has been defined as the culturally based knowledge with a care focus that is used in creative, meaningful, and appropriate ways to provide beneficial and satisfying care to individuals, families, groups, or communities or to help people face death or disabilities. I coined this term in 1962 as the goal of my theory of culture care diversity and universality. The term has caught hold today and is being used by many health care providers. It is now used as a requirement for JCAHO (Joint Commission on Accreditation of Healthcare Organizations) accreditation and with other organizations as essential to work effectively with cultures and their health care needs.

Interviewer: Please describe how a culturally competent nurse's patient care differs from that of one who is not culturally competent.

Dr. Leininger: A culturally competent nurse demonstrates the following attributes and skills: (1) Uses transcultural nursing concepts, principles, and available research findings to assess and guide care practices; (2) understands and values the cultural beliefs and practices of designated cultures so that nursing care is tailor-made or fits individuals' needs in meaningful ways; (3) knows how to prevent major kinds of cultural conflicts, clashes, or hurtful care practices; (4) demonstrates reasonable confidence to work effectively and knowingly with clients of different cultures and can also evaluate transcultural nursing care outcomes.

The nurse who is unable to demonstrate these culturally competent attributes often shows signs of being frustrated and impatient with people of different cultures. Moreover, the nurse who does not practice cultural competencies often shows signs of excessive ethnocentrism, biases, and related problems that impede client recovery and well-being.

Interviewer: How do patients respond differently when nurses take their cultural patterns into consideration when planning and implementing care?

Dr. Leininger: It is most encouraging to observe and listen to clients who have received culturally based nursing care. These clients often exhibit the following behaviors: (1) They show signs of being satisfied and very pleased with nurse's actions and decisions. (2) They make comments such as, "This is the best care I or my family members have received from health care providers." Frequently they say, "How did you know about my values, my culture and how to use these ideas in my care? You anticipated my needs well." (3) They appreciate the different ways the nurse incorporates their cultural needs. They express their gratitude to the nurse. (4) Clients appreciate respect for their culture shown by the nurse in care decisions and practices. (5) The clients do not experience racial biases and

Continued

negative comments about their cultures or familiar lifeways.

Interviewer: With so many cultural groups in this country, knowing all one needs to know about other cultures seems overwhelming. How do you advise nurses to begin the process of becoming culturally competent?

Dr. Leininger: The nurse should first enroll in a substantive transcultural nursing course to learn the basic and important concepts, principles, and practices of transcultural nursing. This knowledge base is essential so the nurse becomes aware of common cultural needs and ways to work with a few cultures that are different. A few cultures are studied in-depth, focusing on common and unique cultural features. The most frequently occurring cultures in the nurse's home or local region are studied first and then one learns about other cultures over time, becoming sensitive and knowledgeable about these cultures. The nurse can greatly increase her or his knowledge of several cultures or sub-cultures by reading the literature, or by studying specific cultures when caring for people under transcultural mentors. Gradually, the nurse learns several cultures in a general way and a few in-depth. As the nurse becomes increasingly knowledgeable about several cultures, comparative knowledge and competencies become evident.

There is no expectation that professional nurses can know all human cultures, as this would be impossible. An open learning attitude and mind with a sincere desire to learn as much as possible about a few cultures will help the nurse in becoming culturally knowledgeable, competent, and sensitive.

Interviewer: What signs can students look for to determine whether their nursing programs are preparing them to provide culturally competent care?

Dr. Leininger: Nursing students will find they are able to provide culturally competent care when (or if) the following signs are evident:

- They consistently know, understand, and respect specific cultures and appreciate commonalities and differences among cultures.
- They feel a sense of confidence, creativity, and competence in their nursing care practices, see how their care fits specific cultures, and accommodate cultural differences in meaningful and creative ways.
- They go beyond common sense to actual use of culture-specific knowledge in patient care as shown in the Sunrise Model (see Figure 13-5).
- They creatively use the clients' beliefs, values, and patterns along with appropriate professional knowledge and skills that meet clients' needs.
- They prevent racial discrimination practices in nursing and in other places; they avoid cultural imposition, ethnocentrism, cultural conflicts, cultural pain, and related negative practices.
- They value and know how to use Leininger's Culture Care Theory and basic transcultural care concepts, principles, and research findings in their nursing practices to provide culturally congruent care for people's health and well-being.
- They appreciate a global perspective of nursing and value transcultural nursing to meet a growing and intense multicultural world.
- They markedly grow in their professional knowledge and sensitivities, developing a global worldview of transcultural nursing. They reach out to help cultural strangers in different living contexts.

Courtesy Dr. Madeleine Leininger.

Figure 10-1
The culturally competent nurse recognizes that in today's diverse society performing a cultural assessment is an increasingly important measure that improves the effectiveness of nursing care. *(Photo by Wilson Baker.)*

care, the nurse must take into consideration how the family both influences and is influenced by the illness of a family member.

Impact of Illness on Patients

Illness creates a variety of emotional responses. Among the more common responses are guilt, anger, anxiety, and stress.

Guilt

Individuals may experience guilt about becoming ill, particularly if the illness is related to lifestyle choices, such as smoking. Guilt may also be associated with the inability to perform usual activities because of illness. A mother who is unable to perform childcare tasks or a father who has to take a lower-paying job because of illness may experience considerable guilt. Some cultures view certain illnesses as shameful and people suffering from them as guilty of cultural transgressions. Nurses who identify and encourage patients to discuss guilt feelings may help prevent the depression that can be a consequence of illness-induced alterations in lifestyle.

Anger

Anger is another common emotional response to illness, particularly in the Anglo-American culture. When patients must make sacrifices to manage their illnesses, such as giving up favorite foods or activities, they may experience anger about the changes. At times, they may feel that their bodies have betrayed them, which results in self-directed anger. Anger may also be directed toward caregivers for their inability to produce a cure, reduce pain, or prevent negative consequences of the illness. Nurses must be prepared to accept such angry feelings, to refrain from rejecting or avoiding patients who express their fears through anger, and to encourage the adaptive expression of angry feelings.

Anxiety

Anxiety is a common and universal experience. It is also a common emotional response to illness and hospitalization. **Anxiety** is an ill-defined, diffuse feeling of apprehension and uncertainty (Ellis and Nowlis, 1994). Anxiety occurs as a result of some threat to an individual's selfhood, self-esteem, or identity.

A number of threats are associated with illness. Illness may alter the way people view themselves. Some illnesses result in a change in physical appearance. Often, ability to function is affected, altering relationships, work performance, and abilities to meet others' expectations. In addition, there may be concern about pain and discomfort associated with illness or treatment. Because of real and potential threats and changes arising from illness, nurses must develop skills that enable them to help patients recognize and manage anxiety.

Although the responses are similar, there is general agreement that anxiety and fear are different. Fear results from specific known causes, whereas with anxiety the cause of the feelings is unknown (Ellis and Nowlis, 1994). For example, if you are home alone at night and you hear an unusual noise outside, most likely your heartbeat and respirations increase, your stomach tightens, and you perspire. The emotion in this situation is fear of an intruder. If you begin to have the same feelings but have heard no noises and cannot identify a source of fear, you are experiencing anxiety. Both emotions may be present at the same time. The patient who is in the hospital for an operation may experience anxiety about the unknown consequences of the surgery and fear of pain and disfigurement from the procedure itself.

Symptoms of anxiety. Nurses should be familiar with the numerous symptoms of anxiety. They are classified as physiological, emotional, and cognitive. Signs and symptoms include increased heart rate, respirations, and blood pressure; insomnia; nausea and vomiting; fatigue; sweaty palms; and tremors. Emotional responses include restlessness, irritability, feelings of helplessness, crying, and depression. Cognitive symptoms include inability to concentrate, forgetfulness, inattention to surroundings, and preoccupation.

Responses to anxiety. Responses to anxiety occur on a continuum. Peplau (1963) described four levels: mild, moderate, severe, and panic. A mild level is characterized by increased alertness and ability to focus attention and concentrate. There is an expanded capacity for learning at this stage.

A person with a moderate level of anxiety is able to concentrate on only one thing at a time. Frequently, there is increased body movement (restlessness), more rapid speech, and a subjective awareness of discomfort.

At the severe level, thoughts become scattered. The severely anxious person may not be able to communicate verbally, and there is considerable discomfort accompanied by purposeless movements such as hand-wringing and pacing.

At the panic level, the person becomes completely disorganized and loses the ability to differentiate between reality and unreality. There are constant random and purposeless movements. The individual experiencing panic levels of anxiety is unable to function without assistance. Panic levels of anxiety cannot be continued indefinitely, because the body will become exhausted, and death may occur if the anxiety is

not reduced. Box 10-5 lists the characteristics of each level of anxiety.

Because anxiety is such a common response to illness and hospitalization, nurses often encounter patients who are experiencing mild or moderate anxiety and, occasionally, patients who are severely anxious. When interacting with an anxious patient, the nurse should carefully assess the level of anxiety before attempting to develop the plan of care.

According to Peplau (1963), anxiety is communicated interpersonally. In other words, it is "contagious." For this reason, it is crucial that the nurse be aware of and manage personal anxiety so that it is not inadvertently transferred to patients. Likewise, self-awareness is essential to prevent absorbing patients' anxiety.

Stress

Stress is another internal variable that affects patients. **Stress** is both a response to illness and

---

Box **10-5** **Levels of Anxiety**

Mild Anxiety
- Increased alertness, increased ability to focus, improved concentration, expanded capacity for learning

Moderate Anxiety
- Concentration limited to one thing, increased body movement, rapid speech, subjective awareness of discomfort

Severe Anxiety
- Scattered thoughts, difficulty with verbal communication, considerable discomfort, purposeless movements

Panic
- Complete disorganization, difficulty differentiating reality from unreality, constant random movements, unable to function without assistance

an important factor in the development of illness. Because illness and hospitalization involve so many alterations in lifestyle, they tend to cause a great deal of stress.

Stress is an unavoidable and essential part of life. To survive and grow, individuals must cope adaptively with constantly changing demands. The stress related to examinations, for example, motivates most students to grow by studying and learning. Although stress is unavoidable, and even sometimes desirable, some control can be exerted over the number and types of **stressors** (factors that create stress) encountered, and responses to the stressors can often be managed.

Hospitalized patients are removed from their usual support systems. They lose much of their control because nurses and other care providers make decisions for them. Being ill often means that they are no longer able to perform activities as they did before the illness occurred. Some patients find themselves in the role of comforting other family members rather than being comforted to avoid increasing family members' distress. Stress is a common response to all these circumstances.

Differentiating between stress and anxiety. Stress and anxiety have some characteristics in common. The physiological responses are similar. Anxiety is a response to some real or perceived threat to the individual, whereas stress is an interaction between the individual and the environment. Stress includes all the responses the body makes while striving to maintain equilibrium and deal with demands. Case Study 10-3 describes one example of stress and anxiety.

Internal, external, and interpersonal stressors. Selye (1956) defined stress as the nonspecific response of the body to any demand made upon it. He named this response the *general adaptation syndrome* and identified three stages through which the body progresses while responding to stress.

Stressors trigger the body's stress response. Stressors are agents, or stimuli, that an individual perceives as posing a threat to homeostasis. Stressors may come from external, interpersonal,

Case Study 10-3

Stress and Anxiety

Mary S is a 32-year-old single mother and a lawyer who was recently hired by an established law firm. One morning as she prepares to take her 2-year-old daughter to the child care center, she receives a phone call informing her that the day care center owner was severely injured in an accident and the center will be closed indefinitely. Ms. S experiences both stress and anxiety in this situation. She has a number of demands placed on her from her workplace and from her family that lead to stress. The additional demands caused by the sudden change in her plans result in even higher levels of stress. In addition, even though none of the male lawyers has responsibility for child care, Ms. S has placed the expectation on herself that she will perform her job exactly like the men in the firm. Being late or missing work as a result of making new arrangements for child care conflicts with her self-expectations and poses a threat to her self-esteem. This threat leads to feelings of anxiety.

or internal sources. External stressors include such things as noise, heat, cold, malfunctioning equipment (such as a car that will not run), or organizational rules and expectations. Interpersonal sources of stress include the demands made by others and conflicts with others. Placing unrealistic expectations on oneself is an example of an internal stressor. In the example of Mary S, an internal stressor is her expectation that her child care responsibilities will not affect the hours she works. It is an unrealistic expectation for any single parent of a small child to expect that the child's needs will never interfere with work.

Responses to stress. Outward responses to stress are determined by the individual's perception of the stressor. Cognitive appraisal, or the way one thinks about a specific situation, determines the degree to which the situation is considered stressful. Loud music at a rock concert, for example, might seem less stressful to adolescents than it would to their parents.

Another factor related to the assessment of threat is whether the individual feels capable of handling the threat, that is, whether the person exhibits hardiness. The person who feels capable can be expected to feel less stress than the person who does not generally feel competent.

Stress affects the physical, emotional, and cognitive areas of functioning just as anxiety does. Physically, there is a feeling of fatigue; muscles are tight and tense. There is an increase in heart rate and respiration. The person who is under prolonged stress may be unable to sleep or eat, or there may be excessive sleeping or eating in an attempt to avoid or cope with the stress.

Emotionally, people under stress feel drained and unable to care for themselves or others. This can result in social isolation and distancing from others. They experience difficulty with enjoying life. They may have feelings of hopelessness and of being out of control. Irritability and impatience often occur.

Cognitively, stress causes decreased mental capacity and problem-solving skills. Therefore there is a tendency to have difficulty making decisions.

Stress and illness.   It has been known for some time that stress plays a major role in the development of illness. More recent research has provided better understanding of the links between prolonged stress and body functioning.

The person who is under stress for long periods of time is at risk for a number of physical problems. The exhaustion that results from excessive, unmanaged stress leads to physiological breakdowns and predisposition to a number of problems. Disorders such as gastric ulcers, hypertension, and autoimmune disorders have been termed stress-related diseases because they frequently occur in individuals who have been severely stressed.

Stress has been found to be related to a reduction in the immune response, which can delay healing and result in greater susceptibility to infectious disorders such as colds and flu. Long-term studies of persons with medical illnesses revealed that the more stress people experienced in a given year, the more likely they were to develop physical illness.

Coping with stress.   Nurses have a role in helping patients modify their stressors. They should assess patients' abilities to recognize symptoms of stress and their usual methods of coping.

Coping with stress can be direct or indirect. In assisting patients to use direct coping, nurses help patients to identify those situations that can be changed and to take responsibility for changing them. The focus is on using problem-solving skills and planning to eliminate or avoid as many stressors as possible. It is important to realize that completely eliminating stress from one's life is neither possible nor desirable.

In helping patients use indirect coping, nurses' actions are aimed at reducing the affective (feelings) and physiological (body) disturbances resulting from stress. Patients are taught techniques such as deep breathing, muscle relaxation, and imagery, which help them cope more effectively with stress (Boxes 10-6 and 10-7).

Box 10-6 **Breathing Exercises**

1. Sit comfortably with feet on the floor and eyes closed.
2. Inhale slowly and deeply through the nose and fill the lungs completely. As you breathe in, imagine the oxygen flowing to all your cells. Hold your breath while slowly counting to 4.
3. Slowly release all the air while thinking the word *calm*. As you breathe out, imagine the air taking all the tension out with it.
4. Repeat the cycle four times. Try to banish all thoughts except those related to your breathing, but do not fight them if other thoughts creep in.
5. When you have completed the exercise, open your eyes slowly and sit for a moment before resuming your regular activities.

To help patients to manage stress, nurses must be skilled in assessing and managing their own personal stress. Nurses who are feeling stressed themselves have difficulty assisting patients in dealing with similar problems. The questions in Box 10-8 can help you identify your own sources of stress and develop self-awareness so that you can be effective in helping patients deal with their stress. For further exploration of stress management approaches, complete the University of Chicago Hospitals' self-study module online (www.nsweb.nursingspectrum.com/ce/ce88.htm).

Coping with stress through learning. Patient education is a major part of nursing practice, and nurses have a professional responsibility to ensure that their patients' learning needs are met. When patients are competent in the knowledge and skills they need to manage their illnesses, they tend to feel more masterful and less stressed.

Nurses who embrace the teaching aspects of the role can assist patients in acquiring new methods of coping with stressors through learning. Historically, nurses considered patient teaching as an integral part of the nursing role. Changes in the health care system have led to a diminution of this aspect of nursing for several reasons. These reasons include lack of time; the short-term nature of many nurse-patient relationships; poor preparation in teaching-learning principles and techniques; the attitude that

---

Box **10-7** | **Relaxation Exercises**

Get into a comfortable position in a place where you will not be interrupted. First focus on slow, deep breathing. Close your eyes and begin to think about the muscle sensations in your body. Identify where you are feeling tense. Slowly inhale as you stretch like a cat; then exhale and allow the tension to flow out.

Neck and Shoulders

- Slowly bend your head forward and backward, then side to side three times. Bring your shoulders up as if you were trying to touch them to your ears. Slowly relax and feel the difference in tension.

Arms and Hands

- Make a tight fist in one hand and tighten the muscles throughout your arm. Slowly release the muscles from the shoulder to the hand. Repeat with the other arm and hand.

Head

- Make a wide smile and hold for a count of five. Slowly relax your face muscles and let your jaw go loose. Tightly close your eyes and feel the tension. Slowly give up the tension and allow your eyes to remain gently closed.

Stomach

- Make your abdominal muscles tight by pushing them out as far as possible. Make your abdomen hard and feel the tension. Slowly relax your muscles and notice the difference.

Legs and Feet

- Holding your leg still, curl your toes down to point to the floor. Do first one leg and then the other. As you tighten your muscles, feel the tension. Then slowly relax.
- Sit quietly for a few moments and feel the relaxation in your body before you resume your activities.

Box 10-8 Personal Stress Inventory

	Very Often	Sometimes	Rarely or Never
1. I feel tense and anxious and have some nervous indigestion.			
2. People at home, school, or work make me feel tense.			
3. I eat, drink, or smoke in response to tension.			
4. I have tension or pain in my neck or shoulders.			
5. I have headaches or insomnia.			
6. I have trouble turning off my thoughts long enough to feel relaxed.			
7. I find it difficult to concentrate on what I am doing because I worry about other things.			
8. I use alcohol, tranquilizers, or other medications to relax or sleep.			
9. I feel a lot of pressure at work or school.			
10. I do not feel that my work is appreciated.			
11. My family does not appreciate what I do for them.			
12. I feel I do not have enough time for myself.			
13. I have difficulty saying "no."			
14. I wish I had more friends with whom to share experiences.			
15. I do not have enough time for physical exercise.			

Scoring: Give yourself 2 points for every check in the Very Often column, 1 point for every check in the Sometimes column, and 0 points for every check in the Rarely or Never column. Total the number of points. A score of 20 to 30 represents a high level of stress. If you scored in this range, you should take steps to reduce your stress level. A score from 10 to 19 means that you are experiencing midlevel stress. You should monitor your stress and begin relaxation exercises. A score of 9 or under means that you are experiencing relatively low stress at the present time.

teaching is a low-priority nursing intervention; lack of emphasis on patient teaching as an indicator of quality care; lack of privacy; refusal of third-party insurers to pay for patient teaching; and lack of confidence that patients really want to be compliant, among others. Nevertheless, nurses have information that can make a positive impact in how patients and their families cope with the stresses of illness. Professional nurses consider patient and family teaching an important, high-priority nursing intervention.

As a first step, nurses must identify factors that can create barriers to learning (Box 10-9). One factor is anxiety. Mild anxiety improves learning by increasing the ability to focus on the task. As anxiety increases, however, the ability to listen, pay attention, and concentrate decreases. Information is not retained, and the patient is unable to make the cognitive connections required for learning to take place.

Physiological factors may also impede learning. For instance, visual or hearing deficits must be

Box **10-9** Barriers to Patient Learning

High anxiety
Sensory deficits (e.g., vision, hearing)
Pain
Fatigue
Hunger/thirst
Shortness of breath
Language differences
Differing health values
Low literacy
Lack of motivation
Environmental factors (e.g., noise, lack of privacy

overcome. Unmet physiological needs, such as fatigue, shortness of breath, hunger, and thirst, decrease the patient's attention to learning. Pain dramatically impairs the ability to learn, and fatigue diminishes the energy required to learn. Nurses who assess and ensure that patients' physiological needs are met enhance their readiness to learn.

Culture also influences learning. This is especially true when patient and nurse have different languages and patterns of learning. When the nurse works toward an educational goal that is not seen as desirable by a patient of a different culture, their cultural values may be in conflict. Understanding the meaning of illness in the patient's culture is necessary. Communicating orally and with handouts that the patient can understand (written in the patient's native language and at an appropriate reading level) is important. Learning a few words of the patient's language and obtaining the services of an interpreter also show sensitivity to cultural differences. Nurses must recognize that low literacy rates are a problem among patients of all cultures, including native-born Americans.

Lack of motivation and readiness are often significant barriers to education. The patient may still be reeling from an unexpected adverse diagnosis and may not be able to focus on learning. The patient may not be motivated to learn what

the nurse believes is important to teach. Patients with an external locus of control, for example, believe that nothing they can do will make a difference and may not be motivated to learn about their own illnesses. Often, nurses believe that simply pointing out what patients need to know is sufficient to motivate them. It is usually more effective to assist patients to make their own decisions about the knowledge they need. This approach may require greater effort initially, but it is ultimately more efficient to assess patient motivation and readiness first, before engaging in patient teaching.

The nurse who is preparing to teach should also assess and manage the environment. A setting that is private, comfortable, and free of distractions is beneficial to the learning process. Once barriers have been identified and removed to the extent possible, nurses must plan patient education using sound principles of learning and teaching-learning concepts. While it goes beyond the scope of this text to review all the complexities of learning, certain basic ideas should be considered. The patient's prior experiences, gender, culture, cognitive style, and motivation are all important determinants of learning. The nurse-teacher's knowledge, flexibility, creativity, communication skills, confidence in the patient's ability to learn, and ability to motivate all facilitate or impede learning. Boxes 10-10 and 10-11 review simple principles of adult learning and teaching-learning concepts that are useful in working with patients.

Impact of Illness on Families

Families are best understood as systems, which means that change in one member changes the functioning of the total family. It is important to remember that the entire family system is affected by a member's illness. Whether the ill family member is hospitalized or cared for in the home, illness drastically increases stress in a family and disrupts usual family function.

The most important factor in how a family tolerates stress is the individual and group coping abilities. Families already experiencing difficul-

Box **10-10** **Principles of Adult Learning**

- Prior experiences are resources for learning.
  Example: If the patient enjoys gardening, try to link health maintenance suggestions to preventive maintenance of indoor/outdoor plants.
- Readiness to learn is usually related to a social role or developmental task.
  Example: New parents are usually eager to learn how to care for their first infants.
- Motivation to learn is greater when the material is seen as immediately useful.
  Example: The same new parents are more motivated to learn care of the small infant than they are to learn about disciplining toddlers.
- The learning environment must be arranged to facilitate learning.
  Example: The room is quiet, kept at a comfortable temperature, with adequate lighting, privacy, and seating.
- Physical needs are met before the teaching session.
  Example: The patient has his or her reading glasses and/or hearing aid, has been given the opportunity to toilet, and is relatively pain free.

Box **10-11** **Basic Teaching Tips for Patients and Families**

- Identify and remove, if possible, barriers to learning.
- Evaluate what the patient and family already know.
- When possible, frequent, short sessions work better than long ones.
- Goals for each session must be realistic.
- Be respectful of cultural differences, for example, in diet planning.
- Avoid medical jargon, acronyms such as PRN, and slang.
- The presentation should proceed from simple to complex concepts.
- Present complex concepts only after there is mastery of simpler ones.
- Patients learn best when they are actively engaged.
- Learning is enhanced when multiple senses are used: seeing, hearing, telling, and doing make the best combination.
- Practice, or frequent repetition, reinforces skill acquisition.
- Reinforce learning with return demonstrations of skills.
- When you give feedback, be sure to include positives as well as negatives.
- Written materials should be at a fourth-grade reading level and, if possible, in the patient's native language to make reading easier for the patient.
- Evaluate patient's understanding of the information presented; provide time to clarify misunderstandings and answer questions.
- Remember to document the teaching session and your evaluation of the outcome.

ties may find that their problems are intensified to the point of disruption when acute or chronic illness occurs.

A sick family member has to give up responsibility to other family members. The family must continue to fulfill its usual functions while dealing with the alterations imposed by the illness or absence of a member. Family members who are able to shift and assume different roles, who can share their feelings, and who seek assistance can be expected to adjust to changes better than those who are inflexible.

Both acute and chronic illness cause changes in family functioning. Chronic illness can be particularly stressful because it is never completely cured. Families experience emotional highs and lows as the patient has remissions and exacerbations. Resentment may be experienced. Family members who must take over the sick person's responsibilities may be angry and then feel guilty about their anger. If they cannot deal with feelings of anger, they may displace them onto nurses by becoming critical and demanding. Similarly, patients may feel guilty about creating hardships for loved ones. They may become convinced that they are no longer essential because others are capably taking over their roles.

Family members sometimes withdraw from each other because they fear that their negative feelings may not be understood and accepted. This mutual withdrawal leads to feelings of isolation for both patients and family members.

Families are often confused or uncertain about how to treat the sick member. They may have problems accepting and responding appropriately to the patients' dependency needs. As discussed earlier, patients may react to illness with either overly dependent or overly independent behaviors. Nurses need to monitor whether family members foster dependence, thereby keeping the patient from becoming more independent. Nurses should also be aware that some families are uncomfortable with the ill person being in a dependent role and do not allow the necessary dependency for recovery. For example, if a man who is very much in control in a family has a heart attack and is in the coronary care unit, family members may have difficulty seeing the usually strong father in a helpless position. They may continue to bring family problems to him. Other families may find it difficult to shift responsibilities back to the formerly ill member as he or she becomes able to resume role functions, thereby fostering dependence. The Evidence-Based Practice Note below shows how illness affects family roles.

The nurse needs to recognize the anxiety in the family and take steps to reduce it. Talking with

 EVIDENCE-BASED PRACTICE

note

Research on how illness affects family roles increases the knowledge base needed to develop effective nursing interventions to meet family needs. Johnson and colleagues undertook a study designed to identify the changes in family roles and responsibilities resulting from the hospitalization of a family member in a critical care unit. They also studied how these changes were affected by the passage of time.

The study involved 52 family members who visited patients in critical care units in a large Midwestern medical center. The subjects completed the Iowa ICU Family Scale each day during the first week and weekly thereafter as long as the patient remained in the unit. Family members were asked to describe changes in family roles and responsibilities. Approximately 59 percent reported that they experienced changes in family roles or responsibilities as a result of the hospitalization. Qualitative analysis of their responses identified seven themes: (1) pulling together, (2) fragmentation, (3) increased dependence, (4) increased independence, (5) increased responsibilities, (6) change in routine, and (7) change in feelings. The researchers recommended that further research be conducted to examine how family roles vary within family systems.

Adapted with permission of Johnson S, Craft M, Titler M et al: Perceived changes in adult family members' roles and responsibilities during critical illness, *Image: J Nurs Scholar* 27(3):238-243, 1995. Copyright 1995 by Sigma Theta Tau International.

family members, explaining what is happening and what to expect, and teaching them how to participate in their loved one's care can help the family considerably. Some families find that becoming active in seeking information, such as through the Internet, helps them manage their anxieties. Support groups and chat rooms, where family members can express their concerns and hear from others with similar issues, are also helpful. Nurses can help family members use these adaptive coping activities effectively by assisting them to find credible websites and evaluate the information they find online. Box 10-12 lists seven "levels of evidence" within health care literature, ranging from least reliable and trustworthy to most reliable and trustworthy.

Other families find that activism helps them control their anxiety. The News Note on p. 263 tells how one man's activism has become a powerful force in the search for a cure for a rare form of abdominal cancer.

The nurse should assess family functioning and the ability of the family to provide support for the patient within the family's cultural context. Observe for feelings of anger, resentment, and guilt and assist the family in identifying adaptive methods of expressing these feelings. The nurse needs to determine the level of knowledge of the family members and assist them to identify concerns and make realistic plans. Providing information and including the family in the planning can result in increased support for the patient and in effective care.

Nurses must be prepared to accept the anger and distrust that often is directed toward care providers who are unable to cure disease or relieve the negative consequences of illness. Understanding that anger expressed by patients and families is not personally directed can enable nurses to assess patients objectively and respond to feelings expressed in a nondefensive manner. Box 10-13

Box 10-13 Reactions to Illness in a Family Member

- Frightened
- Resentful
- Angry
- Guilty
- Feelings of uselessness
- Feelings of hopelessness
- Distrust of health care providers
- Critical and demanding behavior
- Withdrawal from the situation
- Confusion
- Deny seriousness of patient's illness
- Promote dependence by patient

Box 10-12 Seven Levels of Evidence

Patients, families, and nurses must bear in mind that not all published material, including material found on the Internet, has merit. It may or may not be based on evidence. Listed below are seven levels of evidence, ranging from least reliable to most reliable.

- Level 1: Ideas, editorials, letters, and opinion papers
- Level 2: Case reports, case studies, and reports of unusual happenings, such as adverse reactions
- Level 3: Information based on laboratory studies
- Level 4: Information based on animal studies
- Levels 5 and 6: Studies involving human subjects with increasing levels of complexity, scope, and rigor (for example, systematic research reviews, research-based protocols, and clinical practice guidelines)
- Level 7: Clinical trials are the "gold standard." Bear in mind that many nursing-related problems are not amenable to clinical trials because of potential risk to research subjects.

Adapted from McKibbon A: *PDQ: evidence-based principles and practice*, Hamilton, Ontario, BC, 1999, Decker, pp 7-12.

newsnote

Norman Scherzer was compelled to look for help on the Internet following his wife Anita's diagnosis with abdominal cancer. In a patient-run chat room he discovered information about another, more aggressive type of cancer that seemed to match her symptoms more closely. This led the Scherzers to a physician who confirmed a different diagnosis: gastrointestinal stromal tumor (GIST). GIST, Mr. Scherzer learned online, is a rare but deadly cancer that seemed to show a positive response to the drug Gleevec, originally made to treat leukemia. He also learned on the Internet that a clinical trial of Gleevec with GIST patients was under way. Anita had not responded to conventional chemotherapy and her husband succeeded in getting her into the new clinical trial in August 2000. As a result her tumors shrank by 75 percent, and the

Scherzers were able to celebrate their fortieth wedding anniversary in the Fall of 2001.

Mr. Scherzer went on to develop a website and newsletter and to establish a group he termed the Life Raft Group (www.liferaftgroup.org). The group grew from three original members to more than 125 GIST patients and their caregivers. They share information about Gleevec with each other, doctors, and the company that makes the drug, Novartis AG. The Life Raft Group studied side effects from the drug and presented their findings to Novartis. They also published the report on their website.

This is a prime example of how patient activists are using the Web in new ways to help others find reliable and comprehensive, yet understandable health information online.

Modified from Landro L: The best way to get reliable health information, *The Wall Street Journal*, Nov 12, 2001, p R10.

summarizes common examples of family feelings and behaviors that nurses need to recognize, acknowledge, and explore sympathetically with the family.

Despite the numerous stresses, role strains, and adjustments necessitated by illness of a family member, many families find that there are also positive experiences. Finding new activities to share and working together to meet challenges can lead to feelings of closeness and teamwork that were not present before. Previously unrecognized individual strengths may be identified as new roles and responsibilities are assumed. New meanings for the entire family may emerge as values are reassessed and priorities are shifted.

IMPACT OF CAREGIVING ON NURSES

Caring is the foundation of professional nursing practice. Caring meets the essential human need for love and belongingness and assists nurses to

provide high-quality nursing care. A caring attitude towards patients, their families, and colleagues begins with the caregiver—the nurse. Most nurses are not accustomed to caring for themselves, tending to put the needs of others before their own. Finding a balance between caring for others and self-care can be a challenging, lifelong pursuit.

Caring for Self While Caring for Others

Nurses often report that the needs of patients and families, as well as their own spouses and children, take priority over their own needs. They are left feeling stretched, overwhelmed, frustrated, unappreciated, and resentful. This has been termed compassion fatigue (Henry and Henry, 2004). Negative feelings interfere with the ability to maintain a caring attitude and drain caring out of our interactions with others. One nurse stated it well: "As a registered nurse, I try to connect with patients the best I can. Trust develops with personal rapport. When I'm busy and over-worked, I become task oriented and don't have time to work on the trust building" (Roy, Turkel, and Marino, 2002, p. 10). Another used the empty pitcher analogy: "When I have given all I can give, I can't give any more until I get my own pitcher refilled" (Wisdom, 2003).

Although the NANDA diagnosis "caregiver role strain" refers to family caregivers, not professional nurses, some of the defining characteristics of this diagnosis are the same for nurses: anger, stress, impatience, increased emotional lability, frustration, lack of time to meet personal needs, low work productivity, gastrointestinal upset, difficulty performing/completing required tasks, lack of support, and insufficient time (NANDA, 2003, pp. 28-30). These descriptors could also be applied to nurses who feel overwhelmed with competing demands in their work and profes-sional lives.

Nursing theorist Jean Watson referred to caring as the essence of nursing practice. Caregivers who are filled with stress and negativity cannot pro-vide an atmosphere conducive to healing. The inescapable conclusion is that we must learn to care for ourselves in order to truly care for others. Dr. Watson is founder of the Center for Human Caring in Colorado and a renowned nurse theo-rist, speaker, and author. She has identified the consequences of caring and noncaring for nurses (Watson, 2005). The consequences of caring for nurses include:

- Emotional: spiritual sense of accomplish-ment, satisfaction, purpose, and gratification
- Preserved integrity, fulfillment, wholeness, and self-esteem
- Living own philosophy
- Respect for life and death
- Reflective; increased knowledge
- Love of nursing

The consequences of noncaring for nurses include:

- Hardened attitude
- Oblivious to needs of patients and co-workers
- Robot-like manner
- Depression

- Fear
- Fatigue; worn-down feeling

Dr. Watson's work also includes the conse-quences of caring and noncaring for patients. She identified the consequences of caring for patients as:

- Emotional-spiritual: well-being, dignity, self-control, personhood
- Physical: enhanced healing, saved lives, safety, energy, fewer costs, more comfort, less loss
- Trust relationships; decrease in alienation, closer family relationships

The consequences of noncaring for patients, according to Dr. Watson, include:

- Humiliation, fear, out of control, despair
- Helplessness, alienation, vulnerability
- Lingering bad memories
- Decreased healing, lack of trust, detachment

Professional nurses must stay tuned to them-selves to avoid the consequences of noncaring for themselves and their patients. This is a lofty goal and a lifelong challenge. How does one go about maintaining the ability to be caring? Diann Uustal (1997) recommends "creating a balanced life rather than merely maintaining a balancing act" (p. 19). She reminds us of the announcement heard before every airline departure, ". . . put on your own oxygen mask first, before assisting others who may need it" (p. 25). That announce-ment has a lot of relevance to our lives as professional caregivers. Just as airline passengers in an emergency depressurization need oxygen before they can help others, nurses need to meet their own needs so that they will have the physical and emotional energy to care for others.

Choosing to work in a milieu that supports caring and professional nursing practice is one strategy to reduce the stress nurses feel while at work. There is probably no more stressful working environment for nurses today than the hospital. Because of the nursing shortage, however, nursing leaders in hospitals are focusing on retention, and they realize that the atmosphere can help nurses cope with stress in the workplace. One example can be seen in the initiatives designed to create a "Caring Practice Environment" at Hamilton

Medical Center in Dalton, Georgia (Wisdom, 2003):

- Development of a caring vision, mission, and philosophy for the department of nursing, involving all the nurses through surveys, focus groups, and interviews.
- Implementation of Caring Groups, monthly meetings with trained facilitators to promote humor, stress reduction, conflict resolution, and focus on care for self and fellow nurses.
- A caring/healing room, open 24 hours a day, that offers massage therapy, paraffin treatments for hands and feet, aromatherapy, and soothing music. These services are available on a rotating and as-needed basis.
- Incorporation of new graduate nurses into a mentoring program with veteran nurses to help them integrate both clinically and socially into the world of nursing and to the caring environment.

Other activities are being planned.

The Magnet Recognition Program

Another program that supports nurses is the American Nurses Credentialing Center's Magnet Recognition Program. This program formally recognizes health care organizations that have a proven level of excellence in nursing care. The Magnet program was developed by the American Nurses Credentialing Center (ANCC) "to recognize health care organizations that provide the very best in nursing care and uphold the tradition of professional nursing practice" (ANCC, 2006). Achieving Magnet designation demon-strates the importance of nursing and nurses to the entire organization. It recognizes the caliber of the nursing staff, which validates nurses for their hard work and elevates the self-esteem of the entire nursing staff.

As of May 2006, there were more than 180 Magnet-designated health care facilities in the United States. These facilities are "nurse friendly" and have low turnover and vacancy rates, demonstrating that they are desirable places for nurses to work. You can find out about Magnet facilities in your state at the ANCC's website (www.nursingworld.org/ancc/magnet/facilities.html).

Developing a Balanced Life

Keeping the balance between work and personal responsibilities takes conscious and continuous effort. Just as nurses use care plans to organize how they care for patients, they can also identify how to create balance in their own lives. Nurses who feel chronically exhausted and irritable at home and at work; who worry more than usual, cannot seem to complete tasks, lack concentration, and/or are forgetful; and who have diminished self-confidence should be aware that these symptoms indicate a need for more self-care.

Diann Uustal, in her book *Caring for Yourself, Caring for Others: The Ultimate Balance* (1997), recommends taking stock periodically using the guidelines listed in Box 10-14. This can be the beginning of a lifelong effort to maintain balance so that you can continue to be the caring person you want to be in all your life roles, personal and professional.

Box **10-14** **Create a Balanced Life Care Plan for Yourself**

Read the following ideas and reflect on their practical application in your life.

- Taking personal responsibility for your health—physically, emotionally, intellectually, socially, and spiritually—is not easy, but it is the first step. Like it or not, there is no one who can do a better job of taking care of yourself than you.
- Start today with the changes you know are healthful. Make your choices one meal at a time or one day at a time. Do not beat yourself up if you do not always stick to the care plan.

Continued

Box 10-14 **Create a Balanced Life Care Plan for Yourself—cont'd**

- Balance. Try to stay in balance from a holistic perspective. What this means is different to each of us and different at various stages in our own lives.
- Increase your happiness quotient. Identify the things that bring you happiness and joy and enhance your quality of life. Try to do something pleasurable or satisfying each day.
- Identify and decrease the stressors in your personal and professional life. Develop strategies for decreasing the overall level of stress in your life. Some situations and habits can be corrected easily; others will take a real commitment and time to change.
- Make sure your goals and expectations are realistic. Unrealistic goals are self-defeating. Make sure the goals are measurable, manageable, and meaningful to you, not to please somebody else.
- Give yourself permission to relax and take some time for yourself each day. Learn to take "mental health breaks," no matter how brief. Enjoy the time without thinking about what you should be doing, so you can return refreshed.
- Prioritize your commitments based on your values. Make sure you give appropriate time and attention to the relationships that have stability and meaning over time.
- Learn to say "no" if you are pressured and overcommitted. Learn to say no without feeling guilty. Practice thinking that every problem is not your sole responsibility.
- Treat yourself like you treat your best friend. Do something special and "be-friend" yourself.
- Be a person of encouragement—to yourself. Be affirming to yourself. Do not "dump" on yourself or put yourself down.
- Make your physical fitness a priority. Commit to a balanced fitness program that includes stretching, aerobic exercise, and strength exercises. Sneak exercise into your daily life and exercise with a friend.
- Nutrition. Eat a balanced diet low in fat and cholesterol; take a multivitamin; drink lots of water and limit refined sugar intake. Practice portion control. If necessary, consult a dietitian.
- Sleep. Know how much you need and plan to get it. A pattern of too little sleep can injure your health. Avoid trying to be more productive by sleeping less. That can be counterproductive.
- Pay attention to your spiritual growth. Is your faith a first resort or a last resort when all else fails? What does it mean to be "spiritual?" Is being a part of a faith community important to you?
- Challenge yourself intellectually and develop your intellectual curiosity. Try to learn something new every day, no matter how small or insignificant it may seem.
- Stay connected with healthy people. Set time aside and plan for fun with people who can help you lighten up and enjoy some free time. Get out and do things you enjoy doing.
- Try a little "creative neglect" with the "basement people" (we all have them) in your life, especially when you are tired or handling too much. Spend as little time as possible with people who affect you negatively.
- Make sure you get enough "alone time." How much time alone each of us needs varies, so find out what is right for you. Most caregivers spend very little time alone. Check out your balance.
- Express your creativity through music, painting, needlework, sports, decorating, acting, or whatever lets you share yourself from the inside out.
- Don't be afraid to talk with a friend or a professional counselor to help you clarify your direction and put you back in balance again.

Reproduced from Uustal DB: *Caring for yourself, caring for others: the ultimate balance,* Jamestown, RI, 1997, Sea Spirit Press, Educational Resources in HealthCare, pp 113-116.

SUMMARY OF *Key Points*

- Illness is a highly personal experience.
- Reactions to illness are culturally determined.
- Sick people may progress through stages of disbelief and denial, irritability and anger, attempting to gain control, depression, and acceptance and participation.
- Although every culture has expectations about how sick people should behave, previous experience and personality characteristics also affect individuals' responses to illness.
- Culturally competent nurses perform cultural assessments to determine how best to work with patients and families.
- Because of the stress and anxiety involved with illness, it is important for the individual to have methods of coping.
- Coping ability is enhanced in people who exhibit personality characteristics of hardiness, learned resourcefulness, and resilience.
- Patients' spiritual beliefs often play a role in stress reduction and can be used in nursing interventions.
- Providing holistic care means that nurses must consider their patients' physical, mental, emotional, spiritual, social, cultural, and family strengths and challenges to personalize care.

- The family is a system in which a change in one member affects all the other members.
- Illness causes alterations in usual family functioning that can result in emotional changes, including anger and guilt.
- The nurse needs to assess both how the family is influencing the patient and how they are being influenced by the member who is ill.
- An understanding of the cultural factors that affect behaviors associated with illness can provide a better framework for the delivery of nursing care that is both effective and satisfying to patients, families, and nurses.
- As nurses view responses to illness in a cultural context, they are better able to understand and accept the unique ways in which individuals and families react to illness, thereby providing more effective nursing care.
- Caring is the emotional cornerstone of professional nursing practice.
- Creating a balanced life, in which caring for self has a high priority, is the key to sustaining a caring approach to others.

Critical Thinking Questions

1. If you or someone close to you has been hospitalized, how did the nurses and family members encourage or discourage dependent behaviors? Independent behaviors?

2. Would it be easy or hard to allow yourself to be bathed and have other intimate needs met by nurses of the same gender? Of the opposite gender? Of your cultural group? Of a different cultural group? Identify the reasons for your comfort or discomfort.

3. If possible, identify your own cultural group's response to illness. What are your family's characteristic responses to illness of a member?

4. Interview someone from another cultural background to learn how he or she perceives illness. Prepare several specific questions to ask about the meaning, causes, treatment, and feelings engendered by both acute and chronic illnesses. How does his or her culture tend to view nurses?

5. In a small group, discuss aspects of spiritual nursing care that you have used, feel comfortable using, or do not feel comfortable using. Appoint a group member to monitor those interventions that primarily benefit the patient and those that primarily benefit the nurse.

Discuss the appropriateness of each. Report back to the larger class and discuss with your professor.

6. Speculate about the potential changes in the family of a husband and father of four small children who has experienced a severe illness and will be unable to work for an extended period. What stresses is this family likely to encounter? How would these stresses be different if his wife (the mother of the four children) were the sick family member?

7. Identify the ways you show a caring attitude toward patients and toward yourself. If you do not often care for yourself, analyze the reasons.

8. Working in a small group, design a nurse-friendly work setting and present it to the entire class. Be prepared to give rationales for your choices.

REFERENCES

American Nurses Credentialing Center: *ANCC magnet program: recognizing excellence in nursing services,* 2006, available online: www.nursingworld.org/ancc/magnet.html.

Andrews MM: Cultural perspectives on nursing in the 21st century, *J Prof Nurs* 8(1):7-15, 1992.

Benson H, Stark M: *Timeless healing,* New York, 1996, Scribner.

Bowsher J, Keep D: Toward an understanding of three control constructs: personal control, self-efficacy, and hardiness, *Issues Ment Health Nurs* 16(1):33-50, 1995.

Carey B: Long-awaited medical study questions the power of prayer, *New York Times,* March 31, 2006, available online: http://www.nytimes.com/2006/03/31/health/31pray.html?ex=1145937600&en=3cd622f0fc1f109b&ei=5070.

Cassidy CA: Using the transtheoretical model to facilitate behavior change in patients with chronic illness, *J Am Acad Nurse Pract* 11(7):281-287, 1999.

Cavendish R, Luise BK, Horne K et al: Opportunities for enhanced spirituality relevant to well adults, *Nurs Diagn* 11(4):151-163, 2000.

Chilton B: Recognizing spirituality, *Image: J Nurs Scholar* 30:400-401, 1998.

Dewar AL, Lee EA: Bearing illness and injury, *West J Nurs Res* 22(8):912-926, 2000.

Ellis J, Nowlis E: *Nursing: a human needs approach,* ed 5, Philadelphia, 1994, JB Lippincott.

Henry J, Henry L: Self-care begets holistic care, *Reflec Nurs Lead* 30(1):26-27, 2004.

Humphreys JC: Turnings and adaptations in resilient daughters of battered women, *Image: J Nurs Scholar* 33(3):245-251, 2001.

Johnson S, Craft M, Titler M et al: Perceived changes in adult family members' roles and responsibilities during critical illness, *Image: J Nurs Scholar* 27(3):238-243, 1995.

Kirkpatrick SM, Deloughery GL: Cultural influences on nursing. In Deloughery GL, editor: *Issues and trends in nursing,* St Louis, 1995, Mosby, pp 173-197.

Kulwicki AD, Miller J, Schim SM: Collaborative partnership for culture care: enhancing health services for the Arab community, *J Transcult Nurs* 11(1):31-39, 2000.

Landro L: The best way to get reliable health information, *The Wall Street Journal,* Nov 12, 2001, p R10.

Larson L: Heaven and hospitals: the role of spirituality in healing, *AHA News* 32(1):7, 1996.

Leininger M: Personal communication, 1999.

Lewis KS: Emotional adjustment to a chronic illness, *Lippincotts Prim Care Pract* 2(1):38-51, 1998.

McEwen M: Spiritual nursing care: state of the art, *Holistic Nurs Pract* 19(4):161-168, 2005.

McKibbon A: *PDQ: evidence-based principles and practice,* Hamilton, Ontario, BC, 1999, Decker.

NANDA: *Nursing diagnoses: definitions and classification, 2003-2004,* Philadelphia, 2003, NANDA International.

Narayan MC: Cultural assessment in home health care, *Home Healthcare Nurse* 15(10):663-672, 1997.

Parsons T: *The social system,* New York, 1964, Free Press.

Peplau H: A working definition of anxiety. In Burd SF, Marshall MA, editors: *Some clinical approaches to psychiatric nursing,* New York, 1963, Macmillan.

Roy MA, Turkel MC, Marino F: The transformative process for nursing in workforce redevelopment, *Nurs Admin Quart* 26(2):1-14, 2002.

Selye H: *The stress of life,* New York, 1956, McGraw-Hill.

Taylor R: Addressing barriers to cultural competence, *J Nurs Staff Dev* 21(4):135-142, 2005.

Uustal DB: *Caring for yourself, caring for others: the ultimate balance,* East Greenwich, RI, 1997, Educational Resources in HealthCare.

Villaire M: Toni Tripp-Reimer: crossing over the boundaries, *Crit Care Nurse* 14(3):134-141, 1994.

Watson J: *Caring science as sacred science: caritas/love and caring-healing,* presentation at the American Holistic Nurses Association 25th Annual Conference, June 16-19, 2005, King of Prussia, PA.

Whiting SA: A Delphi study to determine defining characteristics of interdependence and dysfunctional independence as potential nursing diagnoses, *Issues Ment Health Nurs* 15(1):37-47, 1994.

Wisdom K: Personal communication, 2003.

Wolin SJ, Wolin S: *The resilient self: how survivors of troubled families rise above adversity,* New York, 1993, Villard.

Zauszniewski JA: Learned resourcefulness: a conceptual analysis, *Issues Ment Health Nurs* 16(1):13-31, 1995.

The Science of Nursing and Evidence-Based Practice

Beth Perry Black

After studying this chapter, students will be able to:

- Differentiate between pure and applied science.
- Describe the historical development of the scientific method.
- Give examples of inductive and deductive reasoning.
- Discuss the limitations of the scientific method when applied to nursing.
- Differentiate between problem solving and research.
- List the steps in the research process.
- Describe the phases in the design of a qualitative study.

- Discuss contributions nursing research has made to nursing practice and to health care.
- Describe the relationship of nursing research to nursing theory and practice.
- Identify sources of support for nursing research.
- Discuss the roles of nurses in research.
- Define evidence-based practice.
- Differentiate between research and evidence-based practice.
- Discuss the pros and cons of evidence-based practice in nursing.

tThe word "science" often conjures up images of laboratories, white lab coats, test tubes, and molecules that leave many students a little apprehensive at the thought. In fact, you are working toward completion of a bachelor of science in nursing (BSN) degree, and you are using nursing science to shape your practice. The purpose of this chapter is to help you understand the links between nursing practice, research, and nursing's scientific base—the science of nursing.

In the mid-twentieth century, the nursing profession was prepared to achieve a higher level of scientific development. Mature professions have a strong scientific base, which was lacking in nursing at the time. Scholars and researchers realized that nursing could achieve a high level of professional status only to the extent that the discipline was based on a scientific body of knowledge unique to nursing. As a result, nursing researchers began developing knowledge unique to nursing, and nursing theorists began developing theories and testing them. Theory and research are the foundations of scientifically based nursing practice.

At the same time, nurses realized that a similar professionalization of patient care practices was needed. Until that time, nurses relied on traditional techniques to manage common patient problems and on trial and error or intuition to manage unusual problems. However, these were no longer acceptable ways to care for patients. The impetus toward evidenced-based practice began to emerge, which required nurses to base their care and activities on research-based knowledge. This requires making a strong link between the work of nurse researchers and nurses in practice. The development of the nursing process became a means of adapting a scientific framework to the management of patient care, so that nurses were no longer depending on hit-or-miss techniques but were shaping care in direct response to the individual needs of the patient. The nursing process is presented in depth in Chapter 8. An understanding of the scientific method is helpful in appreciating both nursing research and the nursing process.

SCIENCE AND THE SCIENTIFIC METHOD

Science is research based on one or more past scientific achievements or accomplishments that are acknowledged by the scientific (academic) community as providing a foundation for further study or practice (Kuhn, 1970). It is important to understand that science requires that research is based on the previous work of others in the same academic discipline or is related to work of others from other disciplines. This is a safeguard that ensures that knowledge development is based on sound principles and theory rather than simply the product of a creative idea that is not based on any known science. Sound science and creativity are not mutually exclusive; creativity has led to many interesting and useful research developments that in turn guide nursing practice.

The scientific community is specific to each academic discipline, meaning that nurse researchers and scholars acknowledge and judge scientific developments in nursing, just as the chemistry academic community establishes the parameters of what constitutes good research and science in chemistry. Social scientists such as sociologists and anthropologists have their own theoretical foundations and foci of research. Common to research in all disciplines, however, is the use of an orderly, systematic way of thinking about and solving problems. This systematic way of thinking is traditionally known as the **scientific method,** used by scientists for centuries to discover and test facts and principles.

The more traditional form of "doing science" required standardized experimental designs, measurable variables and outcomes, and statistical analyses; this form is often referred to as **quantitative research.** Because nursing is interested in phenomena that may not be amenable to traditional quantitative research, a significant number of noted researchers in nursing use qualitative techniques to explore human responses in health and illness. Techniques falling under the rubric of **qualitative research** include ethnography, unstructured interviews, and participant observation, among others (Denzin and Lincoln, 1994). A more recent development in nursing research is the use of mixed methods, a means of examining phenomena of interest using both qualitative and quantitative methods. Regardless of whether a researcher uses quantitative, qualitative, or mixed methods, all good research has a theoretical basis and is carried out in a systematic, disciplined way that furthers the development of a discipline's knowledge base.

Pure and Applied Science and Research

Scientists divide scientific knowledge into two categories: pure and applied. **Pure science** or pure research, sometimes called basic science or basic research, summarizes and explains the universe without regard for whether the information is immediately useful. When Joseph Priestly discovered oxygen in 1774, he did not have an immediate use for that information. Therefore that discovery could be classified as pure science, that is, information gathered solely for the sake of obtaining new knowledge. **Applied science** or applied research seeks to use scientific theory and laws in some practical way. How supplemental oxygen is best used in the care of premature infants with respiratory distress syndrome is an example of applied science. The testing of this method to refine treatment guidelines is applied research. Today's pure science can lead to tomorrow's applied science. Nursing makes use of applied scientific principles and is most effective in conducting applied research to improve patient outcomes through nursing care.

Inductive and Deductive Reasoning

Research requires the use of one of two kinds of logic: inductive reasoning or deductive reasoning. In **inductive reasoning,** the process begins with a particular experience and proceeds to generalizations. Repeated observations of an experiment or event enable the observer to draw general conclusions. For example, a researcher may be interested in the responses of the families of hospice patients to ongoing bereavement support for one year after the death of the patient. After interviewing 10 family members and finding a generally positive response to the support, inductive reasoning may lead the researcher to infer that this is an effective intervention based on this group's response. In other words, the particular experience of 10 families leads to a generalization that everyone would benefit from this sort of support. This type of inference leads to the development of probabilities but not certainties, unless every single member of all families of every hospice patient who died was studied—a study that would be impossible to conduct.

Scientists also use deductive reasoning, a process through which conclusions are drawn by logical inference from given premises. **Deductive reasoning** proceeds from the general case to the specific. For example, if the premises "All families of hospice patients benefit from bereavement support for one year" and "Mrs. Compton is the wife of a hospice patient" are accepted, the conclusion "Mrs. Compton will benefit from hospice support for one year" can be drawn. It may be entirely possible, however, that Mrs. Compton,

although a family member of a hospice patient, will not benefit from bereavement support at all. In deductive reasoning, the premises used must be correct or the conclusions will not be. Conclusions drawn through deductive processes are called valid rather than true. *Valid* is a term meaning "soundly founded," whereas true means "in accordance with the fact or reality" (Flexner, Stein, and Su, 1980). It is possible for a conclusion to be solidly founded without being true for everyone. There is a subtle but real difference in the two terms.

As seen by these examples, neither inductive nor deductive processes alone are adequate. If scientists used only deductive logic, experience would be ignored. If they used only inductive logic, relationships between facts and principles could be overlooked. A combination of both types of reasoning processes in science unifies the theoretical and the practical, which is the basis for the scientific method and research.

Limitations of the Strict Definition of Scientific Method in Nursing

Polit and Beck (2004, p. 16) asserted that the "traditional scientific approach used by quantitative researchers has enjoyed considerable stature as a method of inquiry and it has been used productively by nurse researchers studying a wide range of nursing problems. This is not to say, however, that this approach can solve all nursing problems." There are at least three reasons why the scientific method as implemented exclusively with quantitative techniques has limitations when applied to phenomena of interest to nursing.

The first and most obvious drawback is that health care settings are not comparable to laboratories. Certain phenomena of interest to nurses are simply not amenable to study in a lab setting and in fact are not amenable to study in tightly controlled circumstances. For instance, in the discussion of inductive/deductive logic regarding bereavement support, measurement of the family members' grief and distress in response to the intervention of bereavement support for a year is not possible in the lab setting by conventional measures. The phenomenon of grief may be of great interest to hospice nurses; the systematic examination of an intervention and the measurement of outcomes is not a particularly good fit with the laboratory setting. Grief subsequent to death of a family member is a human response that occurs in real world settings. Research techniques generic to qualitative research may be more appropriate to the aims of this research.

Second, human beings are far more than collections of parts that can be dissected and subjected to examination or experimentation. A strength of nursing is its ability to view patients holistically, whereas the basis of the scientific method is to reduce a problem into manageable problem statements, each of which can be tested. Because humans are complex organisms with interrelated parts and systems, the classic scientific method loses much of its usefulness in the examination of complex human phenomena.

A third limitation of the scientific method as the only approach to solving patient problems is its claim to objectivity; it fails to consider the meaning of patients' own experiences, that is, their subjective view of reality. Nurses are keenly aware, however, that patients' perceptions of their experiences, or subjective data, are just as important as objective data and may have significant effects on their health behaviors. Again, referring to the bereavement example, let us state that Mrs. Compton's grief can be measured by a well-designed, reliable, and valid instrument. After one year, her grief scores are lower and it appears that she has benefited from bereavement support during this time. However, this approach fails to take into consideration Mrs. Compton's own experience of grief and her perception of the support intervention. If she still feels sadder than she believes she should after a year of support, the intervention may be a failure although her "grief scores" are lower. Her perception of her grief and her response are key elements of her experience that cannot be measured objectively and retain the meaning of her situation.

WHAT IS NURSING RESEARCH?

If you are a college or university student, you may have been introduced to research through your basic psychology or sociology courses, in which you may have been required to participate in some way in your professor's research project. While some of these experiments are interesting, in some cases, the only research to which you may have been exposed were surveys or questionnaires. This kind of orientation may lead you to wonder what research has to do with your ability to care for patients.

Nursing research, however, has a different focus that you will likely find more clinically applicable and therefore more valuable than the experiments that you participated in while studying Psychology 101. The National Institutes of Health's (NIH) National Institute of Nursing Research (NINR) describes **nursing research** as "seeking to understand and ease the symptoms of acute and chronic illness, to prevent or delay the onset of disease or disability or slow its progression, to find effective approaches to achieving and sustaining good health, and to improve the clinical settings in which care is provided. Nursing research involves clinical care in a variety of settings including the community and home in addition to more traditional health care sites" (www.nih.gov/ninr/research/themes.doc).

The rest of this chapter describes some basic concepts of nursing research. The purpose is to introduce nursing research, demonstrate its merit, and provide a basic vocabulary. The ultimate goal is for nurses to participate in the research process and apply research findings to clinical practice. This is what is known as evidence-based practice.

Nursing research is the systematic investigation of **phenomena** (events or circumstances) related to improving patient care. Much nursing research arises out of clinical observations. Although a research topic may be in a new area of investigation, much can be gained from choosing research problems that are connected to work already done, thereby building the body of knowledge of nursing. A problem may be amenable to research if these criteria are met:

1. A conceptual framework exists or can be constructed from research that already has been done; that is, the researcher's ideas about the problem fit logically and dovetail with what is already known about the topic.
2. The proposed research project is based on related research findings published in professional journals or is supported by similar ongoing research in other settings, thereby building nursing knowledge.
3. The proposed research is carefully designed so that the results will be applicable in similar situations or will generate hypotheses for further research and testing.

In addition to building nursing knowledge, studies that build on previous work are more likely to receive financial support. Research is expensive and often requires funding beyond what one nurse, hospital, or university can supply. Nurses who want to do research usually find it necessary to obtain outside funding or compete with other aspiring researchers for limited internal (from within the agency) funding. Therefore to receive funding, nurses must do research that interests others, has demonstrated significance, and has support from reviewers who examine the proposed research for the specific funding agency.

Furthermore, research that is not based on or is not related to previous foundational work may have inadvertent violations of human participants' rights. In other words, it is hard to justify asking people to participate in research if there is no real connection to previous work or theory that supports the idea that an intervention works or a problem is significant. Researching or testing an intervention on humans just to see if it works or that seemed like a "good idea" ignores potential shortcomings or may fail to anticipate problems if adequate foundational work is not done before instituting the research. In fact, such research will not receive approval from a federal human participants' review board if significant linkages with previous research are not demonstrated.

Thus although nursing research may be broadly defined as anything that interests nurses and helps them provide better care, controversy exists over what can legitimately be included. When choosing a research question, the wise nurse researcher considers the practical issues of background and financial support. An important source of funding and support for nursing research is the National Institutes of Health's National Institute of Nursing Research (NINR), created in 1992 from what had previously been known as the National Center for Nursing Research. NINR supports clinical and basic research aimed at establishing a scientific basis for nursing practice. Although its budget has quadrupled since NCNR was first created, NINR is still able to fund only a small portion of the proposals it receives. To establish priorities for funding, the National Nursing Research Agenda (NNRA) was launched in 1987. In 2006 NINR published its plan for the next 5 years that was built on past progress in nursing research. The priorities of current research efforts that NINR anticipates continuing to support are listed in Box 11-1.

Research is different from problem solving. **Problem solving** is specific to a given situation and is designed for immediate action, whereas research is **generalizable** (transferable) to other situations and deals with long-term solutions rather than immediate ones. For example, Mrs. Abney is an elderly patient who frequently is found wandering in the halls of the nursing home, unable to find her way back to her room. This is quite distressing to her and time-consuming for the nursing staff who help her find her way "home." A nurse notices that Mrs. Abney has no difficulty recognizing her daughter, so she tapes a photograph of the daughter to Mrs. Abney's door. Now Mrs. Abney can find her room easily. She is less agitated, and the nursing staff time can be spent on other priorities.

Mrs. Abney's case is an example of problem solving, an effective intervention in one set of circumstances that has immediate application. However, the solution that worked for Mrs. Abney may not work for all confused patients. In fact, it may not continue to work for Mrs. Abney if her cognitive abilities decline further. Remember that nursing research was developed in response to the professional and scientific mandate that nursing care be based in evidence and not simply on trial and error. On an occasional basis, creative problem solving such as that of Mrs. Abney's nurse is required on a per-case, situational basis. But this sort of trial and error problem-solving approach is not adequate to base one's professional practice in a substantial and sustained way. Table 11-1 contrasts problem solving and research.

EVIDENCE-BASED PRACTICE: BRIDGING THE GAP BETWEEN RESEARCH AND PRACTICE

The best efforts of nurse researchers are fruitless unless nurses make use of their research findings

Box **11-1**	**National Institute of Nursing Research (NINR) Priorities, 2006**

Chronic Illness
Quality and Cost Effectiveness of Care
Health Promotion and Disease Prevention
Management of Symptoms
Adaptation to New Technologies
Health Disparities
Palliative Care at the End of Life

National Institute of Nursing Research: *Strategic planning for the 21st century*, Bethesda, Md, National Institutes of Health, 2005, available online: http://ninr.nih.gov/ninr/research/diversity/mission.html.

to improve patient care in their day-to-day practices. Patients have become more knowledgeable consumers of health care and nurses must ensure that they provide the latest and best available care. One way to ensure positive patient outcomes is through evidence-based practice.

Evidence-based practice (EBP) means using the best available research findings "to make clinical decisions that are most effective and beneficial for patients" (Cope, 2003, p. 97). EBP was originally created in the 1980s by a Canadian university as an approach to clinical learning. The Centre for Evidence-Based Medicine (EBM) at Oxford University in England defines EBM as "the conscientious, explicit, and judicious use of current best evidence in making decisions about the care of individual patients. The practice of evidence-based medicine means integrating individual clinical expertise with the best available external clinical evidence from systematic research" (Sackett, Rosenberg, Gray et al, 1996, p. 71). The motivation behind EBP was the belief that most of health care practice was based on intuition, experience, clinical skills, and guesswork, rather than science. The value of EBP in clinical practice, as well as in learning situations, was recognized, and its study and use spread rapidly to the nursing profession.

For nursing, EBP requires that you "be aware of research that supports the use of interventions" (Alfaro-LeFevre, 2006). Basing one's practice on evidence cited in the literature or in reliable texts is an element of critical thinking and a good

Table 11-1 COMPARISON OF PROBLEM SOLVING AND RESEARCH

Characteristic	Research	Problem Solving
Type of problems addressed	Widely experienced	Situation-specific
Conceptual basis	Theoretical framework	Often none; trial and error
Knowledge base needed	Extensive review of literature to determine latest thinking and research	Practical knowledge, common sense, and experience
Scope of application	Generalizable to similar situations	Useful in immediate situation; transferability must be determined

means of improving clinical judgment. Focusing on evidence of effective interventions is a good means of preventing one's practice from deteriorating into routine or traditional care based on what has always been done without concern for advances in care. Pursuing continuing education, attending professional conferences, reading journals, and obtaining membership in professional organizations are good means of staying current and keeping aware of new evidence of best practices.

Questions regarding best practices are raised daily by nurses in direct patient care roles. Nurses in practice commonly question procedures and routines, asking if there is a better way to achieve the outcomes of patient care. Most nurses in bedside practice are not equipped to study those questions; however, answers may already be available in the nursing literature. An important focus of professional nursing education is to learn how to seek out and critique research findings in order to implement best practices in one's own nursing practice. EBP represents a formalized process to using the substantial body of nursing research compiled during the past several decades. The seven steps of this process are (Cope, 2003, p. 97):

1. Precise definition of a patient problem
2. Identification of information necessary to solve the problem
3. Efficient and thorough search of the literature
4. Critical appraisal of the evidence
5. Extraction of the clinical answer as it applies to the patient problem
6. Clinical guideline or protocol development and implementation
7. Evaluation

Not surprisingly, EBP in nursing has aroused some controversy (Salazar, 2003). Differences of opinion exist among nurses regarding what types of studies constitute the strongest evidence and what weight to give to each. The use of systematic review of clinical research regarding a particular patient problem poses certain obstacles in examining published reports of research. Some nurses disagree, for example, about the relative merits of randomized controlled trials, long considered the

gold standard in research, versus descriptive and qualitative studies.

Systematic reviews of the research and clinical literature—such as those that can be done on databases like the Cumulative Index of Nursing and Allied Health Literature (CINAHL), the Educational Resources Information Center (ERIC), and PubMed—require that the reviewer has some idea of what type of research method best captures the phenomenon of interest (Macnee, 2004). Remember that evidence-based practice means that best practices are in use; astute use of the literature may result in the decision to forgo certain practices, even when tradition suggests that "this is how it's always been done." Research is used to both support certain practices and discourage others.

Where do clinical expertise, intuition, and patient preference come into the hierarchy of importance in planning care? These issues are being debated in numerous evidence-based practice conferences and symposia. Each of these has significance in planning care for patients; however, basing practice on clinical expertise, intuition, and patient preference without having a thorough knowledge of research that supports care is unprofessional, demonstrating evidence of a lack of critical thinking about the management of one's own practice.

Sigma Theta Tau International, Honor Society of Nursing, has a long history of support of nursing research and dissemination of research findings through its publications. This association has adopted a position statement on evidence-based nursing that demonstrates its importance to the members of that organization. You can read this position statement in Box 11-2.

THE RESEARCH PROCESS

The nursing **research process** is the same as the research process in any other academic discipline; nursing research, however, focuses on a nursing-related problem. Research starts with a problem or stimulus. The stimulus for a research project may be an observation that something related to practice or patients' responses needs to

Box **11-2** Sigma Theta Tau International's Position Statement on Evidence-Based Nursing

As a leader in the development and dissemination of knowledge to improve nursing practice, the Honor Society of Nursing, Sigma Theta Tau International, supports the development and implementation of evidence-based nursing (EBN). The society defines EBN as an integration of the best evidence available, nursing expertise, and the values and preferences of the individuals, families, and communities who are served. This assumes that optimal nursing care is provided when nurses and health care decision makers have access to a synthesis of the latest research, a consensus of expert opinion, and are thus able to exercise their judgment as they plan and provide care that takes into account cultural and personal values and preferences. This approach to nursing care bridges the gap between the best evidence available and the most appropriate nursing care of individuals, groups, and populations with varied needs. The society, working closely with key partners who provide information to support nursing research and EBN around the world, will be a leading source of information on EBN with an integrated cluster of resources, products, and services that will foster optimal nursing care globally. The society, along with its strategic partners, will provide nurses with the most current and comprehensive resources to translate the best evidence into the best nursing research, education, administration, policy, and practice.

Sigma Theta Tau International: *Position statement on evidence-based nursing*, 2005, available online: www.nursingsociety.org/research/main.html#ebp.

be addressed. There may be insufficient data for resolving a problem, or the literature is unclear, or the data presented in the literature are conflicting. When there is a need for more information and no adequate information or conflicting information exists, research is in order.

Whether using quantitative or qualitative techniques or mixed methods, all research must be rigorously planned, carefully implemented, and scrupulously analyzed. Therefore most research follows a formal order known as the research process. Students in baccalaureate nursing programs often take a semester-long course in nursing research in which both qualitative and quantitative methods are described, so this chapter will attempt only a brief introduction to the research process. Steps in the research process include the following:

1. Identification of a research problem
2. Review of literature
3. Formulation of the research question or hypothesis
4. Design of the study
5. Implementation
6. Drawing conclusions based on findings
7. Discussion of implications
8. Dissemination of findings
   Each step will be discussed briefly.

Identification of a Research Problem

Research problems generally come from three sources: clinical situations, the literature, or theories. Clinical situations are rich sources for research problems. Nurses are in a prime position for identifying problems and issues for research. For instance, a common issue among nurses in gerontological settings is the propensity for some elderly patients to wander and get lost. There are several issues related to this problem, including characteristics of patients that tend to wander, time of day this occurs, staffing issues, and medications. Is the nurse seeking to identify patients at high risk for wandering, or is the nurse more interested in preventing nighttime wandering, specifically? A nurse who has identified a clinical problem that may lead to research will have a number of questions to consider as the research is being formulated. Streamlining the problem into a researchable question is a primary goal early in the research process.

Secondly, sometimes researchers become interested in a problem because it has been written about in the literature. They may decide to **replicate** (repeat) the study or may design a similar one to test part of the original study in a new way. For example, suppose that the nurses in the previous scenario read an article in their professional journal about an innovative means of minimizing wandering among elderly patients. In a discussion at their staff meeting about the article, one of the nurses suggests that this approach may not work on this unit for several reasons. The nurses decide to consult with a nurse researcher at the local university to discuss replicating the study on their unit to determine if in fact this innovative intervention will work under the conditions that are in place here or to determine what prevents the intervention from working.

The third source of research problems, theory, relates to testing theoretical models. In Chapter 13 you will read about several models of nursing theory that have been developed. Theoretical models are designed to predict patients' responses to nursing actions; whether or not a model actually does predict patients' responses can be tested through research. The researcher can create certain conditions and determine whether, in fact, the events happen as the theoretical model predicted. Again, consider the nurses on the gerontology nursing unit. Suppose that one of the nurses who has a psychiatric nursing background noted that some psychiatric patients will wander, but using Peplau's theory of interpersonal relations as basis for their psychiatric practice, found that patients who formed excellent relationships with their primary nurses were the least likely to wander. The nursing staff decided to test this theory on their elderly patients, using Peplau's theoretical model as a basis for their intervention, predicting that the formation of a trusting relationship between patient and primary nurse would result in less nighttime wandering among patients without cognitive impairment. A "real life" example of the use of Peplau's theory to guide an ongoing research project is found in Box 11-3.

This study also illustrated the interrelationship between nursing theory, research, and practice.

Review of the Literature (ROL)

Once a problem is identified, the research literature must be reviewed. A review of the literature (ROL) is comprehensive and covers all relevant research and supporting documents to support the research. Doing a thorough ROL requires a great deal of library time or computer search efforts and detective work. Computer-generated searches of the literature can assist tremendously with this step but cannot totally replace the efforts of a dedicated researcher. A major study with many parts requires huge review efforts and usually involves multiple investigators (researchers) in the work to make sure that the literature review is complete.

The ROL is essential to locate similar or related studies that have already been completed and upon which a new study can build. The review is helpful in creating a **conceptual framework,** or organization of supporting ideas, on which to base the study. The ROL answers the question, "What have other researchers and theorists written about this problem?" Sometimes the literature review causes the researcher to rethink or reconceptualize the initial problem, especially if the problem has been studied a variety of ways or if findings in other work are unimpressive or statistically insignificant.

Nursing is a relatively new discipline with a growing but limited knowledge base, especially in comparison to other disciplines such as medicine and some of the humanities. Because nursing has a holistic view of patients and problems, and the nursing literature may not be sufficiently broad, often the ROL has to include research outside of the discipline of nursing. For instance, if a researcher is interested in a phenomenon such as perinatal loss, an ROL must include what has been written in nursing about the phenomenon of perinatal loss, including all aspects such as early and late miscarriage, stillbirth, and elective termination. However, because this is a subject that has many social, ethical, and psychological issues

Box **11-3** A Research Study of a Nursing Intervention Guided by Theory

Hildegard Peplau has been called the "Founder of Psychiatric-Mental Health Nursing" because she started the first graduate programs that prepared nurses to do advanced-practice functions such as psychiatric-mental health diagnosis, psychotherapy and care of persons with complex mental health needs. In 1991, I was developing her Interpersonal Theory of Nursing (ITN) to guide intervention for depressive symptoms. We were exchanging letters and she wrote, "Linda, you need to get to mothers as early as possible so that they can create the kind of relationships with their very young children that foster healthy emotional growth." Now, 15 years later, we are scientifically testing a new form of interpersonal psychotherapy done in the home of low-income, depressed mothers of infants and toddlers. The exciting part of this project is to see master's-prepared psychiatric mental health nurses use the incredibly rich "laboratory" of the mother's interpersonal life—her interactions with her child, her exchanges with her significant others and her relationship with the nurse—to help her change the very sources of her depression. We are trying to help these mothers take charge of themselves and their lives, and in doing so, reduce the risk of more depressive episodes for themselves and later, for their children. The ITN gives the interventionists a framework for constructing interventions to help these mothers solve the deeply difficult issues they face and learn new strategies for reducing their depressive symptoms. We would be lost without Dr. Peplau's roadmap. We are so indebted to her work that we call our project "HILDA"!

Linda Beeber, PhD, RN, FAAN
University of North Carolina at Chapel Hill

Courtesy Linda Beeber.

at stake, a thorough ROL would include literature from sociology, anthropology, ethics, and psychology, and may include work from public health (epidemiology). In addition, literature from the medical field (obstetrics and gynecology) would be reviewed.

As the researcher reviews the literature, he or she will find that some specific papers are commonly cited by other researchers. These "classics" in research, despite being older papers, have a place in a new ROL. Otherwise, most researchers find that literature published within the past 5 years tends to be adequate. Although the review of literature is a tedious task, it is a crucial step in ensuring that the research to be undertaken will be scientifically sound and theoretically congruent with work that has already been completed.

A caveat is in order here about the use of Internet resources for scholarly work. Although there is much information available on the Internet about almost any topic you can imagine, much of this work is not peer-reviewed and should be used with caution. The Internet is best used as a tool for disciplined, organized searches of established databases such as CINAHL, MedLine, PubMed, and PsychInfo. These online catalogs will lead you to peer-reviewed papers that have a place in scholarly work. Increasing your informational literacy (Fitzpatrick and Montgomery, 2004) strengthens your review of the literature by allowing you increased access to scientific publications that have met the challenges of peer review. Box 11-4 lists some important measures to take in establishing the credibility and usefulness of Internet resources for research. Even as a student, this information is important as you perform research for your assignments and prepare for clinical activities.

Formulation of the Research Question or Hypothesis

Once researchers have identified a research problem, are intimately acquainted with the relevant literature, and have chosen or created a

Box 11-4 **Evaluating Information Sources on the Internet**

It is often difficult to know when you are accessing credible information on a website and when you are not, particularly in health care, which has many competing commercial interests. Nursing, Midwifery and Allied Health Professions (NMAP) is part of a gateway system created in the United Kingdom to improve the quality of Internet searches for health-related information. NMAP recommends a six-step process in evaluating Internet resources. You may want to adopt some of these practices to ensure that you are retrieving the best available information from credible sources.

1. **Follow any links** as far as you can to find out details about a resource. The home page, help files, and frequently asked questions (FAQs) are good starting places.
2. **Analyze the URL.** This will give you an idea about the source of the information. For instance, .edu is a U.S.-based educational institution, .com is a U.S.-based commercial establishment, and .org is a U.S.-based organization. A country code such as .UK for the United Kingdom is added if the URL is not based in the United States.
3. **Examine the information** in the resource. Check for thoroughness via a site map or search facility on the website. See who the developers of the website consider to be their target audience—professional health care providers, patients, families. Check for links to other credible websites. Then, **assess the accuracy of the information.** This poses a big task for a student who may not yet have the background to assess a site adequately. You should ask a professor or other expert to help you. Remember that some sites have commercial interests whose information may not be entirely accurate or it may be slanted in such a way to increase sales of a product.
4. **Determine how accessible and easy the resource is to use.** How available and reliable is the server? Are there restrictions on its use? Do you have to pay to use the site? Cumbersome websites with poor information are a waste of time, yielding little if any useful data.
5. **Obtain additional information about the resource.** Double-check the reliability of information on the Internet site you are considering using. Is the site sponsored by a credible agency? How much is this site used? A trustworthy site with reliable information should generate substantial Internet traffic.
6. **Compare the resource to other similar sites and materials.** The website should have basic information that is similar to that of other reliable sources. If the information is very different, look for another website. You must trust that the website's basic information is correct.

From Nursing, Midwifery and Allied Health Professions: *How to evaluate an Internet-based information source*, available online: www.vts.intute.ac.uk/he/tutorial/nurse (accessed Nov 2006).

conceptual framework that helps to focus and support the topic, they need to formulate the **research question.** If the researcher is interested in determining and describing certain characteristics of a situation, he or she may simply pose the problem as a question. For example, "What are the characteristics of mothers who have difficulty initiating breastfeeding with their newborns?" is a research question asking about specific characteristics of a population (mothers with breastfeeding difficulties). If comparing the relationship of two variables, a different type of question might be asked, such as "What is the relationship between maternal age, parity and difficulty in initiating breastfeeding?" This question demonstrates that the researcher has some idea that these variables are related (and that the literature supports this idea), but the exact nature of the relationship is not known or hypothesized.

If conducting an experiment, researchers must have a **hypothesis** (an educated or informed "guess") as to what the outcome will be so that hypothesis-testing statistics may later be applied. For example, "Younger mothers with no previous children will demonstrate later initiation of breast-feeding than older and experienced mothers" is a testable hypothesis. The form and content of the research question are key to the development of the rest of the study. Larger, more complex studies will have multiple questions or hypotheses to address.

Design of the Study

Once the research question(s) is (are) identified or hypotheses are generated, if appropriate, the study must be designed. Numerous forms of research designs exist, but experimental and non-experimental designs are the two major categories. If the purpose of the research is to determine the effect of an intervention or to compare the responses of participants to two or more differing treatments, for example, the research should have an **experimental design.** If not, the research should have a **non-experimental design.** The main difference between experimental and non-experimental research is whether or not the researcher manipulates, influences, or changes the participants in any way by the testing of an intervention or medication or other substance.

True experimental designs provide evidence of a cause-and-effect relationship between actions. For example, testing the hypothesis "patients who receive preoperative teaching need less pain medication in the first 72 hours postoperatively than those who do not" would provide evidence of a cause-and-effect relationship between teaching and perception of pain. Experimental designs require quantitative measures to determine if there are statistically significant differences between the conditions being tested.

Sometimes it is impossible to conduct a true experimental study with human beings, because to do so might endanger them in some way. In those instances, modified experimental studies are used. In this case, a new intensive form of educational intervention before surgery might be tested against the usual form of preoperative teaching. Since preoperative teaching of patients regarding pain management is standard care and an expected behavior of all nurses in that setting, denying that care to patients would be unethical

and inappropriate. The experimental design could, however, test a new intervention against the usual care received by preoperative patients.

Nonexperimental designs are occasionally referred to as "descriptive" or "exploratory" research because the investigator is seeking to increase the knowledge base about a nursing phenomenon by doing careful disciplined research. There are many types of nonexperimental designs: surveys, descriptive comparisons, evaluation studies, and historical-documentary research, among others. Nonexperimental designs may be either quantitative or qualitative, or they may use a combination of both.

Whether the researcher chooses an experimental or nonexperimental design influences the data collection process. The data collection process includes selection of data collection instruments, design of the data collection protocol, the data analysis plan, participant selection, and informed consent and institutional review plans.

Data collection instruments

When designing a study, researchers must consider how the **data** will be collected. Data collection instruments, sometimes called data collection tools, range from simple survey forms to complex radiographic scanning devices. The selected instrument used must be **reliable,** or accurate. A reliable instrument is one that yields the same values dependably each time the instrument is used to measure the same thing. The tool must also be **valid,** which means that it must measure what it is supposed to be measuring. The ideal instrument is highly reliable and provides a valid measure of the condition, such as weight, temperature, or depression.

If body temperature is being measured, a thermometer is an obvious data collection tool. When measuring an abstract factor, such as anxiety or depression, the best data collection tool is not as clear. The selection of a data collection instrument answers the question, "What tool(s) will we use to collect the data?" To minimize measurement errors, beginning researchers should choose instruments with established reliability and validity that have been published and widely used, rather than designing their own. Inexperienced researchers will occasionally make the mistake of designing a questionnaire that they believe is a valid measure of the construct (condition) they want to study. However, this is a serious flaw in the research and must be avoided.

Data collection protocol

Another aspect of designing the study is deciding on the data collection protocol (procedure). The quality of the data depends on strict adherence to the plan. If, for example, the plan calls for administering a questionnaire to renal dialysis patients after dialysis, the data collectors must be sure to give the questionnaire to all participants—and only after their treatments. The protocol for data collection must be carefully explicated and recorded and used by everyone who is collecting data for the study. Data collected in the wrong way or at the wrong time are unusable, introducing error into the study that must be avoided.

Data analysis plan

It may seem premature to decide how the data will be analyzed before they are even collected, but careful planning for the analysis is important. The research design is developed with data analysis in mind. The analysis must be part of the planning process, because the data and the protocols for collecting them depend on how the data will be analyzed. Unless the nurse researcher is an expert in statistics or there is already a statistician on the research team, consultation with a statistician well versed in human participant research is recommended in designing the data analysis plan, which answers the question, "What will we do with the data once we gather them?"

Qualitative analysis, notably, begins immediately with the collection of data, because the data themselves often drive the shape and design of the research. Qualitative analysis is a very difficult and exacting procedure that requires extensive training. Although some researchers believe that qualitative research is "easier" than quantitative research, in fact they are similar in

the disciplined approach to data analysis that is required to produce usable, meaningful results.

Participant selection

Once the researcher knows what is to be done, the specifics of who will be included are decided. The individual people being studied are referred to as **participants,** a newer preferred term for the term formerly used, "subjects." If the researchers plan to study pain control in postoperative patients, for example, they have to decide the specific type of surgery and the age, sex, ethnicity, and geographic location of the patients, as well as a variety of other factors in planning the participant selection (Figure 11-1).

Informed Consent and Institutional Review

Next, researchers who use human participants must plan to protect their rights by asking them to sign an **informed consent** form that describes

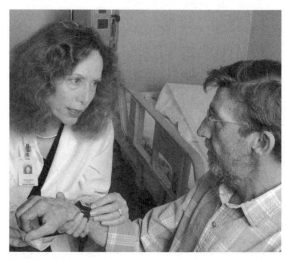

Figure 11-1
Research participants are selected based on factors such as age, gender, condition, and location. They must then be informed about certain aspects of the proposed research in order to make a decision about participating. That decision, which is written and signed, is known as "informed consent." (*Courtesy Memorial Health Care System, Chattanooga, Tenn.*)

the details of the study and what participation means. Any risks involved in participating must be explained. No one should be pressured in any way to participate, and the **confidentiality** (privacy) of participants must be ensured.

A related step when studying humans is the submission of the proposal to the institution, such as a hospital or clinic, where the research will take place for review by a federally approved board known as the IRB—**Institutional Review Board.** An IRB is composed of individuals from different disciplines and exists to ensure that research is well designed and ethical and does not violate the policies and procedures of the institution or the rights of the participants. Only after the institutional review board approves the proposal can the study begin. All persons conducting research or assisting with the management of data must demonstrate evidence that they have taken an online course on the protection of the rights of human participants (www.citiprogram.org). The protection of the rights of participants is the primary consideration of all research involving humans. Modification of any aspect of the research requires that the IRB be notified and approval procured before the change is implemented.

Implementation

Up until this point, only planning has taken place. Careful planning is, however, the key to a successful study. In the implementation phase, the actual study is conducted. The two main tasks during this phase are data collection and data analysis.

Data collection

Data (research-generated information) should be collected only by those who are thoroughly familiar with the study. All research assistants should understand the purpose of the data and the importance of accuracy and careful record keeping. No matter who is collecting the data, the integrity of the project is ultimately the responsibility of the primary researcher.

Data analysis

If all goes well, the data are analyzed exactly as proposed. In analyzing the data, most researchers use the same statistical consultants who assisted in planning the study. The researcher is well advised to work closely with the statistician in interpreting as well as analyzing the data. The nurse researcher is in charge, however, and he or she has the final word on what interpretations are made from the data.

Analyzing the findings of qualitative research presents formidable challenges for several reasons. First, the data are voluminous, often consisting of lengthy dialogues between researchers and participants. Next, dialogues must be transcribed verbatim, yielding hefty stacks of pages. The investigator then faces the task of organizing the transcripts, identifying themes, and arranging the themes into meaningful patterns. Fortunately, computer programs are now available to assist in this process; however, nothing substitutes for contemplation (by humans!) in determining the nuances of meanings in narrative data such as those assimilated in qualitative designs.

✦ *Cultural Considerations* Challenge

Informed Consent

If researchers who use human participants must plan to protect their rights by asking them to sign an informed consent form that describes the details of the study and what participation means, what measures would researchers need to consider when participants are recent immigrants? How might potential risks involved in participating best be explained? How might researchers ensure that these participants do not feel pressured to participate? What assurances might they desire concerning confidentiality that other participants might not need?

Drawing Conclusions Based on Findings

In writing the research report, the findings directly related to the research question are presented first. Findings are presented factually—without value judgments. The facts must speak for themselves. Accurate presentation of the facts is the only requirement. After findings related to the research question are reported, unexpected findings can be reported. Conclusions are then drawn. Conclusions answer the question, "What do these findings mean?" Here researchers can be more reflective about the findings, discussing what was anticipated versus what was found in the study, and suggesting alternative work to clarify findings.

Discussion of Implications

Researchers are always alert to the implications of their studies. Implications are suggestions of things that should be done in the future. Every good study raises more questions than it answers. In nursing studies, there may be indications for modifications in nursing education or nursing practice. Nearly every study has implications for further research, and if the findings turn out as expected, almost all studies should be carefully replicated. Replication can answer these and other questions: "What needs to be known to develop more confidence in the findings? Will the research instrument produce similar results in a similar population in a different geographic location? Will the procedure be effective with patients having a slightly different diagnosis, condition, or type of surgery? Will age make a difference? Will cultural beliefs make a difference? What else do we need to know to improve the care of patients?"

Dissemination of Findings

Findings from a research study must be disseminated so that others can learn from the work that was done. **Dissemination** refers to the process of publication and presentation of findings. Most funding agencies want to know in advance how the researcher plans to disseminate findings because letting others know about the findings is very essential. The two major vehicles for dissemination of knowledge are articles published in professional journals and presentations given at conferences. Prominent nursing research journals include *Research in Nursing and Health (RINAH)*, *Nursing Research (NR)*, *Journal of Nursing Scholarship* (published by Sigma Theta Tau International), and the *Western Journal of Nursing Research*. These journals are not specific to any particular type of nursing, but publish papers of wide interest in nursing. Professional nursing organizations may have their own research journals targeting specific nursing interests, such as *JOGNN: Journal of Obstetric, Gynecologic and Neonatal Nursing*, published by AWHONN (Association of Women's Health, Obstetric and Neonatal Nurses); and *Journal of the Association of Nurses in AIDS Care (JANAC)*, published by ANAC (Association of Nurses in AIDS Care).

A review process, called **peer review**, is the method most journals use to determine whether or not to publish a research report. During peer review, a manuscript is circulated anonymously to a review panel consisting of one or more experts in the area of study. They evaluate its appropriateness and accuracy and recommend that it be published, that it be revised and then resubmitted with changes, or that it be rejected. Most research that is carefully conceived, conducted, and presented can get published, although the researcher must be persistent and resilient in taking criticism and reworking manuscripts.

A somewhat easier, yet still discriminating, route to dissemination is presentation at one or more of the numerous nursing research conferences. Many research conferences also use the peer-review process. In general, however, the proportion of **abstracts** (summaries of research) selected for presentation at conferences is higher than the proportion of manuscripts chosen for publication. In addition to oral presentation of research papers, conferences offer the opportunity for nurses to present their findings in poster sessions, especially appropriate when work is preliminary or is still in progress. Posters allow for brief explanations of the research method and findings in written form, usually a 3 × 4-foot poster that is professionally designed.

Whether research is published or presented at conferences, it is important to disseminate research results to other nurses, who may choose to use the results either to improve patient care practices or to replicate the study (Figure 11-2).

PROGRAMS OF RESEARCH: THE LONG-TERM WORK OF NURSE RESEARCHERS

Numerous nurse researchers have made careers as professors in college or university settings with ongoing funding that supports their long-term research efforts. These researchers develop what is known as programs of research, where they base their later work on previous studies that they have completed. They publish widely in nursing and other disciplines, as their work may cross interdisciplinary lines of interest. Each year since 1982, Springer Publishing Company publishes the *Annual Review of Nursing Research (ARNR)*. Several more recent volumes have focused en-

tirely on a particular area of nursing research, such as chronic illness (Vol. 18), women's health (Vol. 19), and geriatrics (Vol. 20). These volumes are useful to students and to new researchers who are trying to identify those persons that are doing research in an area of specific interest.

Box 11-5 contains a list of programs of research on care of preterm infants and their relationship to developmental science published in *ARNR*, Vol. 21 (Holditch-Davis and Black, 2003). The nurse researchers that are listed are from a variety of universities and colleges throughout the United States, although many of them are doing collaborative research. For example, in 2006 Diane Holditch-Davis, PhD, RN (Duke University), and Rosemary White-Traut, PhD, RN (University of Illinois, Chicago), began a collaborative study in which kangaroo care and an infant massage intervention for premature infants are being compared against an educational control intervention. Outcome measures include certain interactions between mother and infants. This is a combination of expertise between two well-known nurse researchers with the care of preterm infants in common.

Many nurse researchers have found that research on premature infants and their families have proven to be fertile ground for nursing research. Advances in neonatology (the science of the care of premature infants) over the past two decades have raised many issues related to the care of increasingly small preterm infants that face long hospitalizations and numerous health problems. Nurses provide the vast majority of hands-on care of these tiny infants. It is not surprising that the care of preterm infants has been an area of substantial research interest to nurses who are often the first to identify problems in patient care in the neonatal intensive care setting.

Figure 11-2
Large research studies require a team approach. In this photo, Paula Anderson is assigning behavioral codes to a video of a mother interacting with her prematurely born infant. Ms. Anderson is a research associate trained in behavioral coding by Diane Holditch-Davis, PhD, RN, whose program of research includes several studies that examine maternal-infant interactions. Dr. Holditch-Davis is a professor of nursing at Duke University in Durham, NC. *(Courtesy Paula Anderson.)*

RELATIONSHIP OF NURSING RESEARCH TO NURSING THEORY AND PRACTICE

Relationships among nursing research, practice, and theory are circular. As mentioned earlier, research ideas are generated from three sources: (1) clinical practice, (2) literature, and (3) theory.

Questions about how best to deal with patient problems regularly arise in clinical situations. As shown in the earlier example of Mrs. Abney, the elderly lady who could not find her room, problems often can be "solved" for the present. However, when the same questions recur, long-term answers may be needed. Research develops solutions that can be used with confidence in different situations.

Published articles about nursing research often generate interest in further studies. If there is published research on a particular nursing care problem, other researchers may be stimulated to investigate the subject further and refine the solutions. This is how nursing knowledge builds.

Nursing theorists also generate research ideas. They piece together postulates or premises that "explain" what has been discovered. The explanation is "tested" to determine whether it is robust or strong enough to be useful. If so, there may be more implications for applications in clinical practice.

Nursing research journals are filled with clinical studies that have made a difference in patient care.

Box **11-5**	Selected Nurse Researchers and Their Programs of Research on the Care of Preterm Infants

NICU Environment:

Jane Evans: Effects of NICU nursing care; behavioral and physiological responses of preterm infants to procedures

Lina Zahr: Sleep-wake states of preterm infants; physiological responses to noise and nursing intervention; developmental care for preterm infants

Shyang-Yun Pamela Shiao: Sucking, swallowing, and feeding issues; effects of non-nutritive sucking

Karen Pridham: Feeding and growth of preterm infants

Patricia Becker: Modifying the NICU to reduce infant distress

Pain Management:

C. Celeste Johnston: Infant responses to painful procedures

Bonnie Stevens: Infant behavioral and physiological responses to painful procedures

Linda Franck: Use of analgesia for pain management in the NICU; use of comfort measures

Infant Stimulation:

Lynda Law Harrison: Effects of touch on preterm infants

Susan Luddington-Hoe: Effects of kangaroo care (skin-to-skin holding) of preterm infants

Rosemary White-Traut: Effects of infant massage and auditory stimulation

Infant Behavior and Development:

Barbara Medoff-Cooper: Neurobehavioral assessment of preterm infants; nutritive sucking

Gail McCain: Effect of nursing care on infant sleep-wake states

Diane Holditch-Davis: Development of self-wake states in preterm infants and infant interactive behaviors

Barbara Schraeder: Factors related to developmental outcomes of preterm infants

Margaret McGrath: Effects of environmental and medical risks on premature infants' development

JoAnne Youngblut: Effects of maternal employment on development of infants born prematurely

From Holditch-Davis D, Black BP: Care of preterm infants: programs of research and their relationship to developmental science. In Fitzpatrick JJ, Miles MS, Holditch-Davis D, editors: *Annual review of nursing research*, Vol 21, New York, 2003, Springer.

A few examples of changes in nursing practice stimulated by research include the following:

1. Improved care of patients with skin breakdown from pressure ulcers
2. Decreasing light and noise in critical care units to prevent sleep deprivation
3. Using caps on newborns to decrease heat loss and stabilize body temperature
4. Positioning patients following chest surgery to facilitate respiration
5. Scheduling pain medication more frequently following surgery
6. Preoperative teaching to facilitate postoperative recovery

Nursing research findings not only improve patient care but also affect the health care system itself. For example, research studies have demonstrated the cost-effectiveness of nurses as health care providers. This is discussed further in Chapter 14.

A final point about the influence of research on practice is a reminder about the relationship of research and professionalism. In Chapter 3, the characteristics of professions were presented. One of the criteria commonly mentioned is a scientific body of knowledge that is expanded through research. Nursing research enhances the status of nursing as a profession by expanding nursing's

scientific knowledge base. Refer back to Box 11-3 for an example that may clarify the interplay between nursing research, practice, and theory; then take this chapter's Critical Thinking Challenge 11-1.

SUPPORT FOR NURSING RESEARCH

Nursing research is expensive, and support takes many forms. It can include encouragement, consultation, computer and library resources, money, and release time from researchers' regular teaching responsibilities. Each of these forms of support is important, but none alone is adequate. Early in the development of nursing research, encouragement was often the only support available, and not all nurse researchers had that. Gradually over the years, more sources of funding have been identified, but financial support can still be difficult to obtain, particularly for new researchers.

In additional to the National Institute of Nursing Research discussed earlier in this chapter, several other federal agencies accept proposals that meet their funding guidelines when submitted by qualified nurse researchers. These include the National Institute on Aging, the National Cancer Institute, the National Institute

CRITICAL THINKING *Challenge 11-1*

Evidence-based practice is a movement in nursing that is gaining widespread support. Well-informed nurses are likely to provide better care than those who are not well-informed. Yet the mention of the word "research" is likely to send many novice (and experienced) nurses running for cover!

Some nursing journals are heavily research oriented, while others are more clinically oriented. For example, the Association of Women's Health, Obstetric and Neonatal Nurses (AWHONN), a large professional nursing association, publishes two journals: *JOGNN*, which generally publishes research-based articles; and *Lifelines*, which is oriented toward clinical issues in women's health. Your school's library is likely to subscribe to these journals and others like them.

Sit down with back issues of each of these journals or others of interest to you, making sure that one is research based and the other is clinically based. Read the table of contents of each and assess your interest in each topic. Which ones appeal to you? Why? Do you find yourself drawn to one type of journal over another? How hard will it be to maintain evidence-based practice once you are out of school and in the work setting? What can you do to ensure that you remain current in your practice and up-to-date with research findings once you no longer have easy access to a school library?

of Mental Health, the National Institute of Alcohol Abuse and Addiction, the National Institute on Drug Addiction, and the Centers for Disease Control and Prevention. Competition with researchers from other disciplines is keen, however, and generally only experienced nurse researchers are successful in obtaining funding from these sources.

Nursing associations also fund nursing research. The American Nurses Foundation, Sigma Theta Tau, and many clinical specialty organizations provide research awards, even for novice researchers. State and local nursing associations sometimes have seed money for pilot projects. Universities, schools of nursing, and large hospitals also may provide small amounts of research funds. Generally, however, finding adequate funding for large-scale studies continues to be a problem faced by researchers.

ROLES OF NURSES IN RESEARCH

The *Code of Ethics for Nurses* states: "The nurse participates in the advancement of the profession through contributions to practice, education, administration, and knowledge development" (American Nurses Association, 2001). Ideally, every nurse should be involved in research, but practically, all nurses should, as a minimum, use research results to improve their practices. Evidence-based nursing practice requires staying informed about current literature, especially studies done in one's own specific area of clinical practice.

As seen in Table 11-2, in addition to using research to improve practice, all professional nurses can contribute to one or more aspects of the research process. Baccalaureate nurses can read, interpret, and evaluate research for applicability to nursing practice. Through clinical practice they can identify nursing problems that need to be investigated. They can also participate in the implementation of scientific studies by helping principal researchers collect data in clinical settings or elsewhere. These beginning researchers must know enough about the pur-

pose of the research to follow the research protocols explicitly or know when it is necessary to deviate from the protocol for a patient's well-being. Baccalaureate nurses also can help disseminate research-based knowledge by sharing useful research findings with colleagues.

The master's-prepared nurse may be ready to replicate studies that have been previously conducted. Researchers cannot be sure that their findings are true until studies are repeated with similar results. Nurse researchers have learned that it is not necessary (or even desirable) always to generate a totally new and disconnected idea to do research. As mentioned earlier, to be most useful, research must be based on a conceptual framework and related to previous research.

Depending on education, clinical and research experiences, and interests, some nurses at the master's level are better prepared to conduct research than others. In addition to education and experience, a crucial factor is the support system the nurse has available. To do research, nurses need time, money, consultation, and participants. With rich resources in a research environment, master's-prepared nurses can and do make vital research contributions.

Nurses with PhDs (doctor of philosophy) or other doctoral degrees are more favorably positioned to receive research funding than are

Table 11-2 LEVELS OF EDUCATIONAL PREPARATION AND PARTICIPATION IN NURSING RESEARCH

Level of Preparation	Level of Research Participation
Student nurse	Consumer
BSN* nurse	Problem identifier
	Data collector
MSN nurse	Replicator
	Concept tester
Doctoral nurse	Theory generator
Postdoctoral nurse	Funded program director

*Abbreviations: BSN, bachelor of science in nursing; MSN, master of science in nursing.

nurses without doctorates. Researchers across the United States in all professions and academic disciplines compete for a limited pool of research dollars available each year. Only those nurses with strong academic and experiential backgrounds and the best proposals succeed in obtaining federal funding.

Research in nursing provides the avenue for creative, scholarly endeavors driven by a desire to improve the care for patients. It is our hope that you will find research to be an important part of your professional practice both as a consumer of research and as an adherent to evidence-based practice, and in the future, you will conduct research of your own.

SUMMARY OF *Key Points*

- The scientific method is a systematic, orderly process of solving problems. It has been used for centuries and is applicable in many different situations.
- Research can generate pure knowledge (knowledge that is not immediately useful) or applied knowledge (knowledge that can be used in a practical way).
- Both inductive reasoning and deductive reasoning are necessary to combine the theoretical and the practical aspects of the scientific method.
- For safety and ethical reasons, there are limitations on the use of the scientific method with human beings.
- Nursing research is defined as the systematic investigation of phenomena of interest to nursing with the goal of improving care.
- The major steps in the research process are identification of a research problem, review of the literature, formulation of the research question, design of the study, implementation, drawing conclusions based on findings, discussion of implications, and dissemination of findings.

- Nurse researchers have made significant contributions to improvements in nursing care practices.
- Nursing research is related to and informed by nursing theory and nursing practice and in turn influences them.
- Nurses of all educational backgrounds have a role in research.
- Evidence-based nursing practice is the goal of nursing research.

CRITICAL THINKING QUESTIONS

1. Why is nursing called an applied science? Explain why you agree or disagree with this description.
2. Name and describe the two types of reasoning used in the scientific method. Explain why neither alone is adequate to advance knowledge.
3. List and discuss each step of the research process.
4. Explain why a purely experimental model is an inadequate one for nursing.
5. Go to your college library or online and see which nursing research journals are in the collection. Scan through some recent issues and notice the types of studies reported. Compare them with studies done 20 years ago. What similarities and differences do you note?
6. Read a research article that interests you. See whether you can identify each of the steps in the research process. If not, what is missing? Discuss with your teacher and classmates what the significance of the missing steps might be.
7. Find out what research is being done in your school or hospital. If possible, talk with those involved, including data collectors, data analysts, research directors, participants, families of participants, and nurses who work on units where research is being conducted. What do they know about the research? What are their concerns? What do they hope will be learned from the research?

8. Obtain job descriptions for nurses at varying experience levels at different agencies. Are research functions included in the job descriptions? If not, what research functions do you think might be appropriate to include?

9. As a class, explore the evidence-based practice websites and debate the pros and cons of evidence-based practice.

REFERENCES

Alfaro-LeFevre R: *Applying the nursing process: a tool for critical thinking,* Philadelphia, 2006, Lippincott Williams & Wilkins.

American Nurses Association: *Code of ethics for nurses with interpretive statements,* Washington, DC, 2001, American Nurses Publishing.

Cope D: Evidence-based practice: making it happen in your clinical setting, *Clin J Oncol Nurs* 7(1):97-98, 2003.

Denzin NK, Lincoln YS, editors: *Handbook of qualitative research,* Thousand Oaks, Calif, 1994, Sage Publications.

Fitzpatrick JJ, Montgomery KS, editors: *Internet for nursing research: a guide to strategies, skills and resources,* New York, 2004, Springer.

Flexner SB, Stein J, Su PY, editors: *The Random House dictionary,* New York, 1980, Random House.

Holditch-Davis D, Black BP: Care of preterm infants: programs of research and their relationship to developmental science. In Fitzpatrick JJ, Miles MS, Holditch-Davis D, editors: *Annual review of nursing research,* Vol 21, New York, 2003, Springer.

Kuhn TS: The structure of scientific revolutions. In Nurath O, editor: *International encyclopedia of unified science,* ed 2, Vol 2, Chicago, 1970, University of Chicago Press.

Macnee CL: *Understanding nursing research: reading and using research in practice,* Philadelphia, 2004, Lippincott Williams & Wilkins.

National Institute of Nursing Research: *Strategic planning for the 21st century,* Bethesda, Md, 2005, National Institutes of Health, available online: http://ninr.nih.gov/ninr/research/diversity/mission.html.

Nursing, Midwifery and Allied Health Professions: *How to evaluate an Internet-based information source,* available online: www.vts.intute.ac.uk/he/tutorial/nurse/ (accessed Nov 2006).

Polit DF, Beck CT: *Nursing research: principles and methods,* ed 7, Baltimore, 2004, Lippincott Williams & Wilkins.

Sackett DL, Rosenberg WM, Gray JA et al: Evidence-based medicine: what it is and what it isn't, *BMJ* 312:71-72, 1996.

Salazar MK: Evidence-based practice: relevance to occupational health nurses, *AAOHN J* 51(3):109-112, 2003.

Sigma Theta Tau International: *Position statement on evidence-based nursing,* 2005, available online: www.nursingsociety.org/research/main.html#ebp.

12

Conceptual and Philosophical Bases of Nursing

Kay Kittrell Chitty

Learning Outcomes

After studying this chapter, students will be able to:

- Describe the components and processes of systems.
- Explain Maslow's hierarchy of human needs and its relationship to motivation.
- Recognize how environmental factors such as family, culture, social support, the Internet, and community influence health.
- Explain the significance of a holistic approach to nursing care.
- Apply Rosenstock's health beliefs model and Bandura's theory of perceived self-efficacy to personal health behaviors and health behaviors of others.

- Devise a personal plan for achieving high-level wellness.
- Define and give examples of beliefs.
- Define and give examples of values.
- Cite examples of nursing philosophies.
- Discuss the impact of beliefs and values on nurses' professional behaviors.
- Explain how nurses and organizations educating and employing nurses can use a philosophy of nursing.
- Identify personal beliefs, values, and philosophies as they relate to nursing.

There are certain basic concepts, or ideas, that are essential to an understanding of professional nursing practice; they are the building blocks of nursing. These concepts are person, environment, and health. Everything professional nurses do is in some way related to one of these basic interrelated concepts, and is guided by beliefs, values, and statements of philosophy. In this chapter we will explore how these concepts relate to each other and to nursing.

SYSTEMS

An understanding of systems will assist you in understanding the interplay among nursing's basic concepts. General systems theory was originally developed by Ludwig von Bertalanffy in 1936 (von Bertalanffy, 1968). Von Bertalanffy, a biologist, believed that a common framework for studying several similar disciplines would allow scientists and scholars to organize and communicate findings and more readily build upon the work of others. He described a **system** as a set of inter-related parts that come together to form a whole that performs a function. Each part is a necessary or integral component required to make a complete, meaningful whole. These parts are input, throughput, output, evaluation, and feedback.

Components of Systems

The first component of a system is **input,** which is the raw material, such as information, energy, or matter, that enters a system and is transformed by it. For a system to work well, input should contribute to achieving the purpose of the system.

A second component of a system is through-put. **Throughput** consists of the processes a system uses to convert raw materials into a form that can be used, either by the system itself or by the environment or suprasystem. **Output** is the end result or product of the system. Outputs vary widely, depending on the type and purpose of the system.

Evaluation is the fourth component of a system. **Evaluation** means measuring the success or failure of the output and consequently the effectiveness of the system. For evaluation to be meaningful in any system, outcome criteria, against which performance or product quality is measured, must be identified.

The process of communicating what is found in evaluation of the system is called **feedback,** the final component of a system. Feedback is the information given back into the system to determine whether or not the purpose, or end result, of the system has been achieved. Figure 12-1 depicts the components of systems and illustrates how they relate to one another.

Examples of Systems

It may be helpful to use a familiar example to clarify the components of systems. In a college system, input consists of students, faculty, ideas, the desire to learn, and knowledge. Because the purpose of the system is to educate, the students need to be ready to learn, and the faculty should be prepared to teach. The processes (throughput) whereby ideas, knowledge, and skills are transmitted must be clear and understandable. The

Figure 12-1
Major components of a general systems model.

output, or product, of the system is educated graduates. For evaluation of the output, a standardized examination of reading comprehension, mathematics, and analytical skills may be used. Student scores on the comprehensive examination provide feedback to the faculty and administrators. If students score well, the system has achieved its purpose. If not, changes need to be made in the input or in the system itself—for example, admitting brighter students, hiring more talented faculty, or designing more effective courses and curricula.

Systems are usually complex and consist of several parts called **subsystems.** Let us examine a hospital as a system. Technically, it is a system for providing health care, but the success of the system depends on the functioning of many subsystems. The subsystems include the laboratory, radiology, housekeeping, laundry, central supply, medical records, dietetics, nursing, pharmacy, and medical staffs. Each of these subsystems is a system itself. All the subsystems function collaboratively to make the health care system—the hospital—work.

Open and Closed Systems

Continuing with the example, the hospital and all its subsystems are open systems. An **open system** promotes the exchange of matter, energy, and information with other systems and the environment. The larger environment outside the hospital is called the **suprasystem.** A **closed system** does not interact with other systems or with the surrounding environment. Matter, energy, and information do not flow into or out of a closed system. There are few totally closed systems. Even a completely balanced aquarium, for example, often thought of as approaching a closed system, needs light and additional water and nutrients from time to time.

Two more points are essential to a beginning understanding of systems. First, the whole is different from and greater than the sum of its parts. Stated another way, the system is different from and greater than the sum of its subsystems. Anyone who has ever been in a hospital, for example, knows that what happens there is different from and more than the sum of the following equation: laundry + pharmacy + nurses + physicians = hospital. The second point involves synergy. **Synergy** occurs when all the various subsystems and the people who compose them collaborate to work with patients and their families.

Dynamic Nature of Systems

The final point to be made about systems is that change in one part of the system creates change in other parts. If the hospital admissions office, for example, decides to admit patients only between the hours of 8:00 AM and 10:00 AM, that decision creates changes in the nursing units, housekeeping, the business office, surgery, the laboratory, and other hospital subsystems. If that change was implemented without prior communication to the other subsystems and coordinated planning, it could create chaos in the system.

The exchange of energy and information within open systems and between open systems and their suprasystems is continuous. The dynamic balance within and between the subsystems, the system, and the suprasystems helps create and maintain **homeostasis,** or internal stability.

All living systems are open systems. The internal environment is in constant interaction with a changing environment external to the organism. As change occurs in one, the other is affected. For example, walking into a cold room (change in the external environment) affects a variety of physiological and psychological subsystems of a person's internal environment. These, in turn, affect a person's blood flow, ability to concentrate, and feeling of comfort, for example (changes in internal environment).

Application of the Systems Model to Nursing

Why is it necessary for nurses to understand systems? Nurses work within systems every day. Using the hospital example, nurses work within the nursing department's system, a particular unit's system, and with a team system, among others. All three are open systems interacting with one another and the environment. If nurses are to work effectively in such complex systems, they need to have an understanding of how systems operate.

At the individual patient level, the openness of human systems makes nursing intervention possible. Understanding systems helps nurses assess relationships among all the factors that affect patients, including the influence of nurses themselves. Nurses who understand systems view patients holistically, including the subsystems (such as respiratory system and gastrointestinal system) and suprasystem (for example, family, culture, and community). These nurses appreciate the influence of change in any part of the system. For instance, when a diabetic patient has pneumonia (change in subsystem), the infection increases the blood glucose level and may result in hospitalization. Hospitalization may in turn adversely affect the patient's role in the family and community (change in suprasystem). Key concepts of systems are summarized in Box 12-1, and an excellent review of general systems theory and its relationship to nursing can be found online (www.bsn-gn.eku.edu/BEGLEY/GSThand1.htm). With this brief introduction to systems as a foundation, we can now examine the three basic concepts that are fundamental to the practice of professional nursing.

- A system is a set of interrelated parts.
- The parts form a meaningful whole.
- The whole is different from and greater than the sum of its parts.
- Systems may be open or closed.
- All living systems are open systems.
- Systems strive for homeostasis (internal stability).
- Systems are part of suprasystems.
- Systems have subsystems.

PERSON

The term **person** is used to describe each individual man, woman, or child. There are a number of different approaches to the study of person. This chapter briefly examines the concept of people as systems with human needs.

As mentioned previously, each individual is an open system with numerous subsystems that make up the whole person. For example, there are circulatory, musculoskeletal, respiratory, gastro-intestinal, genitourinary, and neurological subsystems that compose the physiological subsystem. There are also psychological, social, cultural, and spiritual subsystems that combine with the physiological subsystem to make up the whole person. Each person is unique and different from all other persons. This uniqueness is determined both genetically and environmentally and is the basis for holistic nursing care—that is, nursing care that takes all the aspects of the person into consideration.

Certain personal characteristics are determined before birth by the genes received from one's parents. Genetically determined characteristics include eye, skin, and hair color; height; gender; and a variety of other features. Other characteristics about persons are determined by the environment. The availability of loving parents or parent substitutes, availability of sufficient nutritious foods, cultural beliefs, degree of educational opportunities, adequacy of housing, quality and quantity of parental supervision, and safety are all examples of environmental factors that influence how a person develops.

Human Needs

In addition to having personal characteristics, people have needs. A human need is a requirement for a person's well-being. In 1954 psychologist Abraham Maslow published *Motivation and Personality*. In this classic book, Maslow rejected earlier ideas of Freud, who believed that people are motivated by unconscious instincts, and Pavlov, who believed humans were driven by conditioned reflexes. Instead, Maslow presented his **human needs theory** and explained that human behavior is motivated by intrinsic human needs. He identified five levels of needs and organized them into a hierarchical order, as shown in Figure 12-2.

Basic needs

The most basic level of needs consists of those necessary for physiological survival: food, oxygen, rest, activity, shelter, and sexual expression. These are needs all human beings, regardless of location or culture, have in common.

Maslow identified the second level of needs as safety and security. These include physical as well as psychological safety and security needs. Psychological safety and security include having a fairly predictable environment with which one has some familiarity and relative freedom from fear and chaos.

The third level of needs consists of love and belonging. To a greater or lesser extent, each person needs close, intimate relationships; social relationships; a place in the social structure; and group affiliations.

Next in Maslow's hierarchy is the need for self-esteem. This includes the need to feel self-worth, self-respect, and self-reliance.

Maslow called the highest level of needs **self-actualization.** Self-actualized people have realized their maximum potential; they use their capabilities to the fullest extent possible and are true to

Figure 12-2
Maslow's hierarchy of needs.

their own nature. People do not stay in a state of self-actualization but may have "peak experiences" during which they realize self-actualization for some period of time. Maslow believed that many people strive for self-actualization, but few consistently reach that level (Maslow, 1987).

Assumptions about needs

Maslow's hierarchy rests on several basic assumptions about human needs. One assumption is that basic needs must be at least partially satisfied before higher-order needs can become relevant to the individual. For example, a starving person can hardly be concerned with self-esteem until a life-sustaining level of nutrition is established.

A second assumption about human needs is that individuals meet their needs in different ways. One person may need 8 or 9 hours of sleep to feel rested, whereas another may require only 5 or 6 hours. Each individual's sleep needs may vary at different stages of life. Older people usually require less sleep than younger people. Individuals also eat different diets in differing quantities and at differing intervals. Some prefer to eat only twice a day, whereas others may snack six or eight times a day to meet their nutritional needs. Sexual energy also varies widely from person to person. The frequency with which normal adults desire sexual activity is determined by a broad range of individual factors.

Even though sleep, food, and sex are considered examples of basic human needs, the manner in which these needs are met, as well as the extent to which any one of them is considered a need, varies according to each individual. It is therefore extremely important to determine a person's perceptions of his or her own needs to be able to provide appropriate, individualized nursing care. If a patient is uncomfortable eating three large meals, such as those served in most hospitals, nurses can help that person by saving parts of the large meals in the refrigerator on the nursing unit and serving them to the patient between regularly scheduled meals. This is a simple example of what is meant by the term *individualized nursing care,* which recognizes each individual's unique needs and tailors the plan of nursing care to take that uniqueness into consideration.

Adaptation and human needs

Another aspect of human needs that must be considered is the nature of people to change, grow, and develop. Carl Rogers, a well-known psychologist, built a theory of personhood based on the idea that people are constantly adapting, discovering, and rediscovering themselves. His book *On Becoming a Person* (Rogers, 1961) is considered a classic in psychological literature. Rogers' idea that a person's needs change as the person changes is important for nurses to remember. The human potential to grow and develop can be used by nurses to assist patients to change unhealthy behaviors and to reach the highest level of wellness possible.

The concept of **adaptation** is also helpful in understanding that people admitted to hospitals and removed from their customary, familiar environments frequently become anxious. Even the most confident person can become fearful when in an uncertain, perhaps threatening, situation. Under these circumstances, nurses have learned to expect people to regress slightly and to become more concerned with basic needs and less focused on the higher needs in Maslow's hierarchy. A "take-charge" professional person, for example, may become somewhat demanding and self-absorbed when hospitalized. As you will see in Chapter 13, several nursing theorists based their theoretical models on adaptation.

Homeostasis

When a person's needs are not met, homeostasis is threatened. Remember that homeostasis is a dynamic balance achieved by effectively functioning open systems. It is a state of equilibrium, a tendency to maintain internal stability. In humans, homeostasis is attained by coordinated responses of organ systems that automatically compensate for environmental changes. When someone goes for a brisk walk, for example, heart rate and respiratory rate automatically increase to keep vital organs supplied with oxygen. When the individual comes home and sits down to read the newspaper, heart rate and breathing slow down. No conscious decision to speed up or slow down these physiological functions has to be made. Adjustments occur automatically to maintain homeostasis.

Individuals, as open systems, also endeavor to maintain balance between external and internal forces. When that balance is achieved, the person is healthy, or at least is resistant to disease. When environmental factors affect the homeostasis of a person, the person attempts to adapt to the change. If adaptation is unsuccessful, disequilibrium may occur, setting the stage for the development of illness or disease. How individuals respond to stress is a major factor in the development of illness. Stress and illness are discussed more fully in Chapter 10.

ENVIRONMENT/SUPRASYSTEM

The second major concept basic to professional nursing practice is environment, or the suprasystem. **Environment** includes all the circumstances, influences, and conditions that surround and affect individuals, families, and groups. The environment can be as small and controlled as a premature infant's isolette or as large and uncontrollable as the universe. Included in environment are the social and cultural attitudes that profoundly shape human experience.

The environment can either promote or interfere with homeostasis and well-being of individuals. As seen in Maslow's hierarchy of needs, there is a dynamic interaction between a person's needs, which are internal, and the satisfaction of those needs, which is often environmentally determined.

Nurses have always been aware of the influence of environment on people, beginning with Florence Nightingale, who understood well the elements of a healthful environment in which restoration and preservation of health and prevention of disease and injury were possible. Concerns about the health of the public have led governmental entities at local, state, and national levels to promulgate standards and regulations that ensure the safety of food, water, air, cosmetics, medications, workplaces, and other areas in which health hazards may occur. Environmental systems to be discussed in this section are family systems, cultural systems, social systems, and community systems.

Family Systems

The most direct environmental influence on a person is the family. The quality and amount of parenting provided to infants and growing children constitute a major determinant of health. We call this the **family system.** Children who are nurtured when young and vulnerable, who are allowed to grow in independence and self-determination, and who are taught the skills they need for social living are likely to grow into strong, productive, autonomous adults.

Nuclear and extended families

For most of the history of humankind, immediate and extended families were relatively intact units that lived together or lived within close proximity to one another. In the **extended family,** children were nurtured by a variety of relatives, as well as by their own parents. This closeness was profoundly affected by industrialization, which fostered urbanization. When families ceased farming, which was a family endeavor, and moved to cities where fathers worked in factories, the first dilution of family influence on children began. The **nuclear family** (mother and father and their children) moved away from former sources of nurturing, as older relatives such as grandparents, aunts, and uncles often stayed in rural areas.

During World War II, more women began to work, taking them out of the home and away from young children for hours each day. The increased geographic mobility of families since World War II has also had a destructive effect on the role of extended family in the lives of children, as nuclear families often live half a conti-

nent or more away from grandparents and other family members. The intense attention children traditionally received from adult relatives diminished, sometimes to the detriment of the child's well-being.

Single-parent families

There are more single-parent families in the United States than ever before, most of which are headed by women. As of 2004, U.S. Census data revealed that there were over 12.6 million single-parent families in the United States. Of these there were 10 million single women heading households with children under 18 and no father present. In addition to single mothers, there were also 2.3 million single custodial fathers in the United States in 2004 (U.S. Census Bureau, 2005, 2006).

Life is challenging for single parents of both sexes who must perform the breadwinner role as well as nurturing roles in the family. The combination of bearing multiple roles alone over long periods of time can be extremely stressful, even exhausting, to single parents.

There is increasing evidence that long-term stress affects the mental and physical health of these adults, which, in turn, affects their parenting abilities. A 2000 study by nursing faculty at the University of Kentucky (Peden et al, 2004) found that low-income single mothers with children between the ages of 2 and 6 have a high prevalence of depressive symptoms, with more than 75 percent scoring in the mild to high range of depressive symptoms. These symptoms included negative thinking and chronic stressors, potentially affecting the entire family's quality of life. The researchers concluded that the combination of low income and single parenting of small children increases the risk of depression and that negative thinking, instead of chronic stressors, might be more amenable to nursing intervention (Peden et al, 2004).

Although many single parents manage stress well and are able to provide excellent parenting, some children's needs are neglected. The impact of this neglect can be seen in the behavior and school performance of children who have not learned the skills they need to be successful. With approximately one third of all children in the United States being born to unmarried women (Edin, 2004), the trend to single-parent households is likely to continue.

The examples given here represent only a few of the ways families influence the well-being of individuals. There are many others. Understanding a patient's family and home environment is part of a complete nursing assessment. Modification of the home environment may be needed, particularly when a person is returning home with a physical disability, or where there is neglect or abuse. Nurses, social workers, and others involved in care planning must collaborate to ensure that needed changes occur.

Cultural Systems

Culture is an extremely important environmental influence affecting individuals. **Culture** consists of the attitudes, beliefs, and behaviors of social and ethnic groups that have been perpetuated through generations. Patterns of language, dress, eating habits, activities of daily living, attitudes toward those outside the culture, health beliefs and values, spiritual beliefs or religious orientation, and attitudes toward children, women, men, marriage, education, work, and recreation all are influenced by culture.

According to U.S. Census Bureau estimates, there were 33.5 million foreign-born Americans in 2003, a dramatic increase from less than 28.4 million only 3 years earlier (U.S. Census Bureau, 2005). The United States is fast becoming a truly multicultural society. Because basic beliefs about health and illness vary widely from culture to culture, nurses need to develop cultural competence to meet the needs of culturally diverse patients. For example, "A traditional Vietnamese folk remedy, *ventouse* . . . , involves placing a heated cup on the skin. It's believed that as the cup cools, it draws away excess energy or 'wind' causing the illness" (Grossman, 1994, p. 58). This practice can cause bruising, which can be mistaken for a sign of abuse. This is just one indication that cultural beliefs of patients have great relevance to nurses. Most cultural differences are more subtle than this and can escape the notice of nurses who have not developed cultural competence.

Effective nurses learn to be aware of and to respect cultural influences on patients. Whenever possible, they pay attention to patients' cultural preferences. They recognize that some cultural groups attribute illness to bad fortune. Individuals from cultures with these beliefs do not see themselves as active participants in their own health status. This attitude is a challenge for nurses who value the collaboration of patients in their own health care planning.

These are only two examples of the influence of cultural beliefs on the nurse-patient interaction. Wise nurses realize that integration of a patient's cultural health beliefs into the **indivi-**

✦ *Cultural Considerations* *Challenge*

Working With the "Passive" Patient

Most professional nurses value engaging patients in their own care planning. These nurses encourage participation and independence in their patients. In some cultures, however, patients expect the caregivers to make decisions for them and resist efforts toward self-care. In other cultures

the head of the family (matriarch or patriarch) is the individual who makes decisions, not the patient himself or herself. How will you modify your usual care practices to work effectively with patients who, for cultural reasons, resist working toward self-care? What challenges will this present to your own beliefs?

dualized care plan can make a strong impact on that patient's desire and ability to get well.

Understanding the relationship between culture and health is the basis for "transcultural nursing," a field of nursing practice initiated by nurse-anthropologist Madeline Leininger. Additional discussion of the influence of culture is included in Chapter 10.

Social Systems

In addition to family and cultural systems, individuals are also influenced by the social system in which they live. Social institutions such as families, neighborhoods, schools, churches, professional associations, civic groups, and recreational groups may constitute a form of social support. Social support also includes such factors as family income; presence in the home of a spouse; proximity to neighbors, children, and other supportive individuals; access to medical care; coping abilities; and educational level.

Social change

Holmes and Rahe (1967) published a study of the relationship of social change to the subsequent development of illness. People with many social changes that disrupt social support, such as death of a loved one, divorce, job changes, moving, or unemployment, were much more likely to experience illness in the following 12 months than people with few social changes. Both positive and negative changes created the need for social readjustment. In 1995 this study was updated, and the Recent Life Changes Questionnaire (Box 12-2) was devised to reflect more accurately contemporary concerns (Miller and Rahe, 1997). Numerous

---

Box **12-2** **Recent Life Changes Questionnaire**

The following 74 potential life changes inquire about recent events in a person's life. A 6-month total equal to or greater than 300 Life Change Units (LCU), or a 1-year total equal to or greater than 500 LCU, is considered indicative of high recent life stress.

Life Change Event	Life Change Units
Health	
An injury or illness that:	
kept you in bed 1 week or more or sent you to the hospital	74
was less serious than above	44
Major dental work	26
Major change in eating habits	27
Major change in sleeping habits	26
Major change in your usual type and/or amount of recreation	28
Work	
Change to a new type of work	51
Change in your work hours or conditions	35
Change in your responsibilities at work:	
more responsibilities	29
fewer responsibilities	21
promotion	31
demotion	42
transfer	32

Continued

Box 12-2 Recent Life Changes Questionnaire—cont'd

Life Change Event	Life Change Units
Troubles at work:	
with your boss	29
with co-workers	35
with persons under your supervision	35
other work troubles	28
Major business adjustment	60
Retirement	52
Loss of job:	
laid off from work	68
fired from work	79
Correspondence course to help you in your work	18
Home and Family	
Major change in living conditions	42
Change in residence:	
move within the same town or city	25
move to a different town, city, or state	47
Change in family get-togethers	25
Major change in health or behavior of family member	55
Marriage	50
Pregnancy	67
Miscarriage or abortion	65
Gain of a new family member:	
birth of a child	66
adoption of a child	65
a relative moving in with you	59
Spouse beginning or ending work	46
Child leaving home:	
to attend college	41
because of marriage	41
for other reason	45
Change in arguments with spouse	50
In-law problems	38
Change in the marital status of your parents:	
divorce	59
remarriage	50
Separation from spouse:	
because of work	53
because of marital problems	76
Divorce	96
Birth of grandchild	43
Death of spouse	119

Box 12-2 Recent Life Changes Questionnaire—cont'd	
Death of a family member:	
child	123
brother or sister	102
parent	100
Personal and Social	
Change in personal habits	26
Beginning or ending school or college	38
Change of school or college	35
Change in political beliefs	24
Change in religious beliefs	29
Change in social activities	27
Vacation	24
New, close, personal relationship	37
Engagement to marry	45
Girlfriend or boyfriend problems	39
Sexual difficulties	44
"Falling out" of a close personal relationship	47
An accident	48
Minor violation of the law	20
Being held in jail	75
Death of a close friend	70
Major decision regarding your immediate future	51
Major personal achievement	36
Financial	
Major change in finances:	
increased income	38
decreased income	60
investment and/or credit difficulties	56
Loss or damage of personal property	43
Moderate purchase	20
Major purchase	37
Foreclosure on a mortgage or loan	58

Miller MA, Rahe RH: Life changes scaling for the 1990s, *J Psychosomat Res* 43(3):279-292, 1997. Reprinted with permission.

other researchers have found additional evidence that social support has a direct relationship to health.

Social support

Individuals vary in their need and desire for social support. When assessing patients, nurses need to remember that adequacy of social support should be determined by the patient, not by the nurse. When it is determined that strengthening social support is desirable, nurses can provide information, give positive affirmation, use empathy, be present for patients, serve as advocates, and provide validation and encouragement

(Finfgeld-Connett, 2005). They can also encourage patients to use interest groups, parenting classes, marriage enrichment groups, religious groups, formal and informal educational groups, and self-help groups to develop stronger support from the social environment.

Increasingly, people receive support online—in chat rooms and through other computer-based forums. People with new insulin pumps, for example, can "talk" online with more than 700 others who have similar pumps, ask questions, and get helpful tips to assist them. There are literally hundreds of online support groups, ranging from those for Alzheimer's caregivers to weight loss groups, and these can be a useful source of social support.

Poverty

As the world's wealthiest country, one would expect poverty in the United States to be low. Sadly, this is not the case. The U.S. Census Bureau reported in 2004 that nearly 37 million Americans were living at or below the poverty level (U.S. Census Bureau, 2004). The U.S. Department of Health and Human Services determines the poverty level annually. In 2006 "poverty level" was considered a total income of $9800 or less for a single person, $20,000 or less for a family of 4, and $33,600 or less for a family of 8 (U.S. Department of Health and Human Services, 2006a).

People living in poverty have diminished access to health care for a variety of reasons. In 2003 more than 17.6 percent of all children under the age of 18 were living below the poverty level (U.S. Census Bureau, 2003). The numbers are even more worrisome for different ethnic groups; for example, 34.1 percent of single-parent African-American families and 29.7 percent of Hispanic families were living below the poverty level. Lack of money often means adequate nutrition and health care are not attainable, adversely affecting the health status of all family members. Indeed, the World Health Organization (WHO) now considers poverty to be the most influential determinant of health.

A 2004 study by the U.S. Department of Health and Human Services highlighted some of the hardships experienced by poor and near-poor families. Factors such as food insecurity or hunger, inability to pay mortgage or rent, and disconnection of telephone, gas, and electricity for nonpayment featured prominently in the findings about these families (Center on Budget and Policy Priorities, 2004).

Nurses often do not understand or appreciate the complex societal forces that contribute to poverty and may even blame the poor for their situation. Misconceptions can lead to stereotyping and insensitivity to the feelings and concerns of the poor. This discourages them even further from seeking health care they need.

A study conducted by Canadian nursing professors (Reutter et al, 2004) revealed that only 13 percent of the 740 basic baccalaureate students surveyed had ever lived in a poor neighborhood and only 7 percent had ever received public assistance. One third of these students reported receiving most of their information about poverty from the news media. They felt they had limited exposure to poverty. The researchers recommended that colleges of nursing increase coursework related to poverty, provide opportunities for students to work with people living in poverty, and facilitate student involvement with groups and organizations that advocate for public policy and societal solutions to poverty (Reutter et al, 2004).

Community, National, and World Systems

The health status of people is also influenced by the larger systems in which they live. The types and availability of jobs, housing, schools, and health care, as well as the overall economic well-being, profoundly affect the citizens in a community. Although nurses may not think they have an obvious role, they can be instrumental in improving the community systems. Identifying health needs and bringing these to the attention of community planners, offering screening programs, serving on health-related committees and advisory boards, and lobbying political leaders can bring about positive change in a community. Nurses have also become politically active by running for elected offices at local, state, and national levels. They can energetically support political candidates who have sound environmental platforms. More information about political activism in nursing is provided in Chapter 15.

On a broader perspective, environment also includes the nation, the world, and the universe. A seemingly isolated incident such as an earthquake in Turkey or an outbreak of influenza in a wild bird flock in Southeast Asia can have worldwide health repercussions. Nurses can contribute to a healthier world environment by supporting, promoting, and, when possible, participating in humanitarian responses to international disasters.

Nurses' potential impact on the environment/suprasystem

Individual nurses, in the interest of world health, may choose to engage in a variety of environmentally sound practices in their personal lives and encourage others to do the same. These include recycling of household trash and hazardous materials such as batteries and paint, using pump rather than aerosol sprayers, avoiding insecticides and unnecessary use of gardening chemicals, buying energy-efficient appliances and automobiles, walking when possible instead of driving, and refusing to buy from or invest in companies that engage in environmentally unsound practices such as polluting air and water or cutting down rain forests.

Professionally, nurses need to be aware that hospitals are among the highest producers of waste, including biohazardous waste. For example, hospitals are a major source of mercury pollution. This highly toxic substance, used in thermometers, blood pressure measuring devices, and other medical devices, ultimately flows into the environment, where it contaminates water. It then is concentrated in the bodies of predator fish such as tuna and swordfish, which are eventually consumed by humans. Mercury, even in small doses, poses serious health risks to pregnant women and young children. Nurses can be instrumental in encouraging their employers to avoid purchasing and using mercury-containing devices and to dispose of them properly when they are discarded.

In an effort to reduce environmental pollution, some health care facilities have committees dedicated to identifying and recommending environmentally sound products. Nurses can volunteer to serve on these committees or recommend the purchase of fewer disposable products and products with wasteful packaging. The News Note on p. 304 discusses the initiatives of a health-related group, Health Care Without Harm, to reduce hazardous waste, specifically mercury, emanating from health care facilities.

HEALTH

Health is the third major concept fundamental to the practice of professional nursing. Health is best viewed as a continuum rather than as an absolute state. Each individual's health status varies from day to day, depending on a variety of factors, such as rest, nutrition, and stressors. Illness is also not an absolute state. People can have chronic illnesses such as diabetes or seizure disorders and still work, take part in recreational activities, and maintain acceptably healthy lives. Figure 12-3 depicts the health-illness continuum.

Defining Health

There are numerous definitions of health. The World Health Organization (WHO) defined **health** as "a state of complete physical, mental, and social well-being and not merely the absence of disease or infirmity" (WHO, 1947, p. 29). This definition was the first modern recognition of health as multidimensional. The WHO definition presented a holistic view of health that reflected the interplay between the psychological, social, spiritual, and physical aspects of human life.

A holistic view of health focuses on the interrelationship of all the parts that make up a whole person. Jan Christian Smuts (1926) first introduced the concept of **holism** in modern Western thought by emphasizing the harmony between people and nature. When viewing health holistically, individual health practices must be taken into account. Health practices are culturally determined and include nutritional habits, type and amount of exercise and rest, how one copes

Study Shows Mercury in Tuna Threatens Developing Babies and Young Children: Hospitals Will Reduce Threat by Eliminating Mercury from Health Care

According to a report released today, some of the most commonly eaten fish contain levels of mercury that pose a risk to pregnant women and young children. In response to the problem of mercury pollution, health care providers such as Kaiser Permanente; Dartmouth-Hitchcock Medical Center in Lebanon, New Hampshire; and New York's Beth Israel Medical Centers are creating model programs for mercury elimination. By phasing out the purchase and use of mercury-containing products and devices, hospitals will eventually decrease the amount of mercury moving up the food chain until it reaches its highest concentrations in top predator fish such as tuna, swordfish, and shark.

These findings are included in the report *Protecting by Degrees*, written by the Environmental Working Group for Health Care Without Harm, a coalition of more than 170 groups dedicated to environmentally responsible health care.

Test results reported in *Protecting by Degrees* are consistent with studies done by the U.S. Food and Drug Administration (FDA) in 1993. In both instances, chunk light tuna contained levels of mercury that create serious health risks:

■ A 140-pound pregnant woman risks subtle but permanent brain damage to her fetus by eating less than half of a 6-ounce can of tuna per day.

■ An average 4-year-old exceeds the EPA's "safe" dose if he or she eats one 6-ounce can per week.

"Tuna fish has too much mercury to be eaten regularly by pregnant women and young children. But that's not the fault of the tuna or the people who caught or canned it," explained Charlotte Brody, RN, co-coordinator of Health Care Without Harm." Industries that use mercury and the governments that regulate them must take responsibility for getting mercury out of our fish and out of our children's developing brains."

"Health care groups like Kaiser Permanente, Dartmouth-Hitchcock, and New York's Beth Israel Medical Center are leaders in developing a cure for the mercury problem," said Todd Hettenbach, EWG policy analyst and primary author of the report. "These hospitals are voluntarily eliminating mercury because of the threat to public health and showing other health care providers and other industries that it can be done."

Safe, cost-comparable alternatives exist for most of the mercury use in hospitals. Thermometers and blood pressure–measuring devices are two of the most commonly used mercury-containing devices. A mercury fever thermometer, such as the kind used in the home, contains enough mercury to potentially contaminate 9000 cans of tuna fish. A desk-mounted sphygmomanometer (used for measuring blood pressure) contains enough mercury to potentially contaminate 492,000 6-ounce cans of chunk light tuna.

"As we learned with mercury instruments, some of the weapons we use to fight disease can also be weapons that compromise a healthy environment," said David Lawrence, MD, chairman and chief executive officer of Kaiser Foundation Health Plan and Kaiser Foundation Hospitals. "We need to address the long-term consequences of treatment options and challenge ourselves to devise effective alternatives that do less environmental harm."

Health Care Without Harm is an international campaign made up of health care professionals, hospitals, environmental advocates, organizations of health-impacted individuals, religious organizations, and labor unions. The campaign's mission is to transform the health care industry so it is no longer a source of environmental harm by eliminating the pollution in health care practices without compromising safety or care. The Environmental Working Group, a member organization of Health Care Without Harm, is an environmental research organization based in Washington, DC.

HCWH press release issued May 6, 1999, available online: www.noharm.org.

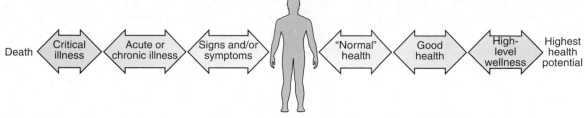

Figure 12-3
The health-illness continuum—a holistic health model.

with stress, quality of interpersonal relationships, expression of spirituality, and numerous other lifestyle factors. As a profession, nurses value a holistic view of health.

Parsons (1959) defined health as "the state of optimum capacity of an individual for the effective performance of his roles and tasks." This definition focused on the roles individuals assume in life and the impact health or illness has on the fulfillment of those roles. A few examples of roles that are familiar may include the student role, the parent role, the breadwinner role, and the friend role. Given the activities inherent in each of these roles, it is easily seen that the state of health profoundly influences how people carry out their roles in life.

Yet another description of health is the opposite of illness (Dunn, 1959). Dunn, in his classic text *High Level Wellness* (Dunn, 1961), described health as a continuum with high-level wellness at one end and death at the other. He described **high-level wellness** as functioning at maximum potential in an integrated way within the environment. A prisoner of war kept in solitary confinement and given a diet of rice for many months certainly would have difficulty maintaining health. If the prisoner keeps active, both physically and mentally, and retains a positive outlook, however, he is likely to be healthier than the prisoner who does none of these things. Using Dunn's definition and taking his environment into consideration, the prisoner may even be said to have attained high-level wellness.

Pender, et al (2006) described health promotion as "approach behavior," whereas prevention is "avoidance behavior" (p. 5). This may be a useful concept for nurses to keep in mind when seeking to help patients expand their positive potential for health.

A National Health Initiative: *Healthy People 2000/2010*

A remarkable national initiative to improve the health of the nation is now in its third decade. The *Healthy People* initiative was an unprecedented cooperative effort that grew out of the 1979 surgeon general's report on health promotion and disease prevention titled *Healthy People*. That report laid the foundation for a national prevention agenda. Federal, state, and territorial governments as well as hundreds of private, public, and nonprofit organizations and concerned individuals worked together for the first time ever. These partnerships resulted in *Healthy People 2000*, an effort designed to stimulate a national disease prevention and **health promotion** agenda to improve significantly the health of all Americans in the last decade of the twentieth century. On September 6, 1990, former U.S. Secretary of Health and Human Services Louis W. Sullivan released a report to the United States titled *Healthy People 2000*. He reported that progress on priority areas was mixed but enough success was achieved to continue the project.

The second phase of the project, called *Healthy People 2010*, was launched in January 2000. It was developed by the *Healthy People* Consortium, an alliance of more than 350 national membership organizations and 250 state health, mental health, substance abuse, and environmental agencies. In addition, more than 11,000 public comments on the draft document were provided through an interactive website. *Healthy People 2010* consists of a revised set of health objectives for the nation, with two over-arching goals: to increase quality and years of healthy life and to eliminate health disparities. Under these 2 goals are 28 focus areas that provide more specific targets. To measure the health of the nation during the decade, 10 leading health indicators will be used. Each leading health indicator reflects an important health issue and has 1 or more of the 28 objectives linked with it. These indicators reflect the high-priority public health concerns in this country at the beginning of the twenty-first century. Box 12-3 contains the essential elements of *Healthy People 2010*.

> *Healthy People 2010* offers a simple but powerful idea: provide health objectives in a format that enables diverse groups to combine their efforts and work as a team. It is a road map to better health for all and can be used by many different people, states, communities, professional organizations, and groups to improve health. The initiative has partners from all sectors (U.S. Department of Health and Human Services, 2003).

Partners are encouraged to integrate *Healthy People* objectives into their programs, special events, publications, and meetings. An example is provided by the Division of Public Health Nursing of the Los Angeles County Health Department, which has shifted its focus from providing care for individuals within families to improving the health of entire communities. Nurses in this department integrated the 10 leading health indicators of *Healthy People 2010* into their public health nursing practice model. This means that these nurses consider the leading health indicators as they assess and diagnose communities with which they work. This ensures consistency within the division and with national priorities (Smith and Bazini-Barakat, 2003)—a perfect example of how the *Healthy People* initiative can be implemented at the local level.

When federal, state, and local health entities combine their efforts, improvements in the health of citizens can be made. Convincing individual Americans to change their lifestyles, however, even when to do so would result in improved health, remains a challenge. As can be seen from this review of the *Healthy People* project over nearly 30 years, changing health beliefs and health behaviors is a slow process. You can learn more about *Healthy People 2010* and check progress toward its goals online (www.healthy-people.gov).

Health Beliefs and Health Behaviors

Health is affected by health beliefs and health behaviors. **Health behaviors** include those choices and habitual actions that promote or diminish health, such as eating habits, frequency of exercise, use of tobacco products and alcohol, sexual practices, and adequacy of rest and sleep (Figure 12-4). Much is known about health-promoting behaviors, and this information is readily available to the public. Yet people do not readily change their behaviors. We will examine several theories about why people change their health behaviors—or why they do not.

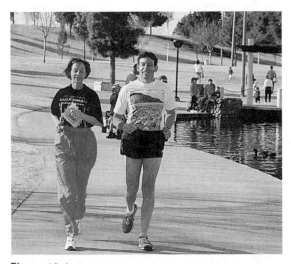

Figure 12-4
More Americans are engaging in health behaviors such as regular exercise, yet obesity is still on the rise.

Box 12-3 *Healthy People 2010* at a Glance

Healthy People 2010 is a comprehensive set of disease prevention and health promotion objectives for the nation to achieve over the first decade of the new century. Created by scientists both inside and outside of government, it identifies a wide range of public health priorities and specific, measurable objectives.

Overarching Goals

1. Increase quality and years of healthy life
2. Eliminate health disparities

Focus Areas

- Access to Quality Health Services
- Arthritis, Osteoporosis, and Chronic Back Conditions
- Cancer
- Chronic Kidney Disease
- Diabetes
- Disability and Secondary Conditions
- Educational and Community-Based Programs
- Environmental Health
- Family Planning
- Food Safety
- Health Communication
- Heart Disease and Stroke
- HIV
- Immunization and Infectious Diseases
- Injury and Violence Prevention
- Maternal, Infant, and Child Health
- Medical Product Safety
- Mental Health and Mental Disorders
- Nutrition and Overweight
- Occupational Safety and Health
- Oral Health
- Physical Activity and Fitness
- Public Health Infrastructure
- Respiratory Diseases
- Sexually Transmitted Diseases
- Substance Abuse
- Tobacco Use
- Vision and Hearing
- Physical Activity
- Overweight and Obesity
- Tobacco Use
- Substance Abuse
- Responsible Sexual Behavior

Continued

- Mental Health
- Injury and Violence
- Environmental Quality
- Immunization
- Access to Health Care

From U.S. Department of Health and Human Services: *Healthy People 2010: fact sheet*, 2006b, available online: http://www.healthypeople.gov/About/hpfact.htmwww.healthypeople.gov/About/hpfact.htm.

Health beliefs model

Rosenstock (1966, 1990) was one of the first scholars interested in determining why some people change their health behaviors whereas others do not. For example, when the surgeon general's report on smoking first came out in 1960, some people immediately quit smoking. Over the years, evidence condemning smoking has accumulated and been widely communicated, yet many intelligent people still smoke. Rosenstock wondered why. He formulated a model of health beliefs that illustrates how people behave in relationship to health maintenance activities and has worked to refine it for three decades. Rosenstock's **health beliefs model** (HBM) included three components:

1. An evaluation of one's vulnerability to a condition and the seriousness of that condition
2. An evaluation of how effective the health maintenance behavior might be
3. The presence of a trigger event that precipitates the health maintenance behavior

Using Rosenstock's health beliefs model, a man chooses to participate in a stop-smoking program depending on his perception of smoking-related heart disease and his personal susceptibility to it. If, because of family history, he believes he is susceptible to heart disease and that it may cause his death prematurely and if he believes that not smoking will substantially reduce his risk, he is likely to participate in the program. If, however, the stop-smoking program is at an inconvenient location, scheduled at an inconvenient time, or not affordable, he is less likely to participate. If his sibling, who smokes, has a massive heart attack, he may be motivated to attend the stop-smoking program despite the inconvenience and cost. The illness of his sibling is what Rosenstock termed "a cue to action," or a trigger event. A trigger event propels a previously unmotivated individual into changing health behaviors.

Self-efficacy and health-related behaviors

Albert Bandura (1997), a cognitive psychologist, developed an approach designed to assist people to exercise influence over their own health-related behaviors. He observed that whether or not people considered altering detrimental health habits depended on their belief in themselves as having the ability to modify their own behavior. He called this belief in their own abilities perceived **self-efficacy.** High belief in one's self-efficacy leads to efforts to change, whereas low perceived self-efficacy leads to a fatalistic lack of change.

Bandura identified four components needed for an effective program of lifestyle change: information, skill development, skill enhancement through guided practice and feedback, and creating social supports for change (Bandura, 1992). Using Bandura's model, a man wishing to stop smoking needs knowledge of the potential dangers of smoking; guidance on how to translate concern into action; extensive practice and opportunities to perfect new, nonsmoking skills; and strong involvement in a social network supportive of nonsmoking.

Locus of control and health-related behaviors

The **locus of control** concept proposed that people tend to be influenced by either an internal or external view of control. People who believe that their health is internally controlled, that is, by what they themselves do, are said to have an internal locus of control. Those who believe their health is determined by outside factors or chance are said to have an external locus of control. A number of studies have hypothesized that internally controlled people tend to see themselves as responsible for their own health status and are therefore more amenable to change. Research findings have been inconsistent, however. Although health locus of control is a concept of general relevance to health, it requires continued attention in research aimed at better understanding behavior and health (Steptoe and Wardle, 2001).

Nurses and health beliefs models

There are numerous other models of health beliefs and health behavior ranging from simple to complex. Many are being tested through empirical studies in attempts to identify the key to motivating people to improve their health choices and behaviors. No single theory of behavior has yet fully explained the complex state called health. It is important for nurses to recognize the following:

- Health is relative, ever changing, and affected by genetics, environment, personal beliefs, and cultural beliefs.
- Health affects the entire person—physically, socially, psychologically, and spiritually.
- Individuals' health beliefs are powerful and influence how they respond to efforts to change their health behaviors.
- Individuals needing or desiring change may lack knowledge, motivation, and support.
- Various models of health beliefs can be used to assess individual, family, and group readiness to change.
- The burden of action is mutually shared by patient, health care providers, and population-focused entities such as public health programs.

Influence of the Internet on Health

With nearly two thirds of adult Americans having online access, the Internet has an impact on every aspect of life. People shop; make travel reservations; check out the latest music, movies, plays, and books; and meet potential spouses online. Is it any wonder, then, that they also seek information about health online? The Internet, with its ready availability of information, ranging from the latest clinical trials and research studies to the most popular herbal remedies and diet fads, has changed the way we learn about health.

With the proliferation of health information sites, Americans are now armed with more information than has ever before been available to consumers. Patients are demanding to be equal partners in making health care decisions once decided only by the professionals they consulted. Health care practitioners encounter numerous patients each day who enter examining rooms with printouts of the latest research and advice, culled from the mountains of data available.

Support groups are available by the score. There is no need to dress, drive across town, or even leave the comforts of home to be in touch with dozens of people who share similar concerns or health problems. Cyberspace support groups have another advantage not shared by face-to-face groups: anonymity.

Some people are concerned about the validity of information available on the Internet (Chase, 1999). In fact, there is a lot of misinformation transmitted along with well-founded information from respected sources. The difficulty for the average citizen is telling the difference. Box 12-4 contains some helpful hints to improve the likelihood of obtaining valid health information from online sources.

Increased reliance on the Internet for health information is expected to continue. This is understandable, since the Internet is readily available, day or night, whereas getting an appointment with a primary care provider can take days or weeks. Nurses have an obligation to adapt to this new influence on health by helping their patients obtain sound advice from online sources. Sharing legitimate websites and guidelines for assessing the quality of information is a way to help patients become better consumers of online health data. This means that nurses themselves must be knowledgeable and stay up to date on both helpful and unhelpful websites. Nurses also should be nondefensive when patients question traditional advice, citing the Internet as their source. Use these exchanges as opportunities to correct misinformation, if needed. Perhaps you will learn something new yourself. Visit Evolve for WebLinks related to the content of this chapter: http://evolve.elsevier.com/Chitty/professional/.

Devising a Personal Plan for High-Level Wellness

Each individual nurse has a personal definition of health, certain health beliefs, and individual health behaviors. How nurses view health behaviors in their own lives affects nursing practice, both directly and indirectly. The personal health practices of nurses play a direct role in their effectiveness in counseling patients on health-related matters. Patients are more likely to adopt health-related behaviors such as not smoking and maintaining a healthy weight when the caregiver promoting these behaviors also engages in them. Yet nurses' own health behaviors are far from exemplary. Studies have shown that in spite of nurses' knowledge, no difference exists between the health behaviors of nurses and those of the general population (Pratt, Overfield, and Gill-Hilton, 1994).

Box **12-4** **Assessing Health-Related Sites on the Internet**

- Determine who sponsors the site. This should be disclosed on the site itself.
- Be skeptical. Evaluate the source to determine whether there is self-interest on the part of the sponsor.
- Make sure the author's name is clearly indicated, including credentials. Is the author qualified on this topic? Who does the author work for?
- What is the purpose of the site—to inform or to sell something?
- Is the material dated and revised frequently to ensure it is current?
- Is there editorial review of the content by a reputable authority or professional peers?
- Does the material consist of scientific information rather than testimonials?
- Determine who runs the website. University, government, and reputable medical organization sites may prove objective and less commercial than those run by companies or individuals wishing to profit.
- Is the information unbiased, and are you referred to other sources that can validate it?
- For chat rooms, go online and "lurk" before getting involved. Monitor conversations or read postings before deciding whether you want to participate.
- Find out whether the group has a moderator who can control monopolizers, commercial pitches, and inappropriate behavior by other participants.
- For interactive sites, be sure to read and understand the privacy policy.
- Until you are confident about the quality of information, cross-check it with print and electronic sources and discuss it with your health care provider.
- Use the Department of Health and Human Services' *Healthfinder* site to find online support groups (www.healthfinder.gov).
- Be highly suspicious of reports of "miracle" cures. Rumors and unsupported claims are rampant on the Internet and cause untold harm. Use *Quackwatch* to check out claims that sound too good to be true (www.quackwatch.com).

From Chase M: Health journal: a guide for patients who turn to the Web for solace and support, *Wall Street Journal*, Sept 17, 1999, p B1; Beyea SC: Evaluating evidence found on the Internet, *AORN J* 72(5):906-910, 2000; and Ahmann E: Supporting families' savvy use of the Internet for health research, *Pediatr Nurs* 26(4):419-423, 2000.

Nurses have a professional responsibility to model positive health behaviors in their own lives, but nurses are individuals too. Being or becoming a healthy role model may require some effort. If you are not the positive role model for health you would like to be, Box 12-5 can help you get started.

PUTTING IT ALL TOGETHER: NURSING

Nursing integrates concepts from person, environment, and health to form a meaningful whole. Figure 12-5 depicts the relationships among nursing's major concepts and illustrates how they overlap to create nursing's sphere of interest and

---

Box 12-5 Self-Assessment: Developing a Personal Plan for High-Level Wellness

Nurses' personal health behaviors send a powerful message to consumers of nursing care. Are you in a position to demonstrate that you practice what you preach? By answering the following questions, you can assess how well you are meeting your responsibilities in this area of nursing.

1. I weigh no more than 10 pounds over or under my ideal weight.
   T F
2. I eat a balanced diet, including breakfast, each day.
   T F
3. Of the total calories in my diet, less than 30 percent come from fat.
   T F
4. I exercise aerobically at least three times each week.
   T F
5. I get at least 7 hours of sleep each night.
   T F
6. I do not smoke or use any other form of tobacco.
   T F
7. I use alcohol in moderation (or not at all) and take mood-altering medication only when prescribed by my physician.
   T F
8. I identify and control the sources of stress in my life.
   T F
9. I have a balanced lifestyle, with work and diversional activities both playing important roles.
   T F
10. I have friends, neighbors, and/or family members who are sources of social support for me.
    T F
11. I practice responsible sex.
    T F

Directions for scoring: If you could not honestly answer "True" to all 11 questions, you need to set goals to enable you to do so.

1. On a piece of paper, begin your personal plan for high-level wellness. Write down at least two things you can do to address each "False" answer you gave to the self-assessment questions.
2. Share your health goals with one other person in your class. Make a contract with that person to serve as your "health coach."
3. Review your progress with your health coach at least once a week for the remainder of the term.
4. Begin your quest for high-level wellness today!

influence. This is termed the holistic approach to nursing.

Holistic Nursing

Holistic nursing care nourishes the whole person, that is, the body, mind, and spirit. Not surprisingly, the root word for nurse and nurture are the same Latin word, *nutrire*, which means "to nourish." Let us look now at eight factors that contribute to a holistic approach to nursing.

1. Nursing is an example of an open system that freely interacts with, influences, and is influenced by external and internal forces.

2. Nursing is the provision of health care services that focus on assisting people in maintaining health, avoiding or minimizing disease and disability, restoring wellness, or achieving a peaceful death.

3. Nursing involves collaborating with patients and their families to help them cope and adapt to situations of disequilibrium in an effort to regain homeostasis.

4. Nursing is integrally involved with people at points along the health-illness continuum.

5. Nursing care is provided regardless of diagnosis, individual differences, age, beliefs,

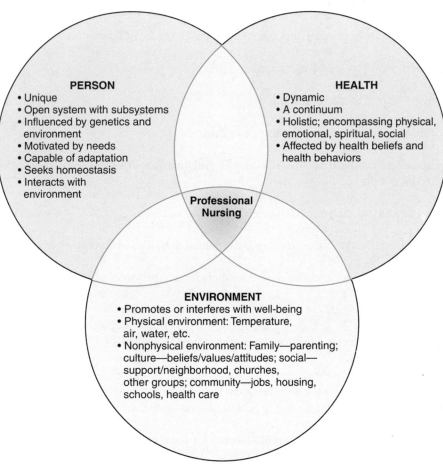

Figure 12-5
Concepts and subconcepts basic to professional nursing.

gender, sexual preference, or other factors. As a profession, nursing supports the value, dignity, and uniqueness of every person and takes their culture and belief system into consideration.

6. Nurses require advanced knowledge and skills; they also must care about their patients.
7. Nursing requires concern, compassion, respect, and warmth, as well as comprehensive, individualized planning of care, to facilitate patients' growth toward wellness.
8. Nursing links theory and research in an effort to answer difficult questions generated during nursing practice.

With an understanding of nursing's major concepts as a backdrop, we will now begin to examine the relationship of nurses' attitudes, beliefs, values, and philosophies to the way they practice; review philosophies of nursing that were developed by an individual, a division of nursing in a hospital, and a school of nursing; and assist readers in beginning to develop their own philosophies of nursing.

BELIEFS

Certain beliefs have evolved during the development of professional nursing. Specific statements of beliefs have been published for more than half a century. The most recent code was generated by the members of the American Nurses Association (ANA) and published in the *Code of Ethics for Nurses with Interpretive Statements* (ANA, 2001). Statements such as the *Code* exist to affirm the beliefs of the profession and to guide the practice of nursing.

A **belief** represents the intellectual acceptance of something as true or correct. Beliefs can also be described as convictions. Groupings of beliefs form codes and creeds. Beliefs are opinions that may be, in reality, true or false. They are based on attitudes that have been acquired and verified by experience. Beliefs are generally transmitted from generation to generation, are stable, and are resistant to change.

Beliefs are organized into **belief systems** that serve as roadmaps for thinking and decision

making (Grube, Mayton, and Ball-Rokeach, 1994). Individuals are not necessarily aware of how their beliefs interrelate or how their beliefs affect their behavior.

Although all people have beliefs, relatively few have spent much time examining their beliefs. In nursing, it is important to know and understand one's beliefs because the practice of nursing frequently challenges a nurse's beliefs. Although this conflict may create temporary discomfort, it is ultimately good because it forces nurses to consider their beliefs carefully. They have to answer the question: "Is this something I really believe, or have I accepted it because some influential person [such as a parent or teacher] said it?" Abortion, advance directives, the right to die, the right to refuse treatment, alternative lifestyles, and similar issues confront all members of contemporary society. Professional nurses must develop and refine their beliefs about these and many other issues. This is often difficult to do, but it pays dividends in self-awareness.

Beliefs are exhibited through attitudes and behaviors. Simply observing how nurses relate to patients, their families, and nursing peers reveals something about those nurses' beliefs. Every day nurses meet people whose beliefs are different from, or even diametrically opposed to, their own. Effective nurses recognize that they need to adopt nonjudgmental attitudes toward patients' beliefs. A nurse with a **nonjudgmental** attitude makes every effort to convey neither approval nor disapproval of patients' beliefs and respects each person's right to his or her beliefs (Figure 12-6).

An example of differences in beliefs that directly affect nursing is the position taken by some religious groups that all healing should be left to a divine power. For members of such groups, seeking medical treatment, even life-saving measures such as blood transfusions or chemotherapy for cancer, is not condoned. From time to time, there have been news reports of parents who are charged with criminal acts because they did not take a sick child to a physician. Typical of such incidents was the one reported in Georgia when the parents of a

19-year-old severely injured in an automobile accident refused to give permission for their unconscious Jehovah's Witness son to continue receiving blood transfusions. He died 2 days later (Eustis, 2002). The courts were involved, but the issue has not been resolved. Cases such as this have an impact on patients, families, the health care professionals involved, and the court system and often create a frenzy of media coverage.

Because you are in a health profession, you clearly have beliefs about the value of modern medicine. Think about how your health care beliefs differ from those of the family just described. What feelings might you have if assigned to work with a family with these beliefs? From this brief consideration, you may be able to appreciate how difficult it can be to maintain a nonjudgmental attitude toward the beliefs of patients. Nevertheless, it is essential.

Three Categories of Beliefs

People often use the terms *beliefs* and *values* interchangeably. Even experts disagree about whether they differ or are the same. Although they are related, beliefs and values are differentiated in this chapter and discussed separately.

Figure 12-6
Professional nurses make every effort to maintain a nonjudgmental attitude toward patients. A nonjudgmental attitude is one of nursing's values. *(Courtesy Emory University, Nell Hodgson Woodruff School of Nursing.)*

Theorists studying belief systems have identified three main categories of beliefs:
1. Descriptive or existential beliefs are those that can be shown to be true or false. An example of a descriptive belief is "The sun will come up tomorrow morning."
2. Evaluative beliefs are those in which there is a judgment about good or bad. The belief "Gambling is immoral" is an example of an evaluative belief.
3. Prescriptive (encouraged) and proscriptive (prohibited) beliefs are those in which certain actions are judged to be desirable or undesirable. The belief "Every citizen of voting age should vote in every election" is a prescriptive belief, whereas the belief "People should not engage in sexual intercourse outside of marriage" is a proscriptive belief. Prescriptive and proscriptive beliefs are closely related to values (Rokeach, 1973, pp. 6-7).

VALUES

Values are the freely chosen principles, ideals, or standards held by an individual, class, or group that give meaning and direction to life. A value is an abstract representation of what is right, worthwhile, or desirable. Values define ideal modes of conduct and reflect what the individual or group endorse and try to emulate. Values, like beliefs, are relatively stable and resistant to change.

Although many people are unaware of it, values help them make small, day-to-day choices, as well as important life decisions. Just as beliefs influence nursing practice, values also influence how nurses practice their profession, often without their conscious awareness. Diann B. Uustal (1985), a contemporary nurse who has written and spoken extensively about values, said, "Everything we do, every decision we make and course of action we take is based on our consciously and unconsciously chosen beliefs, attitudes and values" (Uustal, 1985, p. 100). Uustal also asserts, "Nursing is a behavioral manifestation of the nurse's value system. It is not merely a career, a job, an assignment; it is a ministry" (Uustal, 1993,

p. 10). She believes that nurses must give "caring attentiveness and presence" to their patients and to do otherwise "is equivalent to psychological and spiritual abandonment" (Uustal, 1993, p. 10). Do you agree or disagree with these statements?

Nature of Human Values

Values evolve as people mature. An individual's values today are undoubtedly different from those of 10, or even 5, years ago. Rokeach (1973, p. 3) made several assertions about the nature of human values:

1. Each person has a relatively small number of values.
2. All human beings, regardless of location or culture, possess basically the same values to differing degrees.
3. People organize their values into value systems.
4. People develop values in response to culture, society, and even individual personality traits.
5. Most observable human behaviors are manifestations or consequences of human values.

Authorities agree that values influence behavior and that people with unclear values lack direction, persistence, and decision-making skills (Raths, Harmin, and Simon, 1978). Because much of nursing involves having a clear sense of direction, the ability to persevere, and the ability to make sound decisions quickly and frequently, effective nurses must have a strong set of professional nursing values. A number of professional nursing values are listed in Box 12-6.

Process of Valuing

Valuing is the process by which values are determined. There are three identified steps in the process of valuing: choosing, prizing, and acting.

1. Choosing is the cognitive (intellectual) aspect of valuing. Ideally, people choose their values freely from all alternatives after considering the possible consequences of their choices.
2. Prizing is the affective (emotional) aspect of valuing. People usually feel good about their values and cherish the choices they make.
3. Acting is the kinesthetic (behavioral) aspect of valuing. When people affirm their values

publicly by acting on their choices, they make their values part of their behavior. A real value is acted upon consistently in behavior.

All three steps must be taken, or the process of valuing is incomplete (Uustal, 1998). For example, a professional nurse might believe that learning is a lifelong process and that nurses have an obligation to keep up with new developments in the profession. This nurse would choose continued learning and appreciate the consequences of the choice. He or she might even publicly affirm this choice and feel good about it. If the nurse follows through consistently with behaviors such as reading journals, attending conferences, and seeking out other learning opportunities, continued learning can be seen as a true value in his or her life.

Values Clarification

Nurses, as well as people in other helping professions, need to understand their values. This is the first step in self-awareness, which is important in maintaining a nonjudgmental approach to patients.

Considering your reactions to the following statements can help in beginning to identify some nursing values you hold:

1. Patients should always be told the truth about their diagnoses.
2. Nurses, if asked, should assist terminally ill patients to die.
3. Severely impaired infants should be kept alive, regardless of their future quality of life.
4. Nurses should never accept gifts from patients.
5. A college professor should receive a heart transplant before a homeless person does.
6. Nurses should be role models of healthy behavior.

As you react both emotionally and intellectually to these statements, something about your personal and professional values is revealed. Determining where you stand on these and other nursing issues is an important step in clarifying your values. A variety of values clarification exercises have been developed to stimulate self-reflection and help people understand their

Box 12-6 Professional Nursing Values

- Accountability and responsibility for own actions
- Balancing cure and care
- Benevolence
- Caring as a foundation for relationships
- Collaborative multidisciplinary practice
- Compassion
- Competence
- Concern
- Continuous improvement of service
- Cooperative work relationships
- Courage
- Dependability
- Empathy
- Ethical conduct
- Flexibility
- Focus on patient-defined quality of life
- Health promotion
- Holistic, person-centered care
- Honesty and authenticity in communication
- Humaneness
- Humility
- Illness prevention
- Individualized patient care
- Integrity—personal and professional
- Involvement with families
- Kindness
- Knowledge

- Listening attentively
- Nonjudgmental attitude
- Objectivity
- Openness to learning
- Partnerships with patients
- Patient advocacy
- Patient education
- Presence (being fully present)
- Promotion of health
- Promotion of patient self-determination and patient preferences
- Providing care regardless of patient's ability to pay
- Quality care (physical, emotional, spiritual, social, intellectual)
- Reliability
- Respect for each person's dignity and worth
- Responsibility
- Responsiveness
- Sensitivity
- Sharing decision making
- Sharing self through nursing interventions
- Stewardship; responsible use of resources
- Subordination of self-interest
- Support of fellow nurses
- Teamwork
- Trust in self, others, and the institution

Courtesy Diann B. Uustal (2006).

values. Box 12-7 contains a values clarification exercise you may want to complete to assist you further in understanding the valuing process.

Values Undergirding Nursing's Social Policy Statement

Professional groups, such as nursing, "have collective identities that are evidenced by their actions. These actions stem from a set of values and choices. … [B]y examining the actions of groups…, their basic values can be logically inferred" (Mohr, 1995, p. 30).

Organized nursing, through the ANA, sets forth the values that undergird the profession. This is done in a document published from time to time that is designed to explain "professional nursing's relationship with society and its obligation to those who receive nursing care" (American Nurses Association, 2003, p. 1). The most recent version, titled *Nursing's Social Policy Statement*, was published in 2003. It set forth several underlying values and assumptions on which the statement is based (American Nurses Association, 2003, p. 3):

Box **12-7** **Clarifying Your Values**

Once you have identified a value, it is important to assess its significance to you and to clarify your willingness to act on the value. The following clarifying questions are organized based on the steps of the valuing process and can help you answer questions about what you value. First, identify a value (or values) that is (are) important to you. Write your value(s) below:

_____

_____

_____

_____

   Next, use the questions below to assess the importance of a belief or attitude and to determine whether it is a value. Rephrase the questions to suit your own style of conversation.

Choosing Freely

   1. Am I sure I've thought about this value and chosen to believe it myself?
   2. Who first taught me this value?
   3. How do I know I'm "right"?

Choosing Among Alternatives

   4. What other alternatives are possible?
   5. Which alternative has the most appeal for me and why?
   6. Have I thought much about this value/alternative?

Choosing After Considering the Consequences

   7. What consequences do I think might occur as a result of my holding this value?
   8. What "price" will I pay for my position?
   9. Is this value worth the "price" I might pay?

Complement to Other Values

   10. Does this value "fit" with my other values, and is it consistent with them?
   11. Am I sure this value doesn't conflict with other values I deem important to me?

Prize and Cherish

   12. Am I proud of my position and value? Is this something I feel good about?
   13. How important is this value to me?
   14. If this were not one of my values, how different would my life be?

Public Affirmation

   15. Am I willing to speak out for this value?

Action

   16. Am I willing to put this value into action?
   17. Do I act on this value? When? How consistently?
   18. Is this a value that can guide me in other situations?
   19. Would I want others who are important to me to follow this value?
   20. Do I think I'll always believe this? How committed to this value am I?
   21. Am I willing to do anything about this value?
   22. How do I know this value is "right"? Are my values ethical?

From Uustal DB: *Clinical ethics and values: issues and insights in a changing healthcare environment*, East Greenwich, RI, 1993, Educational Resources in Healthcare. Reprinted with permission.

- Humans manifest an essential unity of mind, body, and spirit.
- Human experience is contextually and culturally defined.
- Health and illness are human experiences. The presence of illness does not preclude health nor does optimal health preclude illness.
- The relationship between nurse and patient involves participation of both in the process of care.
- The interaction between nurse and patient occurs within the context of the values and beliefs of the patient and the nurse.

Chapter 5 contains more about values and their relationship to nursing practice.

PHILOSOPHIES AND THEIR RELATIONSHIP TO NURSING CARE

Philosophy is defined as the study of the principles underlying conduct, thought, and the nature of the universe. A simple explanation of philosophy is that it entails a search for meaning in the universe. You may have learned about philosophers such as Plato, Aristotle, Bacon, Kant, Hegel, Kierkegaard, Nietzsche, Locke, Descartes, and others in nonnursing classes. These philosophers were searching for the underlying principles of reality and truth. Nursing philosophies and theories often derive from or build upon the concepts identified by these and other philosophers.

Philosophy begins when someone contemplates, or wonders, about something. If a group of friends sometimes sits and discusses the relationship between men and women and ponders the differences in men's and women's natures and approaches to life, one might say that they were developing a philosophy about male and female ways of being. It is important to remember that philosophy is not the exclusive domain of a few erudite individuals; everyone has a personal philosophy of life that is unique.

People develop personal philosophies as they mature, usually without being aware of it. These philosophies serve as blueprints or guides and incorporate each individual's value and belief systems. Nurses' personal philosophies interact directly with their philosophies of nursing and influence professional behaviors.

Branches of Philosophy

Before examining professional philosophies, we briefly explore the discipline of philosophy itself. Philosophy has been divided into specific areas of study. This section reviews six branches: epistemology, logic, aesthetics, ethics, politics, and metaphysics.

1. **Epistemology** is the branch of philosophy dealing with the theory of knowledge itself. The epistemologist attempts to answer such questions as "What can be known?" and "What constitutes knowledge?" Epistemology attempts to determine how we can know whether our beliefs about the world are true.

2. **Logic** is the study of proper and improper methods of reasoning. In logic, the nature of reasoning itself is the subject. Logic attempts to answer the question, "What should our thinking methods be in order to reach true conclusions?" Chapter 8 presents a method of logical thinking that nurses use to plan and implement effective patient care, called the nursing process.

3. **Aesthetics** is the study of what is beautiful. It attempts to answer the question, "Why do we find things beautiful?" Painting, sculpture, music, dance, and literature are all associated with beauty. Judgments about what is beautiful, however, differ from individual to individual and culture to culture. For example, Eastern music may sound discordant to the Western ear and vice versa.

4. **Ethics** is the branch of philosophy that studies standards of conduct. It attempts to answer the question, "What is the nature of good and evil?" Moral principles and values make up a system of ethics. Behavior depends on moral principles and values. Ethics, therefore, underlie the standards of behavior that govern us as individuals and as nurses. **Bioethics** is a term

describing the branch of ethics that deals with biological issues. Bioethics and nursing ethics are complex areas of study that are explored in Chapter 5.

5. **Politics,** in the context of a discussion of philosophy, means the area of philosophy that deals with the regulation and control of people living in society. Political philosophers study the conditions of society and suggest recommendations for improving them. They attempt to answer the question, "What makes good governments?"

6. **Metaphysics** is the consideration of the ultimate nature of existence, reality, human experience, and the universe. Metaphysicians believe that through contemplation we can come to a more complete understanding of reality than even science can provide. They ask the question, "What is the meaning of life?" and explore the fundamental nature of all reality.

This brief review of the major branches of philosophy is presented as a backdrop for the discussion of philosophies of nursing.

Philosophies of Nursing

Philosophies of nursing are statements of beliefs about nursing and expressions of values in nursing that are used as bases for thinking and acting. Most philosophies of nursing are built on a foundation of beliefs about people, environment, health, and nursing. Each of these four foundational concepts of nursing is discussed in some detail earlier in this chapter.

Individual philosophies

If asked, most nurses could list their beliefs about nursing, but it is doubtful that many have written a formal philosophy of nursing. They are influenced on a day-to-day basis, however, by their unwritten, informal philosophies. It is useful to go through the process of writing down one's own professional philosophy and revising it from time to time. Comparing recent and earlier versions can reveal professional and personal growth over time. It is also helpful to read one's

philosophy of nursing from time to time to make sure daily behaviors are consistent with deeply held beliefs. Box 12-8 contains one nurse's philosophy of nursing.

Collective philosophies

Although few individuals write down their nursing philosophies, it is common for hospitals and schools of nursing to express their collective beliefs about nursing in written philosophies. In fact, both hospitals and schools of nursing are required by their accrediting bodies to develop statements of philosophy. Philosophical statements should be relevant to the setting. They are intended to guide the practice of nurses employed in that setting. Examining some of these statements clarifies what constitutes a collective philosophy of nursing.

Philosophy of nursing in a hospital setting. First, look at the philosophy of nursing of Memorial Health Care System in Chattanooga, Tennessee, found in Box 12-9. This philosophy describes a commitment to excellence in nursing service, practice, and leadership. Notice statements with which you might agree or disagree. Remember that this is the philosophy of nursing in a hospital setting. Before taking a position in a hospital or health care agency, it is a good idea to ask for a copy of the philosophy of nursing of that institution. Read it carefully and make sure you accept the beliefs and values it contains, for it will influence nursing care in that setting.

Philosophy of a school of nursing. Now examine philosophical statements of a school of nursing. The philosophy of the faculty in the Department of Nursing at the University of North Florida is printed in Box 12-10. After reading this, identify the similarities and differences between the philosophy of nursing in the hospital setting and the one in this school of nursing. What differences in focus can you identify?

An important point about philosophies of nursing is that they are dynamic; they change over time. When a collective philosophy is written, it reflects the existing values and beliefs of the particular group of people who wrote it.

Box **12-8** One Nurse's Philosophy

I believe that the essence of nursing is caring about and caring for human beings who are unable to care for themselves. I believe that the central core of nursing is the nurse-patient relationship and that through that relationship I can make a difference in the lives of others at a time when they are most vulnerable.

Human beings generally do the best they can. When they are uncooperative, critical, or otherwise unpleasant, it is usually because they are frightened; therefore, I will remain pleasant and non-defensive and try to understand the patient's perception of the situation. I pledge to be trustworthy and an advocate for my patients.

I realize that my cultural background affects how I deliver nursing care and that my patients' cultural backgrounds affect how they receive my care. I try to learn as much as I can about each individual's cultural beliefs and preferences and individualize care accordingly.

My vision for myself as a nurse is that I will provide the best care I can to all patients, regardless of their financial situation, social status, lifestyle choices, or spiritual beliefs. I will collaborate with my patients, their families, and my health care colleagues and work cooperatively with them, valuing and respecting what each brings to the situation.

I am individually accountable for the care I provide, for what I fail to do and to know. Therefore, I pledge to remain a learner all my life and actively seek opportunities to learn how to be a more effective nurse.

I will strive for a balance of personal and professional responsibilities. This means I will take care of myself physically, emotionally, socially, and spiritually so I can continue to be a productive caregiver.

Box **12-9** Memorial Health Care System Philosophy of Nursing

Philosophy of Nursing

Nursing care throughout the Memorial Health Care System is committed to upholding the corporate values and the mission of Catholic Health Initiatives. We affirm that the corporate values of Reverence, Compassion, Integrity, and Excellence are in congruence with our professional values. Therefore, we believe that these principles must characterize nursing care.

Reverence
We believe …
■ that each of our patients, regardless of circumstances, possesses intrinsic value from God and should be treated with dignity and respect.
■ that meeting the needs of patients and other customers should always be our number-one priority.
■ that nurses should collaborate with other health care team members to meet the holistic needs of our patients, which include physical, psychosocial, and spiritual aspects of care.
■ that patient confidentiality and privacy should be preserved.
■ that we should be sensitive to individual needs and give support, praise, and recognition to encourage professional and personal development.

Compassion
We believe …
■ that each encounter with patients and families should portray compassion and concern.

Box 12-9 **Memorial Health Care System Philosophy of Nursing—cont'd**

- that our profession is a science and an art, the essence of which is nurturing and caring.
- that our primary duty is to restore and maintain the health of our patients in a spirit of compassion and concern.
- that compassion should be characterized in our day-to-day personal interactions, as well as being a motivating factor in management decisions.

Integrity
We believe …
- that the nursing process is an integral part of our practice as professional nurses.
- that we should aggressively promote patient and family education to allow each individual the opportunity to prevent illness and/or achieve optimal health.
- that we should encourage and support collaborative decision making by those who are closest to the situation, even at the risk of failure.
- that we are accountable to our patients, patients' families, and to each other for our professional practice.
- that we should possess an energy level and personal style that empowers and inspires enthusiasm in others.
- that justice should be applied equitably in all employment practices and personnel policies.

Excellence
We believe …
- that monitoring and evaluating nursing practice is our responsibility and is necessary to continuously improve care.
- that we should pursue professional growth and development through education, participating in professional organizations, and support of research.
- that we should provide a progressive environment, utilizing current technology guided by responsible stewardship, to promote the highest quality patient care and employee satisfaction.
- that we should consider suggestions and criticisms as challenges for improvement and innovation.
- that each patient should receive quality care that is cost-effective, competitive, and based on the latest technology.

From Memorial Health Care System Department of Nursing: Memorial Health Care System philosophy of nursing, Chattanooga, TN, 2003, Memorial Health Care System. Reprinted with permission.

When the group members change, the philosophy may also change. Therefore once a collective philosophy is written, it should be "revisited" regularly and modified to reflect accurately the group's current beliefs about nursing practice.

DEVELOPING A PERSONAL PHILOSOPHY OF NURSING

Your philosophy of life, whether or not you can articulate it, is the basis of your day-to-day behavior. It consists of the principles that underlie your thinking and conduct. Therefore developing a philosophy of nursing is not merely an academic exercise required by accrediting bodies. Having a written philosophy can help guide nurses in the daily decisions they must make in nursing practice.

Writing a philosophy is not a complex, time-consuming task. It simply involves writing down your beliefs and values about nursing. It answers the questions: "What is nursing?" and "Why do I

Box **12-10** Philosophy of the School of Nursing, University of North Florida

The philosophy of the School of Nursing supports the mission of the University of North Florida and the College of Health and reflects the academic goals of the greater university community. The faculty have defined a philosophy of nursing that considers two domains: the patient who is the recipient of care, and the nurse who is the caregiver. The patient domain includes beliefs about persons, environment, and health.

The faculty of the School of Nursing view patients as biopsychosocial beings with inherent dignity and worth who strive to meet a hierarchy of human needs throughout the life span. When unable to satisfy these needs, patients are at risk for alterations in health status. As risks manifest themselves in health problems, patients seek relief in the form of health care from health professionals. Nursing responds to a need for care and support and, in some cases, the need for treatments and curing techniques. Patients of nursing may be individuals, families, groups, or communities.

Patients live in an environment with an internal and external dimension. The internal environment is an open system composed of four subsystems: physical, psychological, spiritual, and cultural. The external environment is composed of groups of individuals and families, each living within their unique sociocultural milieu. These groups function in a universe influenced by political and economic forces. The dynamic relationship between internal and external environments has a profound effect on health status and on how persons adapt to physical, psychological, social, and environmental changes.

Health is viewed as a dynamic state of being on a continuum from optimal wellness to illness. Changes on this continuum are influenced and, in some cases, caused by internal and external environmental stressors. A state of health exists when a person functions as an integrated whole, living and interacting with environments in a productive manner. Movement on the health-illness continuum depends on the severity of stressors, the adaptive mechanisms of the person, and the accessibility to and quality of health care services available.

The nurse/caregiver domain includes beliefs about nursing, education, and professional practice and research. Nursing is a human service that assists patients to achieve optimal wellness and cope with periods of illness and disability. The nurse uses problem-solving skills and caring behaviors to facilitate the patient's adaptive responses in an effort to maintain, promote, and/or restore an optimal state of health or facilitate a peaceful death. Specific caring behaviors are determined by the patient's individual needs and may be assistive, supportive, or facilitative in nature. The nurse assumes independent and interdependent roles at various times, based on mutually identified needs of the patient. Nurses fulfill their professional role as members of a health care team working together in the best interest of the patient.

Nursing education takes place through a planned teaching-learning process. Faculty are responsible for assisting students to achieve their full potential and are sensitive to the individual needs of students. Learning readiness, self-directed learning, recognition of the value of past experience and education, and the development of a problem-solving orientation to learning are important aspects of the teaching-learning process. Students and faculty cooperate in assuming a shared responsibility for planning and implementing learning activities within the context of the curriculum and through individual course offerings. Learning is facilitated when the educational environment provides an open, accepting atmosphere in which the faculty and students work together to achieve mutual goals. Higher education is a process through which the student is afforded opportunities to develop a liberal education, as well as a rich knowledge base on which to build a professional career.

Box 12-10 **Philosophy of the School of Nursing, University of North Florida—cont'd**

Baccalaureate nursing education is specifically concerned with preparation for the first professional degree in nursing. This education prepares the student for professional practice and leadership roles within an ever-changing health care industry. It also serves as a foundation for graduate education and advanced nursing practice.

Graduate nursing education, at the master's level, is specifically concerned with preparing nurses with advanced practice skills. Graduates provide expert nursing care to individuals, families, and communities; contribute to nursing science; serve as mentors and teachers of nurse colleagues; and participate in planning and policy formulations for a variety of patient populations.

Professional nursing practice is based on concepts and theories from the discipline of nursing and from other fields, including the sciences and humanities. Professional nurses use the nursing process, which demands the ability to assess, analyze, plan, implement, and evaluate nursing care. The nursing process is the basis of scientific nursing practice and requires nurses to analyze data from many sources. A strong foundation from the natural sciences and the humanities assists nurses in developing the critical thinking skills essential to the nursing process. The scientific base of practice continues to be developed throughout the nursing curriculum and provides the graduate with the knowledge and skills to practice nursing in a responsible manner.

Nursing is a discipline that uses research as a process to develop a distinct body of knowledge as a basis for scientific practice. Research serves as the basis for changes that influence and improve nursing practice and patient care outcomes. The professional nurse prepared at the baccalaureate level should be an informed consumer of research findings and should be able to collaborate with others to study questions that arise from the practice of nursing and related issues. The professional nurse prepared at the master's level should function as a collaborative member of research teams, evaluate the clinical usefulness of research findings, and assume a leadership role in promoting evidence-based practice.

From University of North Florida, School of Nursing: *Philosophy of the School of Nursing,* Jacksonville, Fla, 2003, University of North Florida. Reprinted with permission.

Box 12-11 **Philosophy of Nursing Work Sheet**

Purpose: To write a beginning philosophy of nursing that reflects the beliefs and values of
_____ [your name].
Today's date is _____.
I chose nursing as my profession because nursing is _____ .
I believe that the core of nursing is_____.
I believe that the focus of nursing is_____.
My vision for myself as a nurse is that I will _____.
To live out my philosophy of nursing, every day I must remember this about:
1. My patients: _____.
2. My patients' families: _____.
3. My fellow health care professionals: _____.
4. My own health: _____.

practice nursing the way I do?" Whether individual or collective, a philosophy should provide direction and promote effectiveness.

Box 12-11 is designed to help you begin to develop your own personal philosophy of nursing. After you write a beginning philosophy, save it.

As you progress through your educational program, take it out and revise it regularly, saving each version. After you graduate, look back at all the different versions and see how your values and beliefs about nursing have changed over time.

SUMMARY OF *Key Points*

- Knowledge of systems and human needs can be used to understand nursing's major concepts.
- Persons are viewed as unique open systems who are motivated by needs.
- Maslow organized human needs into a hierarchy consisting of five levels that range from basic physiological needs, which are common to all people, to self-actualization, which is attained by few.
- Environment consists of all the circumstances, influences, and conditions that affect an individual. The physical environment and family, cultural, social, and community systems all have an impact.
- Health is dynamic and viewed as a continuum.
- Nurses view health holistically, including its effect on an individual's physical, emotional, social, and spiritual functioning, as well as its effect on the family.
- Health is affected by health beliefs and health behaviors.
- As an open system, nursing integrates person, environment, and health into a meaningful whole.

- Nursing assists people to achieve health at the highest possible level, given their environmental and genetic constraints.
- People develop beliefs and values that affect their attitudes and behaviors.
- Beliefs and values influence how nurses practice their profession.
- Nurses need to be aware of their beliefs and values to prevent the unintentional intrusion of personal values into nurse-patient relationships.
- A statement of beliefs can be called a philosophy.
- The purpose of developing a philosophy of nursing is to shape and guide nursing practice.
- Philosophies can express either individual beliefs or the collective beliefs of a group, such as a nursing faculty.
- As nurses progress professionally, they develop ideas about the practice of nursing that they agree with and support. From these, they develop their own personal philosophies of nursing.
- As nurses mature in the profession, they may find that their philosophies about nursing also change, even though underlying values may not.

CRITICAL THINKING QUESTIONS

1. Discuss systems in relation to your family. What are the family equivalents of inputs, throughputs, subsystems, suprasystems, outputs, evaluation, and feedback? Does your family tend to be an open or closed system?
2. Describe Maslow's hierarchy of needs and place yourself on the hierarchy today, 1 week

ago, and when you were a senior in high school. Were you at a different level each time? Consider what factors—internal and external—may have been involved in your placement at each of these times. If possible, compare and discuss your findings with at least one other person.

3. Write your own personal definition of health and share it with one other person. Evaluate your definition in terms of holism.

4. What are factors that influence an individual's personal health behaviors? Make a list of your health behaviors, including those that promote health and those that diminish health. Analyze why you continue both the healthy and the nonhealthy behaviors. Identify population-based initiatives that could influence you to make more health-generating choices.

5. Using a search engine, assess the array of support groups online. Enter the discussion group of one group that interests you, and simply observe. How would you evaluate the quality of the support and information being shared?

6. Look through your local Yellow Pages under "Social Services" and "Organizations." What types of social support do you find that might be useful to patients? Compare these with the online choices. Which type of support—face-to-face or online—is more appealing to you? Why?

7. Conduct an assessment of your community in terms of one of the following: availability of jobs, quality of public education, availability of health services, environmental hazards, and quality of air and water. What is the impact of the factor you selected on the health of the community's citizens? What can you do to strengthen the environmental health of your community?

8. Find out what your state and community are doing to link their health objectives to those of the *Healthy People 2010* initiatives. Discuss these in class. Design a project to assist your school of nursing to support the national effort.

9. Name two of your health-related values. How did these become your values? Describe how you expect these values to influence your nursing practice.

10. Read "One Nurse's Philosophy" in Box 12-8. Then identify at least 10 of that nurse's professional values, using the list in Box 12-6, "Professional Nursing Values." Can you identify other values that are not listed?

11. Obtain the philosophy of the department of nursing of a facility where you work or have clinical labs. Compare it with the philosophical statements of Memorial Health Care System. What are three common elements and three differences? Which of the two statements is most congruent with your own beliefs about nursing?

12. Obtain the philosophy statement of the faculty of your school of nursing. What concepts are included? Which beliefs do you agree with and disagree with? Why?

13. Using the work sheet in Box 12-11, write a beginning personal philosophy of nursing. Share your philosophy with one other person.

14. Discuss how the focus on "the bottom line" affects your own and nursing's professional values.

15. Discuss how having or not having a philosophy of nursing might influence a nurse's practice.

REFERENCES

Ahmann E: Supporting families' savvy use of the Internet for health research, *Pediatr Nurs* 26(4):419-423, 2000.

American Nurses Association: *Code of ethics for nurses with interpretive statements,* Silver Spring, Md, 2001, available online: nursesbooks.org.

American Nurses Association: *Nursing's social policy statement,* ed 2, Washington, DC, 2003, available online: nursesbooks.org.

Bandura A: A social cognitive approach to the exercise of control over AIDS infection. In DiClemente RJ, editor: *Adolescents and AIDS: a generation in jeopardy,* Newbury Park, Calif, 1992, Sage Publications.

Bandura A: *Self-efficacy: exercise of control*, New York, 1997, WH Freeman.

Beyea SC: Evaluating evidence found on the Internet, *AORN J* 72(5):906-910, 2000.

Center on Budget and Policy Priorities: *News release: census data show poverty increased, income stagnated, and the number of uninsured rose to a record level in 2003*, 2006, available online: http://www.cbpp.org/8-26-04pov.htm.

Chase M: Health journal: a guide for patients who turn to the Web for solace and support, *Wall Street Journal*, Sept 17, 1999, p B1.

Dunn HL: High-level wellness for man and society, *Am J Pub Health* 49(6):786-792, 1959.

Dunn HL: *High-level wellness*, Thorofare, NJ, 1961, Slack.

Edin KJ: Testimony of Dr. Kathryn J. Edin before the United States Committee on Finance Subcommittee of Social Security and Family Policy, United States Senate, The Benefits of Healthy Marriage Hearing, May 5, Washington, DC: Dirksen Senate Office Building, Room 219, 2004, available online: http://www.finance.senate.gov/hearings/testimony/2004test/050504ketest.pdf.

Eustis R: *Parents: son would have chosen death over blood*, 2002, available online: www.rickross.com/reference/jw/jw90.html.

Finfgeld-Connett D: Clarification of social support, *Image: J Nurs Scholar* 37(1):4-9, 2005.

Grossman D: Enhancing your cultural competence, *Am J Nurs* 94(7):58-62, 1994.

Grube JW, Mayton DM, Ball-Rokeach SJ: Inducing change in values, attitudes, and behaviors: belief system theory, *J Social Issues* 50(4):153-173, 1994.

Holmes TH, Rahe RH: The social readjustment rating scale, *J Psychosomat Res* 11(2):213-218, 1967.

Maslow AH: *Motivation and personality*, ed 3, New York, 1987, Harper & Row.

Memorial Health Care System Department of Nursing: *Memorial Health Care System philosophy of nursing*, Chattanooga, Tenn, 2003, Memorial Health Care System.

Miller MA, Rahe RH: Life changes scaling for the 1990s, *J Psychosomat Res* 43(3):279-292, 1997.

Mohr WK: Values, ideologies, and dilemmas: professional and occupational contradictions, *J Psych Nurs* 33(1):29-34, 1995.

Parsons T: Definitions of health and illness in light of American values and social structure. In Jaco EG, editor: *Patients, physicians and illness*, New York, 1959, Free Press, pp 165-187.

Peden AR, Rayens MK, Hall LA et al: Negative thinking and the mental health of low-income single mothers, *Image: J Nurs Scholar* 36(4):337-344, 2004.

Pender NJ, Murdaugh C, Parsons MA: *Health promotion in nursing practice*, ed 5, Upper Saddle River, NJ, 2006, Prentice-Hall Health.

Pratt JP, Overfield T, Gill-Hilton H: Health behaviors of nurses and general population women, *Health Values* 18(3):41-46, 1994.

Raths L, Harmin M, Simon S: *Values and teaching*, ed 2, Columbus, Ohio, 1978, Charles Merrill.

Reutter L, Sword W, Meagher-Stewart D et al: Nursing students' beliefs about the relationship between poverty and health, *J Adv Nurs* 48:299-309, 2004.

Rogers C: *On becoming a person*, Boston, 1961, Houghton Mifflin.

Rokeach M: *The nature of human values*, New York, 1973, Free Press.

Rosenstock IM: Why people use health services, part II, *Milbank Mem Fund Quart* 44(3):94-124, 1966.

Rosenstock IM: The health belief model: explaining health behavior through expectancies. In Glans K, Lewis FM, Rimer BK, editors: *Health behavior and health education: theory, research, and practice*, San Francisco, 1990, Jossey Bass, pp 39-62.

Smith K, Bazini-Barakat N: A public health nursing practice model: melding public health principles with the nursing process, *Pub Health Nurs* 20(1):42-48, 2003.

Smuts JC: *Holism and evolution*, New York, 1926, Macmillan.

Steptoe A, Wardle J: Locus of control and health behaviour revisited: a multivariate analysis of young adults from 18 countries, *Br J Psychol* 92(4):659-673, 2001.

University of North Florida, School of Nursing: *Philosophy of the School of Nursing*, Jacksonville, Fla, 2003, University of North Florida.

U.S. Census Bureau: Income, poverty and insurance coverage in the U.S., *Curr Population Rep* 2003:60-226, 2003.

U.S. Census Bureau: *Current population survey: annual social and economic supplements*, 2004, available online: http://www.census.gov/hhes/poverty/histpov/hstpov3.html.

U.S. Census Bureau: *America's families and living arrangements*, 2005, available online:

http://www.census.gov/population/www/socdemo/hh-fam/cps2004.html.

U.S. Census Bureau: *Statistical abstract of the United States,* Washington, DC, 2006, Government Printing Office.

U.S. Department of Health and Human Services: *Healthy people 2010: implementation,* 2003, available online: www.healthypeople.gov/Implementation/default.htm#partners.

U.S. Department of Health and Human Services: *HHS poverty guidelines,* 2006a, available online: http://aspe.hhs.gov/poverty/06computations.shtml.

U.S. Department of Health and Human Services: *Healthy People 2010: fact sheet,* 2006b, online: http://www.healthypeople.gov/About/ hpfact.htm.

Uustal DB: *Values and ethics in nursing: from theory to practice,* East Greenwich, RI, 1985, Educational Resources in Nursing and Wholistic Health.

Uustal DB: *Clinical ethics and values: issues and insights in a changing healthcare environment,* East Greenwich, RI, 1993, Educational Resources in Healthcare.

Uustal DB: *Caring for yourself, caring for others: the ultimate balance,* East Greenwich, RI, 1998, Educational Resources in Healthcare.

von Bertalanffy L: *General systems theory: foundations, development, applications,* New York, 1968, George Braziller.

World Health Organization: *Constitution,* Geneva, 1947, World Health Organization.

13

Nursing Theory: The Basis for Professional Nursing

Beth Perry Black

Learning Outcomes

After studying this chapter, students will be able to:

- Explore elements of selected nursing philosophies, nursing conceptual models, and theories of nursing.
- Consider how selected nursing theoretical works guide the practice of nursing.
- Delineate the role of nursing theory for different levels of nursing education.

- Describe the function of nursing theory in research and theory-based practice.
- Relate the role of nursing theory in education, research, and practice to the development of the profession.

"Theory" is a word that is used frequently in daily language, such as "I have a theory about that" or "In theory, this should work." This use of the word *theory* means that the user has some idea about a phenomenon and the way this phenomenon works in the world. When people say, "I have a theory ..." about a certain phenomenon or situation, they are demonstrating something about their own distinct orientation or way of seeing the world.

Nursing as a profession has a distinct theoretical orientation to practice. This means that the practice of nursing is based on a specific body of knowledge that is built on theory. This body of knowledge shapes and is shaped by how nurses see the world. The word **theory** has many definitions, but generally it refers to a group of related concepts, definitions, and statements that describe a certain view of nursing **phenomena** (observable occurrences) from which to describe, explain, or predict outcomes (Chinn and Kramer, 1998; Powers and Knapp, 1995). Theories represent abstract ideas rather than concrete facts. New theories are always being generated, although some theories are useful for many years. When new knowledge becomes available, theories that are no longer useful are modified or discarded. Although nursing theory has been traced back to Florence Nightingale, most nursing theory was developed in the second half of the twentieth century (Alligood, 2002a; Tomey and Alligood, 2002).

So why is theory important? First, nursing as profession is strengthened when nursing knowledge is built on sound theory. As seen in Chapter 3, one criterion for a profession is a distinct body of knowledge as the basis for practice. Nursing has knowledge that is distinct from, although related to, other disciplines such as medicine, social work, sociology, and physiology. The development of nursing knowledge is an important activity for nurse researchers and scholars. The evolution of the profession of nursing depends on continued recognition of nursing as a scholarly academic discipline that contributes to society.

Second, theory is a useful tool for reasoning, critical thinking, and decision making (Alligood, 2002c; Alligood and Tomey, 2002; Tomey and Alligood, 2002). The ultimate goal of nursing theory is to support excellence in practice. Nursing practice settings are complex, and a vast amount of information about each patient is available to nurses. Nurses must analyze this information to make sound clinical judgments and to generate effective interventions. From organization of patient data to the development and evaluation of interventions, theory guides nurses in developing effective care. Box 13-1 shows how theory guides the clinical practice of nursing.

Several words are used to describe abstract thoughts and their linkages. From the most to least abstract, these include metaparadigm, philosophy, conceptual model or framework, and

Box **13-1** **Nursing Theory and the Professional Nurse**

Theory guides the professional nurse in:
- Organizing patient data
- Analyzing patient data
- Understanding connections between pieces of data
- Discriminating between important and less pertinent data
- Making sound clinical judgments based on evidence
- Planning effective nursing interventions
- Predicting outcomes of interventions
- Evaluating outcomes of interventions

theory. **Metaparadigm** refers to the most abstract aspect of the structure of nursing knowledge (Fawcett, 2000; Powers and Knapp, 1995). The metaparadigm of nursing consists of the major concepts of the discipline—person, environment, health, and nursing—that were discussed in Chapter 12. Simply stated, these four concepts comprise the metaparadigm of nursing; that is, these are the **concepts** (abstract notion or idea) of most importance to nursing practice and research. Nursing philosophies, models, and theories contain most or all of these concepts.

A **philosophy** is a set of beliefs about the nature of how things work and how the world should be viewed (Sitzman and Eichelberger, 2004). A nursing philosophy begins to put together some or all concepts of the metaparadigm. For instance, Florence Nightingale, whose work will be considered in more detail later in this chapter, wrote *Notes on Nursing: What It Is and What It Is Not*, in which her basic philosophy of nursing is described in detail. A **conceptual model** or **framework** is a more specific organization of nursing phenomena than philosophies. As the words "model" or "framework" imply, models provide an organizational structure that makes firmer, more concrete connections between concepts.

Theories are more concrete descriptions of concepts that are embedded in propositions. **Propositions** are statements that describe linkages between concepts and are more prescriptive; that is, they propose an outcome that is testable in practice and research (Alligood, 2002c). For example, Peplau's book *Interpersonal Relations in Nursing* (Peplau, 1952) contains a theory that describes very specific elements of effective interaction between the nurse and patient. Using concepts from nursing's metaparadigm, Peplau created a theory delineating elements of excellent and effective practice in psychiatric nursing. She linked abstract concepts such as health and nursing to create a concrete, useful theory for practice.

The **primary source**—the original writings of the theorist—is the best source for in-depth understanding of theoretical works. Explanatory texts written by other scholars can be very helpful in interpreting primary sources. Explanatory texts introduce students to the theoretical basis of the discipline of nursing from a nursing science perspective that is much broader than any one of the primary sources. That is, these explanatory texts trace the historical development of the philosophy, model, or theory and specify **criteria** (standards) by which to analyze, critique, and evaluate them. Texts such as these were first published in the early 1980s with a completely different purpose than the theorists' original writings. They are designed to contribute to the general understanding of nursing theory and theoretical developments in nursing in a unique but complementary way. Undergraduate and graduate students, faculty, and practicing nurses have found that these explanatory texts on nursing theory make a significant contribution to their knowledge and understanding of nursing science in its own right.

In this chapter, three types of nursing theoretical works will be presented: philosophies, conceptual models, and theories. Selected works from each of the three types provide a broad overview of theory within the discipline of nursing. This introduction is designed to help you develop a beginning understanding of nursing theory on which to build as you pursue your nursing education and career in the profession of nursing.

NURSING PHILOSOPHIES

Chapter 12 introduced nursing philosophy and discussed its function in nursing practice and educational institutions. A philosophy provides a broad, general view of nursing that clarifies values and answers broad disciplinary questions such as the following: "What is nursing?" "What is the profession of nursing?" "What do nurses do?" "What is the nature of human caring?" "What is the nature of nursing practice and the development of practice expertise?" Three philosophies representing different positions in the development of nursing theory are presented here.

Figure 13-1 demonstrates different views of the same patient situation among nurses who ascribe to the philosophies of Florence Nightingale, Virginia Henderson, and Jean Watson, whose work is presented here.

Nightingale's Philosophy

Florence Nightingale was born in 1820, in Florence, Italy. She was the daughter of a wealthy English landowner and his wife, Fanny, whose goal in life was to find a suitable husband for her daughters. Florence was very close to her father and he undertook the responsibility for her education, teaching her a classic curriculum of Greek, Latin, French, German, Italian, history, philosophy, and mathematics. At age 25, after rejecting several suitors, Florence announced her decision to go to Kaisersworth, Germany, to study nursing. Her parents were very upset with this choice because nursing was a pursuit of working-class women and Florence was a lady of some social standing and wealth. Her persistence in the face of her parents' opposition is characteristic of the woman. This trait enabled her to accomplish feats most women of the time would not pursue.

Nightingale's work represents the beginning of professional nursing as we know it today. In her

What needs to be adjusted in this environment to protect the patient? (Florence Nightingale)

How can I create an environment of trust, understanding and openness so that the patient and I can work together in meeting his needs? (Jean Watson)

What can I help this patient do that he would do for himself if he could? (Virginia Henderson)

Figure 13-1
Three nurses: three philosophies. *(Dennis G. Perry.)*

most frequently cited work, *Notes on Nursing: What It Is and What It Is Not* (1969, originally published in 1859), Nightingale addressed the philosophical question "What is nursing?" Importantly, she presented a logical distinction between nursing and medicine by clarifying the major concern of nursing as health rather than illness. Her writing about nursing reflected the sociohistorical context in which she lived: she also made a distinction between the work of nursing and the work of household servants, who were common in her day and often cared for the sick.

Though Nightingale's work contained many ideas about nursing, her unique perspective for nursing practice focused on the relationship of patients to their surroundings. She set forth principles that were foundational to nursing and remain relevant to nursing practice today. For example, her description of the importance of observing the patient and accurately recording information and her principles of cleanliness shape hospital-based nursing practice today. Nightingale's work began to sharpen the focus of the profession on what has become known as the metaparadigm of nursing: person (patient), health (as opposed to illness), environment (how the environment affects health and recovery from illness), and nursing (as opposed to medicine).

Using Nightingale's philosophy in practice

Nightingale believed that the health of patients was related to their surroundings. Recognizing the need for pure air and water, efficient drainage, cleanliness, and light, she emphasized the necessity of adequate ventilation and sunlight, encouraging rearranging patients' beds to give them access to direct sunlight. Her discussion of diet addressed not only the necessity of a balanced diet but also the nurse's responsibility to observe and record what was eaten. Cleanliness of the patient, the bed linens, and the room itself were essential points of emphasis. Nightingale recognized the problem of noise in hospital rooms and halls, which foreshadowed the attention given to excess noise in inpatient settings in recent years. Rest is important in the restoration of health;

Nightingale believed that sudden disruption of sleep was a serious problem.

Nightingale recognized the protective role of nurses. She gave nurses the responsibility for protecting patients from possible harm by well-meaning visitors who may provide false hope, discuss upsetting news, or tire the patient with social conversation. Nightingale even suggested that the nurse's responsibility for patients did not end even when the nurse was off duty. This view underpins the system of primary nursing found in some settings today. The patient's primary nurse develops plans and interventions based on the patient's objective and subjective data that are carried out by other nurses even when the primary nurse is not on duty. Interestingly, Nightingale even suggested that patients might benefit from visits by small pets, another idea that speaks to the ongoing relevance of her work.

The nurse whose practice is guided by Nightingale's philosophy is sensitive to the effect of the environment on the patient's health or recovery from illness. Her philosophy provided the foundational work for a theory development that proposed changing patients' environments to effect positive changes in their health. In Nightingale's view, nurses' primary responsibility was for patients and their surroundings.

Henderson's Philosophy

Virginia Henderson was born in 1897 in Kansas City, Missouri, and was named for the state her mother longed for and to which the family returned 4 years later. Although she received an excellent education from a family friend who was a schoolmaster and her father, a former teacher, it was not a traditional education and it did not yield a diploma. This delayed her entry into nursing school. During World War II she studied under Annie Goodrich at Teachers College, Columbia University, where she ultimately—after numerous interruptions—received her bachelor's and master's degrees. By the time of her death in 1996, Virginia Henderson was internationally known and regarded by many as "the Florence Nightingale of the 20th century."

One hundred years after Nightingale, Virginia Henderson's work first appeared. Henderson emerged at a time when efforts to clarify nursing as a profession emphasized the need to define nursing. Henderson's philosophical approach to nursing is contained in her comprehensive definition: the "unique function of the nurse ... is to assist the individual, sick or well, in the performance of those activities contributing to health or its recovery (or a peaceful death) that he would perform unaided if he had the necessary strength, will or knowledge" (Henderson, 1966, p. 15). Although Henderson, seen in Figure 13-2, was recognized for many contributions to nursing throughout her long career, this early work, which defined nursing and specified the role of the nurse in relation to the patient, remains particularly noteworthy and relevant. Henderson's relationship with one of her former students, who recognizes the ongoing contributions of Henderson's work to nursing, is described in Box 13-2.

Henderson's philosophy of nursing linked her definition of nursing, which emphasized the functions of the nurse and the assisting aspects of nursing, with a list of basic patient needs that are the focus of nursing care. Her work proposed an answer to questions similar to those addressed by Nightingale a century earlier: "What is the nursing profession?" and "What do nurses do?" Henderson described the nurse's role as that of a substitute for the patient, a helper to the patient, or a partner with the patient.

Figure 13-2
Virginia Henderson. (*Courtesy of Edward J. Halloran.*)

Henderson identified 14 basic needs (Box 13-3) as a general focus for patient care. She proposed that these needs encompassed the elements of nursing care. The function of nurses was to assist patients if they were unable to perform any of these 14 functions themselves. Although these needs can be categorized as physical, psychological, emotional, sociological, spiritual, or developmental, a more careful analysis reveals a holistic view of human development and health.

The first nine needs emphasize the importance of care of the physical body: breathing, eating and drinking, elimination, movement and positioning, sleep and rest, suitable clothing, maintenance of suitable environment for the body temperature, cleanliness, and avoidance of danger or harm. Next, she included psychosocial needs such as communication and spirituality, including worship and faith. She concluded with three needs that might be viewed as developmental: the need for work and the sense of accomplishment; the need for play and recreation; and the need to learn, discover, and satisfy curiosity. These 14 needs provide a comprehensive view of aspects of patients' lives amenable to nursing care. They continue to be used today in philosophical statements of schools and departments of nursing.

Using Henderson's philosophy in practice

Nurses whose practice is consistent with Henderson's philosophy adopt an orientation to care from the perspective of the 14 basic needs. Henderson's clarity about the role and function of the nurse is a strength of her work. This philosophy is easily applied to a variety of patient care settings, from brief outpatient encounters in which a limited number of needs are addressed to a complex setting such as intensive care where patients are extremely vulnerable. Henderson used her definition of nursing and the basic needs approach in her well-known case study of a young patient who had undergone a leg amputation. Using this case, Henderson demonstrated how the nurse's role changes on a day-to-day, week-to-week, and month-to-month basis in

Box 13-2 Remembering Virginia Henderson

Although I had known Virginia Henderson from the time when I was a graduate student at Yale, geography later brought us more closely together. Knowing her family lived in Virginia [mine was in Connecticut], whenever I traveled by car from North Carolina to Connecticut I called and asked if she wanted a ride back home with me and I could drop her off in Virginia en-route to North Carolina. Six times we made the eight-hour ride together. Our conversations were wide-ranging as we were both world travelers. We talked much about politics; most about nurses—"see a nurse before you go to a doctor" as a solution to health care cost, quality, and access problems; some about patients—"give them their records" as a most important patient education tool; and some about our large extended families. I was introduced to two of Virginia Henderson's sisters when they were all in their 90s. Four brothers and a sister had pre-deceased them but Frances [Fanny] had maintained the old family homestead so all who could come were welcomed to stay. Come they did for over two generations of reunions, weddings, funerals and holidays, especially Christmas.

What was most amazing to me about our time together was that Virginia Henderson never said anything to me about our profession that she had not written down somewhere for all nurses to read. Yale's School of Nursing asked me to address the topic of her writing in their Bellos Lecture the year they celebrated her 90th birthday. I read her textbook, *Principles and Practice of Nursing,* 6th edition, and discovered any number of conversations I had experienced with her over the years. In preparing the *Virginia Henderson Reader: Excellence in Nursing,* I discovered even more. Her writings are conversational, that is, completely without the jargon of the medical and nursing professions. Her description of nursing is best used by nurses to tell patients what can be expected—to paraphrase—I'm here to help you do what you would do for yourself if you had the strength, will or knowledge and do so for you to become free of my help as rapidly as possible. It is quite reassuring for a patient to know what the nurse is going to do.

Virginia Henderson's writings are timeless. The information in the *Nature of Nursing and Basic Principles of Nursing Care* is as relevant today as the day the book was written. Her textbook is the most important document written about nurses and nursing in the 20th century because it provided evidence of effective and efficient nursing. If you read her work, you can have a conversation with her, too.

Edward J. Halloran, RN, MPH, PhD
Fellow, American Academy of Nursing

Courtesy, Edward J. Halloran.

relation to the patient's changing needs and the contributions of other members of the health care delivery team (Henderson, 1966).

Watson's Philosophy

A later contribution to the evolving philosophy of nursing is the work of Jean Watson. Jean Watson was born in West Virginia in the early 1940s. She received her BSN from the University of Colorado in 1964, her MS from the University of Colorado in 1966, and her PhD from the

University of Colorado in 1973. Only 6 years later, she published her first book, *The Philosophy and Science of Caring.* In this initial work, she called for a return to the earlier values of nursing and emphasized the caring aspects of nursing. Watson's work is recognized as human science. Caring as a theme is reflected in her other professional accomplishments, such as the Center for Human Caring at the University of Colorado in Denver, where nurses can incorporate knowledge of human caring as the basis of nursing practice

| Box **13-3** | Henderson's 14 Basic Needs of the Patient |

1. Breathe normally.
2. Eat and drink adequately.
3. Eliminate body wastes.
4. Move and maintain desirable position.
5. Sleep and rest.
6. Select suitable clothes—dress and undress.
7. Maintain body temperature within normal range by adjusting clothing and modifying the environment.
8. Keep the body clean and well groomed and protect the integument (skin).
9. Avoid dangers in the environment and avoid injuring others.
10. Communicate with others in expressing emotions, needs, fears, or opinions.
11. Worship according to one's faith.
12. Work in such a way that there is a sense of accomplishment.
13. Play or participate in various forms of recreation.
14. Learn, discover, or satisfy the curiosity that leads to normal development and health and use the available health facilities.

Reprinted with permission of Henderson V: *The nature of nursing: a definition and its implications for practice, research, and education,* New York, 1996, Macmillan.

and scholarship. Watson proposed 10 factors (Box 13-4), which she labeled *carative* factors, a term she contrasted with *curative* to differentiate nursing from medicine.

Watson's work (1979, 1988, 1999) addressed the philosophical question of the nature of nursing as viewed as a human-to-human relationship. She focused on the relationship of the nurse and the patient, drawing on philosophical sources for a new approach that emphasized how the nurse and patient change together through transpersonal caring. She proposed that nursing be concerned with spiritual matters and the inner knowledge of nurse and patient as they participate together in the transpersonal caring process. She equated health with harmony, resulting from unity of body, mind, and soul, for which the patient is primarily responsible. Illness or disease was equated with lack of harmony within the mind, body, and soul experienced in internal or external environments (Watson, 1979). Nursing is based on human values and interest in the welfare of others, and is concerned with health promotion, health restoration, and illness pre-

vention. Watson's most recent work (1999) interprets her earlier works in light of postmodern thought for the twenty-first century. Watson recognized the scientific method as a tool for systematic solutions to problems and a guide for making decisions.

Using Watson's philosophy in practice

Watson's carative factors guide nurses who use transpersonal caring in practice. Carative factors specify the meaning of the relationship of nurse and patient as human beings. Nurses are encouraged to share their genuine selves with patients. Patients' spiritual strength is recognized, supported, and encouraged for its contribution to health. In the process of transpersonal relationships, nurses develop and encourage openness to understanding of self and others. This leads to the development of trusting, accepting relationships in which feelings are shared freely and confidence is inspired. Even a core element of practice such as patient teaching can be carried out in an interpersonal manner true to the philosophy and nature of the caring relationship.

Box **13-4** Watson's 10 Carative Factors

1. The formation of a humanistic-altruistic system of values
2. The instillation of faith-hope
3. The cultivation of sensitivity to one's self and others
4. The development of a helping-trust relationship
5. The promotion and acceptance of the expression of positive and negative feelings
6. The systematic use of the scientific problem-solving method for decision making
7. The promotion of interpersonal teaching-learning
8. The provision for a supportive, protective, and/or corrective mental, physical, sociocultural, and spiritual environment
9. Assistance with the gratification of human needs
10. The allowance for existential-phenomenological forces

Reprinted with permission of Tomey AM, Alligood MR: *Nursing theorists and their work*, ed 5, St Louis, 2002, Mosby.

The nurse guided by Watson's work has responsibility for creating and maintaining an environment supporting human caring while recognizing and providing for patients' primary human requirements. In the end, this human-to-human caring approach leads the nurse to respect the overall meaning of life from the perspective of the patient. Watson's 1988 work formalized the theory of human caring from this philosophy. Key aspects of nursing's metaparadigm evident in Watson's work are environment (one that supports human caring), person (both the patient and the nurse), health (in terms of health promotion and illness prevention), and nursing (what nurses contribute to the encounter with the patient).

Clinical example: Watson's philosophy of caring

Understanding how philosophy guides practice can be hard, but an example from clinical practice may help. Mary, a hospice nurse, had a patient who was very ill with lung cancer, and who had received both chemotherapy and radiation with the hope of achieving a long remission. The patient, a 60-year-old woman named Mavis, was what some people would refer to as a "character"—full of opinions that she would share with anyone who came close, still smoking, still cursing. Mavis' cancer did not respond and

she developed metastases in her brain. It was clear to everyone that Mavis was terminally ill. Her abrasive personality did not allow many people to get near her, but she had a particular fondness for Mary, who understood Mavis in a way that few did. They connected on a deep level, and although they never talked in great depth about Mavis' illness and impending death, a key conversation between them revealed that one of Mavis' unfulfilled plans was to be baptized. She did not remember her baptism from childhood and did not want to die without having that memory.

Although nothing in the nursing texts says it is a good idea to take a weakened patient who has weeks to live out into the January cold for a full-immersion baptism, it was Mary's human-to-human caring approach that allowed her to respect the meaning of this event from Mavis' point of view. On a bitterly cold night with a howling wind, Mavis was baptized by a friend who was a minister, her family in attendance, her turban covering her bald head. Mavis told Mary that she was free to die now. Within days she took to her bed. On one of her final days, the family called Mary frantically because Mavis had called for her all day. The on-call nurse covering the weekend simply could not console her, and Mavis' cries for her hospice nurse made the family muster the courage to call Mary on her day off. Mary, knowing Mavis as she did, responded, and when she arrived at the bedside, she asked Mavis what she could do to help her. Mavis' response: "I just wanted to see if you would come." Mary said simply, "I am here." Mavis lapsed into a peaceful coma that evening. Her last words had been to Mary.

Mary practiced nursing with the philosophy that human-to-human relationships are primary in professional practice. In the confines of this deeply caring relationship, Mavis found acceptance and peace from her nurse and was guided into a calm death. Although a nurse whose guiding philosophy is based on human relationships must set clear professional boundaries to prevent overextending himself or herself, this philosophical approach to nursing raises the possibility of exquisite experiences between humans that transcend the nurse-patient relationship, just as Mary and Mavis experienced.

NURSING CONCEPTUAL MODELS

Conceptual models (or conceptual frameworks) are the second type of theoretical work that provides organizational structures for critical thinking about the processes of nursing (Alligood, 2002c; Fawcett, 2000). These are broad conceptual structures that provide comprehensive, holistic perspectives of nursing by describing the relationships of specific concepts. Models are less abstract and more formalized than the philosophies just discussed in this chapter; models are more abstract, however, than theories of nursing, which will be discussed later. Theories are built from conceptual models much like buildings are constructed from blueprints. The blueprints show the general relationships between parts of the building and are adaptable; conceptual models provide a preliminary view of the relationship between concepts of nursing that can be used to build theory.

Three conceptual models will be presented in the following section. These models represent different decades in the development of nursing theory: they are models developed by Dorothea Orem, Imogene King, and Sister Callista Roy. The

focus and perspective of each model are discussed, followed by a brief overview of how that model guides nursing practice. Figure 13-3 demonstrates how the same patient situation is viewed differently by three nurses who practice with Orem, King, or Roy as their model.

Orem's Self-Care Model

Dorothea Orem, born in 1914 in Baltimore, Maryland, first received her diploma in nursing in the 1930s, soon followed by a BS in nursing education in 1939. Six years later she earned an MS in nursing education (Sitzman and Eichelberger, 2004, p. 85). Working as a nurse in a number of roles, Orem first published her concept of **self-care** in 1959. She continued to develop her conceptual model over several decades, with the sixth edition of her work *Nursing: Concepts of Practice* published in 2001. Over the years Orem formalized three interrelated theories: theory of self-care, theory of self-care deficit, and theory of nursing system. Her model focuses on the patient's self-care capacities and the process of designing nursing actions to meet the patient's self-care needs. In this model, the nurse prescribes and regulates the nursing system based on the patient's self-care deficit, which is the extent

What deficits does this patient have in providing his own self-care? (Dorothea Orem)

How can I modify this patient's environment to facilitate his adaptation? (Callista Roy)

What goals can we set together to restore him to health? (Imogene King)

Figure 13-3
Three nurses: three models. (*Dennis G. Perry.*)

to which a patient is incapable of providing effective self-care. An underlying assumption of Orem's model is that "ordinary people in contemporary society want to be in control of their lives" (Pearson, Vaughan, and FitzGerald, 2005, p. 104). Nursing is needed in the presence of an actual or potential self-care deficit (Orem, 2001) when persons cannot provide their own care adequately. Orem's work is widely used in nursing education and practice, providing a comprehensive system for nursing practice in a variety of clinical settings.

Orem and nursing practice

In Orem's model, appropriate care for the patient is developed through a series of three operations: diagnostic, prescriptive, and regulatory. To determine the patient's ability to provide effective self-care, the nurse initiates a diagnostic operation that begins with the establishment of the nurse-patient relationship. This includes contracting with the patient to explore current and potential self-care demands. Factors such as age, gender, and developmental status as well as sociocultural and environmental factors are examined in relation to universal, developmental, and health requirements and related self-care actions of the patient. In other words, the patient's baseline ability to provide adequate self-care is assessed by the nurse to determine the extent to which the patient is limited in providing his or her own effective care. These limitations are self-care deficits.

Prescriptive operations occur when therapeutic self-care requisites (based on deficits) are determined and the nurse reviews various methods, actions, and priorities with the patient. This is a planning stage in which the nurse confirms with the patient the nurse's assessment of the patient's needs and begins to formulate a plan of care. In regulatory operations, the nurse designs, plans, and produces a system for care (Berbiglia, 2002). Systems of care range from wholly compensatory, which is the most comprehensive form of care for patients with few (if any) abilities to provide care for self, to supportive-

educative, in which the patient has the ability to provide effective self-care, but needs to work with the nurse to further develop these abilities or acquire additional information to promote self-care (George, 2002).

King's Interacting Systems Framework and Theory of Goal Attainment

Imogene King was born in 1923 and received her basic nursing education from St. John's Hospital School of Nursing in St. Louis, Missouri, in 1945. Three years later she completed her bachelor of science in nursing education from St. Louis University; in 1957 she earned her master of science in nursing degree from St. Louis University. In 1961 she completed her EdD (doctor of education) from Teachers College, Columbia University, in New York City. Much of her career was spent in academic settings including Ohio State University, Loyola University, and the University of South Florida (Johnson and Webber, 2005, p. 158).

Although King first published early forms of her theoretical work in 1971, *A Theory for Nursing: Systems, Concepts, Process,* published 10 years later in 1981, contained her first claim to a nursing theory (King, 1981). This complex theory focused on persons, their interpersonal relationships, and social contexts with three interacting systems: personal, interpersonal, and social. Within each of these three systems King identified concepts that provide a conceptual structure describing the processes in each system. Significantly, the focus of the nurse is on phenomena of importance to the patient; unless attention is paid to concerns of the patient, mutual goal setting is unlikely to happen (Sieloff, Frey, and Killeen, 2006, p. 254).

King's interacting systems form a framework to view whole persons in their family and social contexts: the personal system identifies concepts that provide an understanding of individuals, personally and intrapersonally (within the person); the interpersonal system deals with interactions and transactions between two or more persons; and the social system presents concepts that consider social contacts, such as those at school, at work, or in social settings. King's work is unique because it provides a view of persons from the perspective of their interactions (or communications, both verbal and nonverbal) with other people at three levels of interacting systems.

Using King's model in practice

When using King's work, nurses focus on goal attainment for and by the patient. The traditional steps of the nursing process—assessment, planning, goal setting, intervention, and evaluation—are augmented in several ways. The steps of the process describe the type of action the nurse is taking, and at each step the nurse gathers and uses information to provide care. Like the nursing process, King's model is not linear: steps occur simultaneously as the nurse and patient work to identify goals and the best means to attain those goals.

The focus of nursing care is guided by concepts at each of the system levels. For example, the personal system leads the nurse to pay close attention to the patient's perceptions, the interpersonal system guides the nurse to explore the patient's roles and the stresses in each role, and the social system cues the nurse to consider influences on the patient's decision making. In this model, for instance, the nurse providing care for a young woman who is a mother will recognize that the patient's maternal role will influence her decisions regarding her health, keeping the best interests of her children in addition to her own health in mind as she makes health-related decisions.

Interaction with the patient is an important component of King's goal attainment model. Nurses are aware of their communication with patients, identifying steps from the first encounter to the attainment of the specified goal. King describes these steps as a progression from perception, judgment, action, reaction, and interaction to transaction (King, 1981). These steps involve increasing involvement between the nurse and the patient, requiring a deep understanding of the goals of the patient within the various

contexts of the patient's life in order to plan and provide effective nursing care. King emphasized the importance of joint goal setting by nurse and patient, reminding nurses that this relationship involves mutuality. King's process provided a structure for the nurse to monitor the relationship's progress. King clearly specified the goal of nursing to be health.

Roy's Adaptation Model

Sister Callista Roy was born in Los Angeles, California, in 1939. Her first degree was a bachelor of arts in nursing from Mount St. Mary's College in Los Angeles. She then earned a master's degree in pediatric nursing and sociology, followed by a PhD in sociology from UCLA. She is a member of the order of Sisters of Saint Joseph of Carondelet. Roy is currently on the faculty of the William F. Connell School of Nursing at Boston College. Although the Roy adaptation model has been in use for 35 years, Sister Roy continues to update, revise, and refine it for use in practice, research, theory, and administration (Roy and Zhan, 2006, pp. 268-269).

Sister Callista Roy first presented her model as a conceptual framework for a nursing curriculum in 1970 (Pearson et al, 2005, p. 123). In 1976 she published *Introduction to Nursing: An Adaptation Model,* and followed with a second edition in 1984 (Roy, 1976, 1984). Roy updated all of her writing in a comprehensive text in 1999 (Roy and Andrews, 1999). Her model is widely used for education, research, and nursing practice today. She focused on the individual as a biopsychosocial adaptive system and described nursing as a humanistic discipline that emphasizes the person's adaptive or coping abilities. Roy's work is based on **adaptation** and adaptive behavior, which is produced by altering the environment. According to Roy, the individual and the environment are sources of stimuli that require modification to promote adaptation in the patient. Roy viewed the person as an adaptive system with physiological, self-concept, role function, and interdependent modes.

Roy's model provides a comprehensive understanding of nursing from the perspective of adaptation. When the demands of environmental stimuli are too high or the person's adaptive mechanisms are too low, the person's behavioral responses are ineffective for coping. Effective adaptive responses promote the integrity of the individual by conserving energy and promoting the survival, growth, reproduction, and mastery of the human system. Nursing promotes the patient's adaptation and coping, with progress toward integration as the goal (Phillips, 2002).

Using Roy's model in practice

The nurse using Roy's model focuses on the adaptation of the patient and on the environment. Adaptation, specifically patients' adaptation behavior and stimuli in the internal and external environments, is assessed and facilitated. Based on these assessments, the nurse develops nursing diagnoses to guide goal setting and interventions aimed at promoting adaptation. Simply stated, the nurse modifies the environment to facilitate patient adaptation.

Observable behavior is recognized and understood in the context of Roy's physiological, self-concept, role function, and interdependent modes. Descriptions of the behaviors included in each mode provide the nurse with a means of making evaluative judgments about the patient's progress toward the goal of adaptation (Phillips, 2002). Roy's model is very widely used in nursing practice and comprehensively described in the literature (Alligood, 2002b; Phillips, 2002; Roy and Andrews, 1999).

Clinical example: Roy's adaptation model

A clinical example of Roy's model will help you understand her work in a real-world context. Mr. Elderd was referred to a home health agency for wound management. He had a very large open wound on his forehead as a result of a wide excision of several significant basal cell carcinomas. Robert, his nurse, was surprised to see that the wound extended completely to Mr. Elderd's skull. Mr. Elderd was out of work as a result of this wound, saw friends infrequently, and was somewhat depressed. His wife, although well-meaning, spent hours each day fixing him high-calorie "treats" because she liked to cook and found it was a good way to release her own anxiety about her husband's condition.

Robert's nursing practice was shaped by Roy's adaptation model. In his initial assessment of the home environment, he noticed the cleanliness of the home, the evidence of vigorous family and social ties, adequacy of income, availability of good nutrition, and other indicators of health. What Robert did not understand was why Mr. Elderd's wound was not healing. After Robert's assessment, he believed that there was some "missing link" in Mr. Elderd's adaptive abilities, but he was not sure if the ineffective coping was psychological, environmental, or physiological.

Robert visited Mr. Elderd daily for 3 weeks, and although the wound did not become infected, it showed very little evidence of closure. Robert expressed his concern to Mr. Elderd, and Robert decided to ask Mr. Elderd again some basic questions related to his fundamental health practices, including nutrition, activity, sleep, and elimination. Mr. Elderd commented almost off-handedly that he was sleeping fine except that he had to get up to go to the bathroom several times each night. His wife chimed in from the kitchen, "But that's no different than from the day. He is always going to the bathroom. I told him to quit drinking so much water all the time!" Robert, being the experienced nurse that he is and seeking ways to assist patients with all forms of adaptation, realized the likely problem. He called Mr. Elderd's physician and received an order for a blood chemistry including glucose to be drawn. Sure enough, Mr. Elderd had undiagnosed diabetes. Mrs. Elderd's stream of goodies from the kitchen aggravated the problem to the point that Mr. Elderd was experiencing polyuria and polydipsia, both signs of diabetes. With aggressive blood glucose level management with insulin, a change in diet, and increasing exercise, Mr. Elderd's wound began to heal almost immediately. He did not require a skin graft as had been feared. The use of Roy's adaptation model allowed Robert to see Mr. Elderd's situation as a function of a variety of maladaptive coping efforts. Correcting the diabetic problem became the foundation for

Mr. Elderd's eventual healing and resumption of his usual life activities.

THEORIES OF NURSING

Nursing theories are the third type of theoretical work in the structure of nursing knowledge to be reviewed in this chapter. Fawcett (2000) classified theories according to their breadth and depth. For example, a **grand theory** is a very broad conceptualization of nursing phenomena, while a **middle-range theory** is narrower in focus and makes connections between grand theories and nursing practice (Parker, 2006, p. 7). Theories are less abstract than models and usually propose specific outcomes. Three theories are presented here that are well-known and commonly used to shape nursing practice. Figure 13-4 shows how three nurses using the theories of Hildegard Peplau, Ida Orlando, and Madeleine Leininger may approach the same patient with a different focus of care.

Peplau's Theory of Interpersonal Relations in Nursing

Hildegard Peplau, born in 1909, was one of the earliest nurse theorists who recognized the importance of the work of nursing rather than continuing to define and delineate nursing (Pearson et al, 2005, p. 179). After receiving her basic nursing training at the Pottstown, Pennsylvania Hospital School of Nursing in 1931, Peplau studied interpersonal psychology at Bennington College in Vermont, receiving a bachelor of arts degree. Later she received a master of arts degree in teaching and supervision of psychiatric nursing, followed by an education doctorate (EdD) from Teachers College, Columbia University, in New York City. Although Peplau's first book, *Interpersonal Relations in Nursing,* dates back to 1952, it was published again in 1988, reflecting both the value of her work and nursing's continuing focus on interpersonal relationships. Peplau drew from developmental, interactionist, and human needs theories in developing her work (Pearson et al, 2005, p. 179), which grew from her interest in nursing care of psychiatric patients. Peplau believed, however, that all nursing is based on the interpersonal process and the nurse-patient relationship (Forchuk, 1993).

Peplau's theory is based on the premise that the relationship between patient and nurse is the focus of attention, rather than the patient only as the unit of attention (Forchuk, 1993, p. 7). Nursing care occurs within the context of the patient-nurse relationship. The goals of therapeutic interpersonal relationship are twofold: first is the survival of the patient; second is the patient's understanding of his or her health problems and learning from these problems as he or she develops new behavior patterns. As the nurse assists the patient in developing new behavior patterns, the nurse also grows and develops a greater understanding of the effect of universal stressors on the lives and behaviors of individual patients (Pearson et al, 2005, p. 182).

Using Peplau's theory in practice

Although Peplau's theory grew from her experience as a psychiatric nurse, her work is applicable to a wide variety of practice settings. Peplau describes a four-pronged process similar to the nursing process by which the nurse assists the patient in

| How can I best figure out what my patient needs through my interaction with him? (Ida Orlando) | What are the best ways to provide care to my patient that are culturally congruent? (Madeleine Leininger) | Within the relationship with my patient, how can I best help him understand his health problem and develop new behaviors? (Hildegard Peplau) |

Figure 13-4
Three nurses: three theories. (*Dennis G. Perry.*)

achieving personal growth. Completion of this process involves six roles by the nurse: counselor, resource, teacher, technical expert, surrogate, and leader (Pearson et al, 2005, p. 184). Depending on the setting, the nurse will spend more or less time in each of these roles. For instance, a nurse in a critical care unit will likely spend more time as a technical expert and less time as a counselor, whereas a nurse on a postpartum unit may act as a surrogate, guiding a new mother into independent care of her newborn infant, with less time spent as a leader.

Peplau's theory is multifaceted and complex. Its importance lies in the focus on what happens between the nurse and patient in a therapeutic relationship and not simply on the patient. Furthermore, Peplau was visionary in her recognition of the importance of the relationship between nurse and patient, publishing early her ideas and continuing to refine and expand her work over several decades. In Chapter 11 (p. 279), you will find a description of an ongoing study at the University of North Carolina at Chapel Hill, named the "Hilda Project." It is named after Hildegard Peplau, whose theory provides the therapeutic framework for the intervention being tested.

Orlando's Nursing Process Theory

Ida Orlando was born in New York in 1926, and like many early nurse theorists, received her basic nursing education in a diploma program. She attended nursing school at the New York Medical College School of Nursing, and in 1951 she graduated with a bachelor of science degree in public health nursing from St. John's University in Brooklyn, New York. Three years later, she completed her master's degree in nursing from Columbia University. Her early practice settings included maternity, medicine, and emergency department nursing (Gess, Dombro, Gordon et al, 2006).

Orlando first proposed her theory of effective nursing practice in 1961, publishing her first book, *The Dynamic Nurse-Patient Relationship: Function, Process and Principles*. She later revised it as a nursing process theory (Orlando, 1990).

Her work actually proposed both: it is a theory about how nurses process their observations of patient behavior and also about how they react to patients based on inferences from patients' behavior, including what they say. Orlando's early research revealed that processing observations as specified in her theory led to effective nursing practice and good outcomes.

Orlando's theory is specific to nurse-patient interactions. The goal of the nurse is to determine and meet patients' immediate needs and to improve their situation by relieving distress or discomfort. Orlando emphasized deliberate action (rather than automatic action) based on observation of the patients' verbal and nonverbal behavior, which leads to inferences. Inferences are confirmed or disconfirmed by the patient, leading the nurse to identify the patient's needs and provide effective nursing care.

Using Orlando's theory in practice

As a nursing practice theory, Orlando's theory specified how patients are involved in nurses' decision making. When used in practice, Orlando's theory guides interactions to predictable outcomes, which are different from outcomes that occur when the theory is not used. Nurses individualize care for each patient by attending to behavior, confirming with the patient ideas and inferences the nurse draws from interactions, and identifying pressing needs.

Use of Orlando's theory improves the effectiveness of the nurse by allowing the nurse to get to the "bottom line" more quickly when observing, listening to, and confirming with patients. Therefore use of this theory saves time and energy for both the patient and the nurse. An excellent example of the use of Orlando's theory in nursing practice may be found in Schmeiding (2002).

Leininger's Theory of Culture Care Diversity and Universality

Born in 1924 in Sutton, Nebraska, Madeleine Leininger received her diploma in nursing at St. Anthony's School of Nursing in Denver, Colorado, followed by a bachelor of science degree in biological science from Benedictine

College in Atchison, Kansas, 2 years later. She received her MSN from Catholic University in Washington, DC, in 1954 and her PhD in anthropology from the University of Washington in Seattle in 1965 (Reynolds and Leininger, 1993).

The work of Madeleine Leininger (1978, 1991) in **cultural care** grew out of her early nursing experiences. She observed that children of different cultures had widely varying behaviors and needs. After discussing the parallels between nursing and anthropology with the famed anthropologist Margaret Mead, Leininger pursued doctoral study in cultural anthropology. Through her doctoral work she became more convinced about the relationship of cultural differences and health practices. This led her to begin developing a theory of cultural care for nursing. Leininger's work is formalized as a theory rather than as a conceptual model. It has stimulated the formation of the Transcultural Nursing Society, transcultural nursing conferences, newsletters, and the *Journal of Transpersonal Caring* and the awarding of master's degrees in the specialty area known as transcultural nursing.

Transcultural nursing's goal involves more than simply being aware of different cultures. It involves planning nursing care based on knowledge that is culturally defined, classified, and tested—and then used to provide care that is culturally congruent (Leininger, 1978). Leininger described theory as a creative and systematic way of discovering new knowledge or accounting for phenomena in a more complete way (Leininger, 1991). She encouraged nurses to use creativity to discover cultural aspects of human needs and use these findings to make culturally congruent therapeutic decisions. Her theory is broad, since it considers the impact of culture on all aspects of human life, with particular attention to health and caring practices. Leininger's theory has become increasingly relevant as global migration continues and societies become more diverse.

Using Leininger's theory in practice

Leininger specified caring as the essence of nursing, and nurses who use Leininger's theory of cultural care in their practices view patients in the context of their cultures. Practice from a cultural perspective begins by respecting the culture of the patient and recognizing the importance of its relationship to nursing care. Use of the "sunrise model" (Figure 13-5) guides the assessment of cultural data for an understanding of its influence on the patient's life (Leininger, 1991). The nurse plans nursing care, recognizing the health beliefs and folk practices of the patient's culture as well as the culture of traditional health services. To this end, nursing care is then focused on culture care preservation, accommodations, or repatterning, depending on the patient's need. The nursing outcome of **culturally congruent nursing care** is health and well-being for the patient. Case applications of Leininger's theory in nursing practice may be found in Morgan (2002).

Clinical example: Leininger's theory of culture care diversity and universality

No matter how expert a nurse is in clinical practice, sometimes failure to recognize and appreciate cultural differences can undermine even the best intentions. One such situation occurred when Jan, a nurse with many years of experience providing care for HIV-positive patients in a large urban hospital, decided that she would move to a less chaotic environment. Jan applied for a job with an agency providing nursing care in the homes of low-income rural women with HIV. Jan had grown up and gone to college in a city in the northeast; her new home was in a rural county in the Deep South.

Almost immediately Jan was discontent. She complained at team meetings that her patients were always late for their appointments. Members of the team, each of whom had grown up nearby, explained to her that this was not unusual behavior and that she should plan "waiting time" into her daily schedule. Jan marveled that the rest of the team reported good visits and outcomes with their patients, and almost all seemed to be caught up with their work all the time. Jan always felt like she was running behind. She began to

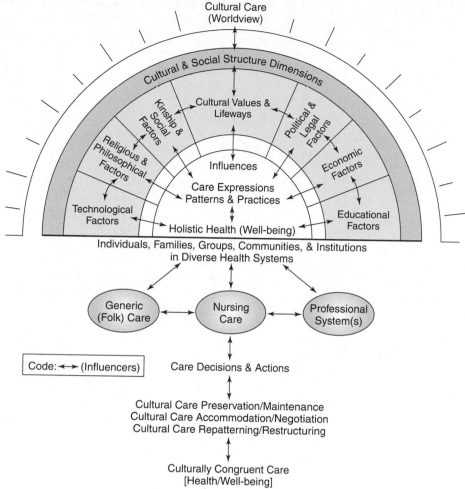

Figure 13-5
Leininger's sunrise model, created to facilitate the application in practice of the Theory of Culture Care Diversity and Universality. *(Courtesy Dr. Madeleine Leininger.)*

question her nursing skills, her knowledge base, and time management behaviors that had served her well in her previous work. Jan described herself as a "fish out of water." She decided that she would spend her "waiting time" by sitting in her car and catching up on paperwork until the patient arrived home.

One day she was invited by the patient's grandmother to wait inside but she declined, saying that she would wait in the car and "get some work done." Her patient arrived home after

20 minutes or so and Jan met with her, reporting to the team later that day that she had a great visit with the patient. Jan's pleasure was short-lived. Her patient called, demanding that she be assigned another nurse because "Jan insulted my grandma." In this community where being invited into the home was considered an honor, Jan's choice to wait instead in the car was interpreted as rude and uncaring. No amount of discussion dissuaded the patient from her insistence that she have a new nurse who "knew how to act." Jan's

team met with her, but they too, as products of the culture, did not understand at first that Jan did not mean to be insulting or rude. Because the other members of the team were deeply accul-turated, they knew the meaning behind the grandmother's invitation: Jan was an honored, trusted guest who was welcomed in their home.

Jan soon realized that her feelings of being a "fish out of water" in this setting were accurate; in fact she did not understand the culture and was not motivated to learn about the cultural norms that so disturbed her. Importantly, she recognized that this prevented her from pro-viding the effective care that she desired. She left the position and moved to a more urban area in which she knew the cultural terrain. While this was a sad chapter in Jan's professional life, she grew from the experience in her understanding of the very deep nature of culture and its influence on the nurse-patient relationship.

THEORETICAL CHALLENGES FOR NURSING EDUCATION, PRACTICE, AND RESEARCH

These examples of nursing theoretical works illustrate the vital position of theory in nursing education, practice, and research. To continue the forward movement of nursing and to improve the quality of nursing care, nurses must engage in theory-based practice, theory-testing research, and theory-generating research. Planning educa-tional curricula based on nursing knowledge and theory is essential to further solidifying the foundations of nursing science.

Theory-Based Education

The curricula of schools of nursing are usually built on one or more specific conceptual models or concepts (McEwen and Brown, 2002). The nursing profession has developed and matured since the early 1950s when Peplau first published her early work that established the modern era of nursing theory development. Schools of nursing have proliferated, preparing nurses from the associate degree level to the doctoral level. Nurses prepared at each level of nursing can be involved with nursing theory, as noted in Box 13-5.

The nursing profession has evolved from an applied vocation dependent on knowledge from other disciplines to its current stage of develop-ment, with its own knowledge base. This period of growth has stimulated—and been stimulated by—the development of the nursing PhD, a research degree that requires the generation of new, discipline-specific knowledge.

At the doctoral level, nurses are concerned with the philosophy of science—that is, the nature of knowledge and how it is known; the philosophy of nursing science and the generation of nursing knowledge; theory testing; and the development of new theory through research. The master's level nurse may be a primary provider in advanced practice, going beyond the generic nursing pro-cess. Master's-prepared nurses use theoretical perspectives focused on the patient for specific nursing outcomes. Many nurses conduct their first research studies as master's students, focusing on nursing practice and the testing of nursing interventions with specific patient groups.

Box **13-5** Levels of Nursing Education and Use of Nursing Theory

PhD in nursing: Conducts theory testing and theory development research for nursing science development; frames practice, administration, or research in nursing works

Master of science in nursing: Frames advanced practice with a nursing model or theory; uses theory to guide research with practice questions

Bachelor of science in nursing: Learns the nursing perspective in a nursing model or theory-based curriculum or courses; uses models, theories, and middle-range theories to guide nursing practice

Associate degree in nursing: May have a nursing model or theory-guided curriculum or courses; may be introduced to middle-range theories for nursing practice

The baccalaureate nurse is introduced to the research process and the use of theory to guide it. The research emphasis for baccalaureate-level students is on learning to critique nursing research, becoming informed consumers of research relevant to evidence-based nursing practice. (See Critical Thinking Challenge 13-1.) Baccalaureate nurses are also introduced to theory through the curriculum (course of study) at their school. Many curricula of bachelor's of science in nursing programs are based on a particular nursing theoretical perspective; others introduce students to a variety of nursing theoretical perspectives. Whether the curriculum is built around one or many nursing theoretical works, the focus for the baccalaureate level is utilization and application of nursing theory as a guide for nursing practice. Associate degree nursing education programs may also use nursing theoretical works to teach the unique perspectives of nursing. Nurses with associate degrees often find middle-range theories, which are specific to patient care, useful in their practice.

Basing nursing education on nursing theory not only benefits nursing students but also con-

tributes to the growth of schools and colleges of nursing. Scholarly discussions about the application of nursing theory in education, research, and practice establish an environment of critical thinking, imagining, questioning, and learning. This does not end with graduation. Practicing nurses are also interested in learning more about nursing theory, as evidenced by the fact that nurse theorists and other distinguished lecturers draw audiences from campuses and surrounding nursing communities, all interested in hearing nursing theorists discuss their work in person.

Theory-Based Practice

How is theory translated into practice? The answer to that question lies with theory-based practice. Theory-based practice occurs when nurses intentionally structure their practice around a particular nursing theory and use it to guide them as they assess, plan, diagnose, intervene, and evaluate nursing care. Theory provides a systematic way of thinking about nursing that is consistent and guides the decision-making process as data are collected, analyzed, and used in the planning and administration of nursing practice. Theory empowers nurses to challenge the conventional views of patients, illness, the health care delivery system, and traditional nursing interventions.

As this chapter on nursing theory comes to a conclusion, we hope that these introductions to some classic nursing theoretical works will lead you to identify works that resonate with your values and that you will select one or two for in-depth study. There are many other nurse theorists

CRITICAL THINKING *Challenge 13-1*

Scan several nursing research studies that are based on nursing theory. Select one article to read carefully; note the theoretical framework it is based upon. Describe how the authors link the study to nursing theory. Does the use of a theoretical framework strengthen the study? How or how not?

✦ *Cultural Considerations Challenge*

Is Nursing Theory Transcultural?

At home and abroad, nurses often work with patients from other cultures. When selecting or creating a nursing theory to guide your practice, envision how useful it might be in the following settings: in a short-term mission team clinic in a remote African village; with

fragile elderly patients displaced by a hurricane and living in a motel; on a Native American reservation working with young adults with substance abuse problems. How can the theories you studied in this chapter be adapted successfully to these settings?

whose works are more recent and complex. In addition, there are substantial numbers of nurse theorists who have developed middle-range theories that may be useful to you in specific areas of your practice as you develop your competence as a practitioner. With increased understanding and education, you can integrate the use of nursing theory in your practice.

Many benefits are gained from theory-based practice. First, you will be able to explain your practice to other members of the health care team. That is, nursing theory provides language for you to explain what you do, how you do it, and why you do it. Second, this language of practice facilitates the transmission of nursing knowledge to you as students who are new to the profession, as well as to other health professionals. Third, theory contributes to professional autonomy by providing a nursing-based guide for practice, education, and research. Finally, nursing theory develops your analytical skills, challenges your thinking, and clarifies your values and assumptions (Holder and Chitty, 1997).

Many nurses have developed their own ideas about nursing and continue to develop nursing assumptions based on education, experience, observation, and reading. Most nurses do not formally develop their own personal theories, even though their ideas certainly influence the way they practice nursing. Wardle and Mandle (1989) studied nurses who believed that their own ideas of practice were "their theories," and they concluded that these nurses' personal theories tended to be incomplete and inconsistent as a basis for nursing practice. When you rely on your personal ideas as a basis for practice or when faculty members use their own ideas as a "framework for curricula," the outcome is ineffective. Wardle and Mandle recommended using a theory that has been tested or developed through nursing research and critiqued, analyzed, and evaluated for usefulness in nursing practice. Each of the philosophies, models, and theories presented in this chapter meets their recommendation. Application of these works in your practice with specific patient groups is an opportunity to test middle-range theories. In addition, many practice areas and patient populations may be addressed in formalized middle-range theories (Alligood, 2002d).

As you engage in theory-based practice, remember to provide feedback to nurse researchers and theorists concerning your experiences. You can do this through the Internet, where you will find groups of nurses using, discussing, and refining the theoretical works that have been discussed in this chapter. You can also assist these scholars and the discipline of nursing by developing manuscripts and submitting your experiences for publication, joining the many nurses who have discovered the benefits of theory-based practice.

Theory-Based Research

Great strides have been made in the last 25 years in nursing research. The expansion of graduate nursing education at the master's level and the proliferation of nursing doctoral programs played a major role, as more nurses than ever before were equipped with the knowledge and skills to conduct research. Nursing research tests and refines the knowledge base of nursing. Ultimately, research findings enable nurses to improve the quality of care and understand how evidence-based nursing actions influence patient outcomes.

Research is vital to the future of nursing, and theory is integral to research. Historically, an emphasis on method has overshadowed the subject of our research and the theory for developing nursing knowledge. In addition, many nurses have continued to use theories that address the phenomena of other disciplines—theories that do not view persons holistically or provide a nursing perspective. Therefore the outcome of their research is often valued by adjunct disciplines as much as by the discipline of nursing. However, more and more nurse researchers have come to understand the vital role of nursing theory in their research for knowledge development in their own discipline. These nurses are meeting the challenge of using nursing theory to structure nursing research that tests theory or that interprets the findings of qualitative research for theory development.

SUMMARY OF *Key Points*

- Theory development is not a mysterious activity restricted to a few nursing scholars. It is an activity that combines education, knowledge, and skill in a sustained effort.
- Nursing philosophies, models, and theories offer many perspectives on nursing, varying in their levels of abstraction and their definitions of four major concepts known as nursing's metaparadigm: person, environment, health, and nursing.
- As nurses devise theories of nursing, present them for review by their colleagues in a peer-review process, publish them in the nursing literature, and test their efficacy in nursing practice, the discipline moves forward in the development of its unique knowledge base.
- Scholarly contributions may be made by nurses at every level of educational preparation. To the extent that nurses question, read, study, network, and write about nursing practice, they contribute to the development of nursing knowledge.

- Nurses in practice settings have invaluable insights and observations, thereby contributing to the knowledge base for nursing. Nursing theorists' early work often grew out of their clinical observations and experiences. Theorists rely on practicing nurses to test clinical interventions and explore the usefulness of their theories.
- Nurse theorists whose works were reviewed in this chapter, as well as others too numerous to include, have made significant contributions to the development of the unique body of nursing knowledge.
- Nurse scholars continue to develop and refine the works of nursing theorists. Each theoretical work has a community of scholars who use the work in their research and practice and continue to expand, clarify, and refine these original works.

Critical Thinking Questions

1. Recognizing that your understanding of the theoretical works of nursing is only beginning, which works introduced in this chapter appeal to you the most? Which ones describe nursing in the way you think about it? What is it about these works that intrigues you?
2. Which of the theoretical works seem the most useful to help you organize your thoughts for critical thinking and decision making in nursing practice?
3. Interview two practicing nurses and ask them which nursing philosophies, models, or theories have influenced their thinking and practice of nursing.
4. Describe the use of nursing theory for nurses at your current level of nursing education.
5. Explain why theory development is important to the profession of nursing.

REFERENCES

Alligood MR: The nature of knowledge needed for nursing practice. In Alligood MR, Tomey AM, editors: *Nursing theory: utilization and application,* ed 2, St Louis, 2002a, Mosby, pp 3-14.

Alligood MR: Nursing models: normal science for nursing practice. In Alligood MR, Tomey AM, editors: *Nursing theory: utilization and application,* ed 2, St Louis, 2002b, Mosby, pp 15-39.

Alligood MR: Philosophies, models and theories: critical thinking structures. In Alligood MR, Tomey AM, editors: *Nursing theory: utilization and application,* ed 2, St Louis, 2002c, Mosby, pp 41-61.

Alligood MR: Areas for further development of theory-based nursing practice. In Alligood MR, Tomey AM, editors: *Nursing theory: utilization and application,* ed 2, St Louis, 2002d, Mosby, pp 453-463.

Alligood MR, Tomey AM: *Nursing theory: utilization and application,* ed 2, St Louis, 2002, Mosby.

Berbiglia V: Orem's self-care deficit theory in nursing practice. In Alligood MR, Tomey AM, editors:

Nursing theory: utilization and application, ed 2, St Louis, 2002, Mosby, pp 239-266.

Chinn P, Kramer M: *Theory and nursing: a systematic approach,* ed 5, St Louis, 1998, Mosby.

Fawcett J: *Analysis and evaluation of contemporary nursing knowledge: models and theories,* Philadelphia, 2000, FA Davis.

Forchuk C: *Hildegard E. Peplau: interpersonal nursing theory,* Newbury Park, Calif, 1993, Sage Publications.

George JB, editor: *Nursing theories: the base for professional nursing practice,* ed 5, Norwalk, Conn, 2002, Appleton & Lange.

Gess T, Dombro M, Gordon SC et al: Part one: twentieth-century nursing. Wiedenbach, Henderson, and Orlando's theories and their applications. In Parker ME, editor: *Nursing theories and nursing practice,* ed 2, Philadelphia, 2006, FA Davis.

Henderson V: *The nature of nursing: a definition and its implications for practice, research, and education,* New York, 1966, Macmillan.

Holder PJ, Chitty KK: Theory as a basis for professional nursing. In Chitty KK, editor: *Professional nursing: concepts and challenges,* ed 2, Philadelphia, 1997, Saunders.

Johnson BM, Webber PB: *An introduction to theory and reasoning in nursing,* ed 2, Philadelphia, 2005, Lippincott Williams & Wilkins.

King IM: *A theory for nursing: systems, concepts, process,* New York, 1981, John Wiley & Sons.

Leininger M: *Transcultural nursing: concepts, theories, and practices,* New York, 1978, John Wiley & Sons.

Leininger M: *Culture care diversity and universality: a theory of nursing,* New York, 1991, National League for Nursing.

McEwen M, Brown SC: Conceptual frameworks in undergraduate nursing curricula: report of a national survey, *J Nurs Educ* 41(1):5-14, 2002.

Morgan MG: Leininger's theory of culture care diversity and universality in nursing practice. In Alligood MR, Tomey AM, editors: *Nursing theory: utilization and application,* ed 2, St Louis, 2002, Mosby, pp 385-402.

Nightingale F: *Notes on nursing: what it is and what it is not,* New York, 1969, Dover Publications (originally published in 1859).

Orem D: *Nursing: concepts of practice,* ed 6, St Louis, 2001, Mosby.

Orlando I: *The dynamic nurse-patient relationship: function, process and principles,* New York, 1990, National League for Nursing (originally published in 1961).

Parker M: *Nursing theories and nursing practice,* Philadelphia, 2006, FA Davis.

Pearson A, Vaughan B, FitzGerald, M: *Nursing models for practice,* Edinburgh, UK, 2005, Butterworth Heinemann.

Peplau HE: *Interpersonal relations in nursing,* New York, 1952/1988, GR Putnam.

Phillips KD: Roy's adaptation model in nursing practice. In Alligood MR, Tomey AM, editors: *Nursing theory: utilization and application,* ed 2, St Louis, 2002, Mosby, pp 289-314.

Powers BA, Knapp TR: *A dictionary of nursing theory and research,* ed 2, Thousand Oaks, Calif, 1995, Sage.

Reynolds CL, Leininger M: *Madeleine Leininger cultural care diversity and universality theory,* Newbury Park, Calif, 1993, Sage Publications.

Roy C Sr: *Introduction to nursing: an adaptation model,* Old Tappan, NJ, 1976, Prentice Hall.

Roy C Sr: *Introduction to nursing: an adaptation model,* ed 2, Englewood Cliffs, NJ, 1984, Prentice Hall.

Roy C Sr, Andrews HA: *The Roy adaptation model,* ed 2, Norwalk, Conn, 1999, Appleton & Lange.

Roy C Sr, Zhan L: Sister Callista Roy's adaptation model and its applications. In Parker ME, editor: *Nursing theories and nursing practice,* ed 2, Philadelphia, 2006, FA Davis.

Schmeiding NJ: Orlando's nursing process theory in nursing practice. In Alligood MR, Tomey AM, editors: *Nursing theory: utilization and application,* ed 2, St Louis, 2002, Mosby, pp 325-337.

Sieloff CL, Frey M, Killeen M: Part two: applications of King's theory of goal attainment. In Parker ME, editor: *Nursing theories and nursing practice,* ed 2, Philadelphia, 2006, FA Davis, pp 244-267.

Sitzman K, Eichelberger LW: *Understanding the work of nurse theorists: a creative beginning,* Sudbury, Mass, 2004, Jones & Bartlett.

Tomey AM, Alligood MR: *Nursing theorists and their work,* ed 5, St Louis, 2002, Mosby.

Wardle MG, Mandle CL: Conceptual models used in clinical practice, *West J Nurs Res* 11(1):108-114, 1989.

Watson J: *Nursing: the philosophy and science of caring,* Boston, 1979, Little, Brown.

Watson J: *Nursing: human science and human care,* New York, 1988, National League for Nursing.

Watson J: *Postmodern nursing and beyond,* Edinburgh, 1999, Churchill Livingstone/WB Saunders/Harcourt Health Sciences.

14

Nursing and Health Care Delivery: System, Roles, and Finance

*Brandi M. Hamlin**

After studying this chapter, students will be able to:

- Describe the four basic types of services provided by the health care delivery system.
- Describe the shared governance model and explain its use in nursing.
- Identify the key members of the interdisciplinary health care team and explain what each contributes.
- Discuss a variety of roles for the nurse in the health care delivery system.
- Differentiate among four nursing care delivery systems.
- Discuss the purpose of differentiated levels of nursing practice.
- Describe how managed care has changed the health care delivery system.

- Relate two major mechanisms used to maintain quality in health care agencies.
- Explain the economic principle of supply and demand and discuss its relevance to health care costs.
- Cite examples of causes of health care cost escalation.
- Explain cost-containment efforts and their impact on nursing practice.
- Describe the impact of managed care on cost containment and health care consumers.
- Describe the relationship between cost containment and quality management initiatives.
- Describe current methods of payment for health care.

THE HEALTH CARE DELIVERY SYSTEM

The term *health care delivery system* as it is used in the United States is a misnomer. Far from providing health care, our system has traditionally provided care for illness. Its complexity,

with multiple types of financing and many different settings where patients can receive services, has resulted in a fragmented system that is difficult to understand and navigate. Although this country has the best technology, the most sophisticated procedures, and the best educated health care providers in the world, many people do not have access to even the most basic care, and even fewer to disease prevention education.

---

*The author wishes to acknowledge the contributions of Jennifer E. Jenkins and Frances A. Maurer in the preparation of this chapter.

The U.S. government has not devised a definitive national health policy. An important first step, however, has been taken. *Healthy People 2010* is "a comprehensive set of disease prevention and health promotion objectives for the nation to achieve over the first decade of the new century" (*Healthy People 2010,* 2005a). The two broad goals of *Healthy People 2010* are to (1) increase quality and years of healthy life and (2) eliminate health disparities. *Healthy People 2010* identified 10 leading health indicators that reflect the major health concerns of the United States at the beginning of the twenty-first century. They are physical activity, overweight and obesity, tobacco use, substance abuse, responsible sexual behavior, mental health, injury and violence, environmental quality, immunization, and access to care (*Healthy People 2010,* 2005b). These indicators will be used to measure the health of the nation over the next several years. You can find more information on the specific focus areas of *Healthy People 2010* online at www.healthy-people.gov.

A health care system that aims to answer the following questions will ensure movement toward meeting the *Healthy People* objectives:

1. What services does the patient need and want?
2. Who can best provide these services (e.g., patient, health care worker, family, others)?
3. Where is the most effective and efficient place to provide these services (e.g., home, community, hospital)?
4. How will these services affect the quality and cost of care, as well as patient and health care worker satisfaction?

Although the nation does not yet have national health care, during the last two decades, the U.S. health care system has undergone major financial and quality reforms. This chapter describes the present health care delivery system, examines nursing's role within this system, and discusses health care finance.

Major Categories of Health Care Services

Regardless of the setting in which services are provided—clinics, hospitals, homes, primary care providers' offices—there are basically four major categories of health services: health promotion and maintenance, illness prevention, diagnosis and treatment, and rehabilitation and long-term care. Each of these categories is briefly explained below.

Health promotion and maintenance

Health promotion and maintenance services assist patients to remain healthy, prevent diseases and injuries, detect diseases early, and promote healthier lifestyles. These services require patients' active participation and cannot be performed solely by a health care provider. Health promotion and maintenance services are based on the assumption that patients who participate in lifestyle changes are likely to avoid lifestyle-related diseases, such as heart attacks, lung cancers, and certain infections.

An example of health promotion and maintenance services is prenatal classes. By learning good nutritional habits, an expectant mother can take care of herself and her baby during pregnancy and after delivery. This increases the chances of a normal pregnancy and the birth of a healthy baby. Other examples include education about aerobic exercise and safe sexual activity.

Health promotion also includes the detection of warning signs indicating the presence of a disease in early stages. Early detection often allows the treatment to be minimal and less costly and results in a good outcome. An example of early detection is breast self-examinations aimed at detecting breast cancer in its early stages and providing a better chance for treatment to be successful.

Illness prevention

With the increasing ability to identify risk factors, such as a family history of heart disease, **illness prevention** services assist patients in reducing the impact of those risk factors on their health and well-being. These services require the patient's active participation.

Prevention services differ from health promotion services in that they address health problems after risk factors are identified, whereas health promotion services seek to prevent development of risk factors. For example, a health promotion program might teach the detrimental effects of alcohol and drugs on a person's health to prevent the person from using alcohol and drugs. Illness prevention services are used when the patient has been using alcohol or drugs and is at risk for developing health problems as a result. The boundary between health promotion and maintenance, early detection, and illness prevention is often blurred. Box 14-1 gives examples of activities in these three areas.

Diagnosis and treatment

Traditionally, in the U.S. health care system, heavy emphasis has been put on diagnosis and treatment. Modern technology has enabled the medical profession to refine methods of diagnosing illnesses and disorders and to treat them more effectively than in the past. Scientific advances permit many noninvasive tests and treatments to be performed. Widely available technologies that were unheard of only a few years ago include the use of ultrafast CT scans to detect calcification in coronary arteries and live three-dimensional (3-D) ultrasonography that creates 3-D images of structures such as the fetal face, hand, or spine. The future promises more high-tech noninvasive technologies.

Laparoscopic instruments and "bloodless" surgery techniques have transformed surgical procedures, allowing incisions of 1 inch or less. This technology has reduced postoperative pain, reduced hospital stays from days to hours, and enabled individuals to return to normal function much more rapidly.

Unfortunately, high-tech services can lead patients to feel dehumanized. This occurs when

---

| Box **14-1** | Examples of Health Promotion and Maintenance, Early Detection, and Illness Prevention Activities |

Health Promotion/Maintenance

- Health education programs (e.g., prenatal classes)
- Exercise programs
- Health fairs
- Wellness programs (worksite/school)
- Nutrition education

Early Detection

- Mammograms
- Vision and hearing screening
- Cholesterol screening
- Periodic histories and physical examinations
- Blood glucose screening
- Osteoporosis screening

Illness Prevention

- Community health programs
- Promotion of healthy lifestyles to counteract risk factors
- Occupational safety programs (e.g., use of eye protection for work that endangers the eyes)
- Environmental safety programs (e.g., proper disposal of hazardous waste)
- Legislation that prevents injury or disease (e.g., seat belt/child restraint laws; motorcycle helmet laws)

caregivers focus on machines and techniques rather than on patients. Nurses must remember that patients benefit most when they understand their diagnoses and treatments and can be active participants in the development and implementation of their own treatment plans.

Rehabilitation and long-term care

Rehabilitation services help restore the patient to the fullest possible level of function and independence following injury or illness. Rehabilitation programs also deal with conditions that leave patients with less than full functioning, such as strokes or severe burns. Both patients and their families must be active participants in this care if it is to be successful. Rehabilitation services should begin as soon as the patient's condition has stabilized after an injury or injury. These services may be provided in institutional settings such as hospitals, in special rehabilitation facilities, in long term care facilities such as nursing homes, or in the home and the community. The objectives are to assist patients to achieve their full potential and return to a level of functioning that permits them to be contributing members of society.

Rehabilitation services also include **disease management** services. Disease management services deal with diseases, such as congestive heart failure and diabetes, and conditions, such as low back pain and hypertension, that contribute to higher health care costs and a reduced quality of life, particularly for aging populations. Disease management focuses on helping participants understand and manage their chronic conditions more effectively through phone calls, coaching and education, symptom prevention and management, and collaboration with their providers. These steps give providers information between office visits so that they can proactively manage the participant's condition before emergency or hospital services are required, thus reducing health care costs and improving the quality of life for their patients.

Long-term care is provided in residential facilities such as assisted-living homes, skilled and intermediate nursing homes, and personal care homes. Each facility is tailored to provide services that the patient or family cannot provide but at a level that maintains the individual's independence as long as possible. With the aging of the population, and with more patients surviving severe trauma and disease with impairments in physical or mental functioning or both, long term care facilities are expected to experience rapid growth.

Classifications of Health Care Agencies

There are many agencies involved in the total health care delivery system. Organizations that deliver care can be classified in three major ways: as governmental or voluntary agencies; as not-for-profit or for-profit agencies; or by the level of health care services they provide.

Governmental (public) agencies

Many **governmental (public) agencies** contribute to the health and well-being of U.S. citizens. All of these public agencies are primarily supported by taxes, administered by elected or appointed officials, and tailored to the needs of the communities served.

Federal agencies.   Federal agencies focus on the health of all U.S. citizens. They promote and conduct health and illness research, provide funding to train health care workers, and assist communities in planning health care services. They also develop health programs and services and provide financial and personnel support to staff them. Federal agencies establish standards of practice and safety for health care workers and conduct national health education programs on subjects such as the benefits of not smoking, prevention of acquired immunodeficiency syndrome (AIDS), and the need for prenatal care. Examples of federal agencies are the National Institutes of Health (NIH), the U.S. Department of Health and Human Services (DHHS), the Occupational Safety and Health Administration (OSHA), the Centers for Medicare and Medicaid Services (CMS), and the Centers for Disease Control and Prevention (CDC).

State agencies

State health agencies oversee programs that affect the health of citizens within an individual state. Examples of state agencies include state departments of health and environment, departments that regulate and license health professionals such as state boards of nursing, and agencies that administer Medicaid insurance programs for the poor. These agencies are not typically involved in providing direct patient care but support local agencies that do provide direct care.

Local agencies. Local agencies serve one community, one county, or a few nearby counties. They provide services to both paying and nonpaying citizens. Public health departments are examples of local governmental agencies found in almost every county in the United States. All citizens, whether or not they can pay, are eligible for health care through local public health departments. These services usually include immunizations, prenatal care and counseling, well-baby and well-child clinics, sexually transmitted infection clinics, tuberculosis clinics, and others. Public health nurses sometimes make home visits as well.

Voluntary (private) agencies

Citizens often voluntarily support agencies working to promote or restore health. When private volunteers support an agency providing health care, it is called a **voluntary (private) agency.** Support is generally through private donations, although many of these agencies apply for governmental grants to support some of their activities.

Voluntary agencies often begin when a group of individuals band together to address a health problem. Volunteers may initially perform all their services. Later, they may obtain enough donations to hire personnel, staff an office, and expand services. They may be able to secure ongoing funding through grants or organizations such as the United Way. Examples of voluntary health agencies are the Visiting Nurses Association, the American Heart Association (Figure 14-1), the American Cancer Society, the American Red Cross, and the March of Dimes.

Not-for-profit or for-profit agencies

The second major way to classify health service delivery agencies is by what is done with the income earned by the agency. A **not-for-profit agency** is one that uses profits to pay personnel, improve services, advertise services, provide educational programs, or otherwise contribute to the mission of the agency. A common misconception is that not-for-profit agencies do not ever make a profit. Actually, they may make profits, but the profits must be used on behalf of the agency. Most voluntary agencies, such as the ones listed previously, are also not-for-profit agencies, as are many private hospitals.

For-profit agencies may distribute profits earned to partners or shareholders. The growth in for-profit health care agencies has risen over the past several decades because of the potential for health care to be very profitable.

For-profit agencies include numerous home health care companies that send nurses and other

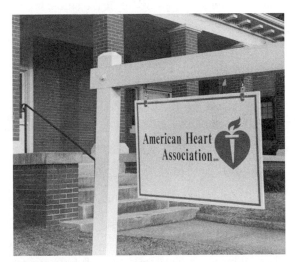

Figure 14-1
Private, not-for-profit agencies, such as the American Heart Association, provide a variety of health-related services to the citizens of their communities. *(Photo by Kelly Whalen.)*

health personnel to care for patients at home. Several large national chains of for-profit health care providers also exist and have demonstrated that it is possible to provide quality patient care and make a profit while doing so. Examples include national nursing home networks, specialty outpatient centers for ambulatory surgery, heart hospitals, and rehabilitation centers. A controversial issue related to for-profit health care organizations is that they do not typically treat nonpaying patients. These people must go to publicly funded facilities that are rapidly becoming overburdened with patients who are unable to pay their bills.

Level of health care services provided

The third way in which health care services can be classified is by the level of health care services they provide. These levels have traditionally been primary care, secondary care, and tertiary care. A new level, subacute care, has recently emerged. These four levels are discussed below.

Primary care services.   Care rendered at the point at which a patient first enters the health care system is considered **primary care.** This care may be provided in a student health clinic, health centers in the community, an emergency department, physicians' offices, nurse practitioners' clinics, or health clinics at worksites. The major goals of the primary health care system are providing the following:

1. Entry into the system
2. Emergency care
3. Health maintenance
4. Long-term and chronic care
5. Treatment of temporary health problems that do not require hospitalization

In addition to treating common health problems, primary care centers are, for many citizens, where much of prevention and health promotion takes place. Unfortunately, these centers are plagued by many problems, such as lack of adequate financing, staffing, space, and community support. However, this pattern is changing, in large part because of the increasing influence of managed care. Access to primary care in the least

costly setting is now mandated by managed care organizations.

Secondary care services. **Secondary care** involves the prevention of complications from disease. It includes such activities as treating temporary dysfunctions requiring medical intervention or hospitalization, evaluating long-term care, evaluating chronic patients who may need treatment changes, and providing counseling or therapies that are not available in primary care settings.

Although hospitals have traditionally been associated with this level of care, other agencies increasingly provide secondary health services. They include home health agencies, ambulatory care agencies, skilled nursing agencies, and surgical centers. These settings offer skilled personnel, easy access, convenient parking, compact equipment and monitoring systems, medications and anesthesia services, and a financial reimbursement program that rewards shorter lengths of stay and home or community care.

A new addition to secondary care is the disease management industry. Health services are provided through outbound/inbound calls with nurses and health professionals, patients' interactive voice responses (using a touchtone phone to respond to questions that are entered into an electronic health record), educational videos/ books sent to the patient, and Internet-based tools. To use these services, patients do not have to leave their homes; they have access to health education, coaching, and tools 24 hours a day, 7 days a week. Another advantage is that patients develop a long-term relationship with their disease management nurse/health professional.

It is expected that the trend toward providing community-based secondary care will continue. However, reimbursement decreased as the terms of the Balanced Budget Act of 1997 were implemented, eliminating many home health services and skilled nursing care previously covered. The full effect of that act on this segment of the health care industry has not yet been evaluated.

Tertiary care services. **Tertiary care** services are those provided to acutely ill patients, to those requiring long-term care, to those needing rehabilitation services, and to terminally ill patients. Tertiary care usually involves many health professionals working together on interdisciplinary teams to design treatment plans.

Examples of tertiary agencies are specialized hospitals such as trauma centers and specialized pediatric centers; long term care facilities offering skilled nursing, intermediate care, and supportive care; rehabilitation centers; and hospices, where care is provided to the terminally ill and their families in the hospital, in the home, or in special hospice "houses."

Subacute care services. A new segment of health care—subacute care services—emerged in the 1990s. **Subacute care** is defined as inpatient care that lies between hospital care and long-term care. It is goal-oriented, comprehensive, inpatient care designed for an individual who has had an acute illness, injury, or exacerbation of a disease process. Generally, the condition of an individual receiving subacute care is such that the care does not depend heavily on high-technology monitoring or complex diagnostic procedures. The goal was to provide lower-cost health care and create a seamless transition for patients moving through the health care system.

Subacute care is generally more intensive than traditional nursing facility care and less intensive than acute inpatient care. It requires frequent (daily to weekly) patient assessment and review of the clinical course and treatment plan for a limited time period (several days to several months), until a condition is stabilized or a predetermined treatment course is completed (Joint Commission on Accreditation of Healthcare Organizations, 1995, p. 3).

Subacute care requires the coordinated services of an interdisciplinary team, including physicians, nurses, and members of other relevant professional disciplines who are knowledgeable and trained to assess and manage these specific conditions and perform the necessary procedures. Growth in subacute care has slowed owing to increasing government regulation and lower third-party reimbursements.

Organizational Structures of Health Care Agencies

The health care delivery system consists of agencies such as hospitals, clinics, associations, long term care facilities, and home health services that provide any of the four major types of health services.

Organizational structure

Organizational structure refers to how an agency is organized to accomplish its mission. The organizational structure of most agencies includes a governing body or board of directors, which may also be called a board of trustees.

Board of directors. In the past, board members were often chosen from two groups: community philanthropists, who were expected to donate generously to the facility; and physicians, who practiced in the institution. Boards were large, met infrequently, and had mainly ceremonial functions.

As the health care environment became more complex, board members were chosen to represent various business and political interests of the community. They were expected to bring knowledge and expertise from the business world, as well as to have an appreciation and understanding of health care agencies and how they operate.

Boards now tend to be smaller and carry significant responsibility for the mission of the organization, the quality of services provided, and the financial status of the organization. Boards are not involved in the day-to-day running of the agency, but they are legally responsible for establishing policies governing operations and for ensuring that the policies are executed. They delegate responsibility for running the agency to the chief executive officer (CEO). Box 14-2 outlines a typical hospital board's primary responsibilities.

Chief executive officer. The **chief executive officer (CEO)** is the individual responsible for the overall operation on a daily basis. He or she usually has a minimum of a master's degree in business or hospital administration. Responsibilities include making sure that the institution runs efficiently and is cost-effective and carrying out policies established by the board. The CEO also has an important external role addressing health care issues in the community and usually sits on the board of directors as well as reports to them. A chief operating officer (COO) often assists the CEO in larger organizations.

Nurses with advanced degrees and experience in administration, business, and health care policy increasingly occupy both of these positions. Boards, who are responsible for hiring CEOs, have found that the broad holistic education and clinical experience of nurses prepares them exceptionally well for these positions.

Medical staff. A medical staff consists of physicians, who may be either employees of the health care organization or independent practitioners. In either case they must be granted privileges by the board of trustees to see patients at that particular institution. They cannot simply decide to admit patients to an institution. A credentials committee, composed of members of the medical staff, performs the credentialing process. This committee is charged with the responsibility of assuring the board of directors that every physician admitted to the medical staff of that facility is a qualified and competent practitioner and that, over time, each one keeps his or her skills and knowledge updated.

The medical staff, through its credentials committee, is often charged with the responsibility

---

Box 14-2 **Board of Directors' Responsibilities**

- Mission development and long-range planning
- Ensuring high-quality care
- Oversight of medical staff credentialing
- Financial oversight
- Selection and evaluation of the hospital chief executive officer
- Board self-evaluation and education

From American Hospital Association: *Welcome to the board: an orientation for the new health care trustee,* Chicago, 1999, AHA Press.

---

for credentialing nonphysician providers who admit or consult with patients. These include advanced practice nurses, psychologists, optometrists, podiatrists, and others.

In large organizations, medical staffs are usually organized by service (e.g., department of surgery, department of medicine, department of obstetrics). The entire medical staff usually elects a chief of staff. The **chief of staff** and the chiefs of the various services work together with the chief executive officer and other administrative representatives through the medical executive committee to make important decisions about medical policy for the institution. The rules and regulations that govern these activities are called bylaws. The board of directors, to whom the physicians are responsible, must approve the credentialing actions of the medical staff.

Service on committees and leadership positions of the medical staff are time-consuming activities; therefore some institutions pay members of the medical staff a fee for special services in recognition that time away from seeing patients reduces their income.

Nursing staff. The senior administrative nurse in an organization is known as the **chief nurse executive (CNE)** or chief nursing officer (CNO), vice president for nursing, or director of nursing. Once excluded from broad institutional decision making, nurse executives today are often members of the board of directors. Many organizations now consider the nurse executive and the chief of the medical staff of equal importance.

The educational preparation of nurse executives usually includes a minimum of a master's degree in nursing, business, or health administration. Some nurse executives hold joint master's of science in nursing and business administration (MSN/MBA) or joint master's of science in health and business administration (MHA/MBA).

Nurse executives are responsible for overseeing all the nursing care provided in the institution and serve as clinical leaders and administrators. Because of the need to coordinate patient care and outcomes among all disciplines, the role may also include administrative responsibilities for departments other than nursing, such as pharmacy, respiratory therapy, and social services.

The nursing staff consists of all the registered nurses, licensed practical nurses/licensed vocational nurses, nursing assistants, and clerical assistants employed by the department of nursing. These staff members are usually organized according to the units on which they work.

Each patient care unit has its own budget and staff, for which the manager is responsible. The manager, who is usually a nurse, is also a communication link between the staff and the next level of management.

In large or networked organizations, there may be an additional level of management between the nurse executive and the manager of a unit. These are middle managers, known as clinical directors or supervisors. In most cases, they are also nurses, but they may come from other clinical disciplines or from a business background. These directors are responsible for multiple units or for specific projects or programs. They ensure that nursing and all other services they manage are integrated with other hospital services. They also serve as the communication link between the unit managers and the executive staff.

Other nurses combine direct patient care responsibilities with research, education, and management responsibilities, such as nurse educators, nurse researchers and clinical nurse specialists, and infection control nurses. Nurses in these roles support direct care nurses and serve as expert resources to them in their areas of specialization.

NURSING ORGANIZATION GOVERNANCE. In most health care agencies, nurses have a nursing staff organization. In some settings it serves mainly as a communication vehicle. In other more enlightened settings, nurses are expected to govern themselves through the organization, much as the medical staff is expected to govern itself through the medical staff organization.

The concept of **shared governance** is founded on the philosophy that employees have both a right and a responsibility to govern their own work and time within a financially secure, patient-centered system. Shared governance promotes decentralization and participation at all levels of nursing. Kerfoot (2005) describes the roles of both the staff and the manager in shared governance. The role of the nursing staff is to be responsible for the professional practice of their nursing unit. The role of the nurse manager and other nurse leaders is to set expectations or standards and partner with the staff in achieving the identified goals. Therefore in order to achieve shared governance, nurse leaders must believe in the ability of their staff (Kerfoot, 2005). An example of shared governance is self-scheduling, in which staff determine their own schedule based on established guidelines set forth by the manager for staffing the unit. Nursing must continue to lead the way in implementing the shared governance model in order to promote improved patient outcomes and enhanced nurse job satisfaction.

Health care organizations are complex facilities. The way they are organized may vary, but each has an organizational chart that shows its unique structure and explains lines of authority. When considering employment in a health care organization, you can learn a great deal by examining its organizational chart to see how nursing is governed and how it relates to senior management and the board of directors. Figure 14-2 shows an example of a basic health care organizational chart.

The Health Care Team

Within the vast array of health care settings discussed in this chapter are the people who provide care to patients—the health care team. At one time, physicians and nurses were the only members of the health care team, but as health care became complex and technology expanded, a number of other health disciplines developed. Today, there are many different health care team members who come from a variety of backgrounds. Physicians, nurses, and all the other individuals who work with patients are called the health care team, or **interdisciplinary team.** They are supported in their work by a number of other departments, such as nutrition services, environmental services, and laundry services. The decision about which of these various personnel should be involved in the care of a patient depends on the desired patient outcomes. Several of the key members who are most likely to be involved in the care of patients are discussed below.

Physicians

Physicians are responsible for the medical diagnosis and interventions designed to restore health. Although physicians have traditionally been involved mainly in restorative care, many are beginning to recognize the value of health promotion and maintenance as well as illness and injury prevention. Some physicians are also integrating nontraditional or alternative treatment choices such as chiropractic medicine, acupuncture, herbal treatments, and massage therapy into their practices.

Physicians have completed college and 3 or 4 years of medical school and are licensed by a state board of medical examiners. Although a hospital residency is not required to practice medicine in all states, most physicians have completed one, and many do postgraduate work in a specialty area and then take examinations to become board-certified in the specialty area.

Physician assistants

Physician assistants (PAs) have emerged in last 30 years as members of the health care team. According to the American Academy of Physician Assistants (AAPA, 2006), physician assistants perform many functions of a physician under the direct supervision of a physician.

Physician assistants must have a bachelor's degree and health care experience before attending a PA educational program, which usually lasts a little over 2 years and results in a certificate. Beyond graduation from this program, PAs are required to be licensed by the state in which they practice. They are required to obtain continuing medical education and regularly be retested on their clinical skills. PAs may also choose to then complete a postgraduate PA program in a clinical specialty area.

Dietitians

Many patients require management of their nutritional intake as part of the healing process. Others need to know how to prepare and eat a healthy diet (Figure 14-3). **Dietitians** understand how the diet (oral or intravenous) can affect a patient's recovery and promote and maintain health. They focus on the therapeutic value of foods and on teaching people about therapeutic diets and healthful nutrition. Dietitians have baccalaureate degrees and may have completed internships in specialty areas, such as pediatrics.

Pharmacists

Pharmacists prepare and dispense medications, instruct patients and other health workers about medications, monitor the use of controlled substances such as narcotics, and work to reduce medication errors. The number and complexity of drugs available today necessitate special education and training in their preparation and dispensing and in monitoring the effects on patients. Clinical pharmacists spend time on

Figure 14-2
A typical health care organizational chart.

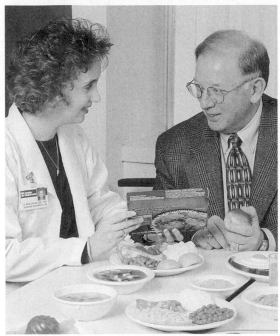

Figure 14-3

Dietitians assist patients to facilitate their own healing and health maintenance through therapeutic diets and healthful nutrition practices. *(Photo courtesy Hamilton Medical Center, Dalton, Ga.)*

hospital units working closely with physicians and nursing case managers to coordinate complex drug administration, such as chemotherapy. They assist in monitoring and minimizing the drug interactions resulting from a patient taking many different medications.

Pharmacists must obtain a doctor of pharmacy (PharmD) degree, which takes 6 years to complete, and pass a state board of pharmacy's licensure examination (U.S. Department of Labor, 2006). Depending on state licensing requirements, they may also be required to complete an internship. Pharmacy technicians assist them.

Technologists

Technologists are personnel who assist health care providers in the diagnosis of patient problems.

Laboratory technologists handle patient specimens—such as blood, sputum, feces, urine, and body tissues—to be examined for abnormalities (Figure 14-4). Laboratory technologists carefully subject these body substances to various tests to determine whether or not the patient needs treatment. Technologists have at least a bachelor's degree and are often assisted by laboratory technicians, who have 2-year degrees. They must pass a state licensing examination to practice.

Radiology technologists perform x-ray procedures. Although patients still need routine x-ray studies, technology in this field has become much more sophisticated. Subspecialties such as computed tomography (CT), magnetic resonance imaging (MRI), and positron emission tomography (PET) have developed. All of these techniques allow practitioners to see what is occurring inside the body without surgery. They also require specially educated technicians who operate multimillion-dollar equipment. Although some radiology technicians are still trained "on the job," most are educated in formal programs lasting from 1 to 4 years. Radiology technologists have a bachelor's degree. They must be registered with the state in which they practice.

Respiratory therapists

Acutely ill or injured patients often require assistance in breathing. Respiratory therapists operate equipment such as ventilators, oxygen therapy devices, and intermittent positive-pressure breathing machines. They also perform some diagnostic procedures, such as pulmonary function tests and, in some facilities, blood gas analysis. With the increase in respiratory care in the home and community, these health care team members are working closely with home health agencies and community health centers. Respiratory therapists must complete either a 2-year or a 4-year educational program and obtain state licensure; in some states they must complete an internship.

Social workers

The social worker is specifically educated and trained to assist patients and their families as they

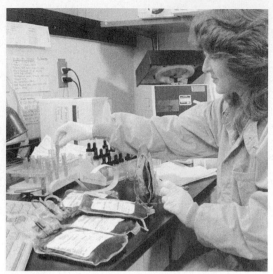

Figure 14-4
This laboratory technologist works in a critically important setting—a blood bank. Here she prepares several units of blood for administration. *(Photo courtesy Hamilton Medical, Center, Dalton, Ga.)*

face the impact of illness and injury. They serve as liaisons between hospitalized patients and the resources and services available in the community. They help patients and their families deal with financial problems caused by interruption of work or inadequate insurance benefits; they also direct them to the appropriate community support systems or facilities for home health care, long-term care, or rehabilitation. In addition to counseling patients and families, social workers are called on to assist other health care personnel to cope more effectively with the stresses associated with caring for patients in crisis. Social workers hold either a bachelor's or a master's degree and are licensed.

Therapists

Therapists help patients with special challenges. Physical therapists, or physiotherapists, assist patients to regain maximum possible physical

activity and strength. They focus on assessing pre-illness or pre-injury function, current damage, and potential for recovery. They then develop a long-term plan for gradual return to function through exercise, rest, heat, and hydrotherapy. Physical therapists, who have a minimum of a master's degree, also supervise physical therapy assistants, who hold associate degrees.

Occupational therapists work with physical therapists to develop plans to assist patients in resuming the activities of daily living after illness or injury. They may help patients learn to cook, carry out their personal hygiene, or drive a specially equipped car. In addition, they assist patients to learn skills to return to their previous jobs or retrain patients for new employment options. Occupational therapists have bachelor's degrees. Other types of therapists include recreational therapists, art and music therapists, speech therapists, and massage therapists.

Administrative support personnel

In all organizations, administrative support staff members are needed for clerical jobs such as admitting patients, answering phones, directing visitors, scheduling patient tests, filing insurance claims, filing forms, paying bills, facilitating payroll, and other support functions. These activities require considerable time. Hiring administrative staff members frees the clinical staff to concentrate on direct patient care.

The administrative staff ensures that the operations of the facility run smoothly and that clinicians have the resources necessary to meet patient needs. These staff members also educate the clinical staff on financial constraints and work with the staff to find ways to provide quality care at the lowest possible cost.

Keeping complete and accurate medical records is an extremely important administrative function that ensures proper insurance billing, eligibility for accreditation, and legal protection of the hospital and its staff. Registered records' administrators are vital members of the administrative staff. These professionals staff the medical records department. Many organizations today now refer to the medical records departments as "health information services."

The Nurse's Role on the Health Care Team

Whatever the setting, nurses fulfill a number of roles on the health care team. As the health care delivery system changes, the evolving role of the registered nurse requires new competencies and skills in each of the roles described below.

Provider of care

Nurses provide direct, hands-on care to patients in all health care agencies and settings. As providers, they take an active role in illness prevention and health promotion and maintenance. They offer health screenings, home health services, and an array of health care services in schools, workplaces, churches, clinics, physicians' offices, and other settings. They are instrumental in the high survival rates in trauma centers and newborn intensive care units, among others. Nurses with advanced nursing degrees are increasingly providing care at all levels of the health care system. Managed care has created opportunities for nurses to provide direct care as gatekeepers in primary care settings. Their breadth and depth of knowledge, their ability to care holistically for patients, and their natural partnership with physicians make nurses some of the most sought-after care providers.

Educator

As patient and family educators, nurses provide information about illnesses and teach about medications, treatments, and rehabilitation needs. They also help patients understand how to deal with the life changes necessitated by chronic illnesses and teach how to adapt care to the home or community setting. In the current health care climate, patients are being discharged from hospitals faster than ever before. Patients and their families often must manage complex treatments, such as central lines or feeding tubes, in the home setting. A major role of the nurse as educator in today's hospital setting is to ensure continuity from inpatient to outpatient care

through coordination of home care services and through discharge teaching (Bastable, 2003).

Nurses also act as educators in community settings. The major focus of the nurse in the community setting is health promotion and injury and illness prevention. Often, nurses teach classes jointly with other health care team members. For example, a nutritionist and a nurse may teach a group of expectant parents the benefits of breast-feeding their infants. Nurses also have a responsibility to understand and teach how a healthful or unhealthful environment may affect both the short-term and the long-term health of the community. Another community setting for nurse educators is faith community nursing, discussed in Chapter 1.

Nurses also serve as patient educators in disease management companies. By educating patients about their chronic diseases and coaching them in effective self-care behaviors, nurses work with the patient and the primary care provider to keep the patient healthier. Thus nurses as patient educators help reduce health care utilization and cost.

Nurses are often the key educators on the health care team. They teach other team members about the patient and family and why different interventions may have varying degrees of success. Nurses help other team members find cost-effective, quality interventions that are desired and needed by the patient rather than wasting resources on ineffective, inefficient, undesired, or unneeded services.

Nurses also serve as teachers of the next generation of nurses. Nursing students need educators who set high standards and ideals and who help students understand the ethical choices that all health care providers must make.

The Internet plays a significant role in health education today. It has completely transformed the access and dissemination of information for millions of Americans. Nurses functioning in the role of educator assist patients to use the Internet as an enhancement to traditional education. Tips for nurses to use in helping patients evaluate health information on the Internet are found in Box 14-3.

Counselor

People who experience illness or injury often have strong emotional responses. It is clear that the relationships among the emotions, the mind, and the body are critical to promotion of and restoration to health. As counselors, nurses provide basic counseling and support to patients and their families.

Using therapeutic communication techniques, nurses encourage people to discuss their feelings, to explore possible options and solutions to their unique problems, and to choose for themselves the best alternatives for action. They also serve as bereavement counselors to terminally ill patients and their families. Because nurses spend more time with patients than other professionals, they have opportunities to respond to the emotional needs of patients as they occur. Therefore the nurse's role as counselor often overlaps with the roles of social workers, psychiatrists, spiritual advisers, and mental health specialists. Nurses may, with advanced education and certification, provide psychotherapy services that extend beyond the basic counseling role.

Manager

In their daily work, all nurses are managers. The bedside staff nurse must manage the care of a group of patients, prioritize how to accomplish patient care activities during an 8- or 12-hour period, and determine staff and patient assignments. Nurses are also involved in reviewing patient cases and coordinating services so that quality care can be achieved at the lowest cost.

In addition, nurses serve in the role of managers of patient care units, outpatient clinics,

---

Box 14-3 **Tips for Helping Patients Evaluate Online Health Information**

Nurses should advise patients to apply the following guidelines when searching for health information on the Internet:

1. Identify the sponsor.
   - Government-sponsored sites have .gov in the website address.
   Example: The National Cancer Institute website: www.cancer.gov
   - Professional organization sites have .org in the website address.
   Example: The American Cancer Society website: www.cancer.org
   - Educational institution sites have .edu in the website address.
   Example: The Johns Hopkins University website: www.jhu.edu
   - Commercial sites* have .com in the website address.
   Example: Johnson & Johnson website: www.jnj.com
2. Identify the timeliness.
   - Is the site dated?
   - Is the date current (within the last 3 years or less)?
3. Identify the accuracy.
   - Is the information clear and factual?
   - Can it be verified with a professional source?
   - Who is the author?
   - What are the author's credentials on this topic?
4. Identify the audience.
   - Is this site intended for health care consumers or professionals?

*Commercial sites are most likely sponsored by a company and can have useful health information but also exist to sell products.
From Medical Library Association: *A user's guide to finding and evaluating health information on the Web*, 2005, available online: www.mlanet.org/resources/userguide.html#5.

or home health agencies. The effective management of nursing resources is essential. With budgets ranging from hundreds of thousands to many million dollars, nurse managers manage "businesses" larger than many small companies. Nurse managers must have clinical and administrative expertise, including but not limited to leadership, human resources, financial, organizational behavior, system and program design, outcome research, and marketing skills.

Chief nurse executives may manage more than 1000 employees and multimillion-dollar budgets. They interact with other top executives and community leaders, often sitting on the health care organization's board of directors. Nurse executives must ensure the quality of nursing care within financial, regulatory, and legislative constraints. As noted earlier, nurses may serve as patient care executives, chief operating officers, and chief executive officers. Key responsibilities of nurse managers and nurse executives are listed in Table 14-1.

Researcher

All nurses should be involved in nursing research whether or not research is a nurse's primary responsibility. According to the American Nurses Association's *Scope and Standards of Practice* (ANA, 2004), the registered nurse integrates research findings into practice. Nurse researchers investigate whether current or potential nursing actions achieve their expected outcomes, what options for care may be available, and how best to provide care. Nursing research looks at patient outcomes, the nursing process, and the systems that support nursing services.

Outcomes research has become an integral part of the health care delivery system. Managed care organizations and regulatory agencies require health care organizations to report outcome data related to quality of care, which requires research by nurses. Participation by all nurses in research is essential to the growth and development of the nursing profession.

Collaborator

With so many health care workers involved in providing patient care, **collaboration** among the professions is increasingly important. The collaborator role is a vital one for nurses to ensure that everyone agrees on the same patient outcomes. Multidisciplinary teams require collaborative practice, and nurses play key roles as both team members and team leaders. Collaboration

---

Table 14-1   RESPONSIBILITIES OF NURSE MANAGERS AND NURSE EXECUTIVES

Nurse Managers	Nurse Executives
■ Direct supervision of assigned staff and interdisciplinary collaboration	■ Partner with other disciplines and leaders
■ Manage recruitment, selection, retention, staffing, scheduling, and assigning	■ Acquire resources for function and process and provide leadership in human resources development and management
■ Accept organizational accountability for services provided	■ Lead and direct patient care delivery
■ Evaluate quality and appropriateness of health care delivery for assigned areas	■ Accountable for continuous quality improvement for entire nursing system
■ Budget for assigned areas	■ Budget for entire nursing department and input into system-wide budget planning

From American Nurses Association: *Scope and standards for nurse administrators*, ed 2, Washington, DC, 2004, available online: nursesbooks.org.

requires that nurses understand and appreciate what other health professionals have to offer. Nurses must also interpret to others the nursing needs of patients.

An often-overlooked collaborative function of nurses is collaboration with patients and families. Involving patients and their families in the plan of care from the beginning is the best way to ensure their cooperation, enthusiasm, and willingness to work toward the best patient outcomes.

Entrepreneur

Nurse **entrepreneurs** are becoming more common. Nurses now have businesses of their own that provide direct patient services in hospitals, community settings, businesses, schools, homes, and many other settings. Nurse entrepreneurs provide consultation and educational services to nurses and other health team members. They provide services to businesses by conducting work- site wellness programs and by advising human resource staff on how to provide high-quality health benefits to employees while reducing costs.

Patient advocate

Rules and regulations designed to help a complex hospital run efficiently can often get in the way of a patient's treatment, and an impersonal health care system frequently infringes on the patient's rights. Therefore it is every nurse's responsibility to advocate for patients daily.

Many health care institutions take this concept a step further by employing nurses as **patient advocates.** Patient advocates know how to cut through the levels of bureaucracy and red tape of health care organizations and will stand up for the patient's rights, advocating his or her best interests at all times. They must value patient self-determination, that is, patient independence and decision making. In this role, nurses sometimes help patients bend the rules when it is in the patient's best interests and doing so will harm no one else. Patient advocates are nurses who realize that policies are important and govern most situations well but occasionally can, and should,

be broken. For example, special care units often have strict visiting hours. Family members may be allowed to see the patient for only 10 minutes each hour. If a patient's recovery will be faster if the family is present, the nurse, serving as a patient advocate, will allow the family members more generous visitation than the policy provides.

In conclusion, nurses must be prepared to participate both as leaders and as members of the interdisciplinary team and to assume and relinquish the leadership role to best meet the needs of patients and the team. More information about collaboration with members of interdisciplinary teams is found in Chapter 9.

In order to fully understand the nurse's role on the health care team, it is important to examine the types of nursing care delivery systems and how they have changed over the years.

Types of Nursing Care Delivery Systems Historically Used in Acute Care Settings

Before World War I, nurses visited the sick in their homes to care for them. As hospital care improved and nursing education evolved, more sick people were treated in hospitals. Providing care to groups of patients rather than to individuals required nurses to be efficient and use their time effectively. Various types of care delivery systems were designed to meet the goals of efficient and effective nursing care. Several types of patient care delivery systems have been used in acute care settings. Four systems—functional nursing, team nursing, primary nursing, and case management nursing—are reviewed in this chapter.

Functional nursing

The functional approach to nursing care grew out of a need to provide care to large numbers of patients. It focused on organizing and distributing the tasks, or functions, of care. In **functional nursing,** personnel worked side by side, each performing an assigned task. Trained nurses provided care that required high skill levels, and untrained workers with little skill or education performed many less complex tasks. For example, one nurse may administer medications and another nurse performs assessments while a nursing assistant gives baths and changes linen.

The goal of functional nursing was efficient management of time, tasks, and energy. Although this practice saved hospitals money, patient care was fragmented, because caregivers were focused on individual tasks and not individual patients. A patient could not refer to one person as "my nurse."

Today, functional nursing can still be used in some settings, such as the operating room, where the care is task-oriented (Cherry and Jacob, 1999). It is particularly useful when there are few staff members available, such as at night, on weekends, and on holidays. Box 14-4 lists advantages and disadvantages of functional nursing.

Team Nursing

In response to the frustration some nurses felt when using the functional approach to patient care, Lambertson (1953) designed **team nursing** (Figure 14-5). She envisioned nursing teams as democratic work groups with different skill levels represented by different team members. They were assigned as a team to a group of patients.

Team nursing has been widely used in hospitals and long term care facilities. The team usually consists of a registered nurse (RN), who serves as team leader, a licensed practical nurse (LPN), and one or more certified nursing assistants (NAs).

The team leader, although ultimately responsible for all the care provided, **delegates** (assigns responsibility for) certain patients to each team member. Each member of the team provides the level of care for which he or she is best prepared. The least skilled and experienced members care for the patients who require the least complex care, and the most skilled and experienced members care for the most seriously ill patients who require the most complex care.

In team nursing, the RN team leader oversees all care for a particular shift, makes assessments, and documents responses to care. The licensed practical nurse team member provides direct care by performing treatments and procedures and reporting patient responses to the team leader. The certified nursing assistant provides routine direct, personal care. If multiskilled, nonlicensed workers are used, the role of the licensed practical nurse or certified nursing assistant is often eliminated.

Today, team nursing is still used, but the model is usually modified. Many of the patient-focused care models implemented during patient care redesign use registered nurses as team leaders coordinating care for a group of patients and supervising multiskilled workers who have been trained to perform a variety of comfort measures, such as positioning, and technical procedures, such as taking vital signs or drawing blood.

Box 14-4 **Advantages and Disadvantages of Functional Nursing**

Advantages
- Efficient—can complete many tasks in a reasonable time frame
- Proficient—workers only perform tasks they are educated to do and become very efficient
- Promotes organizational skills—each worker must organize his or her own work
- Promotes worker autonomy

Disadvantages
- Lacks holistic view of patient—emphasis on task, not person
- Lacks continuity—patients often do not know who their nurse is
- Little time for registered nurses to talk with patients or render personal care

As with functional nursing, team nursing has both advantages and disadvantages; these are presented in Box 14-5.

Primary nursing

Developed by Manthey (1980), **primary nursing** was designed to promote the concept of an identified nurse for every patient during the patient's stay on a particular unit. The goal of primary nursing is to deliver consistent, comprehensive care by identifying one nurse who is responsible, has authority, and is accountable for the patient's nursing care outcomes for the period during which the patient is in a unit.

In primary nursing, each newly admitted patient is assigned to a primary nurse. Primary nurses assess their patients, plan their care, and write the plan of care. While on duty, they care for their patients and delegate responsibility to associate nurses when they are off duty. Associate nurses may be other registered nurses or licensed practical nurses.

Patients are divided among primary nurses in such a manner that each nurse is responsible for the care of a group of patients 24 hours a day. Unless there is a compelling reason to transfer a patient, the primary nurse cares for the patient in the unit from the time of admission to the time of discharge. The primary nurse may be assisted by other care providers (such as other nurses, aides, and technicians) but retains **accountability,** or responsibility, for care outcomes 24 hours a day while the patient is in

---

Box 14-5 Advantages and Disadvantages of Team Nursing

Advantages

- Potential for building team spirit
- Provides comprehensive care
- Each worker's abilities used to the fullest
- Promotes job satisfaction
- Decreases nonprofessional duties of registered nurses

Disadvantages

- Constant need to communicate among team members is time-consuming.
- All must promote teamwork, or team nursing is unsuccessful.
- Team composition varies from day to day, which can be confusing and disruptive and decreases continuity of care.
- May result in blurred role boundaries and resulting confusion and resentment.

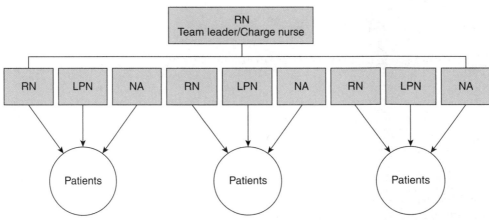

Figure 14-5
Team nursing.

the unit. The primary nurse communicates effectively with associate nurses caring for the patient on other shifts and with primary nurses in other units if the patient is transferred (e.g., to the operating room and intensive care unit).

Primary nursing is used in a variety of settings and is often modified from its original form. Advantages and disadvantages of primary nursing are listed in Box 14-6.

Case management nursing

The most recent evolution in nursing care delivery systems is **case management nursing.** Begun in the late 1980s as another attempt to improve the cost-effectiveness of patient care, case management allows the nurse to oversee patient care and manage the delivery of services from the entire health care team throughout a patient's illness (Cherry and Jacob, 1999). Nursing case management keeps costs down by striving to achieve predetermined patient outcomes within a specified time period.

In 2003 the Case Management Society of America (CMSA) revised its standards of practice for case management. The CMSA has approved the definition of case management as:

> a collaborative process which assesses, plans, implements, coordinates, monitors and evaluates options and services to meet an individual's health needs through communication and available resources to promote quality and cost-effective outcomes (Case Management Society of America, 2003).

Key functions of the case manager role include assessor, planner, facilitator, and advocate (Box 14-7). Key skills for nurses in these roles include critical thinking, communication, advocacy, negotiation, holistic planning and evaluation, and the ability to set both long-term and short-term goals.

Two models of case management nursing have evolved over time. These are characterized by either an "internal" focus, in which the case manager works within a treatment facility, or an "external" approach, in which the case manager oversees patients and the delivery of services over the continuum of an illness or long-term disease. Although different in scope, these two models share the same principles.

Box **14-6** **Advantages and Disadvantages of Primary Nursing**

Advantages
- High patient and family satisfaction
- Promotes registered nurse responsibility, authority, autonomy, and accountability
- Nurse can care for entire patient—physically, emotionally, socially, and spiritually
- Patient knows nurse well, and nurse knows patient well
- Promotes patient-centered decision making
- Increases coordination and continuity of care
- Promotes professionalism
- Promotes job satisfaction and sense of accomplishment for nurses

Disadvantages
- Difficult to hire all registered nurse staff
- Expensive to pay all registered nurse staff
- Nurses do not know other patients—difficult to "cover" for each other
- May create conflicts between primary and associate nurses
- Stress of round-the-clock responsibility
- Heavy responsibility, especially for new nurses

The New England Medical Center and the Center for Case Management in Boston, Massachusetts, developed the internal approach using the nursing case manager to coordinate care for select patients—about 20 percent of the hospital population—whose care is complex or requires the use of many health care resources (Bower, 1992). These nursing case managers are primary nurses on various units, usually medical-surgical units. They not only care for these patients while on their assigned units but also manage the plans of care from admission to discharge, crossing interdepartmental lines. Although nursing case managers do not physically provide care in all units, they actively collaborate with primary nurses assigned to the patients in those units. This model is similar to the one used by a family practice physician who coordinates medical care for a hospitalized patient but defers to the expertise of a specialist physician if the patient is in the intensive care unit.

Box **14-7** **Case Manager Functions**

Assessor
- Gathers all relevant data and obtains information by interviewing patient/family and performing careful evaluation of the entire situation.
- Evaluates all information related to the current treatment plan objectively and critically to identify barriers, clarify or determine realistic goals and objectives, and seek potential alternatives.

Planner
- Works with patient/family to develop a treatment plan that enhances the outcomes and reduces the payer's liability.
- Includes the patient/family as the primary decision maker and goal setter.
- Incorporates contingency plans for each step in the process to anticipate treatment and service complications.
- Initiates and implements plan modifications as necessary through monitoring and reevaluation to accommodate changes in treatment or progress.

Facilitator
- Actively promotes communication among team members, patient, family, provider, and all parties involved.
- Collaborates with the patient and the health care team to maximize outcomes.
- Coordinates the health delivery process by eliminating unnecessary steps and by promoting timely provision of care.

Advocate
- Incorporates the patient's individualized needs and goals throughout the case management process. Supports and educates the patient to become empowered and self-reliant.
- Obtains consensus of all parties to achieve optimal outcomes.
- Promotes early referral to provide optimum care and cost containment.
- Represents the patient's best interest through advocacy for necessary funding, treatment alternatives, coordination of health services, and frequent reevaluation of progress and goals.

In this nursing model, critical paths are used for all patients. A **critical path,** such as the congestive heart failure CareTrac, which can be found on the Evolve website (www.evolve.elsevier.com/Chitty/professional/), is an interdisciplinary agreement showing who will provide care in a given timeframe to achieve agreed-upon outcomes. The use of critical paths is intended to standardize patient care and allow hospitals to plan staffing levels, lengths of stay, and other factors that heretofore could not be anticipated. Variances in the path are identified. Using continuous quality improvement methodology, health care team members review data periodically to determine whether variations are patient-induced, staff-induced, or system-induced. Once the causes are identified, team members attempt to plan solutions to reduce variances.

The external model of case management nursing began at Carondelet St. Mary's Hospital and Health Center in Tucson, Arizona (Bower, 1992). The nurse case managers spend about 30 percent of their work time in the hospital and 70 percent outside the hospital. Similar to their counterparts in New England, the St. Mary's team members are partners with their patients. Other similarities include a professional practice model of nursing that uses principles of shared governance, acuity-based billing for nursing care, and salaried, rather than hourly, pay status for the case managers. The nurse case manager in this "multisetting case management model" is part of a large network (i.e., hospital, clinic, home health agency, long-term care) and may provide services anywhere in the system.

Other case management models may be found in health maintenance organizations (HMOs), managed care organizations (MCOs), third-party payers (e.g., insurance companies), public health departments, physicians' offices, home health agencies, and long term care facilities. As can be seen from the type of activities in which they engage, case managers perform complex and challenging work. Nurses generally need about 5 years of clinical experience to fill this role effectively. Social workers, psychologists, rehabilitation counselors, or other professionals may also serve as case managers. All case managers, regardless of their discipline, work to reduce the cost of providing services through coordination of providers across the continuum of care.

Advantages and disadvantages of case management nursing are shown in Box 14-8.

Differentiating Levels of Practice: An Ongoing Debate

A continuing issue in the delivery of nursing care is differentiating among the levels of nursing practice. Historically, nurses with different levels of education were used interchangeably in hospitals. Nursing graduates qualify for the same license, and in many settings, diploma, associate degree, and baccalaureate nurses all function under the same job description. According to the National League for Nursing Accrediting Commission (NLNAC, 2005), **differentiated practice** describes the system of sorting roles, functions, and work of nurses according to education, clinical experience, and defines competence and decision-making skills required by different client needs and settings in which nursing is practiced. The

---

Box 14-8 Advantages and Disadvantages of Case Management Nursing

Advantages

- Promotes interdisciplinary collaboration.
- Increases quality of care.
- Is cost-effective.
- Eases patient's transition from hospital to community services.
- Nurse has increased responsibility.

Disadvantages

- Requires additional training.
- Requires nurses to be off the unit for periods of time.
- Is time-consuming.
- Is most useful only with high-risk/high-cost/high-volume patients.

goal of differentiated practice is to define two levels of practice, implying two levels of education and possibly leading ultimately to two levels of licensure.

Clearly, differentiating two levels of practice would promote understanding of nursing practice in terms of technical skills needed to provide care, interpersonal skills needed to facilitate care, and leadership skills needed to manage care. In the mid-1980s a group of donors, including the Kellogg Foundation, funded the South Dakota Statewide Project for Nursing and Nursing Education, which lasted 2 years. The project participants differentiated the competencies for the associate degree in nursing (ADN) and the bachelor of science in nursing (BSN) as follows:

> The BSN cares for focal clients who are identified as individuals, families, aggregate, and community groups. The level of responsibility of the BSN is from admission to post discharge. The unstructured setting is a geographical and/or situational environment that may not have established policies, procedures, and protocols and has the potential for variation requiring independent nursing decisions. The ADN cares for focal clients who are identified as individuals and members of a family. The level of responsibility of the ADN is for a specified work period and is consistent with the identified goals of care. The ADN is prepared to function in a structured health care setting. The structured setting is a geographical and/or situational environment where the policies, procedures, and protocols for the provision of health care are established and there is recourse to assistance and support from the full scope of nursing expertise (Primm, 1988, p. 2).

Though the work of this group in defining the differences between BSN and ADN nurses is more than 20 years old, little progress has been made toward applying these differences to different levels of practice despite recent research that shows differences in patient outcomes based on nurse education levels (Aiken, Clarke, Cheung et al, 2003). Box 14-9 compares selected competencies of nurses with associate degrees in nursing and those with a bachelor of science in nursing.

FORCES CHANGING THE HEALTH CARE DELIVERY SYSTEM

The U.S. health care system changed dramatically in the twentieth century, and the 1990s have been described as the most turbulent time of transition and reform that the U.S. health care system ever experienced. Total expenditures on health care in the United States exceeded $1 trillion for the first time in the 1990s according to a report by the National Center for Health Statistics (2005). Hospital spending and prescription drug expenditures fueled this increase. As escalating costs of delivery of services hit record levels, a major change in reimbursement for services took place. During that same period, the explosion of information technology contributed to a revolution in consumer knowledge and changing expectations for involvement in treatment options.

Managed Care

The term **managed care** is used to describe a wide variety of organizations and activities that attempt to control health care costs. Issues of access and quality are key factors in determining the success of various managed care strategies. It is interesting

---

Box 14-9 Comparison of Differentiated ADN and BSN Competencies

Clients
- ADN: Individuals and family members
- BSN: Individuals, families, aggregates, and community groups

Level of Responsibility
- ADN: For a specified work period
- BSN: From admission to after discharge

Type of Setting
- ADN: Structured; other personnel available
- BSN: Unstructured; other personnel may not be available

ADN, Associate degree in nursing; *BSN*, bachelor of science in nursing.
From Primm P: Differentiated practice for ADN and BSN prepared nurses, *J Prof Nurs* 3(4):218-225, 1987.

to note that managed care has health promotion, not illness treatment, as one of its primary goals. As the 1990s progressed, several factors led to the development of a variety of managed care models (Figure 14-6), which included the rising cost of providing health care benefits, growing taxpayer unrest about the expense of tax-funded health care programs, unequal access to services, and concerns about quality.

Types of managed care organizations

Managed care organizations (MCOs) can be categorized into four basic models: health maintenance organizations (HMOs), preferred provider organizations (PPOs), point-of-service (POS) plans, and physician hospital organizations (PHOs).

Health maintenance organizations. In contrast to the traditional fee-for-service system, the **health maintenance organization (HMO)** is a system in which a defined group of people receives health care services for a predetermined fixed fee. This method of financing is called **capitation,** and it is paid on a per-member per-month basis. The same amount is paid to the provider each month regardless of whether services were provided or how much the services cost. The fee is usually negotiated for a period of 1 to 3 years. The patient's access to services is coordinated and managed by a primary care provider. The primary care provider, sometimes called a **gatekeeper,** is responsible for all referrals for tests and to specialists. Keeping patients healthy means that the primary care provider gets to keep more of the fee. Some people worry that this will discourage gatekeepers from ordering diagnostic tests and referring patients to specialists, even when indicated.

Preferred provider organizations. The **preferred provider organization (PPO)** contracts with independent providers such as physicians and hospitals for a negotiated discount for the services provided to its members.

Point-of-service organizations. The **point-of-service (POS) organization** is a form of MCO with more options. Members may choose to receive services within the defined network, or they may go outside the network and pay a higher deductible or copayment.

Physician hospital organizations. As managed care organizations penetrated the market and threatened the financial viability of hospitals and many physicians' practices, the providers of health services created another type of organization, **physician hospital organizations (PHOs).** The PHO is a separate corporation formed by a hospital and a group of its medical staff for the purpose of joint contracting with managed care organizations. This structure allows hospitals and physicians to work together to negotiate fees for services directly with self-insured employers and managed care organizations.

Nurse's role in managed care

Registered nurses are used extensively throughout managed care systems. Many HMOs use advanced practice nurses in the primary care role in ambulatory and community settings. Another key role for the registered nurse is that of case manager, discussed earlier in this chapter. Nurses also serve in a triage role, deciding the most appropriate course of intervention. Nurses are often employed as utilization reviewers to determine the most appropriate and cost-efficient level of care. This role often facilitates moving a

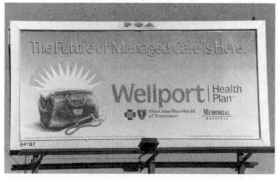

Figure 14-6
Managed care has created a highly competitive health care market, as this billboard illustrates. *(Photo by Kelly Whalen.)*

patient out of the hospital and into a rehabilitation center, a nursing home, or home, with home health services.

The consumers' perspective toward managed care and their experiences with it vary. Some consumers have good access, a full range of services, providers they trust, and lower costs. Others have experienced access problems, denial of treatment, and limited coverage. As consumers became more educated, they began to fight for their rights to health care through political reform and the legal system. The collective power of consumers has created changes in the health care system, mainly in terms of safeguards to protect patients.

Changes in consumers' expectations

The computer age has afforded access to global information at explosive rates. Society has embraced the information technology age and has become increasingly dependent on instant global news, information, and service. The proliferation of Internet websites has dramatically affected the knowledge and expectations of health care consumers.

In 2004 95 million U.S. adults reported using the Internet to obtain health information, compared to 22 million in 1998 (Fox, 2005). According to the Pew Internet & American Life Project, 80 percent of Internet users in 2005 had searched online for information on at least one major health topic. Most of these Internet users searched for five major health topics or more. In fact, 58 percent of health information users report that they have found the Internet to be their most important source of information when dealing with a loved one's health crisis (Madden and Fox, 2006). Thus more and more Americans rely on the Internet when making health decisions.

Health-related websites offer a wide range of topics, such as wellness, nutrition, general health information, live surgery and births, women's health, medication reference books, government health agencies, professional associations, referrals; information about hospitals, physicians, managed care, patient rights; and libraries filled with medical textbooks and journals. Live interactive websites even offer diagnosis, treatment, and medication prescription services without a hands-on assessment and examination. As the number of Latinos in the United States continues to rise, many health-related websites offer information in English and Spanish. As mentioned earlier, nurses have a responsibility to assist patients to find reliable health information online. Box 14-10 highlights the top 10 most useful consumer health websites.

Health Care's Response to Managed Care and Consumer Expectations

The impact of managed care and advanced information technology has forced the health care system to undergo massive transformation to meet the demands of new reimbursement structures and consumer expectations. The reengineering of health care organizations has included the redesign not only of patient care delivery but also of the organizational structures necessary to support the changes.

Reengineering

During the 1990s health care organizations recognized the full impact of managed care and changes in consumer expectations. Hospitals were so complex and bureaucratic that many were failing to deliver high-quality services consistently. In health care, for example, it was not unusual for a patient staying 5 to 7 days in a typical hospital to travel by wheelchair or stretcher 8 or 9 miles during that stay. A simple laboratory test might require 40 to 60 separate activities or steps before results could be reported. Excessive and duplicative paperwork and trivial tasks burdened care providers and left patients dissatisfied and angry. The patient was no longer the center of the system. At times, it seemed patients and families were nuisances that got in the way of bureaucratic activities and record keeping.

Health care organizations recognized that becoming more efficient through reengineering while focusing on patient-centered care was

Box 14-10 MLA's "Top Ten" Most Useful Consumer Health Websites (Listed Alphabetically)

www.cancer.gov—National Cancer Institute (available in Spanish)
www.cdc.gov—Centers for Disease Control and Prevention (available in Spanish)
www.familydoctor.org—American Academy of Family Physicians (available in Spanish)
www.healthfinder.gov—Office of Disease Prevention and Health Promotion (available in Spanish)
www.hivinsite.ucsf.edu—HIV InSite University of California, San Francisco, School of Medicine
www.kidshealth.org—Kidshealth® Nemours Foundation's Center for Children's Health Media
www.mayoclinic.com—Mayo Foundation for Medical Education and Research
www.medem.com/medLB/medlib_entry.cfm—Medem: an information partnership of medical societies
www.MEDLINEplus.gov—United States National Library of Medicine and National Institutes of Health (available in Spanish)
www.noah-health.org—NOAH: New York Online Access to Health (available in Spanish)

From Medical Library Association: *MLA's "top ten" most useful consumer health websites*, 2005, available online: www.mlanet.org/resources/userguide.html#5.

imperative for survival. **Reengineering** is the "fundamental rethinking and radical redesign of business processes to bring about dramatic improvement in performance" (Hammer and Stanton, 1995). **Patient-centered care,** also known as patient-focused care, means placing the patient at the center of activity and designing processes that efficiently and effectively attain desired patient outcomes.

Management experts believe that reducing layers of management is an essential component of any reengineering initiative. One key to the new organization and structure is decentralization. **Decentralization** empowers staff, allowing them to exercise their own good judgment rather than waiting to be told what to do. Decision-making authority is given to those most affected by the decision, rather than being limited to a few executives or managers. This means fewer layers in an organizational chart and is in agreement with the philosophy of shared governance that all professionals should be encouraged to use their talents fully. For empowerment to be effective, the board of directors and top executives must clearly articulate their vision, goals, and expectations so that all employees understand the direction of the organization and their roles in it.

Reengineering and patient-centered care are also accomplished by cross-functional teams, who are involved with all aspects of achieving a specific patient-centered outcome. **Cross-functional teams** are composed of people from all areas of the organization who contribute to a particular process and outcome. They redesign, from scratch, how the work will be done and who will do it and in what time frame and location. In some new models, staff members are cross-trained to be able to complete several different tasks, each of which was formerly performed by a different worker. Workers who are cross-trained to perform different tasks are known as **multiskilled workers.** For example, a single worker may be trained to collect admission demographic information, draw blood for tests ordered, and perform an electrocardiogram. With these changes, patient satisfaction is typically higher than with the older fragmented bureaucratic methods.

When done well, reengineering addresses the purpose of the business; the organizational culture needed for success, processes, and performance; and the people, knowledge, and skills needed to accomplish the redesigned work. When done poorly, reengineering is often a euphemism for downsizing or staff reductions or layoffs. Although it is true that as the work is redesigned fewer people may be needed, staff reduction is not the main goal of reengineering. Box 14-11 lists key components for successful reengineering.

New organizational models

After more than 20 years of restructuring efforts in hospitals, there are several basic organizational models in use, each with numerous variations. Five representative structures are described below. These models overlap and few "pure" models are in use.

Functional model. The traditional functional model clearly defines each major function of the organization and establishes clear lines of managerial authority. Examples of the major functions are inpatient care, outpatient care, surgery, professional services, facility operations, marketing and planning, and human resources.

Service line model. The service line model establishes management responsibilities around specific types of services wherever they occur in the hospital or in its associated clinics and offices. Examples of major service lines include cardiology, orthopedics, oncology, obstetrics, ambulatory services, and behavioral health.

Matrix model. The matrix model is a complex model with multiple authority and support systems. This model is a blend of the functional and service line models. In the matrix model there is one overall manager who directs dual lines of authority. It is a team concept with one manager overseeing the specialized functional areas and another manager providing the expertise to the particular service. In this model some employees report to two managers. For example, the housekeeping supervisor in the surgical department would report to both the head of housekeeping and the director of the surgical services.

Process model. The process model is a newer approach that organizes management of care around phases in the process of health care delivery. These phases include access, treatment, transition, and evaluation. Responsibilities of managers in the process model span all departments.

Regional model. The regional model is another new organizational model appropriate for complex health care systems that grew from acquisitions made by hospitals. It is organized by type of service provider. Examples include home health, nursing homes, managed care organizations, rehabilitation centers, and smaller hospitals all of which may be part of a larger health care system.

Maintaining Quality in Health Care Agencies

Maintaining high-quality services should be the goal of every health care agency. As pressure increases to control costs, it becomes evenmore important to ensure that quality is not sacrificed simply to save dollars. This can be accomplished in a variety of ways, chiefly through accreditation and quality care initiatives.

Box **14-11** **Keys to Successful Reengineering**

- Strong leadership
- Support from the top (e.g., financial, cultural, time, resources)
- Team members who love ambiguity, creativity, risk taking, and holism
- An irreverence for the past
- Optimism, persistence
- Ability to answer these questions: What is our business? What culture do we want? How do we need to do our work? What people do we want to work with?

Accreditation of health care agencies

Health care organizations such as hospitals, home health agencies, and long term care facilities seek accreditation through one of two accrediting bodies approved by the Centers for Medicare and Medicaid Services (CMS). They are the Joint Commission on the Accreditation of Healthcare Organizations (JCAHO), a not-for-profit organization that serves as the nation's predominant standards-setting and accrediting body in health care (JCAHO, 2006), and the Healthcare Facilities Accreditation Program (HFAP). The goal of accreditation is to improve patient outcomes. Accreditation is important and requires that a number of standards be met in every department. Considerable resources of time and money are spent making sure accreditation criteria, set by these external accrediting bodies, are met. An additional strategy through which most organizations choose to work internally toward improvement in patient outcomes is continuous quality improvement.

Continuous quality improvement/total quality management

The concept of **continuous quality improvement (CQI)** was first developed by management expert W. Edwards Deming in the 1940s when he suggested that managers in industry should rely on groups of employees, which he called quality circles, as they made decisions about how work was to be done. In today's health care systems, CQI, also called total quality management (TQM), is one of the most important concepts borrowed from industry. Rather than trying to identify mistakes after they have occurred, these systems focus on establishing procedures for ensuring high-quality patient care. Using quality improvement concepts, groups of employees from different departments decide how care will be provided. They decide what outcomes are desired and design systems and assign roles and activities to create those outcomes. Every effort is made to anticipate potential problems and prevent their occurrence. Management delegates authority to the providers of services to plan and carry out quality improvement programs. Programs in CQI/TQM reinforce the belief that quality is everyone's responsibility.

Recently **performance improvement (PI)** has been used to describe organizational efforts to improve corporate performance. Incorporating aspects of quality management, PI focuses efforts on increasing individual and group competence and productivity. When done well, the company and its employees and customers gain many advantages. Employees who are more efficient may find job enrichment opportunities. When done poorly, however, quality can be compromised in the process of increasing productivity. Reduction in labor force is often a result of these efforts and can lead to lowered employee morale.

Nurses are actively involved in quality and performance improvement and in accreditation processes, but these activities are not the responsibility of nursing alone. They are institution-wide initiatives, and everyone, at all levels, gets involved. Working together to improve patient care builds cooperation among departments and clinical disciplines and boosts morale.

Tomorrow's health care workers are facing an ever-changing work environment. They will probably have 7 to 10 different jobs during an average work career rather than the 3 jobs or fewer held by previous generations. Even when employed in the same position, they should expect that position to undergo major evolution and change. You may ask yourself, "How can I thrive in this constantly changing environment?" The following suggestions should help you keep your options open, even as the health care system and nursing's role within the system change:

- Take every opportunity to learn new skills.
- Read extensively both inside and outside your field.
- Identify emerging trends and new opportunities.
- Find new ways to apply your knowledge and skills.
- Volunteer for community activities that will stretch your skills, help you learn new ones, and allow you to meet people who can be helpful to you.

- Keep your resume current, but do not change jobs too often because this implies instability.
- Develop flexibility, including openness to new challenges.
- Actively participate in professional organizations.

FINANCING HEALTH CARE

The United States health care delivery system continues to experience dramatic reform early in the twenty-first century, particularly in the area of health care finance. There is renewed vigor to the public debate over financing health care in this country. Health care costs continue to climb, as does the number of uninsured citizens. Legislative reforms and managed care efforts have had mixed success at cutting health care costs and increasing access to health care. The nation's dilemma remains: how to provide high-quality health care services to all citizens while keeping costs down.

In 2004 the nation's health care expenditures reached $1.9 trillion and consumed 16 percent of the gross domestic product (GDP) (Centers for Medicare and Medicaid Services, 2006b). This represents a 7.9 percent increase in health care spending from the previous year. If this trend is allowed to continue until the year 2010, 40 percent of all national resources will be spent on health care. Estimates for the year 2015 indicate that health care costs are expected to reach $4 trillion. Yet the health of American citizens is not as good as it should be. As a result, almost everyone agrees that there is a crisis in health care and that reform is needed.

Americans are concerned about rising health care costs. Today the public's concern is about the ability of our health care system to maintain the Medicare program, provide for the growing number of uninsured, and ensure the quality of managed care. It seems that at a time when health care breakthroughs are at an all-time high, public support for the system that created those breakthroughs is eroding.

Financial issues profoundly affect nurses and nursing practice. The financial component of health care affects nurses professionally, in their nursing practice, and personally, in the type of insurance and health services they and their families are able to afford. Therefore students of professional nursing need to understand the overall economic context in which nursing care is provided. Several major concepts necessary to understanding health care finance will be explored, including basic economic theory, the economics of nursing care, a brief historical review of the causes of health care cost escalation, cost-containment efforts, current methods of payment, and the impact of cost containment on nursing care. Criteria to evaluate health reform proposals are summarized.

Basic Economic Theory

Nursing school curricula do not typically require undergraduates to take courses in economics, yet there is an urgent need for nurses to understand the economic context in which they practice. Economics influences the type and quality of health services provided, as well as employment opportunities for nurses.

Supply and demand

A basic economic theory is the law of supply and demand. According to this theory, a normal economic system consists of two parts: suppliers, who provide goods and services; and consumers, who demand and use goods and services. In a monetary environment, that is, one in which money is used as a unit of exchange, consumers exchange money for desired goods and services.

In an efficient marketplace, the market price of goods and services serves to create an equilibrium in which supply roughly equals demand, and demand roughly equals supply. When demand exceeds supply, prices rise. When supply exceeds demand, prices fall. The relationship between price and equilibrium can be illustrated by a clothing store. During an unusually mild winter, for example, the demand for heavy coats is likely to be low. Because demand is low, manufacturers cut back on production, and retailers stop ordering coats and place their current stock of coats on sale. If the sale price is low enough, however, people will continue to buy coats. Through fluctuations in supply and demand, created by price, equilibrium is approached. This example illustrates the principle of price sensitivity; that is, a change in demand for goods or services is a function of the change in the price of those goods or services (Finkler, 2000). Figure 14-7 illustrates the relationships among price, supply, and demand.

Is Basic Economic Theory Applicable to Health Care?

Health care as a right or privilege

In a free-market economy, consumption of any good or service is determined by an individual's ability to pay. In a pure free market, a portion of the population would be denied health care if they were unable to pay. People who support this position consider health care a privilege. Others believe that everyone should have access to basic health care and consider health care a right.

Despite the United States' leanings toward a free-market economy in general, most Americans consider health care a right, not a privilege. Rather than allowing economically disadvantaged citizens to do without health services, the federal government has taken steps to ensure certain groups have access to health care services through publicly funded programs such as Medicare and Medicaid. Although this is generally considered an ethical policy, it is nevertheless a policy decision that interferes with the functioning of free-market principles.

Price sensitivity in health care

In the days before health insurance existed, people paid their own medical bills, and providers set their fees with some sensitivity to what patients could pay. When costs were high, patients complained. Health insurance created an indirect payment structure, **third-party payment,** that removed price sensitivity from the concern of most health care consumers because they pay only a small portion of the actual costs. A third party (the employer, insurance company, or government) pays the rest. If someone other than the consumer pays, demand can increase because the consumer is insensitive to cost. This is an important point to keep in mind when reviewing the history of health care finance. History has demonstrated that when there is little or no out-of-pocket expense to the consumer, economic equilibrium is upset because consumers use more health care services (Jacob and Rapoport, 2002).

Additional influences on the health care market

Economists have identified a number of other factors that affect the health care market in ways that violate the assumptions surrounding an

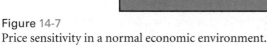

Figure 14-7
Price sensitivity in a normal economic environment.

effective free-market system. For example, consumers cannot always control demand for health care services. With ordinary products, a consumer can delay a purchase until there is a sale or forego the purchase altogether. Health care is different because often health care needs are immediate. The consumer might suffer serious harm or even death by a delay in seeking services. Thus the health care market differs from the free market system in several key ways. Box 14-12 summarizes some of the factors that reduce the efficient functioning of free-market economics in the health care market.

Economics of Nursing Care

Historically, nurses were unconcerned with the cost of care, believing all patients were entitled to high-quality nursing care regardless of ability to pay. Until fairly recently, few efforts were made to determine the actual cost of nursing care. The average hospital bill included the cost of nursing services in the general category of "room rate," just as housekeeping services are included in the room rate. In the past, the hospital census (number of patients) was used to determine the number of nurses needed. This worked fairly well when payment was retrospective. With the advent of prospective payment, however, it was imperative for hospitals to determine their staffing needs more efficiently.

In the past, it was assumed that the cost of nurses was a major part of hospital expenses. During tough economic times, the first cost reduction efforts were therefore aimed at nursing. Studies in the mid-1980s found that nursing accounted for only 20 to 28 percent of the costs of hospitalization for two thirds of the diagnosis-related groups (DRGs) examined (McKibben, 1985). Costing nursing services and developing standardized reimbursements based on costs were expected to enhance the ability of nurse managers to control nursing resources and negotiate for a fair share of hospital financial resources.

Not knowing the exact costs of nursing services limits nurses' ability to determine what high-quality nursing care costs and to calculate the number of hours of nursing care it takes to provide service for each DRG. Determining the best **skill mix,** the ratio of registered nurses to licensed practical nurses and nursing assistants in each hospital unit, is also impaired when the cost of nursing care is unknown. It has long been recognized that different patients require different amounts of nursing time, depending in large part on how sick they are. Therefore **patient classification systems (PCS)** have been developed to identify patients' needs for nursing care in quantitative terms in order to help hospitals determine the need for nursing resources.

When the drive to provide high-quality nursing care meets the constraints of cost containment head-on, it creates a very difficult situation. What nurses hope, as both providers and consumers of health care, is that quality will not suffer because of the emphasis on "the bottom line." The financial realities that affect the institutions in which 56.2 percent of nurses practice—hospitals—cannot be ignored. To stay in business, hospitals must make at least enough money to pay personnel, maintain buildings and equipment, and pay suppliers of goods and services.

The leadership of the American Nurses Association (ANA) has been outspoken in their assertion that overzealous cost-containment efforts have led to lower quality hospital care. A strong boost to their contention that the number and mix of nurses in a hospital make a difference in patient outcomes came early in the twenty-first century with research that showed an increased patient death rate with higher nurse:patient ratios (Aiken, Clarke, Sloane et al, 2002). Other recent research focused on comparing the cost of nurse staffing in hospitals to the cost savings gained through improved patient care (Needleman, Buerhaus, Stewart et al, 2006). As research continues to demonstrate the link between nursing and quality of care, the demand for nursing services will continue to flourish.

History of Health Care Finance

Before 1940 more than 90 percent of Americans either paid directly from their own pockets for

---

Box **14-12** Barriers to a Free Market Economy in Health Care

Poor Consumer Information

Individual consumers are not accustomed to "shopping" for the best available prices for medical services, supplies, and equipment. Even when the consumer is motivated to compare costs, getting that information from the suppliers of health care is difficult and time-consuming. Most consumers require services quickly and cannot afford long delays to seek information, even if they have the expertise to search out the needed information.

Ineffective Pricing System

When the price of services is based on "reasonable and customary costs of similar services" in an area, health care providers have an incentive to continue to increase their prices rather than compete by lowering prices. Eventually the new, higher price becomes the "reasonable and customary" price. Reform efforts have had some success at reducing the impact of this phenomenon by establishing prospective funding and capping reimbursement for the cost of selected services.

Health Care Providers' Interests May Conflict With Consumers' Interests

Health care providers have economic interests that can be in opposition to consumer interests. Physicians, for example, act both as suppliers of health care and as demanders of patient services. When physicians are partners or stockholders in services, such as laboratories or radiographic facilities, they are more likely to order such tests, according to studies by the Department of Health and Human Services. Conversely, HMO or PPO physicians who receive incentives for not referring patients to specialists are less likely to do so.

Cost Efficiency Is Not Always a Motivator for Suppliers

Although businesses are expected to operate with cost-efficiency, others, particularly some nonprofit organizations, may be influenced by other factors. By law, nonprofits cannot keep or distribute profit or surplus of funds at the end of the fiscal year, but there is no law that dictates how they spend that money. Most nonprofits operate efficiently and at the lowest cost to consumers; others have been found to use their funds to provide amenities and perks for staff and board members, such as plush exercise facilities, all-expense-paid trips, or purchases of private boxes at sports stadiums.

Modified from Maurer FA: Financing of health care: context for community health nursing. In Smith C, Maurer FA, editors: *Community health nursing: theory and practice*, ed 2, Philadelphia, 2000, WB Saunders.

health care or depended on charity care. Few had private health insurance. Public insurance programs, such as Medicare and Medicaid, did not exist. Following World War II, most industrialized countries began publicly financed health care systems that provided care for all citizens. The United States, however, did not adopt a public, universal access system, choosing instead to continue the private, fee-for-service system.

Growth of private insurance

In 1943 the Internal Revenue Service (IRS) ruled that health benefits paid by employers were not taxable as income. Employers began to offer health benefits as compensation to employees. At the same time, states granted tax-exempt status to private insurance companies, such as Blue Cross and Blue Shield, and private insurers grew dramatically. By 1960 two thirds of non-elderly

Americans had private health insurance, mostly paid for by employers.

Hill-Burton Act

In 1946 the U.S. Congress passed the Hospital Survey and Construction Act, also known as the **Hill-Burton Act.** This law called for and funded surveys of states' needs for hospitals, paid for planning hospitals and public health centers, and provided partial funding for constructing and equipping them. The Hill-Burton Act spurred community hospital construction. With accessible, new, well-equipped hospitals in many towns and employer-paid health insurance a standard job benefit, the stage was set for increased consumer demand, leading to dramatic increases in the utilization of hospitals and health care services.

Rise of public insurance programs

The problem of paying for health care for the unemployed and the elderly was not solved by the advent of private insurance, and many continued to receive inadequate care. In 1965 Congress responded by approving two public insurance programs to cover these groups: Medicare for the elderly and certain disabled people, and Medicaid for the poor. These programs were designed to ensure that citizens who were uninsured by employers and unable to afford their own private health insurance would be protected. Medicare and Medicaid will be discussed in detail later in this chapter.

With the formation of these public insurance programs, a unique public/private partnership system of insurance that would care for all seemed to be in place. Unfortunately, that partnership has not lived up to anyone's expectations and, more than 40 years later, the United States still does not have a system that guarantees **universal care** for all Americans.

Retrospective reimbursement

Originally, both public and private insurance plans were based on **retrospective** (after-the-fact) **reimbursement.** This meant that when a patient was admitted to the hospital with pneumonia, for example, a request was sent to the insurer for reimbursement for whatever services were rendered (such as chest x-rays, blood work, physical examinations, and antibiotic therapy). Depending on the terms of the patient's insurance policy and the level of the patient's **deductible** (the portion paid yearly before insurance coverage begins), the hospital was reimbursed for much, or even most, of the charges. **Copayments** (the percentage of charges the patient pays) were low, often as low as 10 percent. Using retrospective reimbursement, the cost of services to insured consumers of health care was extremely low or zero. Because neither the providers of health care nor the consumers (patients) were concerned about cost, the demand for health care services became virtually insatiable, driving costs up dramatically (Jacob and Rapoport, 2002).

Early cost-containment initiatives

In an attempt to contain costs, new federal legislation in the 1960s required states to develop comprehensive health planning. At least one agency per state was established and empowered to review the health care needs of communities in order to reduce costs and duplication of service. A **certificate of need (CON)** had to be approved by the health planning agency before new construction, expansion of existing facilities, or major equipment purchases were permitted. Even today, CONs are only issued to projects that can demonstrate a real need in a community.

By 1975 additional serious **cost-containment** efforts were under way, stimulated by the concerns of politicians, consumer groups, and employers about costs. Some states initiated rate setting, which placed limits on reimbursement to health care providers for services. One important strategy was a move toward replacing retrospective payment for services with **prospective payment systems (PPS).** In prospective payment systems, providers, such as physicians and hospitals, receive payment on a per-case basis, regardless of the cost to the provider to deliver the services. Prospective payment systems were developed because of escalating costs in the

Medicare and Medicaid programs. It became apparent that basic changes in payment mechanisms were needed.

The passage of the Tax Equity and Fiscal Responsibility Act (TEFRA) in 1982 dramatically restructured the payment method for Medicare to a prospective payment system based on diagnosis-related groups (DRGs), which are described later in this chapter. Prospective payment stimulated competition among health care providers by awarding incentives to those who operated in a cost-effective manner. Because prospective payment has the potential to encourage providers to undertreat patients to reduce costs, quality management initiatives were implemented to protect consumers.

Continued Escalation of Health Care Costs

Despite those early comprehensive cost-planning efforts, health care costs continued to rise in the 1980s and 1990s. Factors that have affected costs include inflation, new technologies and drugs, increased demand for health care services, and the impact of fraud and abuse.

Inflation

Inflation generally affects all business sectors but has tended to escalate faster in health care than in other segments of the economy. Even during economic climates of low to moderate inflation, health care costs continue to consume a greater portion of the GDP, limiting what can be spent on other segments of the economy.

New technologies and drugs

Another reason for the rise in costs is related to the demand for and development of new technologies and new drugs. In fact, prescription drug spending is growing faster than any other segment of health care costs (Cowan, Catlin, Smith et al, 2004). Modern medical care depends on advanced technologies that were not even dreamed of a few decades ago. Equipment such as magnetic resonance imaging (MRI) and procedures such as angioplasty and hip replacement are now commonplace. New technologies are extremely costly: A single x-ray machine can cost up to $250,000, and more advanced types of diagnostic imaging machines can cost more than $2 million. Health care costs are also driven upward by new lifestyle drugs, such as Viagra, a male potency drug, and Zoloft, an antidepressant, which had revenues of $1.6 billion and $3.3 billion, respectively, in 2005 (Pfizer, 2005).

Increased demand for health care services

Demographics also play a role in escalating health care costs. The United States has experienced rapid growth in both the elderly and the uninsured nonelderly populations. Medicare and Medicaid have improved access for the poor and elderly, two groups that previously had limited access because of inability to pay. Because older persons are more likely to have chronic illnesses, their demand for health care services exceeds that of younger segments of the population. The elderly population is expected to continue to rise, thus increasing the demand for services. In 2005 more than 36 million Americans were older than 65 years of age. By 2020 this figure will increase to greater than 54 million, or 16.3 percent of the population (U.S. Census Bureau, 2006). Furthermore, with the total population of the United States reaching 300 million, overall population growth will continue to fuel the demand for health care services.

Fraud and abuse of payment systems

Fraud and abuse of payment systems account for continued cost escalation. An estimated $75 billion of the United States' annual health expenditures may be attributable to fraud, including as much as 20 percent of all workers' compensation claims and up to 10 percent in Medicare losses.

Health care providers such as physicians, clinics, and hospitals are on the honor system, but some intentionally cheat the system. In response, the Department of Health and Human Services developed Operation Restore Trust in 1995 to combat fraud in the Medicare program. This program's stringent oversight of health care charges has successfully reduced unnecessary costs by about half. Despite these efforts, problems continue.

The result of upwardly spiraling costs—fueled by technology, demand for services, and fraud—is that health care costs accounted for an increasing portion of U.S. resources. Most economists believe that this trend cannot continue without further damaging the nation's economy.

Cost-Containment Measures Revisited

Both public and private health care entities have a vested interest in containing costs. The continuous escalation in health care costs during the 1980s and 1990s caused both public and private insurers to rethink past containment strategies and to institute a variety of newer measures designed to reduce costs. Sometimes alone, sometimes in tandem with one another, and frequently with one sector leading and the other following, new initiatives have been developed and older ones revitalized. Several cost-containment entities and legislative efforts of which students should be aware are described below.

Centers for Medicare and Medicaid Services (CMS)

The **Centers for Medicare and Medicaid Services (CMS),** formerly the Health Care Financing Administration (HCFA), is a federal cost-containment program. Its purpose is to establish and enforce standards and monitor care in both programs. It has the authority to enforce these standards for hospitals, nursing homes and other long term care facilities, laboratories, clinics, and other health entities that care for Medicare and Medicaid patients. It is also responsible for establishing regulation and oversight of any changes legislated by Congress to either program.

The CMS does not directly administer Medicare or Medicaid. It contracts private insurance agencies, such as Blue Cross and Blue Shield, to service the Medicare program. When patients or their families have questions about coverage or payments, nurses advise them to contact the insurer who administers the program in their area, not the CMS. While retaining oversight of the Medicaid program, the CMS has ceded administration of that program to the states. CMS publications are a good source of information on health care costs, government share of funding, descriptions of the populations served by both programs, and evaluations of program effectiveness (www.cms.gov).

Professional review organizations (PROs)

Professional review organizations (PROs) are designed to monitor the quality of care received by health care consumers and to ensure that care meets professional standards. The peer review process is a combined public and private effort. These organizations are usually private, but their functions in certain situations are a requirement of federal regulation.

Peer review started as a voluntary review process that brought prestige to hospitals passing review. Professional review organizations became mandatory as a result of Medicare regulations, which stipulated that all hospitals receiving Medicare payments had to submit to peer review. Medicare required that hospital admissions and lengths of stay be examined to ensure that a patient's health and treatment needs were best met in a hospital environment. If a patient is hospitalized unnecessarily or for a period of time longer than the PRO determines to be appropriate or if procedures are performed that the PRO determines are unnecessary, the hospital is denied Medicare reimbursement for the extra days and the unnecessary procedures. This causes hospitals and providers to be careful about whom they admit, how long they allow patients to stay, and what procedures are performed while patients are hospitalized.

Professional review organizations first concentrated on care delivered in hospitals because of Medicare regulations. Private-sector insurance companies expanded the peer review process into other areas, such as outpatient and community-based services. In addition, managed care organizations (MCOs) developed a peer review process. The National Committee for Quality Assurance (NCQA) is a not-for-profit organization that measures quality through a set of quality measurements (HEDIS) based on clinical outcomes and patient satisfaction (National Committee for Quality Assurance, 2006). Though peer review is voluntary, more than half of the MCOs in the United States, including Medicare and Medicaid programs, participate in NCQA review. What started as a voluntary annual review process became a required protocol for Medicare, Medicaid, and private insurance reimbursement contracts.

Diagnosis-related groups (DRGs)

Diagnosis-related groups (DRGs) were developed as part of the reform of Medicare payments into a prospective payment system. They place diagnoses with similar resource consumptions and length-of-stay patterns into a single category. Diseases are grouped into 495 DRGs, or categories, for reimbursement purposes. An example of a DRG is pneumonia. For each DRG, the Medicare system has predetermined a fair price for hospital services based on averages. This represents the amount the hospital is paid by Medicare to treat patients in that particular DRG. If the hospital's costs exceed the preestablished reimbursement rate, it loses money. If the hospital is able to treat the patient successfully for less than the established reimbursement rate, it may keep the excess.

Private insurers have benefited from this cost-containment initiative because they tend to establish private reimbursement rates at the same level the federal government uses for reimbursing hospitals for Medicare DRGs.

Block grants

Combined with the enactment of DRGs and prospective payment, federal reform efforts in the 1980s included block grants to states. Block grants changed the funding mechanism the federal government employed to supply monies for combined federal-state programs. Instead of sharing the expense of a program, such as matching a state's expenditures on Medicaid, the block grant program gave the state a set amount of money, depending on several factors, including

caseload. The state government then decided how to spend the federal and state dollars on behalf of Medicaid patients.

Since inception, block grants have reduced the proportion of health program costs paid by the federal government, while the states' shares have increased. At the same time, states have been mandated by federal requirements to provide specific health services to Medicaid patients, such as poor children and the elderly. Block grants have dramatically increased the number of dollars state budgets have been required to expend on health care, thereby forcing either tax increases or reductions in other state-funded programs.

Reform proposals in the mid-1990s brought further reductions in federal block grants and frequent proposals to lower federal standards for mandated care, such as in nursing homes. There are added concerns for the Medicaid program related to budget crises that most states have experienced in recent years resulting from reduced tax revenues and increased health care costs. Concerned health professionals believe that increased state budget constraints will leave the poor, especially children and the elderly, at greater risk for reduced access to care and lower quality of care.

Continued expansion of managed care

Private insurers and employers have increasingly relied on the managed care concept to lower their health care costs. By 2001 managed care had become the largest provider of health care in the United States. More than 100 million Americans are enrolled either in private-sector or in public-sector managed care programs (U.S. Census Bureau, 2006). Managed care programs limit consumers' choices of treatment options or provider of care (or both) but are not intended to reduce quality of care.

Although the private sector initiated managed care, the public sector soon followed. The Medicare program has allowed seniors to use managed care organizations for some time and in 1998 unveiled several new health care options for seniors with a managed care emphasis. Federal legislation allowed states to pilot the use of managed care in the Medicaid program, and legislation in 1997 expanded that use to most of the clients in Medicaid programs. For the foreseeable future, managed care is here to stay in both public and private sectors.

Current Methods of Payment for Health Care

There are four major methods of payment for health care in use today: private insurance, Medicare, Medicaid, and personal payment. Workers' compensation is an additional mechanism for financing some health care services. Each of these is briefly explained in the following paragraphs.

Private insurance

Private insurance, also called voluntary insurance, is a system wherein insurance premiums either are paid by insured individuals or their employers or are shared between individuals and employers. Periodic payments (**premiums**) are paid into the insurance plan, and certain health care benefits are covered as long as the premiums are paid. Early in the development of private insurance, many treatments were covered only if they were performed in an inpatient (hospital) setting. This was one of the features that tended to drive up the cost of services. Today most insurers stipulate that costs of hospitalization are reimbursable only if treatment cannot be performed on an outpatient basis.

Medicare

Medicare, or Title XVIII of the Social Security Act, is a nationwide federal health insurance program established in 1965. Medicare is available to people ages 65 and older, regardless of the recipient's income. It also covers certain disabled individuals and people requiring dialysis or kidney transplants. Medicare has four basic programs. The first program, known as Part A, covers inpatient hospitalization, skilled care in nursing facilities, hospice care, and some home health care. Part B is a supplementary medical insurance program that covers visits to physicians' offices and other outpatient services. Part C offers a variety of managed care options instead of the fee-for-service programs of Parts A and B (Harris, 2003). The Prescription Drug Plan is the latest addition to Medicare and is an additional supplementary insurance program to cover prescription drug costs. In addition to the four basic parts of Medicare, the Medigap and Medicare Advantage programs are available to Medicare-eligible individuals as supplemental insurance sold by private insurance companies to help fill the "gap" between Medicare and out-of-pocket costs. Thus Medicare offers several choices to its recipients.

Originally intended to be a no-cost or low-cost program for the elderly, the cost of participating in Medicare has risen steadily. By 2006 Part A required participants to pay a deductible of $942 for hospitalization, and Part B required an annual $124 deductible and a monthly premium of $88.50 (Centers for Medicare and Medicaid Services, 2006). Although the program was originally designed to be all-inclusive, many elderly people now find they cannot afford to participate in Medicare. Ironically, some elderly are so poor that they qualify for Medicaid assistance in paying their Medicare premiums. For the most recent updates on Medicare, online resources include www.cdc.gov and www.medicare.gov.

Medicaid

Medicaid, or Title XIX of the Social Security Act, is a group of jointly funded federal-state programs for low-income, elderly, blind, and disabled individuals. It, too, was established in 1965. There are broad federal guidelines, but states have some flexibility in how they administer the program. People must meet eligibility requirements determined by each state. Eligibility depends on income and varies from state to state. Rates of payment also vary, with some states providing far higher payments than others. The amount the federal government contributes to Medicaid varies from a minimum of 50 percent of total costs to a maximum of 76.8 percent. The differences in eligibility and payment rates lead to wide variations in the level of care provided to the poor in different states. In contrast to those on Medicare, people who receive Medicaid are not required to pay any fees to participate. Table 14-2 highlights the similarities and differences in the Medicare and Medicaid programs.

Personal (out-of-pocket) payment

Personal payment for health care services is the least common method. The last several years have seen an increase in personal payments resulting from rising costs in copayments and deductibles determined by insurers. Few people can afford **out-of-pocket payment** for more than the most basic health services. At today's prices, an illness or injury severe enough to require hospitalization can quickly exhaust a family's financial reserves, forcing them into bankruptcy. Generally, only those people without access to some form of private group insurance or public insurance rely on personal payment. It sometimes takes years to pay a single, large medical bill.

Workers' compensation

Workers' compensation constitutes a small proportion of insurance coverage. The program varies from state to state but generally covers only workers who are injured on the job. It usually covers treatment for injuries and weekly payments during the time the worker is absent from work for injury-related causes. In the case of accidental death, the worker's family receives compensation. Companies are required by law to contribute to a compensation fund from which money is withdrawn when accidental injuries or deaths occur at work.

Figure 14-8 represents the proportion each of the major payment methods contributed to the funding of health care services in the United States in 2004.

Health Care Finance Challenges

Current challenges related to health care finance include the number of uninsured Americans, quality of care, limits and restrictions imposed by managed care, prescription drug costs, and malpractice costs. Each of these issues is explored in the following paragraphs.

Continuing crisis: uninsured Americans

The number of uninsured Americans continues to grow at an alarming rate. In 2004 an estimated 45.8 million or 15.7 percent of Americans had no health insurance (DeNavas-Walt, Proctor, and Lee, 2004). When the temporarily uninsured are added to the count, the number of persons without health insurance is even greater. Of the number of uninsured Americans, 8.3 million are children (under 18 years old), representing 11.2

Table 14-2   FACTS ABOUT MEDICARE AND MEDICAID

	Medicare	Medicaid
Funding	Federal government	Federal and state governments
Administration	Federal government	State governments
Eligibility	People ≥ 65 and certain others	Selected poor and disabled (includes some elderly)
Level of benefits	Same nationwide	Varies from state to state
Payment by recipients	Required	Usually not required; copayments may be required in Medicaid managed care
Coverage	Inpatient care; outpatient care; optional prescriptions	Comprehensive inpatient and outpatient care

From Centers for Medicare and Medicaid Services: *Medicare program—general information*, 2006a, available online: www.cms.hhs.gov/MedicareGenInfo/; Centers for Medicare and Medicaid Services: *Medicaid at-a-glance 2005, a Medicaid information source*, 2005, available online: www.chs.hhs.gov/MedicaidGenInfo/Downloads/MedicaidAtAGlance2005.pdf.

percent of the total number of uninsured. The poor, near poor, foreign-born, and young adults (between 18 and 24) are in greatest danger of having no health insurance.

Because most non-elderly Americans are insured by job-related policies, they are at risk if they change or lose their jobs or if their employer chooses not to offer health insurance benefits. It is a myth that people do not have health insurance because they do not work. Some uninsured people do not work, but most have part-time or full-time jobs. The U.S. Census Bureau (2006) estimates that of the 45 million uninsured Americans, only 30.7 percent live below the poverty level. Thus most of the uninsured are employed or have employed workers in their family (Kaiser Commission on Medicaid and the

Uninsured, 2006). Ironically, poor workers are less likely to be insured than poor nonworkers, perhaps because many poor nonworkers may be eligible for government-sponsored health care such as Medicaid.

The number of uninsured Americans is expected to continue to rise. This should be a concern for all, because being uninsured affects the health and well-being of a major segment of our population. Studies have revealed major disparities in access to care between people with health insurance and those without. According to a 2003 Kaiser Foundation health insurance survey, 47 percent of the uninsured reported postponing care because of cost while 35 percent decided to forgo care altogether. Not filling a prescription because of cost was reported by 37 percent of the uninsured. In addition, 36 percent of uninsured reported problems paying medical bills, and 23 percent had been contacted by collection agencies about their medical bills (Kaiser Commission on Medicaid and the Uninsured, 2006).

A major reason for the growth of the uninsured population is change in employer-provided health insurance. Because of increased costs, some employers have left the system and insured their own employees (called **self-insurance**), scaled back or eliminated health benefits, limited the employees' choice of insurance plans, or passed more of the costs of insurance on to employees.

Employers led the charge to managed care, and now many employers limit their health insurance plan to managed care options. At the same time employers have increased the employee share of premium costs, making health insurance unaffordable to many workers. As health care costs increase, health insurance programs sponsored by employers continue to decline.

In an effort to cut costs, employers are also dropping health care coverage for their retirees. This is particularly burdensome for those retirees younger than age 65. They are not yet eligible for Medicare and must either pay for individual health coverage, often only available at very high costs, or go without coverage.

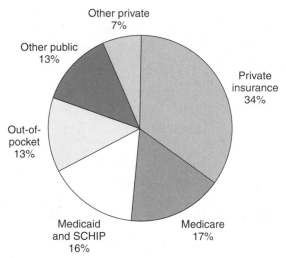

Figure 14-8
Funding sources for health care, 2004. Centers for Medicare and Medicaid Services, Office of the Actuary, National Health Statistics Group: *The nation's health dollar, calendar year 2004: where it came from,* 2004, available online: www.cms.hhs.gov/National-HealthExpendData/downloads/PieChartSources-Expenditures/2004.

Quality of care

Most people agree that there is potential for disaster if cost reduction is the only outcome that matters in the health care system. The challenge is to balance the cost-effectiveness and quality of patient care. The rapid growth of HMOs and related managed care organizations has raised concerns that quality of care might suffer. Care decisions, formerly based on the needs of the patient, have become increasingly influenced by business interests. Physicians, hospitals, and other providers are being forced to provide services for less. These conditions have created shock waves in the health care industry, resulting in limits on choice and services, provider restrictions, and financial incentives for providers to limit services. As discussed earlier, concern for maintaining high-quality services in the face of cost constraints has led to the development of quality management health care initiatives. Quality management continues to grow and create change within acute care, community, and extended health care settings.

Limits on choice and services

Since the mid-1990s, many employers have limited employees' choice of health plans. Some managed care plans increased the cost (co-payments or deductibles) to consumers who used out-of-plan providers and services. Some plans refused to pay any part of out-of-plan services. In addition, managed care plans set stricter limits than other health insurance plans on the types of services covered. For example, previously covered routine services, certain expensive therapies, and referrals (especially outside the plan) are often denied by today's managed care plans.

Provider restrictions and financial incentives to limit services

Managed care has made efforts to regulate information supplied to patients by their providers. Providers were sometimes discouraged or forbidden by their managed care contracts to mention treatment options that were expensive or not covered by a patient's managed care plan. These attempts to restrict providers' autonomy have been voluntarily discontinued because of intense negative publicity or, in some cases, by state regulation. Other influences to limit service persist.

Some managed care plans offered providers bonuses for providing less costly care. For example, physicians were offered bonuses if they were able to reduce hospital admissions and referrals to specialists (Harris, 2003). Physicians who called attention to bonus plans or exceeded average costs for services could be terminated by the plans. These practices evoked concern by health care interest groups in medicine and nursing, consumer groups, and the U.S. Congress, because such bonuses placed physicians in conflict between the best interests of patients and their own economic best interests.

Costs of prescription drugs

The rising cost of prescription medication is a concern, especially for seniors. The elderly use more prescription drugs than any other segment of the population, and before 2006 Medicare did not routinely pay for medications. Consumers of prescription drugs have resorted to various methods to reduce the cost of prescription drugs, ranging from importing drugs from other countries to using less medicine than prescribed, or discontinuing medication altogether. In fact, 37 percent of seniors with no prescription drug coverage report not filling a prescription or skipping doses or taking smaller doses so that the medicine lasts longer (Kaiser Family Foundation, 2005). The impact of the Medicare Prescription Drug plan, implemented in 2006, on prescription drug costs has not yet been determined.

Malpractice costs and the impact on access to care

Physicians and hospitals have recently experienced increases in the cost of malpractice insurance. In 2003 malpractice insurance premiums increased more than 20 percent, according to the Medical Liability Monitor Reporter (MLMR) (Rodwin, Chang, and Claussen, 2006). There is some concern these increases will limit access to health care services as physicians limit or discontinue practicing as a result of the financial burden of insurance. Despite this widespread belief, a recent study showed that the rising cost of malpractice insurance premiums has actually had a relatively small impact on physicians' net income (Rodwin, Chang, and Claussen, 2006).

The Government Accounting Office (GAO) conducted a study (GAO, 2003) in response to these access concerns. They measured the impact of rising malpractice costs on access in the nine states most affected. The GAO found no widespread access problems. It did find limited sporadic access problems in some rural and isolated communities. Unless the malpractice crisis becomes more widespread or severe, it appears malpractice costs will not endanger access to services for most people. Meanwhile, there is discussion of congressional action on tort reform, which would limit the amounts juries could award in medical malpractice cases. This is vigorously opposed by consumer advocacy groups and trial attorneys' associations.

HEALTH CARE REFORM AND UNIVERSAL ACCESS—THE FUTURE?

The United States and South Africa are the two only industrialized nations that do not provide universal access to health care to all of its citizens. Despite the fact that in 2005 U.S. health care expenditures totaled more than any other country in the world, the U.S. infant death rate was ranked 43 of all nations (Central Intelligence Agency, 2006).

Concerns about health care in the United States are not new. In the 1992 presidential campaign, candidates in both political parties, as well as nonpartisan groups, advocated some type of health care reform. These groups included nursing organizations, the American Association of Retired Persons, labor unions, the American College of Physicians, the National Leadership Coalition for Health Care Reform, and members of the U.S. Congress. Most of these groups put forward specific plans for reform, including

Nursing's Agenda for Health Care Reform by the American Nurses Association (1993). Despite widespread public support for reform, the effort failed. Lobbying against legislation on health care reform were powerful interest groups such as the pharmaceutical, health insurance, and health equipment industries, as well as the American Medical Association and the American Hospital Association.

Today, concerns about access to health care, the quality of care, and limits on consumer choice in managed care have fueled a new debate about health care in this country. There is the question about what to do with the millions of people who have no insurance and limited access to health care. In addition, growing concern exists about consumer choice restrictions in MCOs.

In the present political climate, it seems unlikely that a systematic and comprehensive reform of the entire health care system is possible. Instead, we can expect to see state-by-state efforts to address the specific current issues of concern discussed earlier. Most experts agree that reform efforts must be projected to reduce, or at least not increase, the cost of health care if they are to be supported by Congress. Despite wide-ranging differences of opinion about the specifics of health care reform proposals, some general questions should be asked in evaluating reform proposals:

1. Is there a uniform minimum set of benefits for all citizens, otherwise known as universal care?
2. Are coverage and benefits continuous and not dependent on where people live or work?
3. Are there mechanisms for controlling costs, especially administrative expenses?
4. Are provisions made for care to be provided by the most cost-effective personnel, taking quality issues and patient outcomes into consideration?
5. Are the issues of adequate facilities and personnel to ensure access for all addressed?
6. Is there an emphasis on quality care?
7. Are there incentives for healthy lifestyles and preventive care?

Further changes in nursing and health care delivery and finance are certain to be on the horizon. Most likely they will be gradual, rather than revolutionary. It remains to be seen whether these changes will improve access and quality of health care for all Americans.

SUMMARY OF *Key Points*

- The health care delivery system in the United States is a complex system that provides health promotion, illness prevention, diagnosis and treatment, and rehabilitation and long-term care.
- Health care agencies may be classified as governmental or voluntary, as for-profit or not-for-profit, or according to level of care provided. A single agency may fit into all three categories.
- Health care agencies have traditionally been structured with boards of directors, chief executive officers, medical and nursing staffs, and members of a variety of other disciplines.
- An interdisciplinary health care team consists of an array of professionals, including physicians and physician assistants, nurses, dietitians, pharmacists, technologists and technicians, social workers, various therapists, and administrative support personnel. Each member has an important part to play in ensuring the best patient outcomes.
- Historically, there have been a number of systems of nursing care delivery, each of which has advantages and disadvantages.
- Many variations and combinations of the major nursing care delivery systems are in use today.
- Nurses use a variety of roles, such as provider of care, teacher, counselor, manager, researcher, collaborator, entrepreneur, and patient advocate, in meeting patients' needs.
- Managed care has forced major changes in the health care delivery system.
- Information technology, leading to increased consumer expectations, has contributed to revolutionary change that will continue in the future and will affect professional nursing in many ways, most of which are yet unknown.
- As a result of managed care and changes in consumer expectations, organizations have

gone through reengineering, reducing layers of management and empowering the workforce to take part in decision making.
- Accreditation and continuous quality improvement are efforts to ensure public safety and institutional effectiveness and accountability.
- Health care financing in the United States is directly influenced by a basic economic disequilibrium in health care because people who do not pay directly for health care are not sensitive to the price of care.
- The entire health care system, including nurses and nursing services, has been profoundly affected by health care financing principles.
- Medicare and Medicaid programs, begun in 1965, quickly created a serious financial drain on federal and state budgets that continues today. In response, cost-containment efforts were begun by the federal government in the 1970s and persist in various old and new forms.
- Initial cost-containment efforts were unsuccessful, so in 1982 more sweeping reforms were initiated. Retrospective payment was replaced by prospective payment.
- System-wide health reform efforts were supported by public opinion but failed to pass the U.S. Congress. Even without governmental action, many Americans have seen substantial changes in their health care plans, stimulated by business interests and employers.

CRITICAL THINKING QUESTIONS

1. Using the yellow pages of your telephone directory or a directory of social services, identify local health services in the following areas: health promotion, illness prevention, diagnosis and treatment, rehabilitation, and

long-term care. Judging from the number of agencies for each service, where does the health care emphasis seem to be? What implications does this have for citizens of your community?

2. Obtain the organizational chart of a health care facility. Determine how it compares with one of the organizational structures described. Examine it to see how nursing fits into the overall structure. Who reports to the nurse executive, and to whom does the nurse executive report? What other administrative staff members are on the same level with the nurse executive?

3. Hold a panel discussion on reimbursement. Invite representatives from government, a managed care organization, a hospital, a major employer, and a nonprofit charity to discuss how managed care has affected their organizations.

4. Interview nurses in the hospital, home health, disease management, and case management settings. Look for the similarities and the differences in their work and interactions with patients. How do they work together to provide seamless care for the patient?

5. Interview a nurse and one or more nonnurse health professionals. Ask them to share some of their experiences as members of interdisciplinary health care teams during reengineering or restructuring of their institutions. What impact have these initiatives had on the way they care for patients?

6. Go to the patient websites identified in Box 14-12. Analyze the information on these websites using the guidelines in Box 14-3.

7. Compare and contrast the four types of nursing care delivery systems from the viewpoint of the patient. If you were a consumer of nursing care, which system would you prefer? Why?

8. Look at the same question from the standpoint of the nurse. Which system would you find most satisfying in terms of your practice? Which would you like least?

9. Interview nurses in practice in an acute care setting in your community to determine what type of governance structure is used by the nursing staff. What do they see as the positive and negative aspects of the type identified?

10. In your view, is access to health care a basic right? Who should pay for it? Be prepared to defend your opinions.

11. List the basic health care services that should be provided to all citizens. Compare your list with the lists of classmates and discuss the rationale for your priorities.

12. Should there be a limit on the percentage of national resources expended on health care? If so, how should the limit be established? Who should be responsible for determining the limit?

13. What process should be used to determine how health care resources are allocated? List criteria you would suggest to determine whether or not a person should receive a kidney transplant, a hip replacement, or a bone marrow transplant.

14. Should people with healthy lifestyles pay the same for care or insurance as those whose habits result in a greater likelihood of illness? How could such a differentiation be determined?

15. Should there be rationing of extremely expensive procedures, such as heart transplants, even if the patient is able to pay? Give a rationale for your answer.

REFERENCES

Aiken LH, Clarke SP, Sloane DM et al: Hospital nurse staffing and patient mortality, nurse burnout and job dissatisfaction, *JAMA* 288:1987-1993, 2002.

Aiken LH, Clarke SP, Cheung RB et al: Educational levels of hospital nurses and surgical patient mortality, *JAMA* 290:1617-1623, 2003.

American Academy of Physician Assistants: *Information about PAs and the PA profession*, 2006, available online: www.aapa.org/geninfo1.html.

American Hospital Association: *Welcome to the board: an orientation for the new health care trustee*, Chicago, 1999, AHA Press.

American Nurses Association: *Nursing: scope and standards of practice*, Washington, DC, 2004, available online: nursesbooks.org.

American Nurses Association: *Scope and standards for nurse administrators*, ed 2, Washington, DC, 2004, available online: nursesbooks.org.

American Nurses Association: *Nursing's agenda for health care reform*, Washington, DC, 2003, American Nurses Publishing.

Bastable SB: *Nurse as educator*, Sudbury, Mass, 2003, Jones & Bartlett.

Bower FA: *Case management by nurses*, Washington, DC, 1992, American Nurses Publishing.

Case Management Society of America: *Standards of practice for case management*, Little Rock, Ark, 2003, Case Management Society of America, pp 8-12.

Centers for Medicare and Medicaid Services, Office of the Actuary, National Health Statistics Group: *The nation's health dollar, calendar year 2004: where it came from*, 2004, available online: www.cms.hhs.gov/NationalHealthExpendData/downloads/PieChartSourcesExpenditures/2004.

Centers for Medicare and Medicaid Services: *Medicaid at-a-glance 2005, a Medicaid information source*, 2005, available online: www.chs.hhs.gov/ MedicaidGenInfo/Downloads/MedicaidAtAGlance2005.pdf.

Centers for Medicare and Medicaid Services: *Medicare and you 2006*, 2006, available online: www.medicare.gov/publications/pubs/pdf/10050.pdf.

Centers for Medicare and Medicaid Services: *Medicare program—general information*, 2006a, available online: www.cms.hhs.gov/MedicareGenInfo/.

Centers for Medicare and Medicaid Services: *National health care expenditures projections: 2005-2015*, 2006b, available online: www.cms.hhs.gov/NationalHealthExpendData/downloads/proj_2005.pdf.

Central Intelligence Agency: *The world factbook: rank order—infant mortality rate*, 2006, available online: http://www.cia.gov/cia/publications/factbook/rankorder/2091rank.html.

Cherry B, Jacob SR: *Contemporary nursing: issues, trends, and management*, St Louis, 1999, Mosby.

Cowan C, Catlin A, Smith C et al: National health expenditures, 2002, *Health Care Financing Rev* 25(4):143-166, 2004.

DeNavas-Walt C, Proctor BD, Lee CH: *U.S. Census Bureau: income, poverty, and health insurance coverage in the United States*, 2004, available online: www.census.gov/prod/2005pubs/p60-229.pdf.

Finkler SA: *Financial management for nurse managers and executives*, ed 2, Philadelphia, 2000, Saunders.

Fox S: *Health information online: eight in ten users have looked for health information online, with increased interest in diet, fitness, drugs, health insurance, experimental treatments, and particular doctors and hospitals*, released May 17, 2005, Pew Internet & American Life Project, available online: www.pewinternet.org/pdfs/PIP_Healthtopics_May05.pdf.

Government Accounting Office: *Medical malpractice: implication of rising premiums on access to health care (GAO-03-836)*, Washington, DC, 2003, Government Printing Office.

Hammer M, Stanton S: *The reengineering revolution*, New York, 1995, Harper Business.

Harris DM: *Contemporary issues in healthcare law and ethics*, ed 2, Chicago, 2003, Health Administration Press.

Healthy People 2010: Healthy People 2010 fact sheet, Rockville, Md, 2005a, available online: www.healthypeople.gov/About/hpfact.htm.

Healthy People 2010: What are the leading health indicators? Rockville, Md, 2005b, available online: www.healthypeople.gov/LHI/lhiwhat.htm.

Jacob P, Rapoport J: *The economics of health and medical care*, Sudbury, Mass, 2002, Jones & Bartlett.

Joint Commission on Accreditation of Healthcare Organizations: *Survey protocol for subacute programs*, Oakbrook Terrace, Ill, 1995, Joint Commission on Accreditation of Healthcare Organizations.

Joint Commission on Accreditation of Healthcare Organizations: *Facts about the Joint Commission on Accreditation of Healthcare Organizations*, 2006, available online: www.jointcommission.org/AboutUs/joint_commission_facts.htm.

Kaiser Commission on Medicaid and the Uninsured: *The uninsured: a primer: key facts about Americans without health insurance*, 2006, available online: www.kff.org/uninsured/upload/7451.pdf.

Kaiser Family Foundation: *Prescription drug trends*, 2005, available online: www.kff.org/insurance/upload/3057-04.pdf.

Kerfoot K: Establishing guardrails in leadership, *Nurs Economic$* 23(6):334-335, 2005.

Lambertson E: *Nursing team organization and functioning*, New York, 1953, Columbia University.

Madden M, Fox S: *Finding answers online in sickness and health,* Released May 2, 2006, Pew Internet & American Life Project, 2006, available online: www.pewinternet.org/pdfs/PIP_Health_Decisions_2006.pdf.

Manthey M: *The practice of primary nursing,* Boston, 1980, Blackwell Scientific Publications.

Maurer FA: Financing of health care: context for community health nursing. In Smith C, Maurer FA, editors: *Community health nursing: theory and practice,* ed 2, Philadelphia, 2000, Saunders.

McKibben RC: *DRGs and nursing care,* Kansas City, Mo, 1985, American Nurses Association Center for Research.

Medical Library Association: *A user's guide to finding and evaluating health information on the Web,* 2005, online: www.mlanet.org/resources/userguide.html#5.

Medical Library Association: *MLA's "top ten" most useful consumer health websites,* 2005, available online: www.mlanet.org/resurces/userguide.html#5.

National Center for Health Statistics: *Health, United States, 2005 with chartbook on trends in the health of Americans,* 2005, available online: www.cdc.gov/nchs/data/hus/hus05.pdf.

National Committee for Quality Assurance: *NCQA overview,* 2006, available online: www.ncqa.org/Communications/Publications/overviewncqa.pdf.

National League for Nursing Accrediting Commission, Inc: *Accreditation manual with interpretive guidelines by program type for post secondary and higher degree programs in nursing,* 2005, available online: www.nlnac.org/manuals/NLNACManual2005.pdf.

Needleman J, Buerhaus PI, Stewart M et al: Market watch. Nurse staffing in hospitals: is there a business case for quality? *Health Affairs* 25(1):204-211, 2006.

Pfizer: *Annual report, 2005,* 2005, available online: www.pfizer.com/pfizer/annualreport/2005/annual/renew2005.pdf.

Primm PL: Differentiated practice for ADN and BSN prepared nurses, *J Prof Nurs* 3(4):218-225, 1987.

Primm PL: Differentiated nursing care management/patient care delivery system, *Kansas Nurse,* April 1988, p. 2.

Rodwin MA, Chang HJ, Claussen J: Malpractice premiums and physicians' income: perceptions of a crisis conflict with empirical evidence, *Health Affairs* 25(3):750-758, 2006.

U.S. Census Bureau: *Statistical abstract of the United States: 2006,* 2006, available online: www.census.gov/prod/www/statistical-abstract.html.

U.S. Department of Labor, Bureau of Labor Statistics: *Occupational outlook handbook,* 2006, available online: www.bls.gov/oco/ocos079.htm.

15

The Political Activism of Nursing—In Organizations and the Government

*Judith K. Leavitt**

- Differentiate between politics and policy.
- Explain why professions have associations.
- Demonstrate an understanding of the complex role that associations play in the profession and in society.
- Recognize the opportunities that associations offer to increase the leadership capacity of nursing students and registered nurses.
- Explain the concept of personalizing the political process.

- Cite examples of sources of both personal and professional power.
- Describe how nurses can become involved in politics and policy development at the levels of citizen, activist, and politician.
- Explain how organized nursing is involved in political activities designed to strengthen professional nursing and influence health policy.

Did you ever know a nurse member of Congress or a state legislator? Did you know that a former president of the American Nurses Association, Virginia Trotter Betts, became a special adviser to the former U.S. Secretary of Health and Human Services and currently serves as commissioner of the Tennessee Department of Mental Health and Developmental Disabilities? Did you know that the former head of the Social Security Administration, Shirley Chater, was a nurse and president

of Texas Women's University? And did you know that a former president of the National Student Nurses Association, Sheila Burke, was considered the most powerful staff person in Congress (Leavitt, 1998)? Before assuming these impressive positions, all of these nurses first served in leadership positions in nursing professional organizations and associations. They become widely known for their expertise, and this led to their powerful positions in government.

Nursing has a rich history of leaders who have influenced policy in both government and professional associations as well as in their communities and workplaces. This chapter will focus

*The author wishes to acknowledge the prior contributions of Diane Mancino and Virginia Trotter Betts in the preparation of this chapter.

on why and how nurses have been able to do this and explore issues about how you can become involved—and why your voice and your talent are needed.

POLICY AND POLITICS: WHAT IT IS AND IS NOT

Policy and politics are more than what is happening in Washington, DC. They encompass what happens to us in our daily lives, in the workplace, and in our organizations, as well as in government. **Politics,** the art of influencing decisions, is part of every aspect of our lives, both personal and professional. People often speak of politics with negative overtones. In fact, politics is neither good nor bad. It is the outcome of the political process that may be judged as positive or negative.

Policy is defined as principles that govern actions directed toward given ends; policy statements set forth a plan, direction, or goal for action. Policies may be laws, regulations, or guidelines that govern behavior in the public arena (such as in government) or in the private arena (such as in workplaces, schools, organizations, and communities). Health policy refers to public or private rules, regulations, laws, or guidelines that relate to the pursuit of health and the delivery of health services. Policy reflects the choices that an entity (government or organization) makes regarding its goals and priorities and how it will allocate its resources.

Policy decisions (e.g., laws or regulations) reflect the values and beliefs of those making the decisions. As values and beliefs change, so do policy decisions. For instance, laws limiting smoking in public buildings or private restaurants were nonexistent 40 years ago because smoking was considered to be "cool" and sexy at that time. The harmful effects of smoking were not as well-known as they are today. As the public became more aware of the dangers of smoking, values about smoking changed. Changes in laws followed the change in values. Laws limiting smoking and the sale and use of tobacco products have now become commonplace. Elected officials responded to the changing values of the public and recognized that the public supported the passage of laws limiting smoking.

In professional organizations, policy focuses on the rules and guidelines established by the governing body of the organization, usually a board of directors. Those guidelines or policies also reflect the values of the organization. For instance, one would expect a nursing organization to focus on issues of health, prevention, and practice guidelines. That would be quite different for an organization like the National Rifle Association, where the values of the members would be reflected in policies and recommendations that support the ownership and recreational use of guns.

Politics is the process of influencing the allocation of scarce resources. Allocation assumes that there are not enough resources for all who may want them. Those resources might be money, people, time, supplies, or equipment. Who gets what, or how those resources are allocated, is determined through the political process. Policies are the decisions; politics is influencing those decisions. There are always **stakeholders,** individuals with a vested interest, who try to influence those with the power to make the final decisions. In organizations, stakeholders are the members, the larger community served by the work of the organization, and other groups or individuals affected by those decisions. For example, an organization started by a nurse, Patients Out of Time, has worked for years to educate the public and health care professionals about the therapeutic use of cannabis and to advocate for the medicinal use of marijuana (www.medical-cannabis.com). Stakeholders for this organization would be affected patients and families, health care providers, and those who make decisions about the laws and regulations about cannabis use. These include state and federal legislators as well as the Food and Drug Administration (FDA), the Secretary of Health and Human Services (who oversees the policies of the Food and Drug Administration), and organizations like the American

Nurses Association and the American Public Health Association, both of which have been supportive of the issue (Mather, 2007).

Politics works similarly in the public arena. For example, to garner support from state legislators to increase funding for nursing scholarships, an organization or coalition of organizations must have a plan to mobilize stakeholders to lobby legislators. Such stakeholders would include administrators of nursing organizations, colleges of nursing, hospitals, nursing homes, and other health care organizations, as well as physician groups and others who know the necessity of having a competent and adequate nursing workforce. The more stakeholder support that can be mustered, the more likely it is that policymakers will appreciate the broad constituent support for the issue and the more likely they will be to vote for increased funding for nursing education and scholarships.

Linking Practice, Policy, and Politics

Leaders in nursing, from Florence Nightingale to Lavinia Dock, saw and understood the connection between their work and the larger world in which policy decisions affected what they were able to do. "Flo" could not have been successful in the Crimea without the support of Sir Sidney Herbert, Secretary of War. Lavinia Dock joined with other nurses to found the American Nurses Association, pressure hospital administrators to improve working conditions for nurses, and galvanize support for nursing registration (Lewenson, 2007, p. 23). A recent example is Karen Daley, a modern nurse who went public with her needlestick injury in order to influence legislation requiring protective devices. In each instance these leaders knew that nursing practice could only be improved through legislation, regulation, or unification to create a formidable national organization. The larger world of public policy and the work of organizations become the arena in which someone with a vision for improved health or working conditions can change the way health is delivered and improve the health of populations. With these examples in mind, we

now turn our attention to professional organizations as a means of activism.

PROFESSIONAL ORGANIZATIONS

Professionals create organizations to work collectively on behalf of issues that enhance their work and their involvement in communities, ensure continued learning and competence, and use political action to influence policymakers to support the mission of the organization. Professional organizations offer a supportive way to learn leadership skills, to test ideas, and to follow these ideas to completion. Nursing has a national organization open to all graduate nurses, the American Nurses Association (www.nursingworld.org); a national student nurses organization, the National Student Nurses Association (www.nasn.org); and many other specialty organizations developed around particular practice areas.

What do nursing organizations do and how are they involved in influencing public policy? We will answer that question by looking at the role and function of organizations, examining why nurses do or do not join organizations, and discussing examples of collective action. Because organizations are often the catalyst for involvement in political action, we will also explore the broader area of political action in the public arena.

Joining a Professional Organization

Nurses join organizations to network with colleagues, to pursue continuing education and certification opportunities, to stay informed on professional issues, to develop leadership skills, to influence health policy, and to work collectively for job security. Yet less than 10 percent of the nation's registered nurses are members of the American Nurses Association (Kany, 2007) and only about 20 percent of nurses belong to 1 of the 100 or more specialty nursing organizations.

Nurses cite issues of high cost of dues, lack of time, and lack of interest as reasons that they do not join. There are also different expectations and interests among the generations. While baby boomers and older members accepted organizational structures and volunteer tasks, generation Xers prefer short-term projects, using technology such as blogs and chat rooms rather than face-to-face meetings. They expect to assume leadership positions quickly without having to work up through the ranks, as required in the past (Holland, 2005). As older members retire, organizations are becoming more responsive to incorporating processes and products that appeal to younger members.

Types of Associations

As mentioned, there are more than 100 national nursing organizations and many more state and local groups. Understandably, individual nurses often express confusion about which group to join. In general, associations can be classified as one of three main types:

1. Broad purpose professional associations
2. Specialty practice associations
3. Special interest associations

ANA is an example of a broad purpose association. Individual nurses can belong directly to the ANA or to 1 of its 54 constituent member (state and territorial) nurses associations.

As the nursing profession's body of knowledge and research grows and diversifies, many nurses limit their practices to specialty practice areas such as maternal/infant care, school or community health, critical care, or perioperative or emergency/trauma nursing. They often join the specialty organization for their area of clinical interest. Members of specialty practice nursing associations also may choose to belong to the ANA or one of its constituent member associations (at the state level) to support the entire profession because specialty associations focus only on standards of practice or professional needs of the particular specialty. Sixty-six specialty organizations are represented in the Nursing Organizations Alliance.

Examples of special interest organizations include Sigma Theta Tau International (the Honor Society of Nursing), which one must be invited to join, and the American Association for the History of Nursing, which focuses on a particular area of study in nursing. Comprehensive and frequently updated lists of nursing organizations are available online (www.nurse.org/orgs.shtml).

Nurses are connected internationally through the International Council of Nurses (ICN). The ICN is a federation of national nurse associations (NNAs) representing nurses in 118 countries. The ANA represents U.S. registered nurses in the ICN, and the National Student Nurses Association (NSNA) represents U.S. nursing students in the ICN.

Founded in 1899, the ICN is the world's first and widest-reaching international organization for health professionals. Operated by nurses for nurses, the ICN works to ensure quality nursing care for all, sound health policies globally, the advancement of nursing knowledge, the presence worldwide of a respected nursing profession, and a competent and satisfied nursing workforce. For additional details about the ICN's activities in professional nursing practice, nursing regulation, and the socioeconomic welfare of nurses, visit the ICN home page (www.icn.ch).

PURPOSE AND ACTIVITIES OF ORGANIZATIONS

Organizational activities are derived from their mission statements. The mission statement is generated by the membership and defines the purpose and who is served by the organization. For instance, the mission of the ANA is "to work for the improvement of health standards and availability of health care services for all people, foster high standards for nursing, stimulate and promote the professional development of nurses, and advance their economic and general welfare." This defines the association's areas of focus as practice standards, a code of ethical conduct, continuing education and conferences, and collective action around workplace issues. In 1999 the ANA House of Delegates, the elected representatives from the constituent member associations (CMAs), approved the creation of two divisions for economic and employment issues:

the Center for American Nurses (CAN) (http://centerforamericannurses.org) and a collective bargaining unit, the United American Nurses (UAN) (www.uannurse.org/). CAN's mission is to promote safe workplace environments and to advocate for issues of appropriate staffing, generational workplace issues, and patient and provider safety. The UAN (www.uannurse.org) focuses on collective bargaining and is the only national union of nurses. It provides guidance, information, and support for state nursing association affiliates. The UAN is an affiliate of the largest labor organization in the country, the AFL-CIO.

Nurses and Unions

Why do some nurses join unions and what purpose do they serve? Nurses may choose to join unions to work collectively, to have control over their practice, and to try to equalize the power between management and staff. This can be an effective approach if the health care organization is willing to work collaboratively with unions. Union affiliation is a highly complex process, one that is defined by rules and regulations under the National Labor Act and overseen by the National Labor Relations Board. There are limits on what issues unions can bargain about; for instance, hours, pay, and benefits are included in all contracts for all unionized workers.

For nurses there are additional issues that are increasingly part of contract negotiations. These include issues like staffing, work assignments, and shared governance responsibilities. The national nursing shortage is creating an environment in which both management and nurses themselves have a desire to create work environments that decrease turnover and ensure a competent workforce.

United American Nurses represents only nurses, but there are many nursing units affiliated with nonnursing unions. The Service Employees International Union (SEIU); the American Federation of Teachers (AFT); the Association of Federal, State, County, and Municipal Employees (AFSCME); and the United Mine Workers (UMW) are all examples of organizations that have nursing units, but also represent larger, nonnursing constituencies.

Should nurses join unions? Much of that depends on where they work. If seeking a staff job in an institution in which a nursing union already exits, a nurse may be required to join the union as a condition of employment. This is called a "closed shop," meaning that management is required to bargain with the union and union membership is required as a condition of employment. An "open shop" is one in which employees are not required to join but in which an individual's contract will be dependent on what union and management have negotiated. Most nurses work in nonunion facilities. Some states are more "union friendly" than others. States in which labor unions flourish, such as in the Northeast, Northwest, and the Midwest, have the vast majority of nursing unions. Smaller states, particularly in the Southeast (other than Florida) and the Southwest, have few or no nurse unions. These are known as "right to work states." Though unions have made numerous attempts to organize nurses in these states, the value system of the work culture is less supportive of union affiliation by professionals.

BENEFITS OF BELONGING TO PROFESSIONAL ASSOCIATIONS

Whether or not a nurse engages in collective bargaining, a variety of benefits result from membership in professional associations. These range from certification and discounts on travel, products, and services, to opportunities to engage in research projects and learn political action strategies.

Developing Leadership Skills

Students who join the NSNA have opportunities to learn from and socialize with their peers in school and at the state and national levels (Figure 15-1). As NSNA members, they benefit from developing leadership and organizational skills that can be vital in their professional careers and

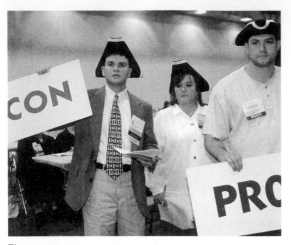

Figure 15-1
Students serving as delegates to the National Student Nurses Association House of Delegates learn leadership and political skills while having fun and meeting others from around the United States, Puerto Rico, and Guam. In this photo, students voice their views about resolutions being considered by the delegates. *(Courtesy National Student Nurses Association.)*

personal lives. Through the NSNA Leadership University, the NSNA recognizes students for their leadership and management competencies with a certificate presented at the annual NSNA convention. The NSNA Leadership University provides an opportunity for nursing students to earn academic credit for their participation in NSNA's many leadership activities. From the school chapter level to the state and national levels, nursing students learn how to work in shared governance and cooperative relationships with peers, faculty, students in other disciplines, community service organizations, and the public. In addition to preparing students to participate in professional organizations, practicing shared governance also prepares students to work in health care delivery settings that incorporate unit-based decision making, such as magnet hospitals. By participating in the NSNA Leadership University, students learn and practice the skills needed for future leadership. A list of those skills and competencies is provided in Box 15-1. For com-

plete details about the NSNA Leadership University and all of the NSNA's programs, visit their websites (http://www.nsna.org and www.nsna-leadershipu.org).

Leadership skills are foundation blocks for nursing professional practice. Nurses have multiple opportunities to exercise leadership at the bedside, in clinical teams, and in management teams. The Nursing Alliance Leadership Academy (Nursing Organizations Alliance, 2005) was created to help nurses enhance leadership skills and focus on patients and care issues. The academy also focuses on developing political skills and policy awareness (http://www.nursing-alliance.org/events.cfm).

Professional associations offer a supportive environment in which members can practice the acquisition of important leadership skills. Speaking publicly, planning projects, managing resources, and developing resolutions and position papers are opportunities to practice skills essential to formal leadership roles. It is no accident that nurses who are active in associations also tend to be recognized leaders in their work settings—and many, like Virginia Trotter Betts and Sheila Burke, mentioned earlier, have gone on to achieve national and international leadership positions.

Certification and Continuing Education

Practicing nurses want to be recognized, through both compensation and position, for their level of professional expertise. Toward those ends, they may pursue certification in a specialty area. Certification is granted through professional associations. As discussed in Chapter 7, certification is a formal but voluntary process of demonstrating expertise in a particular area of nursing. Certified nurses may receive salary supplements and special opportunities. For information about credentials in nursing, visit the website of the ANA's subsidiary, the American Nurses Credentialing Center (ANCC), which offers a range of certification credentials (http://www.nursingworld.org/ancc). Links to additional websites of specialty nursing organizations that also offer certification can be

| Box 15-1 | **Attributes and Competencies Needed by Future Nurse Leaders and Managers*** |

- Demonstrates intellectual and analytical capacity
- Develops critical thinking ability
- Develops systems thinking
- Comprehends interdisciplinary models
- Communicates effectively
- Demonstrates effective interpersonal skills
- Listens empathetically and actively
- Adapts quickly to new situations
- Identifies global, national, and local trends
- Accepts high moral and ethical standards
- Manages conflict and masters conflict resolution skills
- Facilitates collaboration and group process
- Motivates others to participate in decision making
- Demonstrates capacity to interchange leadership/followership roles
- Mentors future leaders
- Empowers others
- Functions as a team player
- Understands strategic/tactical planning, implementation, and outcome evaluation
- Treats all human beings with respect and acceptance
- Strives for an inclusive society
- Balances professional responsibilities and personal life
- Accepts responsibility and accountability for decisions
- Demonstrates a commitment to lifelong learning
- Practices the spirit of cooperation
- Balances "high tech" with "high touch"
- Solves problems creatively
- Demonstrates the capacity for introspection and reflection
- Demonstrates the capacity to connect with the spiritual nature of human beings

Compiled by Dr. Diane J. Mancino, Executive Director, NSNA.
*These competencies and attributes are developed during participation in NSNA's leadership activities at the school, state, and national levels of the association. Visit http://www.nsnaleadershipu.org for more details.

found online (http://www.nsna.org/resources/index.asp).

Political Activism

As their careers develop, nurses may obtain master's-level and doctoral-level preparation or become nurse practitioners and practice independently outside an institution. These nurses desire and deserve direct reimbursement for their work, and they need state laws that mandate direct reimbursement of nurses. Others work in settings in which there are not enough registered nurses available to provide the quality of care the residents need. These nurses need laws that ensure appropriate RN staffing and control educational requirements for unlicensed assistive personnel.

In each of these instances, the ANA, labor unions, and specialty organizations are involved in political action with legislators and regulators in the government arena. However, who are the people in the organizations who advocate for the legislation and regulation needed to support nursing's position and who develop the stance that nursing organizations take? The process of political action and policy recommendations involves both paid staff, usually in the government affairs department, and volunteer members of the organizations, usually practicing nurses. The legislative agenda, that is, the public policy issues the organization supports, is developed by members appointed by the board of directors as well as by staff who are experts in political and policy issues. The board of directors approves the legislative agenda. Organizations with legislative agendas depend on members to lobby legislators. They provide members with background information and also create "talking points" to use when lobbying for the selected issue. For example, ANA has been trying to garner congressional support for safe staffing levels by means of two bills: the Safe Staffing Act and the Quality Nursing Care Act (http://www.nursingworld.org/gova). As part of the process of encouraging nurses to lobby, information is given on the website about the bill along with talking points for writing or speaking with congressional representatives. Members can be very influential in lobbying legislators, particularly when the constituency is nationwide and representative of different stakeholders. Learning how to be politically active increases the power of both the individual and the organization represented. Figure 15-2 shows a group of Maryland nurses participating in the American Nurses Association's 2005 Lobby Day on Capitol Hill.

Nursing organizations also work collaboratively through coalitions with other health professional and consumer groups. Such coalitions are focused on specific issues. For example, Health Care Without Harm (http://www.noharm.org) is a group of 443 organizations in 52 countries whose mission is to protect health by reducing pollution in the health care industry. It was founded when one nurse, Hollie Shaner McRae of Vermont, became concerned about the waste created by disposable instruments in an operating room (Shaner McRae, 2002). The organization is now a significant national and international force advocating for the recycling and safe disposal of

Figure 15-2
Maryland nurses turned out in force to lobby their members of Congress on behalf of issues important to nurses. This photograph was taken during the American Nurses Association's 2005 Lobby Day on Capitol Hill. Notice that the nurses are attired to clearly identify them as professional nurses. *(Courtesy American Nurses Association.)*

dangerous materials, such as mercury. This example clearly demonstrates how one individual, working through organizations and coalitions of organizations, can have worldwide positive impact.

Practice Guidelines and Position Statements

Organizations serve an important function by defining practice standards, taking positions on practice issues, and developing ethical guidelines. For example, the American Nurses Association has positions on Blood-borne and Airborne Diseases (http://www.nursingworld.org/readroom/position/blood) that include statements about HIV infection and nursing students. It defines ANA's recommendation of requiring educational content about such infections by qualified faculty, mandating universal precautions, and providing post-exposure support for students who may sustain a needlestick injury. These statements serve to guide the organization's work in both the practice and the policy arenas and help individual nurses within workplaces to implement the policy. Guidelines and position statements emanate from research on the issue as well as opinions of nurse experts in the field. For example, ANA was involved in national coalitions and with the Occupational Safety and Health Administration (OSHA) when developing the brochure, *Blood-Borne Diseases.*

Another example is the recent revision of the *Code of Ethics for Nurses,* found inside the back cover of this book. A task force was appointed by the board of directors to review the previous *Code* and create revisions and recommendations. The revisions went through a process of approval by many entities within the ANA: the Congress of Nursing Practice, the Board of Directors, and the House of Delegates, which speaks on behalf of all the members. Approval from so many groups within an organization assures "buy-in" by the membership. Buy-in is important because the *Code* serves as an ethical standard for all practicing nurses, whether they are ANA members or not, and is therefore of critical importance.

The National Student Nurses Association also has a *Code of Conduct* (Box 15-2), which provides guidance for nursing students. This *Code* serves as the ethical foundation of student practice.

Other Benefits

There are many other benefits of membership, such as access to journals, newsletters, and action alerts about particular topics that need immediate response; eligibility for group health and life insurance; networking with peers; continuing education opportunities; and discounts on products and services, such as car rentals, computers, or books.

Deciding Which Associations to Join

As you decide whether to belong to an association, visit the group's website to find out more about its activities. Then ask yourself the following questions:

1. What is the mission and what are the purposes of this association?
2. Are the association's purposes compatible with my own?
3. How many members are there nationally, statewide, and locally?
4. What activities does the association undertake?
5. How active is the local chapter?
6. What opportunities does the association offer for involvement and leadership development?
7. What are the benefits of membership?
8. Does the association offer continuing education programs?
9. Does this organization lobby for improved health care legislation? How successful is it?
10. Is membership in this association cost-effective?
11. Even if I am not active, what benefit will I derive from the legislative agenda and other activities that the association undertakes to advocate for nurses and patients?

Answering these questions and speaking with current association members should provide nurses with adequate information to make reasoned decisions.

POLITICAL ACTIVISM IN THE GOVERNMENT ARENA

Now that you understand how professional organizations use collective power to influence policy decisions, let us examine how policy influences the practice of nursing. The ability of the individual nurse to provide care is significantly affected by public policy decisions. Yet too few nurses are aware of the importance of their role in influencing such policy outcomes, because they miss the connection between their own practice and the world of public policy.

As discussed in Chapter 4, state licensure of a registered nurse derives from legislation that defines the scope of nursing practice. The defined scope determines what a nurse legally can and cannot do. For example, giving intravenous medication and performing physical assessments are now accepted as actions within the scope of nursing practice. Forty years ago such activities

Box 15-2 **National Student Nurses Association's Code of Academic and Clinical Conduct**

Preamble

Students of nursing have a responsibility to society in learning the academic theory and clinical skills needed to provide nursing care. The clinical setting presents unique challenges and responsibilities while caring for human beings in a variety of health care environments.

The Code of Academic and Clinical Conduct is based on an understanding that to practice nursing as a student is an agreement to uphold the trust that society has placed in us. The statements of the Code provide guidance for the nursing student in the personal development of an ethical foundation and need not be limited strictly to the academic or clinical environment but can assist in the holistic development of the person.

A Code for Nursing Students

As students are involved in the clinical and academic environments, we believe that ethical principles are a necessary guide to professional development. Therefore within these environments we:

1. Advocate for the rights of all clients.
2. Maintain client confidentiality.
3. Take appropriate action to ensure the safety of clients, self, and others.
4. Provide care for the client in a timely, compassionate, and professional manner.
5. Communicate client care in a truthful, timely, and accurate manner.
6. Actively promote the highest level of moral and ethical principles and accept responsibility for our actions.
7. Promote excellence in nursing by encouraging lifelong learning and professional development.
8. Treat others with respect and promote an environment that respects human rights, values, and choice of cultural and spiritual beliefs.
9. Collaborate in every reasonable manner with the academic faculty and clinical staff to ensure the highest quality of client care.
10. Use every opportunity to improve faculty and clinical staff understanding of the learning needs of nursing students.
11. Encourage faculty, clinical staff, and peers to mentor nursing students.
12. Refrain from performing any technique or procedure for which the student has not been adequately trained.
13. Refrain from any deliberate action or omission of care in the academic or clinical setting that creates unnecessary risk for injury to the client, self, or others.
14. Assist the staff nurse or preceptor in ensuring that there is full disclosure and that proper authorizations are obtained from clients regarding any form of treatment or research.
15. Abstain from the use of alcoholic beverages or any substances that impair judgment in the academic and clinical setting.
16. Strive to achieve and maintain an optimal level of personal health.
17. Support access to treatment and rehabilitation for students who are experiencing impairments related to substance abuse and mental or physical health issues.
18. Uphold school policies and regulations related to academic and clinical performance, reserving the right to challenge and critique rules and regulations according to school grievance policy.

Adopted by the NSNA House of Delegates, Nashville, Tenn, on April 6, 2001.

were within the scope of the medical practice act rather than the nursing practice act. As a result of changes in education and clinical practice, nursing organizations influenced legislators to change state nurse practice acts to reflect what nurses were qualified to do.

Regulations are developed to guide the implementation of legislation. They affect practicing nurses and their work environments. For example, the rules for administering and documenting the administration of narcotic drugs are promulgated by a regulatory agency of the federal government, the Food and Drug Administration, a division of the Department of Health and Human Services. The way in which such regulations are written can greatly affect nurses' ability to practice.

The regulations in each state governing nursing practice flow from the state's nurse practice act. When the regulations change, for example, adding a requirement for continuing education for license renewal, it affects all nurses in the state. For advanced practice nurses, there are a variety of regulations related to prescription writing and autonomy issues. These change from time to time, and if nurses do not actively participate in changes, new regulations can restrict rather than enhance nursing authority for regulated activities.

A specific example of the impact regulatory changes can have involves advanced practice nurses, such as nurse practitioners and certified registered nurse anesthetists (CRNAs). A November 2001 federal ruling from the Centers for Medicare and Medicaid Services (CMS) required that CRNAs must practice under the supervision of a surgeon or anesthesiologist in order to receive Medicare reimbursement. This change limits what many states had previously allowed nurses to do—practice "collaboratively" rather than "under the supervision of." CRNAs are working with governors in each state to get an exception (known as an "opt-out") and enable previous state laws to take precedence (http://www.aana.com/). Without such political involvement, CRNAs will have their practices, and their reimbursement, restricted (AANA, 2006).

Broader issues affecting the nursing profession are also political in nature. Issues of pay equity, or equal pay for work of comparable value, are of concern to nurses, because they have historically been underpaid for their services. One of the earliest cases demonstrating the inequality of nursing salaries involved public health nurses in Colorado. These nurses brought a case against the city of Denver, stating that they were paid considerably less than city tree trimmers and garbage collectors. The nurses demanded just compensation for their work by demonstrating that nursing requires more complex knowledge and is of greater value to society than the other occupations.

As a result of this suit, recognition of nursing's low pay was brought to public attention; this in turn mobilized public support for increasing nursing salaries. This is an example of political action by nurses that resulted in both policy outcomes (regulations that expanded comparable pay issues to other jobs) and professional outcomes (salary increases for the individual nurse). More recently, the nursing shortage has caused concern among the public that the number of nurses available to provide care in hospitals and other agencies is inadequate. Nurses in California mobilized the public and other constituency groups to get the first legislation requiring specific nurse-to-patient ratios passed in 1999. However, the regulations were not implemented until 2004. Massachusetts is expected to be the second state to mandate minimum nurse:patient ratios.

An unfortunate example of the problems that can result when nurses do not work together in a politically savvy manner is found in Box 15-3.

"The Personal Is Political"

Women involved in the feminist movement in the 1960s coined the phrase "The personal is political." This statement recognized that each individual—woman or man—could use personal experience to understand and become involved in broader social and political issues. This concept enabled individuals who did not consider themselves political to gain insight into what needed to be changed in society and how they could help bring

Box 15-3 **Politics Gone Wrong: A Painful Lesson for Nurses**

An unfortunate event that dramatically illustrates how politics can influence policy occurred in the state of North Dakota in 2003. For about 15 years, North Dakota was the only state requiring the baccalaureate degree as the minimum educational requirement for registered nurse licensure. When a group of well-intentioned nurses attempted to get the oversight of nursing education moved from the Board of Nursing's jurisdiction to the Board of Higher Education's jurisdiction, those opposed to the mandatory BSN lobbied hard for a reversal. Community colleges were opposed to the BSN, and representatives of long term care agencies, long opposed to the BSN requirement, testified that they "needed the economic benefit that would result from having a lesser-educated nursing work force" (Mooney, 2003, p. 9). Unfortunately, nurses were divided and testified on both sides, confusing legislators. "Opponents to higher standards for nursing education used the dissent in the ranks of nurses to fuel their agenda and achieve their goals" (Mooney, 2003, p. 9).

As a result, the bill that ultimately passed and was signed into law removed the requirement for the baccalaureate degree, among other provisions. North Dakota's strong history of support for nursing education and high-quality health care ended with a very painful lesson for the nurses of the state and the rest of the nation lost a role model. Those with vested interests aligned against a divided nursing profession—and nursing lost. According to a professor at the North Dakota State University Department of Nursing, nurses must "strengthen the bonds of trust among ourselves, disagree without being disagreeable, discern which fights to keep in the family and which to advance to the public forum, and hone the political and negotiation skills of our future leaders" (Mooney, 2003, p. 9).

From Mooney MM: Hog-housed! *Reflect Nurs Leadership* 29(4):8-9, 2003.

about the change. It gave power to each individual and resulted in people becoming involved in the political process—usually for the first time.

This premise of personalizing the political process has become a fundamental activity for organized nursing. Nurses at the grassroots level become involved in advocating for legislation and supporting candidates for elective office because they understand the relationship between public policy and their professional and personal lives. Most associations, such as the American Nurses Association, American Association of Colleges of Nursing, the American Hospital Association, and numerous specialty nursing organizations, actively engage in lobbying to advocate for the professional concerns of their members. Contemporary nursing leaders recognize that "being political," both through professional associations and as individuals, is a professional responsibility essential to the practice and promotion of the nursing profession.

Politics and Power

Politics connotes power. Power is the ability to make something happen. Without power, there cannot be influence. To be effective in influencing the outcome of decisions, an individual must ask the following questions: "Who has the power?" "How is it used?" "How can it be mobilized?"

There are different types of power. **Position power** is that which is inherent in a position such as that of a dean, vice-president for nursing, or chief executive of a company. **Expert power** comes from the knowledge a person has that can influence an outcome. Nurses have expert power because of their knowledge about health care. There is **power in numbers**; a group is almost always more influential than an individual. There is power related to wealth. Wealth itself is a resource and provides access to other significant resources. Also, there has always been power accorded to whomever belongs to the dominant race, gender, or class in a community or nation.

Latent power is power that is untapped and underused. As the largest group of health care providers, nurses have had latent power. Although there are more than 2.9 million nurses in the United States, nurses are only recently recognizing the potential power that such numbers suggest. Of all women voters in the Unitcd States, 1 in 44 is a nurse. Imagine how influential nursing could be if that power were used collectively. Nurses could be pivotal in getting laws passed to improve health care and getting policymakers elected to office who would support nursing's agenda. The power of nursing knowledge has also been underused. No other group of health care providers spends as much time as nurses in direct patient contact. Nurses know what patients need, and they can use this knowledge to develop workplace and community policies. More nurses than ever are using their expertise to participate in the development of health policy, by sharing knowledge with legislators and regulators (Figure 15-3). In addition, they are using nursing research to substantiate the need for public policies that have been shown to affect positive health outcomes and provide needed public health services.

Power, like politics, is neither good nor bad; how it is used gives it value. If, for example, nurses use the power of persuasion to motivate patients to take prescribed medication, they are using the power of position and knowledge positively.

Power is not given; it must be taken. The taking of power converts latent power into action. Nurses are beginning to recognize that to have power they must want it, and they must use it. Use of power is a hallmark of political activity.

There are differences in the ways people have traditionally used power. One traditional model of power has been described as **power grabbing.** It involves hoarding power and control, taking it from others, or wielding it over others. Another model is **power sharing**, which is a process of equalizing resources, knowledge, or control. The most effective power brokers are those who can use both methods and know which is most likely to be effective in a given situation.

The Power of the Media

The *Woodhull Study on Nursing and the Media* (Sigma Theta Tau, 1997), described in Chapter 2, analyzed more than 2000 health-related articles from 16 major news publications. Recognizing that communication media are the most effective ways in which to send a message to a large audience, this study recommended that the nursing profession be proactive in promoting and establishing ongoing dialogue with representatives of these media. Effective utilization of media is a powerful political tool for influencing both the public and those who hold elective offices. The *American Journal of Nursing* has the largest circulation of any health professional journal in the world. Many of their research articles are picked up in the national press. Such media coverage is critical for nurses' expertise to be recognized by the public and ultimately by the policymakers who make the laws and regulations that affect nursing practice.

Different kinds of media provide different ways to influence opinions. For example, talk radio has

Figure 15-3
Testifying before congress is a way to educate elected officials about issues affecting nursing and health care. Here Patricia Yoder-Wise testifies before a congressional committee. *(Courtesy American Nurses Association.)*

become very influential. Talk radio hosts advocate certain opinions, often with little factual information. By controlling who gets to talk, these radio hosts can control the kinds of information and the values expressed by callers and eliminate those that are in opposition to the host. Before the 2000 elections, when the Republican party had control of both houses of Congress, the majority of talk radio supported the Republican agenda. It is believed that their collective messages influenced the outcomes of the elections. More recently, the Internet has become a powerful medium to generate support for political candidates. Although he was initially not well-known, 2004 Democratic presidential candidate Howard Dean used the Internet to raise more money than any other Democratic candidate during the primary elections. His campaign used MeetUp.com, a Web tool for forming social groups, and bloggers (Wolf, 2004). This marked the first time a candidate fully utilized the power of the Internet, and it was highly successful, especially among young people who had grown up using the Web.

This electronic strategy is now being called a **distributed campaign.** A distributed campaign is "a Web-based campaign that contains a viral aspect, and whose success depends on the viability of three important online campaign components: websites, networks, and message delivery methods" (Ozimek, 2007, p. 171). This may become one of the most important campaign strategies in the future in generating responses, eliciting ideas for candidates' positions on issues, and raising money.

Television is also a forceful medium for visual influence, and is particularly useful for political advertisements. In 2004 Senator John Kerry ran against incumbent President George Bush. Kerry was a decorated Vietnam veteran. To garner support for his candidacy, Kerry's ads asserted that Bush had avoided the draft by enlisting in the National Guard. However, the ad backfired when a group of veterans who served with Kerry formed a group called the Swift Boat Veterans for Truth. In their own ad campaign, they questioned whether Kerry's medals were deserved and sug-

gested that his antiwar stance upon his return jeopardized the safety of those still serving in Vietnam. Regardless of the truth of the matter, the power of those ads was partially credited with Kerry's defeat and Bush's win.

The print media are also effective in disclosing information about health issues. For example, the nursing shortage became major news in 1999 when numerous articles about the absence of qualified nurses appeared in newspapers throughout the country. The public grew alarmed by inadequate nurse staffing in hospitals and other facilities and wanted policymakers and others to ensure that there would be a qualified and adequate workforce. Both the private sector and the public sector responded with ad campaigns and public funding to recruit more people into nursing. Johnson & Johnson, the giant health care company, donated more than $25 million in public service announcements and created community coalitions to sponsor nursing scholarships (www.discovernursing.com). State legislatures allocated increased funding for nursing scholarships and loan repayment programs, and the federal government passed legislation, the Nurse Reinvestment Act, to increase funding for baccalaureate and graduate education. The media response, as well as a downturn in the economy, resulted in a significant increase in applicants to nursing programs. Through support of private foundations, such as the Robert Wood Johnson Foundation, and funding from state legislatures, many states established centers to study workforce issues and collect data about workforce needs. The media were a significant factor in getting legislators to support the efforts. The power of the media affects both legislators and the public. It is a tool that nurses must use to affect public policy.

A LESSON IN CIVICS COMES ALIVE

It is essential that nurses and other health professionals clearly understand how government works before they can successfully influence the process. Americans have the greatest system of democracy in the world but it cannot run without citizen involvement; too few appreciate how vital it is to participate in the running of government. Take voter turnout, for example. In 1964 Americans had the highest turnout ever for a presidential election: 69 percent of the voting age population voted. In 2004 only 58 percent voted and that was a higher turnout than had been seen since 1984 (U.S. Census Bureau, 2006). In midterm elections, the turnout rarely exceeds one fourth to one third of the electorate. Most telling is the fact that the United States ranks twentieth out of 21 democracies in voter participation. Most countries have more than 80 percent turnout, and some require citizens to vote (The Center for Voting and Democracy, n.d.).

How one vote can make a difference in the outcome of a presidential race was made clear in the 2000 presidential election between Republican George W. Bush and Democrat Albert Gore, Jr., which resulted in the closest and most bizarre vote count in the country. Although Gore won the popular vote with 50,996,582 votes over Bush's 50,456,062, according to the electoral college system, Bush had been elected. After the Democrats charged that votes were undercounted and miscounted (the so-called "hanging chads") in Florida, the case went to the Florida Supreme Court, which ordered a recount of undercounted districts (Posner, 2001). The U.S. Supreme Court reversed the decision and refused to allow any recounts. As a result, Bush was declared the winner in Florida by 537 votes out of 6 million votes cast. The election was not decided until January 6, 2001, when the electoral college votes were officially counted and Bush and running mate Cheney were declared the winners with 271 electoral votes, compared with 267 for Gore and Leiberman (Eagleton Institute of Politics, 2000).

Imagine if you were a registered voter who did not vote in Florida. Think how much your vote might have changed the outcome of the electoral votes and thus the outcome of the presidential election. This example demonstrates the importance of every single vote.

Three Branches of Government

The framers of the U.S. Constitution had a major objective—the separation of powers—to prevent the aggregation of power in any one person or branch of government. Thus they set up a government with three branches—legislative, executive, and judicial—along with a mechanism of checks and balances for each. U.S. history reveals a waxing and waning of the powers of each branch, depending on the personalities of incumbents, contemporary social problems, and world events.

Under the Constitution, each branch of the federal government has separate and distinct functions and powers. The function of the **legislative branch**, which includes the House of Representatives and the Senate, is to deliberate and enact laws. Examples of legislative powers include setting and collecting taxes, overseeing commerce, declaring war, defining criminal offenses, coining money, and amending the Constitution. The legislative branch, particularly the House of Representatives, is assumed to be the government's closest link to the people and more susceptible to change through elections and social pressure. Figure 15-4 shows how a bill progresses through the legislative process to become a law.

The chief function of the **executive branch** of government is to administer the laws of the land. At the federal level, power is vested with the president, who has a wide variety of governmental departments (the cabinet) and employees (the bureaucracy) to carry out executive functions. The president has extensive powers of appointment (judges, ambassadors, agency heads) and is commander-in-chief of the armed forces. The president recommends legislation, gives the State of the Union report, and approves or vetoes the legislation of Congress, contributing to the balance of power.

The role of the **judicial branch** is to adjudicate, or decide, "cases or controversies" of particular matters. The judicial branch is divided into the federal and state court systems. The greatest power of the courts is to provide judicial review over governmental activities to uphold the

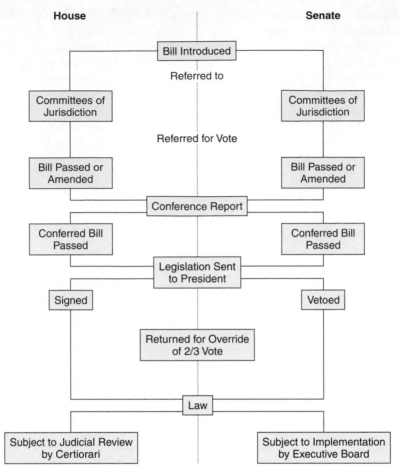

House   **Senate**

Figure 15-4

This flow chart shows how a bill progresses through the legislative process to become a law. Notice that both sides of Congress (the House of Representatives and the Senate) and the executive branch (the President and his administration) are involved and that laws are subject to judicial review.

privileges of the Constitution. The Supreme Court is the ultimate legal authority of the land and reviews decisions from lower courts.

Refer to Figure 15-4 again and notice that all three branches of government—legislative, executive, and judicial—are involved in the passage and interpretation of federal legislation.

Three Levels of Government

Government in the United States is organized at federal, state, and local levels. The Constitution established the relative powers of federal and

state governments and the rights of the individual. The Constitution identified specific powers of the federal government as matters of national interest needing uniform policies and reserved all other powers for the states. States, in turn, have developed their own constitutions and delineated power relationships with local communities and between branches of state government.

Exclusive powers of the federal government include declaring war, making treaties, administering public health services, and developing relationships with foreign powers. State and local governments maintain internal order, regulate domestic relationships, and protect the people. Currently, both the federal and the state governments can tax and spend and promote health. In times of shrinking resources, programs that are considered to be costly, such as health services, may be shifted to state control, calling into question the federal government's role in ensuring uniform access to health services throughout the United States.

All levels of government are expected to maintain their activities within the parameters of the Constitution. The Bill of Rights serves to promote and protect the rights of the individual from governmental intrusion.

Electoral Process

The process of electing public officials to office is known as the electoral process. Governmental elections generally focus on selecting local, state, and federal legislators and executive branch leaders such as the president, governor, and mayor. Federal judges are appointed, although in some states the people elect judges.

During the 1994 elections, members of third parties, such as United We Stand America, not only affected the outcome of the elections but also shaped the issues that were discussed as part of a "change agenda." Up until this point, the process of getting elected to office had occurred primarily through the two major parties—the Democratic and Republican parties. Third parties have become active in different regions at different times. Besides the Reform party (formerly United We Stand America), some of the more familiar third parties are the Libertarian, Conservative, Green, Socialist, and Communist. While they have some influence, third parties do not generally play a pivotal role in elections.

In most states, until recently, citizens declared a party affiliation when they registered to vote. This is changing; fewer states now require people to declare a party affiliation. Registered voters may participate in three major types of elections: primary elections, general elections, and referendums.

Primary elections are those in which a party is choosing among several party-affiliated candidates for a particular office. The outcome of primary elections is the selection of a party's candidate for a particular office. For those states that do not require a party designation, voters can choose which party's primary ticket to support. There is no obligation to vote for the same party in the next primary election. In states where voters must declare a party affiliation at the time they register, voters may vote only in the primary of the party in which they are registered. In **general elections,** all registered voters may vote. They are not required to vote a "straight party ticket"—that is, the voter can choose a candidate from any party on the ballot. Unless there is a tie or a challenge to the general election, the winner in a general election is usually the candidate with the highest number of votes. However, some states require a majority for elected office and may have a run-off between the two individuals with the greatest number of votes if a majority is not achieved. Length of service as an elected official depends on the office. For example, U.S. senators serve 6-year terms, and members of the House of Representatives serve 2-year terms; most governors and state legislators serve 4-year terms.

A **referendum** occurs when registered voters are asked to express directly their preferences on a policy issue. Usually, these issues are referred to the public either by a legislative body or by civic activists who have gathered enough signatures to require a vote. For example, a county commission may seek a referendum on raising property taxes to support school reform. Activist groups may seek a state referendum on gay rights, assisted suicide, or other controversial issues. The 2003 recall election of Governor Gray Davis of California (and the concomitant election of Arnold Schwarzenegger) occurred as a result of a referendum to oust Davis because of his unpopular fiscal and energy policies.

Working on a campaign, raising money for a candidate, and running for office require strict adherence to election laws. Rules vary from locality to locality and from state to federal elections. In recent years, Congress has passed legislation to tighten rules for individuals, businesses, labor unions, organizations, and political action committees (PACs) to fund candidates running for office. Running for office is expensive. Election laws for local, state, and federal elections require candidates to file financial reports indicating how much money they receive and spend for elections. The purpose is to prevent any one individual or organization from "buying" an election and to promote fairness for all candidates. Information about election regulations in each state can be obtained from the office of the Secretary of State. Federal election regulations can be obtained from the Federal Election Commission.

HEALTH CARE LEGISLATION AND REGULATION

Many issues facing nursing professionals can best be addressed through public policy, which requires that nurses influence government. The key questions for nurses to ask when seeking governmental intervention to improve nursing practice and health care are "Where can we play?" and "Where can we win?" The options to consider are the judicial, regulatory, or legislative arenas.

There are local, state, and federal courts, all of which require standing (a material interest in the outcome of a case) to seek a judicial remedy. In the executive branch, there are mayors, governors, presidents, and their staffs and department heads who make key decisions about how to implement (or not implement) rules and regulations. Most often, nurses have focused on legislative remedies to change health policy and have learned to be effective with legislative branch relationships. The nursing profession has now broadened its focus to use the regulatory and the judicial branches more effectively.

During the last 50 years of changing national and state health policies, nurses have increased their political savvy. Through the well-orchestrated efforts of the ANA, other professional organizations, constituent member associations, and

political action committees (PACs), nurses are now participating more effectively in both governmental and electoral politics than in the past. Nursing PACs raise and distribute money to candidates who support the profession's stand on certain issues. Nurses' endorsements of candidates have become a valued political asset for many local, state, and federal candidates.

Influencing Public Policy

Nurses can make a difference in health policy outcomes. Through the political process, nurses influence policy in a variety of ways: by identifying health problems as policy problems; by formulating policy through drafting legislation in collaboration with legislators; by providing formal testimony; by lobbying governmental officials in the executive and legislative branches to make certain health policies a priority for action; and by filing suit as a party or as a friend of the court to implement health policy strategies on behalf of consumers. All the major nursing professional associations engage in these activities. Because the American Nurses Association is the major organization that speaks for all nurses, specific examples of influencing public policy will be drawn largely from ANA's activities.

Capitol Update, an online newsletter published by the ANA, reports on the progress of nursing influence with the president, members of Congress and their staffs, and the regulatory agencies that set policy for health programs (www.capitolupdate.org/newsletter/). Such activity reflects the work of both ANA members and ANA staff. The ANA's political activity in Washington, DC, is mirrored throughout the United States by other nursing organizations and by ANA constituent member associations conducting similar work with their state governments.

Nurses Strategic Action Teams (N-STAT) is ANA's grassroots network of nurses across the country who keep elected representatives in Congress informed about issues of concern to patients and nurses. By notifying network members, ANA can rapidly mobilize nurses to lobby their federal representatives to support or oppose particular legislation and/or rules and regulations. Through the use of telephones, fax, e-mail, and regular mail, N-STAT members can respond by sending well-timed, well-targeted messages to members of Congress.

Organized activity in identifying, financially supporting, and working for candidates who are committed to nursing and "nurse-friendly" issues has dramatically increased since the early 1990s. The electoral process is an essential function of the professional association. No better example of the interrelationship of nursing, public policy, and political action exists than the 1992 presidential election and its aftermath. ANA became the first national health care organization to support President Clinton's candidacy publicly. As a result, there were an unprecedented number of nurses appointed to federal office. That early and visible political support meant that nursing enjoyed unprecedented access to the White House during the Clinton/Gore administration.

The Nurse Reinvestment Act, passed in 2002, was the culmination of work by many national organizations and individual nurses who lobbied for the federal legislation to ease the nursing shortage (Figure 15-5). The legislation provides loan repayment programs and scholarships for nursing students, public service announcements to encourage people to enter nursing, grants to schools to encourage nurses to enter gerontology, and repayment of loans for nurses to pursue careers in teaching.

Nurses working at the state level are also making their presence felt. In 2005 there were more than 80 nurses elected to state legislatures (http://nursingworld.org/gova/state/nursleg2.htm). Many hold important positions as leaders on health policy issues. For instance, Judith Robson, RN, is Senate minority leader in Wisconsin, and Paula Hollinger, RN, is chair of the Health Committee in the Maryland Senate. In their leadership roles, they have been critical in passing legislation on issues such as prohibiting mandatory overtime and authorizing nurse practitioners and clinical nurse specialists to prescribe medications.

Figure 15-5
A press conference was held during National Nurses Week, May 7, 2002, to announce the passage of the Nurse Reinvestment Act. Pictured are ANA past president Mary Foley, Senator Tim Hutchinson (R-AK), Senator Barbara Mikulski (R-MD), and Senator John D. Dingell (D-MI, 16th). *(Courtesy American Nurses Association.)*

Individual nurses can make a difference in policy development and elections. Either by election or by appointment, nurses need to be making health policy decisions, not just influencing them. Getting elected or appointed requires visibility, expertise, energy, risk taking, and a belief that policy and politics are critically important in achieving nursing's goals.

Getting nurses appointed

How does one get appointed to a powerful position in government? The chief executive of a city, county, state, or the nation makes appointments. Such appointments are to regulatory agencies, such as a state board of nursing, or to specific taskforces or committees focused on particular health issues. Appointments are usually the result of the expertise and visibility of the individual appointee and of the power and influence of that appointee's membership in an organization that supported the elected official.

Nurses at the national level have been appointed to a variety of significant national policymaking positions. To get appointed, a nurse needs to be known to organizations with considerable political influence. As mentioned, ANA worked intensively to help get President Clinton elected, and more nurses were appointed to office during his administration than in any previous administration. The political activism of the appointees, along with the support of ANA and other national organizations, helped secure these important federal appointments.

During the administration of President George W. Bush, who was not supported by the ANA, few nurses were appointed. An exception was the appointment of three nurses to the Federal Advisory Committee on Regulatory Reform for the Centers for Medicare and Medicaid Services (CMS).

The same process for appointments occurs at the state level. The governor makes appointments to many boards, commissions, and key government positions. Thus gubernatorial elections are of critical importance to state associations. Qualified nurses who have supported the election of the governor and are known to their constituent member association are encouraged to seek appointments to regulatory bodies such as state boards of nursing. As previously discussed, state boards of nursing, through rules and regulations, make definitive health policy and are highly important to issues related to nursing practice. For most nurses, appointments at the state level are more attainable than national posts. It is vital that the executive director of the state organization know the nurse, because directors are often consulted in the appointment process.

GETTING INVOLVED

To get involved, a nurse must begin to understand the connections between individual practice and public policy. Once that happens, it is easy to get started. Three levels of political involvement in which nurses can participate are as nurse citizens, nurse activists, and nurse politicians.

Nurse Citizens

A nurse citizen brings the perspective of health care to the voting booth, to public forums that advocate for health and human services, and to involvement in community activities. For example, budget cuts to a school district might involve elimination of school nurses. At a school board meeting, nurses can effectively speak about the vital services that school nurses provide to children and the cost-effectiveness of maintaining the position.

Nurses tend to vote for candidates who advocate for improved health care. Here are some examples of how the nurse citizen can be politically active:

- Register to vote.
- Vote in every election.
- Keep informed about health care issues.
- Speak out when services or working conditions are inadequate.
- Participate in public forums.
- Know your local, state, and federal elected officials.
- Join politically active nursing organizations.
- Participate in community organizations that need health experts.
- Join a political party.

Once nurses make a decision to become involved politically, they need to learn how to get started. One of the best ways is to form a relationship with one or more policymakers. Box 15-4 contains several pointers for influencing policymakers.

Nurse Activists

The nurse activist takes a more active role than the nurse citizen and often does so because an issue arises that directly affects the nurse's professional life (Figure 15-6). The need to respond moves the nurse to a higher level of participation. For example, a nurse in private practice who has difficulty getting insurance companies to honor patients' claims for reimbursement of nursing services may become active in lobbying state legislators for changes in insurance regulations.

Box 15-4	Communication Is the Key to Influence

Cultivate a relationship with policymakers from your home district or state. Communicate by visits, telephone, e-mail, and letters. Letters and other messages need these elements:

- If writing a letter, use personal stationery.
- State who you are (a nursing student or registered nurse and a voter in a specific district).
- Identify the issue by a file number, if possible.
- Be clear on where you stand and why.
- Be positive when possible.
- Be concise.
- Ask for a commitment. State precisely what action you want the policymaker to take.
- Give your return address, e-mail address, and phone number to urge dialogue.
- Be persistent. Follow up with calls or letters.
- If you plan to visit your policymaker on a specific issue, be sure to make your appointment in advance in writing and indicate what issue you are interested in discussing.
- Be quick to thank and praise policymakers when they do something you like.

Figure 15-6
The nurse activist has a high level of involvement in selected political issues. Here she visits with one of her state legislators at the state capitol. *(Courtesy Tennessee Nurses Association. Photograph by Chip Powell.)*

Nurse activists can make changes by:
- Joining politically active nursing organizations.
- Contacting a public official through letters, e-mails, or phone calls.
- Registering people to vote.
- Contributing money to a political campaign.
- Working in a campaign.

- Lobbying decision makers by providing pertinent statistical and anecdotal information.
- Forming or joining coalitions that support an issue of concern.
- Writing letters to the editor of local newspapers.
- Inviting legislators to visit the workplace.
- Holding a media event to publicize an issue.
- Providing or giving testimony to legislators and regulatory bodies.

Box 15-5 includes pointers on how to make a difference in health policy development.

Nurse Politicians

Once a nurse realizes and experiences the empowerment that can come from political activism, he or she may choose to run for office. No longer satisfied to help others get elected, the nurse politician desires to develop the legislation, not just influence it.

As of 2006 there were three nurses serving in Congress. In 1992 Congresswoman Eddie Bernice Johnson (D-TX) was the first nurse elected to the U.S. House of Representatives. She has been consistently reelected since. The second nurse, Carolyn McCarthy (D-NY), an LPN, was elected in 1996 as a result of her stance on gun control. Her husband was killed and her son critically injured

Box **15-5** Key Questions for Nurses Who Want to Make a Difference in Health Policy

1. Know the system. Is it a federal, state, or local issue? Is it in the hands of the executive, legislative, or judicial branch of government?
2. Know the issue. What is wrong? What should happen? Why is it not happening? What is needed: leadership, a plan, pressure, or data?
3. Know the players. Who is on your side, and who is not? Who will make the decision? Who knows whom? Will a coalition be effective? Are you a member of the professional nursing organization?
4. Know the process. Is this a vote? Is this an appropriation? Is this a legislative procedure? Is this a committee or subcommittee report?
5. Know what to do. Should you write, call, arrange a lunch meeting, organize a petition, show up at the hearing, give testimony, demonstrate, or file a suit?

after a lone gunman with a 9-mm semiautomatic pistol walked through a train on the Long Island Railroad and killed 25 people and wounded 19 others. Carolyn was suddenly thrown into the national spotlight when she challenged the incumbent congressman running for office on his stand supporting a repeal on a ban for assault rifles. Her ability to speak passionately about the issue led to her campaign against the incumbent and her election to his seat. She has been a leader in the House of Representatives on gun control, as well as on nursing issues (McCarthy, 2007). In 1998 Congresswoman Lois Capps (D-CA) became the third nurse to be elected to the House of Representatives. Congresswoman Capps was a long-time leader in health care and a school nurse. After her election to Congress, she drew on her extensive health care background to co-chair the House Democratic Task Force on Medicare Reform, and in 2003 she founded the Bipartisan Congressional Caucus on Nursing and the Bipartisan School Health and Safety Caucus.

Nurse politicians use their knowledge about people, their expertise about health, their ability to communicate effectively, and their superb organizational skills in running for office. Because the public places a high value on nurses, nurse politicians tend to be trusted. If nurses know how to run a campaign and can raise money, they stand a good chance of being elected.

Once nurses are elected, they can sponsor legislation that reflects their professional experiences. Many of the laws that expand reimburse-ment for nursing services, funding for services to women and children, occupational safety and health issues, and research on women's health have been sponsored by nurse legislators and supported by nurses working as key legislative staff members.

Political life can be grueling, and the nurse politician must be ready to sacrifice a regular schedule and personal privacy. In addition, adequate financial resources are critical to a successful campaign for office. Fortunately, more nurses today are willing to make this commitment because they believe in their own power and ability to enhance the well-being of the public (Figure 15-7). Individual nurses and nurse-specific PACs are increasingly willing and able to support nurse candidates financially at all levels of government.

The nurse politician can:
- Run for an elected office.
- Seek appointment to a regulatory agency.
- Be appointed to a governing board in the public or private sector.
- Use nursing expertise as a front-line policymaker who can enhance health care and the profession.

We Were All Once Novices

In general, nurses who have achieved success as leaders started with no knowledge of the political process and no expectations of the greatness they would achieve. Instead, they became involved because some issue, injustice, or abuse of power affected their lives. Instead of complaining or

Figure 15-7

Nurse legislators from the state of Washington and representatives of the Washington State Nurses Association celebrate the signing of the Safe Patient Handling Act by Governor Christine Gregoire. The state has eight registered nurses who serve as elected representatives in the state legislature.

feeling helpless, they responded by taking an active role in bringing about change.

The mark of a leader is the ability to identify a problem, have a goal, and know how to join others in reaching that goal. A leader must ask the right questions, analyze the positive and restraining forces toward meeting the goal, and know how to obtain and use power. A leader must know how to ask for help and how to give support to those who join the effort. These are the marks of nursing leaders who have become political experts.

NURSES WHO KNEW HOW TO USE POLITICAL POWER

Diane Carlson Evans is a nurse who made a difference by using her political power. Diane served in Vietnam as an Army nurse. Several years after

returning to the United States she read an article in the newspaper describing a bronze sculpture of three male infantryman that would be erected as part of the Vietnam Memorial. For her it was a wake-up call that the country did not know the women who served alongside the men depicted in the memorial statue. The "personal became political" for Diane, and she was moved to change America's image about who the soldiers were. Her goal became to recognize women, particularly nurses, who served in Vietnam.

She began by speaking to community groups and veterans groups. The more she spoke, the more she realized that women had been invisible in Vietnam. Other than family and friends there was little publicity to inform the public about their role. To change the perception, Diane established a core group of nurse veterans who created a national nonprofit organization. The organization's mission was to raise money to create a sculpture depicting the women who served, to facilitate research about the women, and to educate the public about the contributions of these women.

Diane and her colleagues developed short-term and long-term strategies and engaged in a 10-year effort to get the Vietnam Women's Memorial erected. Their strategies included:

- Developing stakeholder support by creating coalitions of veterans, civilians, humanitarians, and business groups.
- Finding a sculptor to create a depiction that was agreeable to major supporters.
- Getting Congress to pass legislation to erect the memorial alongside the Vietnam Wall.
- Overcoming opposition from the various Washington commissions that had to give their approval.
- Getting President George Herbert Walker Bush to sign the legislation.
- Using the media, especially an extensive interview on *60 Minutes* that was seen by millions of viewers.

On November 11, 1993, Diane's dream was realized when the Vietnam Women's Memorial was dedicated on the National Mall close to the Vietnam Veterans Memorial Wall (Figure 15-8).

Figure 15-8
Vietnam Women's Memorial.

Diane's story is one of responding to a public issue that she believed was important. She displayed vision, leadership, and a willingness to take risks that changed her life. As she says, "It is easy to be intimidated by the mysteries of politics, politicians, and the political process. Yet this is where action, driven by our personal aspirations, values and beliefs can force change—and even alter the way people view the world" (Evans, 2002, p. 197). (For a complete story, read *Transforming Vision into Reality: The Vietnam Women's Memorial* by Diane Evans [Mason, 2007].)

Karen Daley is another living nurse hero. Karen's story about learning to use her power to change both public and workplace policy also began with her own experience. In 1998 Karen sustained a needlestick injury while working as an experienced nurse in one of the busiest hospital ERs in the country. As she held a patient's arm after a venipuncture, Karen turned to drop the used needle into the sharps container on the wall behind her. Unfortunately, there was a second needle wedged inside the box and she sustained a needlestick injury. She learned 5 months later,

after experiencing weight loss and fatigue, that she had contracted both HIV and hepatitis C from the needlestick.

After coping with the reality of how her life had changed, Karen began a mission: to prevent other health care providers from sustaining such injuries. Her story is one of mobilizing state legislatures, Congress, and health organizations to establish safety policies involving equipment, the redesign and placement of sharps containers, and the reporting and detailed follow-up of all injuries, without punitive consequences to anyone. Despite her own illness and resulting symptoms, Karen's willingness to go public with her story brought national media attention to the issue of needlestick injuries and contributed to policy reform at state and national levels. This included:

■ Passage of legislation in Massachusetts, making it the only state that mandates 100 percent sharps surveillance and reporting.

■ Passage of legislation in 20 states to improve protection from needlestick injuries.

■ Revision of the blood-borne pathogen standard to include all private sector employers as well as public; the use of safety devices mandates that direct care providers be involved in selection and evaluation of equipment as well as conducting HIV testing after all contaminated sharps injuries. This resulted in federal legislation—the Needlestick Prevention and Safety Act of 2000.

■ A national needlestick prevention campaign by the ANA and the state nursing associations.

Karen's interview with Mike Wallace on *60 Minutes* as well as meeting the press in at least the 20 states demonstrated her political skills to educate the public about workplace safety. An expert nurse, she used her own story to change national and state policy. The considerable decline in such injuries is testimony to the power of one nurse in changing workplace and public policy (Daley, 2007).

NURSING AWAITS YOUR CONTRIBUTION

You can apply the skills discussed in this chapter. Look to teachers, family, friends, and community leaders whom you admire. What are the leadership qualities they possess that you wish to have? These individuals can offer inspiration and serve as role models for you to imitate.

You may also choose to form a relationship with a political mentor. A mentor not only serves as a role model but also actively teaches, encourages, and critiques the process of growth and change in the learner. All nurses who have become political leaders have found mentors along the way to guide and support their growth. Your mentor could be a faculty member, such as the adviser to the nursing student organization or honor society, who can teach you leadership skills. Ask for help in running for a class office or student council president. If elected office does not appeal to you, use your political skills to develop a school or community project with other nursing students.

You may have a relative or friend involved in a political campaign who could help you learn about the political process. You might find a problem during a clinical experience that inhibits your ability to provide the level of care that you wish to provide. Seek a faculty member or nurse in a clinical facility who can guide you through the process of policy change within the agency or institution.

Watch the communication skills of your role models or mentors. How does your own behavior compare with theirs? What enhances or impedes your progress? Get your friends and peers to join your activity. Seek their help and support. Always thank them and be ready to offer your help and support when they need it.

SUMMARY OF *Key Points*

■ Professional associations are the vehicle through which nursing takes collective action to improve both the nursing profession and health care delivery.

■ There are many nursing associations from which to choose and they offer a variety of benefits to the public, to the nursing profession as a whole, and to individual members.

■ Membership in professional associations is essential for professionals, but selecting which associations to join can be a challenge. Prospective members should ask key questions to help them select wisely.

■ Professional organizations and professional nurses have much to offer in formulating policy decisions at federal, state, and local levels and in each branch of government.

■ Today, organized nursing is involved in politics at many levels in promoting comprehensive health reform and creating a safer workplace.

■ Becoming politically active is as easy as signing your name in support of an issue, registering to vote, organizing a project, or speaking out on an issue.

■ Political involvement is empowering; one person *can* make a difference.

■ The involvement of nurses in the political process benefits nurses, the nursing profession, and the recipients of health care.

CRITICAL THINKING QUESTIONS

1. Look in a local newspaper for articles about federal legislation that support nursing's concerns, such as the Safe Staffing Act, or other nursing-related or patient-related legislation pending in your state. Write a letter to the editor of your local paper about these bills, taking a stand on the issues.

2. Find out whether there is a student nurses association on your campus. If there is, learn all you can about it and consider joining. Get your friends to join with you. If there is not a student nurses association, consider establishing one. (Resources: Go to www.nsna.org; click on "Program Activities.")

3. As a student, attend a local or state nurses association meeting to gain a better sense of the issues in the profession, so that you can be prepared for what lies ahead when you graduate. How is the association addressing these issues? Do they interest you? How can you get involved?

Consider the following hypothetical situations:

4. You read in a local newspaper that students at your university have a high rate of drug and alcohol use. The following week, a story appears about a senior university student who died following a car crash. The student was driving under the influence of alcohol. How can nursing students address the need for education about drug and alcohol use? What collective action can you initiate to address this or another issue of importance to your college or university community? (Resources: Go to www.nsna.org; click on "Publications" to download Guidelines for Planning Community Health Projects.)

5. The demand for nursing services is increasing, but the availability of registered nurses will not meet this demand. The student nurses association chapter has formed a recruitment committee to address this issue and answer the following questions: Why are students not considering nursing as a career? Why are students considering nursing as a career? How many registered nurses will be needed in the future? Why do many nursing programs have waiting lists to enter the program? Plan a collective action project that can be implemented by the student nurses association to increase interest in the nursing profession. (Resources: Go to www.nsna.org; click on "Publications" to download Guidelines for Planning Breakthrough to Nursing Projects.)

6. Students at your school must struggle to pay tuition. Many students work part-time while attending school full-time. They have taken out student loans and have applied for scholarships to help pay for tuition, books, and other school-related expenses. A faculty member announces in class that the Nurse Reinvestment Act is going before Congress for funding authorization. What collective actions can the student nurses association take to ask Congress to increase funding for undergraduate nursing education and for student loan repayment programs? (Resources: Go to www.nsna.org; click on "Publications" to download Guidelines for Planning Legislative Activities.)

7. A classmate asks you to share a paper you prepared for a leadership course she is now taking so that she can see how you handled the assignment. You willingly give her a copy of your "A" paper. At the end of the semester, the faculty member who teaches the leadership course calls you into her office. She shows you the paper you wrote for her course last semester, but it now has your classmate's name on it instead of yours! What collective action can the student nurses association take to prevent plagiarism and cheating? (Resources: Go to www.nsna.org; click on "Publications" to download the NSNA Bill of Rights and Responsibilities for Students of Nursing and the NSNA Code of Academic and Clinical Professional Conduct.)

8. Conduct a class poll. Of those in the class who are eligible to vote, how many are registered? How many voted in the last local, state, or national election? Challenge those not registered to become registered before the end of the current school term.

9. Because nurses have differing personal and political values, it has been a challenge to get them all united behind a single issue or candidate. If you were the president of the American Nurses Association, what techniques would you use to convince the 2.9 million American nurses to use the power of their numbers, their knowledge, and their commitment on behalf of their profession?

10. Find out whether the members of your state board of nursing are elected or appointed. What is the composition of the board (that is, how many registered nurses, licensed practical nurses, and consumers are there, for example)? Do nurses hold most of the seats on the state board? Are there any other health professionals, such as physicians, on the board of nursing? If so, are there any nurses on the state board of medicine?

REFERENCES

American Association of Nurse Anesthetists: *Concerning state opt-outs and November 13, 2001 CMS rule,* 2006, available online: http://www.aana.com/advocacy.aspx?ucNavMenu_TSMenuTargetID=49&ucNavMenu_TSMenuTargetType=4&ucNavMenu_TSMenuID=6&id=1790.

American Nurses Association: Blood-borne diseases, 1993, available online: http://nursingworld.org/dlwa/osh/wp2.htm.

Center for Voting and Democracy: *Voter turnout* (no date given), available online: http://www.fairvote.org/?page=262.

Daley K: Needlestick injuries in the workplace: implications for public policy. In Mason D, Leavitt J, Chaffee M, editors: *Policy and politics in nursing and health care,* ed 5, St Louis, 2007, Saunders.

Eagleton Institute of Politics, Rutgers University: *2000 Presidential election,* 2003, available online: http://www.rci.rutgers.edu/~eagleton/e-gov/e-politicalarchive-2000.htm.

Evans D: Transforming vision into reality: the Vietnam women's memorial. In Mason D, Leavitt J, Chaffee M, editors: *Policy and politics in nursing and health care,* ed 4, St Louis, 2002, Saunders.

Holland K: *Dealing with generational differences: we have always done it that way,* 2005, available online: http://www.alwaysdoneitthatway.com/2005/11/20/dealing-with-generational-differences/.

Kany K: Contemporary issues in nursing organizations. In Mason D, Leavitt J, Chaffee M, editors: *Policy and politics in nursing and health care,* ed 5, St Louis, 2007, Saunders.

Leavitt J: Rising to the top; an interview with Sheila Burke. In Mason D, Leavitt J, editors: *Policy and politics in nursing and health care,* ed 3, Philadelphia, 1998, Saunders.

Lewenson S: An historical perspective on policy, politics and nursing. In Mason D, Leavitt J, Chaffee M, editors: *Policy and politics in nursing and health care,* ed 5, St Louis, 2007, Saunders.

Mason D: Harnessing the power of the media to influence health policy and politics. In Mason D, Leavitt J, Chaffee M, editors: *Policy and politics in nursing and health care,* ed 5, St Louis, 2007, Saunders.

Mather M: Reefer madness: the illogical politics of medical marijuana. In Mason D, Leavitt J, Chaffee M, editors: *Policy and politics in nursing and health care,* ed 5, St Louis, 2007, Saunders.

McCarthy C: A nurse in congress. In Mason D, Leavitt J, Chaffee M, editors: *Policy and politics in nursing and health care,* ed 5, St Louis, 2007, Saunders.

Mooney MM: Hog-housed! *Reflect Nurs Leadership* 29(4):8-9, 2003.

Nursing Organizations Alliance: *Nursing alliance leadership academy,* 2005, available online: http://www.nursing-alliance.org/events.cfm.

Ozimek R: Distributed campaigns: using electronic media to empower activism. In Mason D, Leavitt J, Chaffee M, editors: *Policy and politics in nursing and health care,* ed 5, St Louis, 2007, Saunders.

Posner R: *Breaking the deadlock: the 2000 election, the Constitution and the courts,* Princeton, NJ, 2001, Princeton University Press, p 48.

Shaner McRae H: Environmental advocacy: a nurse's journey. In Mason D, Leavitt J, Chaffee M, editors:

Policy and politics in nursing and health care, ed 4, St Louis, 2002, Saunders.

Sigma Theta Tau International: *Woodhull study on nursing and the media,* Indianapolis, 1997, Center Nursing Press.

U.S. Census Bureau: *Statistical abstract of the United States,* 2006, available online: http://www.census.gov/population/www/socdemo/voting.html.

Wolf G: How the internet invented Howard Dean, *Wired Magazine,* 2004, available online: www.wired.com/wired/archive/12.01/dean.html.

16

Nursing's Future Challenges

Kay Kittrell Chitty

Learning Outcomes

After reading this chapter, students will be able to:

- Review societal influences on the nursing profession anticipated during the next decade.
- Recognize the impact that changes in the health care system will have on the practice of nursing.
- Explain trends in nursing education needed to meet society's future nursing needs.

- Describe major challenges that the nursing profession must resolve to ensure it remains in control of its destiny.
- Describe the major components of Nursing's Agenda for the Future.

As you have seen throughout this textbook, the nursing profession is profoundly affected by a rapidly changing world. The challenges nurses face today relate to a variety of factors: changes in demographics, unhealthy lifestyles of many Americans, the continued deterioration of the environment, rapid change in the health care system, cost-containment pressures, advances in technology (notably in genomics and informatics), bioterrorism, natural and man-made disasters, cultural diversity within both nursing and the population, blurring of professional boundaries, increasing interdisciplinary collaboration, and issues within nursing itself.

It is painfully clear that even in the United States, the wealthiest of the industrialized nations, we fall far short of the goal of having a healthy nation in spite of spending nearly $2 trillion annually on health care in recent years. More than 45 million Americans have no health insurance, and many others have less than enough (Porter, 2005). Infant death rates remain unacceptably high. Among 33 industrialized nations, the United States is tied with Hungary, Malta, Poland, and Slovakia with a death rate of nearly 5 per 1000 babies (Tanner, 2006).

The fitness level of citizens, including young people, continues to decline as obesity increases at an alarming rate. Smoking in youth continues to increase. In addition, the threat of bioterrorism is a new challenge we must face as a profession and as a nation. All these negative trends continue even though the United States spends more of its gross domestic product (16% in 2004) on health than any nation in the world (Porter, 2005). Complete overhaul of the health care system, believed by many Americans to be essential if these problems are to be addressed, has been stalled in Congress since 1994.

Nursing enjoys high levels of respect and public confidence. It is a profession in heavy demand, and its practitioners enjoy more autonomy than ever. As the health care profession with the highest number of practitioners, nursing has enormous but largely untapped political power that would allow nurses to influence societal changes— rather than simply be influenced by them—if they were unified in their efforts. Yet turf issues, lack of focus, and inaction continue to divide nurses, diminishing their influence at every level.

You might wonder what purpose is served by thinking about the future. The purpose of "futures work" is "to study potential developments, using tools and certain attitudinal alignments, to effect change in a desired direction. A deliberated future may be personal, professional or organizational, but the process is the same: creating an image of a desired result to serve as a blueprint for action. It allows us to avert, encourage, or direct the course of events" (Dickenson-Hazard, 2003), rather than simply reacting to them.

This chapter explores some of nursing's challenges and opportunities in the future.

SOCIETAL CHALLENGES

At least six societal influences are expected to have major impact on the future of the nursing profession: demographic changes, environmental deterioration, the recently recognized need to prepare for large-scale public health disasters, unhealthy lifestyles and resulting illnesses, continuing need for cost containment, and regulation of health care. Each of these influences is examined briefly.

Demographics

Demography is the science that studies vital statistics and social trends. Demographers examine vital statistics such as **birthrates** (births per 1000 people in 1 year), **morbidity rates** (illness), **mortality rates** (deaths), marriages, the ages of

various populations, and migration patterns. From this wealth of information, **futurists,** people who try to project what will occur, draw conclusions about what these trends mean for the future.

Four demographic trends are particularly important to the future of nursing: the aging population, poverty, the cultural diversity of the population, and urbanization, including increasing levels of violence. Each has implications for nursing.

Aging population

Estimates vary, but demographers have predicted that the number of people older than age 75 in the United States by the year 2020 will exceed 21.8 million. The number of aging baby boomers will create an additional strain on the U.S. health care system. These "boomers" will be different from patients in the past because they will "expect more and tolerate less" (Wolf, 2003, p. 32). They will be the most knowledgeable health care consumers ever and will keep their caregivers on their toes.

Centenarians, people more than 100 years of age, represent one of the fastest-growing groups in the United States. The World Future Society predicts that by the end of the twenty-first century, the average life span will approach 100 years (Hendrick, 1995). Many elderly people are healthy, but the likelihood of illness becomes greater as people age. For example, indications are that by the age of 90, one of two people will develop Alzheimer's disease (Herbert, Scherr, Beckett et al, 1995). In general, the elderly are greater users of health care than any other population segment (Valentino, 2002). Clearly, nurses of the future must be prepared to work effectively with the rising numbers of elderly patients.

Ethical issues such as **euthanasia** and **assisted suicide** will become increasingly important as technology enables people to sustain life far beyond the point of useful, meaningful existence. Society's views of assisted suicide and euthanasia are changing, as evidenced by the fact that juries acquitted Dr. Jack Kevorkian of charges of murder in the assisted deaths of several terminally ill people before he was ultimately convicted and sentenced to prison. Additionally, the citizens of Oregon passed an assisted suicide referendum. Two countries, The Netherlands and Belgium, have legalized assisted suicide and a number of other nations are considering it. The future will gradually bring further changes in laws and attitudes toward giving individuals control over the timing and manner of their own deaths. As our population ages, **end-of-life care,** particularly pain control and other forms of **palliative care,** will increasingly be a focus of formal and continuing education nursing programs.

Poverty

Even though the United States is considered the world's wealthiest nation, the number of Americans living below the poverty line is increasing. This is particularly true of women, children, and the elderly. Another large group of Americans are employed yet cannot make enough money to provide adequately for their families' needs. They are known as the **working poor.** This group has grown since "welfare reform" legislation passed in 1996. The gap between the "haves" and the "have-nots" in the United States continues to widen, creating discontent and disillusionment. Never was this more clearly seen than following Hurricane Katrina, when the poor residents of New Orleans lived in inhumane conditions for days on end.

When basic needs for food, clothing, and shelter are unmet or uncertain, health care becomes a luxury. Children's immunizations, prenatal care for pregnant women, nutritious meals, dental care, and a variety of other health-maintaining factors are neglected. **Medically indigent** people, those who do not qualify for Medicaid but nevertheless cannot pay for health care, tend to put off seeking care until illness is advanced and thus harder to treat. Conditions that can be prevented often are not because of lack of education, poor sanitation, crowded living conditions, improper shelter, homelessness, and a host of other poverty-related factors.

It is a sad reality that poverty will continue to rise in the future, creating increasing numbers of **disenfranchised** people, that is, people who have no power in the political system, with limited access to health care. As their numbers grow, both federal and state governments will be forced by limited resources to implement more strategies that limit health care expenditures for these **vulnerable populations.**

Nursing, as a profession, values providing care to all people, regardless of social and economic factors. The increasing numbers of medically disenfranchised people and pressure to limit health care expenditures will collide to create an intense values conflict for nurses of the future.

Cultural diversity

Cultural diversity refers to the array of people from different racial, ethnic, religious, social, and geographic backgrounds who make up a particular entity. Some countries, such as Japan, are **homogeneous** in culture. This means that most citizens have similar cultural beliefs and practices. Others, such as the United States, have a **heterogeneous** cultural mix. The cultural beliefs and practices of our citizens are quite different and becoming more so with every passing year.

Immigration to the United States from Southeast Asia, Central America, the Middle East, Mexico, and the islands of the Caribbean has increased in recent years as a result of civil unrest, wars, and poor economic conditions (Figure 16-1). People from these countries are the latest wave of newcomers to the United States and join the European-Americans, African-Americans, and others whose ancestors came to this country in the twentieth century and earlier. Each group has its own nutritional practices, health beliefs, folk remedies, childcare practices, and conventional wisdom about health and illness.

Nurses need to take cultural beliefs, values, and practices into consideration when planning and implementing nursing care for individuals of diverse cultural backgrounds. Culturally competent care will be more important in the future than ever before (see Cultural Considerations Challenge, below). Speaking a second language, particularly Spanish, will be an important skill that will both enhance nurses' ability to communicate with patients and increase nurses' value to health care organizations.

The nursing profession itself will become increasingly diverse as its membership reflects a

Figure 16-1
Immigration to the United States from Southeast Asia, Central America, Mexico, and the Caribbean islands is expected to continue in the next decade, contributing to sweeping demographic changes. Here nursing students and their faculty participate in a farm worker family health program for migrant workers in rural Georgia. *(Courtesy Emory University, Nell Hodgson Woodruff School of Nursing.)*

heterogeneous society. This will create the need for nurses to understand, respect, and value the contributions of co-workers of all cultural backgrounds.

Urbanization

Urbanization, that is, people moving from rural, farming areas to cities, has increased since the time of the Industrial Revolution. That trend continues today and is expected to go on well into the new century.

As cities grow, suburbs flourish, and many people who can afford to do so move away from the business centers of cities. Decaying inner cities with large populations of poor people create major social problems such as homelessness, drugs, gangs, single-parent households, mental illness, violence, and crime. Despite the increase in public-private partnerships designed to revitalize inner cities and programs formulated to deal effectively with urban issues, social problems continue to grow and spill over into the suburbs and rural areas, creating further social changes. Nurses of the future will be increasingly confronted with health problems resulting from these social phenomena.

Violence is of particular concern to members of the nursing profession. Violence is present in our homes, workplaces, schools, and communities, causing untold chaos and loss. Violence is becoming a major public health problem in the

 Cultural Considerations *Challenge*

The Impact of Immigration on Your Nursing Practice

Immigration, especially from Mexico, is a phenomenon expected to continue. In a group setting with classmates, respond to these questions:
- What effects do you anticipate that immigration may have on your own practice?
- What preparations have you made to incorporate immigrants into your practice?

- What do you believe is your professional responsibility in the care of immigrants?
- Does your personal belief system about immigration affect the way that you may react to immigrants in your work as a nurse?
- How is the immigration status (documented or undocumented) of a patient relevant to the care you provide to that patient?
- What adjustments might you need to make to accommodate persons who have migrated to the United States?

United States and elsewhere, and we see the results in offices, clinics, and trauma units. Because the nursing profession cannot turn a blind eye to this problem, we will see nurses as individuals and as a professional group increasingly take action against the rising tide of violence to protect the basic societal principles of safety and security.

Environment

Every newspaper, news magazine, and television news program brings disturbing reports of the deterioration of our environment. There are major environmental tragedies, such as a nuclear power plant incident in Japan and floodwaters spreading effluent from hundreds of hog farms in eastern North Carolina. These overshadow the less dramatic but insidious gradual decline in the quality of the world's air, water, and plant and animal life.

Acute and chronic respiratory diseases are increasing, as are debilitating allergic reactions to chemicals in the environment and cancers of all types (Figure 16-2). Reports of deterioration of the ozone layer, accidental lead and mercury poisonings, toxic shellfish beds, truckloads of pesticides spilling into streams and rivers, and accidental release of radioactive steam from nuclear power plants all occur with distressing regularity. Meanwhile, clear-cutting of forests, destruction of wetlands by development, and relaxing of standards for polluting industries have become "business as usual." Scientists now agree that global warming is accelerating and is attributable to human activity. Still, our government does little to control emissions.

Epidemiologists, who study the origins and spread of diseases, believe that there is a relationship between environmental decline and increases in certain diseases, including avian flu and mad cow disease. Emerging diseases and **multidrug resistant strains** (MDRS) of organisms currently under control, such as tuberculosis, will increasingly challenge health care resources.

Humans are responsible for destroying the environment, and the more human beings there

Figure 16-2

This manufacturing plant, while providing jobs to scores of workers, has polluted the air and the ground around it, as well as a nearby stream. Although the plant is slated for closure, it will take years to clean up the ground and water contaminated during its decades of operation. *(Photo by Kelly Whalin.)*

are, the faster the environment will decline. Overpopulation contributes to the deterioration of the world's environment, yet too few countries are dealing effectively with issues of overpopulation, including the United States.

In June 2006 the world population reached the record number of 6.5 billion people. The U.S. Census Bureau has projected that the world's population will increase to 8.8 billion by the end of 2025 (U.S. Census Bureau, 2006). Feeding, immunizing, providing potable water, and caring for this many human beings threaten to destroy the environmental, economic, social, and medical systems of the world. In the United States alone there is one birth every 8 seconds, one international migrant every 30 seconds, and one death every 13 seconds—for a net gain of one person every 11 seconds (U.S. Census Bureau, 2006).

At the most recent Earth Summit Conference held in Johannesburg, South Africa, in 2002, the analogy of the overloaded lifeboat was frequently used. World overpopulation, overdevelopment, and overconsumption by wealthy nations threaten to deplete the resources and destroy the environment of the entire world, not just overpopulated countries. The related problems of environmental deterioration and overpopulation are health care issues that future nurses will face, and there are no easy answers.

Disasters and Bioterrorism

Since September 11, 2001 and Hurricane Katrina in September 2005, and its aftermath, many professions have reevaluated their disaster preparedness. Nurses are often at the forefront in emergency and disaster situations, but few U.S. schools of nursing include disaster training in their curricula. As we have all so sadly witnessed, this needs to change in the future.

A **disaster** is defined as "an event or situation that is of greater magnitude than an emergency; disrupts essential services such as housing, transportation, communications, sanitation, water, and health care; and requires the response of people outside the community affected" (Gebbie and Qureshi, 2002). Disasters can be natural or man-made and range from earthquakes, hurricanes, and major fires to wars and major environmental contamination. The Southeast Asia tsunami of December 26, 2004, serves as a sad example of a natural disaster on a scale heretofore unseen.

Regardless of the cause of a disaster situation, no two of which are alike, the basic competencies nurses need in disaster preparedness are essentially the same. The Centers for Disease Control and Prevention collaborated with a nurse, Dr. Kristine M. Gebbie, to develop a set of core emergency preparedness competencies for public health workers. This served as a basis upon which Dr. Gebbie and another nurse, Kristin Qureshi, developed core competencies for nurses (Gebbie and Qureshi, 2002). The core disaster preparedness competencies for nurses are found Box 16-1.

Until recently, nurses were not expected to know much about the types of disasters caused by bioterrorism. **Bioterrorism** refers to the use of a biological or chemical agent as a weapon. Now nurses must be able to recognize the signs and symptoms of biological agents such as anthrax and smallpox or chemical agents such as Ricin. They must know how to notify the proper authorities; "assist with diagnosis, postexposure prophylaxis, and treatment; and participate in infection control" (Coleman, 2001).

Nurses are encouraged to keep up with emerging information to improve their readiness for possible bioterrorism by referring to the CDC's bioterrorism website (www.bt.cdc.gov). You can register for the CDC's free e-mail updates and training opportunities via the CDC's Clinician Registry (www.bt.cdc.gov/clinregistry/index.asp).

Nursing organizations are taking an active role in improving the preparedness of professional nurses. The American Nurses Association (ANA) worked with the Office of Emergency Response, U.S. Department of Health and Human Services, in the establishment of the National Nurses Response Team (NNRT). According to the ANA, "The NNRT creates an excellent opportunity for registered nurses who on September 11 were asking themselves, 'What can I do to help my country?'" (American Nurses Association, 2006a). The NNRT will be composed of 10 regionally based teams of 200 registered nurses who could be called on to assist in chemoprophylaxis or vaccination of hundreds of thousands or even millions of Americans, or in other scenarios requiring large numbers of nurses. Team members will be enrolled in the National Disaster Medical System. You can learn more on the ANA website (www.nursingworld.org/news/disaster/biocare.htm).

Unhealthy Lifestyles

Despite the focus on wellness and fitness in contemporary American society, unhealthy lifestyles still predominate; this trend shows no signs of changing; in fact, the number of people with bad habits is increasing.

Obesity

Every year public health officials report that there are more obese Americans than ever, even though

---

Box 16-1 Core Nursing Competencies for Disaster Preparedness

To consider themselves prepared for a major emergency or a disaster, nurses should be able to perform the following:
- Describe the agency's (your place of employment's) role in responding to a range of emergencies that might arise.
- Describe the chain of command in emergency response (to whom you would report).
- Identify and locate the agency's emergency response plan (or the pertinent portion of it).
- Describe emergency response functions or roles and demonstrate them in regularly performed drills.
- Demonstrate the use of equipment (including personal protective equipment) and the skills required in emergency response during regular drills.
- Demonstrate the correct operation of all equipment used for emergency communication.
- Describe communication roles in emergency response within your agency, with news media, with the general public (including patients and families), and with personal contacts (one's own family, friends, and neighbors).
- Identify the limits of your own knowledge, skills, and authority, and identify key system resources for referring matters that exceed these limits.
- Apply creative problem-solving skills and flexible thinking to the situation, within the confines of your role, and evaluate the effectiveness of all actions taken.
- Recognize deviations from the norm that might indicate an emergency and describe appropriate action. Participate in continuing education to maintain up-to-date knowledge in relevant areas.
- Participate in evaluating every drill or response and identify necessary changes to the plan.

  In addition, nurses with managerial or leadership responsibilities should be able to perform the following:
- Ensure that there is a written plan for major categories of emergencies.
- Ensure that all parts of the emergency plan are practiced regularly.
- Ensure that identified gaps in knowledge or skills are filled.

From Gebbie KM, Qureshi K: Emergency and disaster preparedness: core competencies for nurses, *Am J Nurs* 102(1):46-51, 2002.

---

obesity, defined as a body mass index (BMI) of 30 or more, has long been known to predispose people to a number of illnesses, including diabetes, heart disease, high blood pressure, and arthritis. The accompanying News Note 16-1 tells of a distressingly rapid increase in the number of Americans who are more than 100 pounds overweight. You may want to compute your BMI, using the formula found in Box 16-2.

Futurists predict that Americans will eat more meals in restaurants in the future, but ordering a nutritious, well-balanced meal in a restaurant is a major challenge, even to people with a working knowledge of nutritional science. In a distressing sign that indicates acquiescence to the fast-food mentality of many families, nutritional consultants are now being hired by public school districts to teach cafeteria workers how to make nutritious school lunches look and taste more like fast foods. Apparently, many modern children refuse to eat anything else.

As a result of pressure from health-conscious consumers, many of whom are now aging baby boomers, some restaurant chains have introduced grilled foods and other "low-fat" items. On examination, however, the fat content of some of these foods is unacceptably high. Restaurant owners report that even when they include low-fat meals on the menu, few people order them. The majority of regular menu items are still

Extreme Obesity Ballooning: 1 in 50 Adults in U.S.
newsnote *at Least 100 Pounds Too Heavy*

Americans are not just getting fatter; they are ballooning to extremely obese proportions at an alarming rate. The number of extremely obese American adults, those who are at least 100 pounds overweight, has quadrupled since the 1980s to about 4 million. That equates to about 1 in every 50 adults.

Extreme obesity once was thought to be a rare, distinct condition whose prevalence remained relatively steady over time. The new study contradicts that thinking and suggests that it is at least partly attributable to the same kinds of behaviors, overeating and underactivity, that have contributed to the epidemic number of Americans with less severe weight problems.

In fact, the findings by a RAND Corporation researcher show that the number of extremely obese adults has surged twice as fast as the number of less severely obese adults.

On the scale of obesity, "as the whole population shifts to the right, the extreme categories grow the fastest," said RAND economist Roland Sturm. He added, "These people have the highest health costs."

Sturm said health problems associated with obesity—including diabetes, heart disease, high blood pressure, and arthritis—probably affect the extremely obese disproportionately and at young ages. "There is no evidence that it (the obesity rate) is flattening out," Sturm said. "It's full speed ahead." Sturm has completed projections showing that if this problem is not addressed, the number of obese Americans will jump from about 20 percent of adults today to 80 percent by 2040, and the proportion of normal-weight people will drop from 42 percent today to 5 percent in 2040.

Sturm's study, which appeared in the *Archives of Internal Medicine*, is based on nationwide telephone surveys conducted by the U.S. Centers for Disease Control and Prevention, in which people were asked their height and weight. His report covers surveys from 1986 through 2000.

In 1986, 1 in 200 adults reported height and weight measurements reflecting extreme obesity, or a body-mass index of at least 40. By 2000 that number had increased to 1 in 50, Sturm found. Body mass index is a ratio of height to weight.

The prevalence of the most extreme obesity, people with a BMI of at least 50, grew fivefold—from 1 in 2000 to 1 in 400—Sturm said. By contrast, ordinary obesity, a BMI of 30 to 35, doubled—from about 1 in 10 to 1 in 5—based on the same surveys.

Americans tend to understate their weights, and a recent study based on actual measurements found an obesity rate of nearly 1 in 3, or almost 59 million people. Sturm said his findings probably understate the problem for the same reason.

The average man with a BMI of 40 in the study was 5 feet 10 inches and 300 pounds, while the average woman was 5 feet 4 inches and 250 pounds. Sturm said the trend largely is the result of the increasing affordability of calorie-dense food. "We've reached Nirvana," he said. "Food is cheap and plentiful. You can stuff yourself on less than a half-hour of minimum wage."

The trend is also fueled by a substantial reduction in the amount of physical activity that Americans engage in, said Linda Baumann, a nursing professor at the University of Wisconsin, Madison. School physical education budgets have been cut, suburban neighborhoods have been built without sidewalks, and "children are driven instead of walking to school," said Baumann, who is also is president of the Society of Behavioral Medicine.

Obesity researchers say the trend has to be reversed, or the health consequences will be devastating. "How can we put up with having this many people that large?" said James Hill, an obesity expert at the University of Colorado. "We have to do something quick."

From Extreme Obesity Ballooning (2003). The Associated Press, December 19, 2003.

Box 16-2 **Compute Your Body Mass Index (BMI)**

Body mass index (BMI) is a mathematical calculation used to determine whether a patient is overweight. BMI is calculated by dividing body weight in kilograms by height in meters squared (weight [kg] ÷ height [m^2]) or by using the conversion with pounds (lbs) and inches squared (in.^{2}) as shown below. This number can be misleading for very muscular people, or for pregnant or lactating women.

Calculate Your BMI

$$[\text{Weight (lbs)} \div \text{Height (in.}^2)\,] \times 704.5 = BMI$$

For example, if you are 5 feet 5 inches tall and weigh 134 pounds, your formula will look like this:

$$[134 \div (65 \text{ inches} \times 65 \text{ inches})] \times 704.5 = 22.34$$

Being obese and being overweight are not the same condition. A BMI of 30 or more is considered obese and a BMI between 25 and 29.9 is considered overweight. There are many factors that impact a person's health risk relative to their BMI, such as waist size, smoking, the types of foods regularly eaten, exercise, and medical conditions associated with obesity including diabetes, high blood pressure, high cholesterol level, and coronary artery disease.

From American Obesity Association: *AOA fact sheet: what is obesity?* 2006, available online: http://www.obesity.org/subs/fastfacts/obesity_what2.shtml.

loaded with animal fats (long known to cause cardiovascular disease) and sodium (known to aggravate a variety of health conditions). A taco salad, for example, can contain as many as 30 grams of fat.

Tobacco use

Yet another lifestyle issue is tobacco use. Smoking continues to increase among the young, especially females and minorities, both of whom are targeted for higher levels of marketing by tobacco companies. For decades, smoking has been known to cause lung cancer, emphysema and other chronic lung diseases, low–birth-weight babies, and a host of other health problems.

Lung cancer is a leading cancer killer in both men and women. There were an estimated 164,100 new cases of lung cancer and an estimated 156,900 deaths from lung cancer in the United States in 2000. The rate of lung cancer cases appears to be dropping among white and African-American men in the United States, while it continues to rise among both white and African-American women (American Lung Association, 2003).

The use of smokeless tobacco is rising, creating unhealthy oral mucous membranes and predisposing users to oral cancer. All these trends ensure that tobacco-related illnesses and deaths will rise in the future.

Lack of exercise

Lack of exercise is a troubling lifestyle issue for Americans of the future, particularly the young. The ready availability of entertainment on television is at least partly to blame. Studies show that the more television people of all ages watch, the more likely they are to be overweight. Snacking and television watching usually go hand in hand. Entire generations of Americans, raised watching several hours of television each day, are unlikely to give up the habit in the future, especially because more options are added yearly. Others spend hours in front of computer screens, playing video games, or in other sedentary pursuits. These habits are expected to continue in the future.

Lack of exercise is not limited to the young, however. For every jogger seen pounding the roadways, legions of sedentary adults remain unseen at home, gradually becoming less fit and more susceptible to disease. Browsing through mail-order catalogs aimed at the affluent middle-aged population reveals a plethora of labor-saving devices being developed and marketed to make Americans even less active in the future.

Eating disorders

Television and advertising affect yet another lifestyle risk factor. With the emphasis on thinness in fashion advertising, the celebrity culture, and television shows, many girls and young women resort to unhealthy habits such as starving or bingeing and purging. Rather than eating sensibly and engaging in exercise to maintain normal weights, they assume bizarre eating habits in the pursuit of the fashionable, if unnatural, degree of gauntness. Eating disorders also are on the rise in young men. Barring a dramatic change in the fashion industry, eating disorders and their resulting health hazards will continue to increase.

Stress

Another lifestyle issue is stress. The rapid pace of modern life creates stress, yet Americans continue to step up the pace with cellular telephones, fax machines, satellite communications, personal computers, paging devices, call-waiting options, and all the other fruits of modern technology. Although many Americans mourn the loss of leisure time, indications are that when given more leisure time, many people spend it working. This evidence indicates that stress-related diseases are on the increase.

HIV/AIDS and drug abuse

The epidemics of acquired immunodeficiency syndrome (AIDS) and drug abuse are two issues that will affect the future of nursing.

HIV/AIDS.   When the AIDS epidemic began in the United States early in the 1980s, many of those affected were homosexual men. A few years later, infection rates among intravenous drug users began to rise. By the mid-1980s, AIDS moved into the general population of heterosexual adults, a trend already seen in other countries and now well established in the United States. Although HIV/AIDS no longer commands the headlines as it did in the early years of the epidemic, it continues to take a heavy toll on the population at home and abroad. In some African countries, for example, more than half of all adults are infected and the number of orphaned children is increasing rapidly.

Even optimists in the medical community no longer predict a vaccine against human immunodeficiency virus (HIV), believing that it will be many years before a vaccine is discovered, if ever. Meanwhile, millions of Americans are already infected, and no cure is on the horizon. Long-term survival has become commonplace, however, because of the increasing availability of effective chemotherapy.

Due to the widespread incidence of blood-borne diseases, nurses of the future must continue to be vigilant about protecting themselves and their patients from transmission of these diseases.

Drug Abuse.   Drug abuse is a lifestyle choice that continues to plague modern life. Its impact on nursing is multidimensional and brings up issues such as addiction, withdrawal, harm reduction, non-compliance to health care regimens, and appropriate pain management for drug abusers. Because of their lifestyle choices, drug abusers are at increased risk for many diseases such as HIV/AIDS, hepatitis, various resistant bacterial infections, noninfectious liver disorders, and kidney failure.

Substance-abusing people suffer more accidents and illness than their nonabusing counterparts, thus requiring more medical and nursing care. They are also more likely to have unprotected sex, putting them at risk for acquiring HIV and other sexually transmitted diseases. If current trends continue, nurses of the future will be called on to provide intensive nursing care to increasing numbers of substance abusers. Nurses will be involved in the development of public policies concerning drug abuse treatment and prevention.

Given the predominance of unhealthy lifestyle choices, it is clear that nurses will play an increasingly important role in educating people about wellness and self-care in the years ahead. Nurses will also be instrumental in educating the public about how to be informed consumers of health care services. As nurses continue to provide care in acute care settings, hospitals, and clinics, their personal opinions and judgments must be put aside in order to be effective patient advocates and provide equal opportunities for health care to all populations.

Cost Containment

During the last 30 years, governmental budget deficits reached all-time highs. At federal, state, and local levels, governments spent more money than was generated through taxes, and the pressure for health care for the elderly and poor created a significant part of those budgetary problems.

As mentioned earlier, our infant death rate is a national embarrassment and our prescription drug costs are the highest in the world. Society's poor, homeless, elderly, substance abusers, AIDS patients, and mentally ill are increasing in number and will continue to increase. The question yet to be answered is, "How can we pay for health care for these vulnerable populations now and in the future when their numbers are even greater?"

Federal and state governments are seeking to answer that question. In most states, Medicaid is the largest and fastest-growing single state expense. Although welfare reform efforts have effectively removed thousands from welfare rolls, the aging of America will continue to create huge numbers of social security–eligible and Medicare-eligible citizens. The corresponding decrease in the number of those working and paying social security and income taxes will place an additional burden on the federal government's budget.

The future may bring hospital closings, continued pressures from the business community to force changes in health care financing, and significant health care reform, piece by piece if not by sweeping legislative mandate. The nursing profession stands to benefit because nursing has been shown to be a cost-effective yet high-quality alternative to traditional medical care. In addition, nurses are well equipped to provide managed care. As a profession, nursing is expected to benefit from health care woes in the United States by expanding roles in prevention and community-based nursing.

One cost-effective method of providing basic health care to children is through school nurses. As the burden of providing care continues to shift from federal agencies to state and local agencies, local school boards will recognize the economies to be realized through school nursing. Health care reform will likely provoke a dramatic rise in state-mandated health "safety net" services for children. Many of these services will be delivered by nurses.

Regulation of Health Care

Even if the cost of health care can be contained, health care expenses in the United States will continue to rise. This rise is anticipated owing to the large number of aging Americans and the growing number of impoverished ones. As more citizens are covered by government-sponsored medical programs such as Medicare and Medicaid, even greater governmental regulation of health care will be required.

Nurses will become increasingly active in developing health policies that improve access, quality, and value in the delivery of health services. Legislation mandating the direct reimbursement of nurses for their services will be a feature of most government-funded programs, despite the opposition of organized medicine and hospitals. Private **managed care** programs will increasingly use advanced practice registered nurses to provide primary health care.

Nursing, through its professional associations, will continue to be a player in health care politics in the United States. Nurses will form coalitions with consumer groups to influence consumer-friendly legislation at state and national levels. Individual nurses will become more politically active as voters, campaign workers, community health activists, and political candidates. As nursing's public profile becomes higher, public scrutiny of the profession will increase. Consumers of nursing services will exercise their political power to ensure that nurses and other primary care providers consistently offer first-class health care.

CHALLENGES IN NURSING PRACTICE

The societal changes just reviewed will necessarily create changes in nursing practice. Nurses in the next decade will face an ever-widening array of practice opportunities in hospital and community-based health care settings, each of which will bring its own set of challenges.

Differentiating Practice Levels

There has been considerable resistance to differentiating levels of nursing practice, even though visionary nursing leaders have pointed out the need to do so for years. **Differentiated practice** means that nurses prepared in associate degree, baccalaureate degree, and higher degree programs should have different, well-defined roles and possibly even different levels of licensure. The competencies of nurses at each level could be clearly demonstrated, and nurses at each level could be held accountable for practice standards at that level. If differentiated practice became a reality, educational programs could be streamlined, employers and consumers could understand the differences, and patient care delivery systems could be reorganized to capitalize on the strengths of each level.

In the past, nurses prepared in diploma and associate degree programs opposed efforts to differentiate educational and practice levels in nursing, believing that they would be disenfranchised. Nursing leaders have been unwilling to take the risk of tackling such a potentially divisive issue. The result is that nursing is the only health care profession for which entry into practice is less than a baccalaureate degree. Many professions currently require a master's degree as the credential for entry into a profession, and educational standards are rising in all fields but nursing. This has hampered nursing in its quest for professionalism and equal status among the health care professions.

In addition to improving educational standards, differentiated practice could help nurses be more cost-effective by determining who is best suited to perform certain nursing actions. Differentiated practice can be realized in the future only if practicing nurses are willing to give up the notion that "a nurse is a nurse is a nurse" and acknowledge that different educational programs do and should prepare different types of nursing practitioners. Nurses must be willing to see the larger picture and recognize that advances in the profession benefit all nurses. They are being encouraged in these efforts by the American Association of Colleges of Nursing (AACN), which refers to differentiated practice as one of the "hallmarks of the professional nursing practice environment" in its white paper by the same title. You can read the entire document at AACN's website (www.aacn.nche.edu/Publications/positions/hallmarks.htm).

Cost Containment's Impact

During the 1990s, cost-containment initiatives in hospitals eliminated layers of middle-management nurses. This represented a crisis for individual nurse managers but created an opportunity for a stronger voice for nurses involved in direct patient care. Future cost-containment measures such as managed care and capitation will require nurses to demonstrate the cost-effectiveness of the care they provide. The "bottom line" will be an increasing focus of concern in all health care settings, and nurses will need resource management skills more than ever before. Nurses will find that they need business expertise as much as they need clinical expertise.

Increasingly, nurses will work with unlicensed assistive personnel and delegate tasks to deliver patient care. They will need communication, interpersonal, and management skills to make the new partnerships work. **Multiskilled workers** will take their place alongside nurses in all settings. Nurses will be challenged to expand their skills into areas formerly the domain of specialized workers, such as respiratory therapists and physical therapists. This will be essential if nurses are to cope with the periodic variations in supply and demand for traditional nursing positions. In addition, a variety of new health care job opportunities in quality care, case management, advanced practice, and primary care will present themselves as a result of economic pressures of managed care and health reforms (Marrilli, 2006).

Autonomy and Accountability

Shared governance, that is, participation by nurses on strong policymaking hospital committees, is a trend already seen and mandated by accreditation bodies such as the Joint Commission on the Accreditation of Healthcare Organizations (JCAHO). Along with the empowerment of nurses, however, will come increased demand for accountability. Effective nursing care will be measured by patient outcomes. Continuous quality improvement of nursing care will be emphasized more than ever. Nurses must be able to show evidence that the care they provide makes a demonstrable difference in patient outcomes.

As more and more nursing care is provided in community settings, autonomy and accountability will become increasingly important. Nurses who function independently in homes and other community-based practice settings need additional education and experience. When the supervisory guidance of better-prepared colleagues is not readily available, novice or inexperienced nurses must assume responsibility for knowing the limits of their expertise and for seeking consultation to ensure patient safety. Professional nurses of the future will increasingly pursue baccalaureate and advanced degrees to prepare them for autonomous practice. More than ever, **lifelong learning** will be a requirement for professional nurses.

Technology and Nursing Informatics

All types of technology will continue to advance at a dizzying pace, as they have in the first years of the twenty-first century. Areas expected to affect nursing are nursing informatics, telecommunications, genetic engineering, alternative treatments, and the Internet.

Nursing informatics

Nursing informatics, the organization and use of nursing data, continues to change nursing practice dramatically. Computerized health information networks (CHINs) will allow immediate access to all patient data needed in refining the plan of care. The increased access to patient data will reinforce the need for patient confidentiality. Voice-activated bedside computers already allow nurses to record patient information literally "at the bedside," rather than making written notes and transferring them to the patient's chart at a later time. This practice will become widespread.

Telecommunications

Advances in telecommunications will improve access to medical services for rural and elderly Americans. Nurses and physicians will examine and treat patients who are hundreds of miles away using two-way television systems. They will evaluate and prescribe treatments via telephone. Telemedicine will become routine for those who live in remote areas or are homebound. Nurses will be increasingly involved in telehealth and there will be explosive growth in home telemonitoring of patients.

Genetic engineering and the genomic revolution

Genetic engineering has become more common since scientists participating in the **Human Genome Project** completed the initial mapping and sequencing of a composite set of human genes in 2003. This made it potentially possible to treat and prevent many more genetically transmitted and genetically predisposed diseases. It will also create ethical dilemmas of dramatic proportions as the ability to clone individuals and predetermine characteristics of human infants becomes a reality. Genetic research will also make possible individualized medications, or designer medicines. **Designer medicines** are drugs tailor-made to treat patients based on their individual genetic makeup. A new role for nurses, the Genomics Nurse Case Coordinator, has already been proposed (Lea and Monsen, 2003). Programs preparing nurses for basic practice have been encouraged to include knowledge and skills to prepare graduates for "family history assessments, screening, and case coordination for clients receiving genetic testing and gene-based therapies" (Lea and Monsen, 2003, p. 75). Genetic literacy will be a must for nurses of the future.

Complementary and alternative therapies

As disenchantment with traditional medicine grows, more Americans will turn away from mainstream medical care and seek other treatments as they take responsibility for their own health (Figure 16-3, Box 16-3). Nontraditional techniques, such as chiropractic, homeopathy, acupuncture, massage, therapeutic touch, and herbal remedies, among others, are considered complementary or alternative therapies. **Complementary therapies** include these techniques that are used along with standard medical care. **Alternative therapies** are used in place of standard care. Nurses, with their holistic focus, are well positioned to assist in establishing **integrative care,** combining the best of both standard and nontraditional treatments. These therapies will increasingly become a focus of interest, study, research, practice, and publication in nursing.

The Internet

The Internet will create major changes in the way Americans view health care and their role as partners in their own care. The proliferation of websites designed to provide reliable medical and health information to the lay public will continue. Nurses will be called on to educate patients about how to evaluate and appropriately use the information they obtain from these sites.

Figure 16-3
Alternative treatments, such as massage therapy, are appealing to more Americans as they take responsibility for their own health. This trend to natural healing and the use of alternative and complementary therapies is expected to increase in the future. *(Courtesy Memorial Health Care System, Chattanooga, Tenn.)*

As a result of these and other unforeseen technological advances, nurses of the future will continue to fight the dehumanizing tendency of technological advances such as patient monitoring devices while valuing and providing a holistic, "high-touch" environment for patients. Nurses will realize that advanced technology and traditional nursing values are not mutually exclusive. Patients can have both if nurses stay focused on the patient rather than on the machine or monitor. Advances in technology will bring new ethical dilemmas. Nurses will be more active in exploring ethical aspects of patient care, and their unique ethical perspective will be valued by other professionals. As a result, nurses will sit on ethics committees and serve as ethics consultants in greater numbers.

Box 16-3 Complementary and Alternative Therapies

- Nearly 50 percent of Americans use some form of complementary and alternative therapies (CAT).
- About 80 percent of the world's population use herbal medicine.
- Approximately 72 percent of people who use CAT do not tell their health care providers.
- Complementary and alternative therapies can interact with other forms of treatment to create potential risks.
- In a study, more than half of critical care nurses surveyed reported that patients and families requested common therapies (e.g., diet, exercise, relaxation, prayer) as well as massage and counseling.
- Therapies considered legitimate by more than 75 percent of critical care nurses surveyed included diet, exercise, massage, counseling, prayer, relaxation techniques, music therapy, meditation, pet therapy, and behavioral medicine. Those viewed as not legitimate by 25 percent or more of respondents included megavitamin therapy and electromagnetic/magnet therapies.

From Goley A: APNs need to learn more about complementary and alternative medicine, *Top Adv Pract Nurs eJournal* 4(2), 2004, available online: http://www.medscape.com; Tracy MF, Lindquist R, Savik K et al: Use of complementary and alternative therapies: a national survey of critical care nurses, *Am J Crit Care* 14(5):404-415, 2005.

Practice in Community Settings

Community-based primary health care will continue to expand as cost-effectiveness remains a high priority. Nurse-managed clinics will increasingly serve underserved populations in inner city and rural areas. School nurses will be needed in large numbers, as will hospice nurses and those specializing in gerontology and chronic illnesses. For nurses who are willing to work outside traditional settings and their own "comfort zones," there will be no end to the available opportunities.

Flexible scheduling and job sharing will increase in all professions and will become commonplace in nursing. Nurse entrepreneurship will flourish in the future as a result of changes in restrictive legislation, the resourcefulness and self-confidence of better-educated nurses, and the trust the public places in the nursing profession. Increasing numbers of nurses will own clinics and other health-related businesses, such as independent practice associations, free-standing wellness programs, adult day care centers, dialysis care services, and worksite health programs.

Cultural Competence

Providing culturally competent nursing care will become even more important in the future as the nation's demographics change even more drama-

tically than they have in the past. Nurses of the future must recognize that cultural sensitivity begins with one's fellow health care providers. If relationships within the team are strained by insensitivity and prejudice, patient care cannot be culturally sensitive. Meaningful dialogue must become a vehicle for building relationships within the work group. A united team will be capable of providing respectful, understanding, and dignified care to patients.

Effective nursing leaders of the future will provide cultural support groups and mentoring to ensure that "faculty, providers, students, patients, and others can become less inhibited about individuals who are culturally different. They can foster the courage to engage in conversations, to get to know each other, to share our worldviews, to speak out, and to trust that interactions about our specific and particular culture, on a personal level, will make a difference" (Gary, Sigsby, and Campbell, 1998, p. 277). Nurses who are unable or unwilling to become culturally aware, culturally sensitive, and culturally competent will unnecessarily limit their career potential.

Maintaining a Healthy Work Environment

No profession is free from hazards, and no workplace can ever ensure absolute security. Nursing is no exception to this sad fact of contemporary life. Occupational health hazards in nursing include needlestick injuries and possible infection with bloodborne diseases exposure to chemicals such as disinfectants and chemotherapeutic agents; and violence in the workplace, among others.

Additional hazards include latex allergy, a continuing concern for nurses, with a prevalence rate of approximately 8 to 12 percent in frequent glove users (American Nurses Association, 2006b). Injuries from accidents and back strain also occur too frequently, with pain, disability, lost income, absenteeism, and decreased productivity only a few of the results.

Shift work itself is a hazard to nurses, causing a variety of physical and psychological problems, including exhaustion, depression, interpersonal problems, and accidents. Stress from work overload, inadequate staffing, and the intense feelings generated by caring for acutely ill and dying patients add to the mix of workplace hazards faced by nurses.

In addition, nurses increasingly find themselves at risk for violence in the workplace. This is not a new phenomenon, but it is being discussed more openly than in the past, as evidenced by the fall 1999 issue of Sigma Theta Tau International's membership publication *Reflections* (now titled *Reflections on Nursing Leadership*), being devoted entirely to the issue of workplace violence.

Among the articles in that issue of *Reflections* was a report of a 1997 survey by the Colorado Nurses Association's Task Force on Violence, which conducted a seven-state survey examining nurse safety. There were 586 respondents, one third of whom disclosed "that they were victims of workplace violence in 1996." Most nurses indicated patients were the assailants, "yet half of the nurses acknowledged that violence went unreported at work" (Carroll and Goldsmith, 1999, p. 26).

Assuring nurses of a healthy work environment is a major challenge for the next decade. It is not, however, a problem that nurses can expect will be solved by others. Clearly, nurses of the future must themselves take positive, effective, united action to ensure the basic dignity and safety of practicing nurses everywhere. They must demand and use safer needlestick devices and disposal containers; high-efficiency ventilation systems; alternatives to latex gloves and products; adequate housekeeping support; adequate lifting assistance with devices or additional personnel; reduction or elimination of shift rotation; and appropriate occupational safety and health training. Nurses themselves must use impeccable hand washing techniques and personal protective equipment such as gloves, gowns, and masks when needed. In addition, they must demand that adequate security be provided to protect them against violent patients and family members.

CHALLENGES IN NURSING EDUCATION

As the profession of nursing matures, more nurses will recognize the value of bachelor's degrees for beginning professional practice and master's degrees for advanced practice. More nurses will pursue doctoral degrees to prepare for leadership roles in research, theory development, and teaching. In response, colleges of nursing will expand flexible educational programs to improve access. They will also develop differentiated levels of nursing education that correspond to differentiated levels of practice.

Outcome-Based Education

The quality of educational programs will continue to be judged by student competencies—that is, what students can actually do as a result of education. Nursing educational programs will monitor their graduates' activities and achievements as professional nurses. They will be required to report on graduates' accomplishments as part of the accreditation process. The emphasis on accountability of nursing education programs will increase as measures of competence in graduates are refined.

Just as nursing practice is being challenged to measure patient outcomes and adopt evidence-based practice, nursing education will be challenged to develop student outcomes and adopt evidence-based education. Faculty will modify age-old teaching/learning strategies and adopt new pedagogies (teaching methods) proven effective through research (i.e., evidence-based teaching). Passive learning, such as lectures, will be deemphasized. Critical thinking, independent decision making, and creative problem solving will assume even greater importance, fostered by role playing, simulations, and group problem solving (Davidhizar and Shearer, 2005). Faculty will be required to document evidence-based teaching as part of accreditation processes.

Accreditation of nursing education programs will become more difficult to achieve as national accrediting bodies come under increasing pressure to raise standards and to apply standards consistently. Substandard programs will be closed. This will strengthen nursing but will not help the nursing shortage.

Diversity

Students in nursing education programs will reflect the demographics of the United States and become more diverse than ever before. More men, older students, and students with baccalaureate degrees in other fields will come into nursing because of the emotional rewards, economic stability, and professional image it offers. Student bodies will become more culturally diverse, reflecting the diversity of the nation's population. Educational needs of students from different cultures will be unique and will not be adequately met with traditional teaching strategies (Davidhizar and Shearer, 2005). Schools of nursing must strive to offer **culturally competent education.**

Access to education for nontraditional and traditional students will be an even greater issue. Schools will expand nontraditional curricula that enable adults to work and go to school simultaneously. Nursing courses delivered by **distance learning** technologies, such as telecommunications and satellite linkages, will increase access for students living in remote areas. Cost-minded legislators will require that state-supported schools offer fully articulated programs in order to qualify for state funding. Schools that fall behind in distance learning offerings will have difficulty filling their classes as more and more students seek nonresidential education.

Changes in demographics will affect the content of curricula, as well as the methods by which content is delivered. As the population ages, the need for nurses prepared in gerontology, chronic disease management, and hospice care will give emphasis to educational programs at both undergraduate and graduate levels. Curricula will emphasize community-based care instead of traditional hospital-based care. Educational programs will develop and expand multicultural courses. Foreign languages will again become a graduation requirement in baccalaureate programs. International educational opportunities will increase as the global village concept becomes a reality. Every nursing program will have the provision of culturally competent care as an outcome criterion for its graduates.

Technology and Nursing Informatics' Impact

Technological advances and the growth of nursing knowledge will create the need for informatics expertise in nursing education as well as in nursing practice. Computer competence will not suffice for nurses of the future. Students will need to master sophisticated information systems to use the wealth of available knowledge to improve and document patient care.

Faculty will be challenged to keep pace with students' acquisition of knowledge from the World Wide Web. Students of the future will become increasingly active in obtaining information from a vast array of sources available to them at the touch of a computer key. This will enable students to be more engaged in their own learning process and foster active learning.

Nursing faculty will be required to practice the profession actively to keep up with rapidly changing technologies. Maintaining faculty currency will become a greater focus in higher education. Active practice in addition to teaching will become an expected part of the faculty role. Students will be incorporated into faculty practices to obtain clinical experience. In this regard, nursing education will resemble medical education.

It will be impossible for nursing education programs to include in their curricula everything nurses of the future need to know. If, for example, genomics and disaster nursing are to be added to curricula, what will be removed? Nursing students already are overwhelmed with the amount of material they must master.

The solution to this problem is that all nurses must be educated to become **lifelong learners.** They must be taught to expect change and be prepared to adapt or retool their skills quickly to respond to health care marketplace demands (Jenkins, 2005). They must invest in themselves, pursuing knowledge and refreshing their knowledge base through vigorous, self-motivated continuing education efforts.

Licensing examinations will change to reflect the expansion of nursing knowledge and the increase in community-based practice and resulting autonomy. Licensure at multiple levels will become a reality. Employers of new graduates will expect to provide internships designed to enable novices to make the transition from student to practicing nurse effectively.

Collaboration

As nurses acquire more education, the resulting knowledge and self-confidence will enable them to develop collaborative relationships on an equal footing with physicians and other highly educated health care professionals. This will enable nurses to be more assertive in patient advocacy and will improve patient care and strengthen the profession.

Nursing faculty, nurse managers, and practicing nurses will join forces to strengthen educational experiences and mentorships for tomorrow's nurses. They will collaborate on clinical research that demonstrates the effectiveness of nursing care in terms of patient outcomes. They will collaborate with other nurses and consumer groups to remove regulatory restrictions that impede advanced clinical practice. They will

work together to close the gap between education and practice.

Nurse educators will recognize the need to treat students as professionals in training and will transform nursing education attitudes from controlling students to collaborating with them. This will create a new generation of empowered nursing professionals.

Disciplinary boundaries are becoming blurred as knowledge from all disciplines is brought to bear on problems of mutual concern, such as breast cancer, domestic violence, and AIDS. Nursing must become more interdisciplinary in its focus. Only nurses with a strong sense of personal and professional identity will be able to enter fully into multidisciplinary collaboration. Those nurses who understand the value of collaboration will become the managers of care using a case-management model, and they will thrive.

Reforms in Health Care and Higher Education

As a result of health care reforms and cost-containment initiatives, nurses of the future will need to be well versed in the costs, budgeting, and financing of health care. Business education will be increasingly emphasized, particularly at the graduate level, as nurses pursue entrepreneurial roles. Nursing faculty either will return to school to prepare themselves to teach business courses or will create interdisciplinary alliances with business schools to provide nursing students with the necessary business courses.

Higher education will undergo public scrutiny and reform. It already suffers from serious underfunding. As governmental grants are reduced or eliminated to help balance the national budget and state tax revenues decline, educational programs will experience budgetary constraints. Several nursing education programs, including some well-regarded ones, have closed as a result of funding shortfalls. In many universities, autonomous schools and colleges of nursing were combined with health and human service programs into one administrative unit to save money. This often weakened the nursing program's voice on the campus. Budgets for operating expenses, equipment, and faculty salaries are under par in many locations, even though the demand for nursing education remains high.

For a time, it appeared that hospitals could be a source of support for nursing education programs, but with their own significant budgetary constraints, it is unlikely that this will be a long-term solution. Hospitals, however, will support nursing education for as long as possible with financial aid to students, subsidies of faculty salaries, joint appointments of faculty, and other forms of assistance.

Graduate education programs will change to produce practitioners who can meet consumer demands. Changes in hospital-based nursing practice will force a reexamination of the clinical nurse specialist and nurse practitioner roles. The need for efficiency and cost-effectiveness will lead to a revision of advanced practice models, and educational programs will combine the two roles and emphasize community-based practice.

Curricula at all levels will be standardized and streamlined to reduce cost and confusion and improve student mobility. Fast-track curricula will proliferate. The trend toward use of multi-skilled workers will force nursing faculty to identify unique aspects of nursing and to educate students for broader roles in the delivery of patient care.

Faculty Shortage/Student Shortage

In the next decade, many long time nursing faculty members, educated at the master's level during the nurse-traineeship funding heyday of the 1960s, will retire. There will be no one to replace many of them because relatively few younger nurses are entering teaching; this shortage of teachers is attributable to the fact that nursing education salaries lag behind those in practice settings. By the year 2010 there will be a serious shortage of nursing faculty. This will force a major restructuring of nursing education programs and negatively affect the already problematic shortage of nurses.

Colleges of nursing already report turning away qualified applicants, often because of a lack of faculty to teach them. These two problems—too few faculty members and fewer students in the pipeline—combine to create a negative synergy and downward spiral in the number of practicing nurses. The nursing profession, working in collaboration with public and private funding sources and policymakers, and employers of nurses must find a solution to these twin problems in the near future if nursing is to thrive as a profession. Creating a more desirable work environment for practicing nurses, thereby retaining nurses who might otherwise leave the profession, will attain a greater and much needed focus (Valentino, 2002).

As the faculty shortage in nursing is translated into a student shortage—and therefore to a worsening of the nursing shortage—medical schools are increasing their output of physicians. Of particular concern is the trend toward physician role expansion in the area of inpatient care by **hospitalists.** These are physicians who are hospital-based and care for patients only while they are hospitalized. They "are predicted to care for many nonsurgical patients by 2005, thus decreasing demand for advanced practice nurses" (Wolf, 2003, p. 32). Because advanced practice nursing is the goal of many of today's undergraduate nursing students, this is a troubling trend that bears monitoring. Outside the hospital walls, the declining number of primary care physicians entering practice will open opportunities for family nurse practitioners to fill the gap (American College of Physicians, 2006).

A CHALLENGE TO THE ENTIRE NURSING PROFESSION: FOCUS, UNITE, ACT!

Most of the important issues the nursing profession will face in the next decade cannot be resolved by any one group of nurses. These concerns will require the attention of the entire profession, working in a focused, united, active manner through nursing's professional associations. Although collective power is the only way nursing will effectively resolve these issues, less than 10 percent of all nurses belong to their professional association, a sad commentary on the priorities most nurses place on this vital aspect of professionalism.

As the largest health care profession in the United States, with more than 2.9 million registered nurse members, nursing can and should have a powerful voice and presence at every table where substantive health care issues are discussed. However, nurses have historically been unwilling to throw their support behind their professional organizations. They have allowed issues of educational background, political philosophies, right-to-life, and other concerns to divide them.

If you think for a moment about other groups to which you belong—for example, a political party, church, or parent-teacher association—you do not expect to agree with every position taken by the organization or its leaders. Nurses seem to have such an expectation of their professional association, however, and use that as a reason for lack of unity. This is naïve and unrealistic. With nursing and society becoming increasingly diverse, nurses of the future must become more tolerant of differences and work hard to find common ground with their colleagues in the profession. If we fail to do so, nursing will not prosper, nor will its practitioners.

Nursing's Agenda for the Future

An encouraging development was the coming together in 2001 of 19 major nursing organizations at the Nursing Profession Summit. A $100,000 grant from the American Nurses Foundation, a branch of the American Nurses Association, enabled the ANA to convene this group, which formed a steering committee. The steering committee took leadership in identifying 10 domains (areas) that describe the work needed to accomplish the vision they set forth in a document titled *Nursing's Agenda for the Future*. This document identifies what the steering committee envisioned: how nursing should look and where it should be by the year 2010. In other words, this committee developed a desired future

vision for nursing and set forth areas that must be addressed to achieve the desired vision.

The steering committee called on all nurses to review *Nursing's Agenda for the Future* "and to find those objectives that match with the mission, priorities and resources of their own entities. The intent is to involve as many nurses as possible in charting their own future. It is this critical . . . step that will bring the strategic plan to life, move it forward and make progress toward the desired future state" (Nursing's Agenda for the Future Steering Committee, 2002, pp. 6-7). You can download the report in PDF form from the ANA website (www.nursingworld.org/naf). I challenge you to do so to monitor progress toward these goals and to decide how you will participate in achieving the vision.

You, the readers of this book, are the future of the nursing profession. You represent our best hope for building nursing into an even more powerful force for good. Look around at the other members of your class. Whether you have 25 fellow students or 125, you can accomplish far more working together than you can working in isolation. So it is with nursing's future: we can accomplish far more by working collectively. All nurses, individually and as a profession, will benefit from the results. As Mohandas Ghandi said, "Be the change you wish to see in the world."

SUMMARY OF *Key Points*

- Future societal changes will occur in the following areas: demographics, the environment, potential for disasters such as bioterrorism, lifestyles, economics, and governmental regulation of health care.
- Both nursing practice and nursing education will be affected by these changes.
- Nursing roles will be differentiated.
- Nursing practice will become more community-based with new roles continually emerging.
- Today's nurses should be prepared to serve effectively as members of an emergency and disaster response team.

- Nurses will be able to demonstrate that the care they provide makes a positive difference in patient outcomes.
- Nurses will continue to provide a warm, humanizing influence on patient care in potentially dehumanizing high-tech environments.
- Effective nurses will become culturally competent.
- The major challenges for nursing education will be to respond to societal changes rapidly with appropriate curricular modifications; to produce a steady supply of well-prepared graduates in the face of an aging faculty; to adapt to rapidly changing technology; to acquire competency needed to respond to increasing cultural diversity of students and patients; and to address the lack of human and budgetary resources in higher education.
- Active membership in professional associations is the best way for nurses to focus, unite, and act to solve the challenges facing the profession.

CRITICAL THINKING QUESTIONS

1. As the number of elderly Americans rises, the rate of chronic illness also rises. What challenges does this present for nurses of the future?
2. Take a position on the statement "Nurses of the future will have an impact on the environment that exceeds that of the ordinary citizen." Be prepared to defend your position.
3. Describe economic issues that will affect nurses of the future. How can you begin now to prepare yourself to deal with these issues?
4. Initiate a classroom debate on the issue "HIV-positive nurses should not be limited in how they practice nursing."
5. As a class, brainstorm ways a school health nurse could improve pupils' health status. Then design an educational program to prepare school nurses. Compare your curriculum with that of an existing school health nurse program.

6. Interview faculty members to identify components of your educational program that will prepare you for the culturally competent nursing needed in the twenty-first century. Report your findings to the class.
7. Using the core competencies listed in Box 16-1, evaluate your own disaster preparedness and devise a plan to become better prepared.
8. Using the GeneTests website as a resource (www.genetests.org), learn all you can about testing, counseling, and treatment for a genetic condition. These might include albinism, sickle cell disease, hereditary breast or ovarian cancer, hemophilia, hemochromatosis, Marfan syndrome, cystic fibrosis, or others of interest to you or your family. Report your findings to the class.

REFERENCES

American College of Physicians: *The impending collapse of primary care medicine and its implications for the state of the nation's health care*, 2006, available online: www.acponline.org/hpp/statehc06.htm.

American Lung Association: *Facts about lung cancer*, 2003, available online: www.lungusa.org/diseases/lungcanc.html.

American Nurses Association: *Bioterrorism website*, 2006a, available online: www.nursingworld.org/news/disaster/biocare.htm.

American Nurses Association: *Workplace issues: occupational safety and health*, 2006b, available online: www.nursingworld.org/osh/latex.htm.

American Obesity Association: *AOA fact sheet: what is obesity?* 2006, available online: http://www.obesity.org/subs/fastfacts/obesity_what2.shtml.

Carroll V, Goldsmith J: One-third of nurses are abused in the workplace, *Reflections* 25(3):24-27, 1999.

Coleman EA: Anthrax: know the guidelines for management, *Am J Nurs* 101(12):48-52, 2001.

Davidhizar R, Shearer R: When your nursing student is culturally diverse, *Health Care Manag* 24(4):356-363, 2005.

Dickenson-Hazard N: Future study or the Magic 8 Ball? *Reflect Nurs Leadership* 29(4):4, 2003.

Gary FA, Sigsby LM, Campbell D: Preparing for the 21st century: diversity in nursing education, research, and practice, *J Prof Nurs* 14(5):272-279, 1998.

Gebbie KM, Qureshi K: Emergency and disaster preparedness: core competencies for nurses, *Am J Nurs* 102(1):46-51, 2002.

Goley A: APNs need to learn more about complementary and alternative medicine, *Top Adv Pract Nurs eJournal* 4(2), 2004, available online: http://www.medscape.com.

Hendrick B: The coming millennium, *The Atlanta Journal/The Atlanta Constitution,* July 16, 1995, p A12.

Herbert LE, Scherr PA, Beckett LA et al: Alzheimer's disease, *JAMA* 273(17):1354-1359, 1995.

Jenkins A: Invest in yourself, *Nurs Standard* 20(10):69, 2005.

Lea DH, Monsen RB: Preparing nurses for a 21st century role in genomics-based health care, *Nurs Educ Perspect* 24(2):75-80, 2003.

Marrilli T: Nursing in flux: are you ready to meet the challenge of the future? *Am J Nurs* 106(1,suppl):19-25, 2006.

Nursing's Agenda for the Future Steering Committee: *Nursing's agenda for the future: the future vision for nursing,* Washington, DC, 2002, American Nurses Publishing.

Porter E: Health care for all just a (big) step away, *New York Times,* Dec 18, 2005, available online: http://www.nytimes.com/2005/12/18/business/your money/18view.html.

Tanner L: *U.S. scores poorly on infant mortality: shortcomings in basic health care, obesity cited for low rank among modern nations,* Associated Press, 2006, at www.commondreams.org/headlines06/0510-06.htm.

Tracy MF, Lindquist R, Savik K et al: Use of complementary and alternative therapies: a national survey of critical care nurses, *Am J Crit Care* 14(5):404-415, 2005.

U.S. Census Bureau: *Population clock, U.S. and international,* 2006, available online: www.census.gov/main/www/popclock.html.

Valentino LM: Future employment trends in nursing, *AJN 2002 career guide,* New York, 2002, Lippincott Williams & Wilkins.

Wolf G: Coming of age in health care: changes, challenges, choices, *Reflect Nurs Leadership* 29(4):32-34, 2003.

E P I L O G U E

You, our readers, are inheriting a rich legacy of achievement and progress in the nursing profession. While appreciating the accomplishments of those who paved the way for us, we cannot lose sight of the fact that much remains to be done. As health care professionals, you will be challenged to lead your communities in addressing the complex issues of containing health care costs, improving access to health care for the disenfranchised, decreasing health disparities and other not-yet-imagined concerns. You will be part of the solution.

It is the hope of all the nurses who participated in preparing this textbook that you have been inspired to develop values, beliefs, knowledge, professionalism, and desire to become a nursing leader of the future and a positive force for change in the nursing profession.

You can begin to exert your influence to improve the profession by evaluating this book. If you are willing to help in this way, please e-mail us and we will send you a brief questionnaire. You can also tell us anything else you would like to share about the helpful and not-so-helpful aspects of the current edition. With your assistance we will continue to improve this book to better meet the needs of future students.

KayKChitty1@comcast.net
beth_black@unc.edu

GLOSSARY

A

AACN American Association of Colleges of Nursing; a national organization devoted to advancing nursing education at the baccalaureate and graduate levels.

Abstract Summary of a research report or article.

Acceptance See Nonjudgmental acceptance.

Accountability Responsibility for one's behavior.

Accreditation A voluntary review process of educational programs or service agencies by professional organizations.

Action language A developmental phase in language development of older infants. Examples include reaching for or crawling toward a desired object or closing the lips and turning the head when an undesired food is offered.

Active collaborator One who is engaged as a participant with another person.

Active listening A method of communicating interest and attention using such signals as maintaining good eye contact, nodding, and encouraging the speaker.

Acuity Degree of illness.

Acute illness Sudden, steadily progressing symptoms that subside quickly with or without treatment, such as influenza.

Adaptation A change or coping response to stress of any kind.

Adaptation model A conceptual model that focuses on the patient as an adaptive system; that is, one that strives to cope with both internal demands and external demands of the environment.

Adjudicate To decide or sit in judgment, as in a legal case.

Administrative law Law created by a governmental agency to meet the intent of statutory law.

Advance directives Written instructions recognized by state law that describe individuals' preferences in regard to medical intervention should they become incapacitated.

Advanced degrees Degrees beyond the bachelor's degree; master's and doctoral degrees.

Advanced practice Nursing roles that require either a master's degree or specialized education in a specific area.

Advanced practice nurse A registered nurse who has met advanced educational and practice requirements beyond basic nursing education.

Aesthetics Branch of philosophy that studies the nature of beauty.

Affective domain Field of activity dealing with a person's mood, feelings, values, or belief system.

Alternative educational programs Programs other than basic nursing programs, such as baccalaureate programs for registered nurses and the Excelsior Program, formerly known as the New York Regents' External Degree Program.

Alternative therapies Treatments other than traditional Western medical treatments.

Altruism Unselfish concern for the welfare of others.

Ambulatory care Health services provided to those who visit a clinic or hospital as outpatients and depart after treatment on the same day.

American Assembly for Men in Nursing (AAMN) Professional organization that seeks to encourage, support, and advocate for men in nursing.

American Association of Colleges of Nursing (AACN) A national organization devoted to advancing nursing education at the baccalaureate and graduate levels.

American Nurses Association (ANA) A professional organization that addresses ethics, clinical standards, public policy, and the economic and general welfare of nurses. Membership is limited to nurses.

American Organization of Nurse Executives (AONE) An organization for high-level nursing managers, such as chief nurses. Leaders in nursing education can be associate members.

American Nurses Credentialing Center (ANCC) The credentialing arm of the American Nurses Association that deals with certification of individual nurses, and approval of organizations as continuing education providers.

ANA Position Paper A 1965 paper published by the American Nurses Association concluding that baccalaureate education should become the basic foundation for professional practice.

Analysis The second step in the nursing process during which various pieces of patient data are analyzed. The outcome is one or more nursing diagnoses.

Ancillary workers Nonprofessional auxiliary health care workers, such as nursing assistants.

Androcentric Male-centered cultural bias.

Anxiety A diffuse, vague feeling of apprehension and uncertainty. Also a psychiatric condition.

Applied science Use of scientific theory and laws in a practical way that has immediate application.

Appropriateness A criterion for successful communication in which the reply fits the circumstances and matches the message, and the amount is neither too great nor too little.

Articulation An educational mobility system providing for direct movement from a program at one level of nursing education to another without significant loss of credit.

Assault A threat or an attempt to make bodily contact with another person without the person's consent.

Assessment The first step in the nursing process involving the collection of information about the patient.

Assisted suicide Suicide by a person with help from another person, such as a health care provider.

Associate degree in nursing program The newest form of basic nursing education program, leading to the associate degree in nursing (ADN), consisting of 3 or fewer years, and usually offered in technical or community colleges.

Association An organization of members with common interests.

Authority Possessing both the responsibility for making decisions and the accountability for the outcome of those decisions.

Autonomy Self-determination. Control over one's own professional practice.

B

Baccalaureate degree in nursing (BSN) Degree offered by programs that combine nursing courses with general education courses in a 4- or 5-year curriculum in a senior college or university.

Balance of power A distribution of forces among the branches of government so that no one branch is strong enough to dominate the others.

Basic program Any nursing education program preparing beginning practitioners.

Battery The impermissible, unprivileged touching of one person by another.

Belief The intellectual acceptance of something as true or correct.

Belief system Organization of an individual's beliefs into a rational whole.

Beneficence The ethical principle of doing good.

Biases Prejudices, often outside the individual's awareness.

Biculturalism A term used to describe a nurse's ability to balance the ideal nursing culture learned about in school and the real one experienced in practice, using the best of both.

Bioethics An area of ethical inquiry focusing on the dilemmas inherent in modern health care.

Biomedical technology Complex machines or implantable devices used in patient care settings.

Bioterrorism The use of a biological or chemical agent as a weapon.

Birthrate The number of births in a particular place during a specific time period, usually expressed as a quantity per 1000 people in 1 year.

BRN Baccalaureate registered nurse, a term sometimes used to describe a registered nurse who has returned to school to earn a bachelor's degree.

Brown Report A 1948 report recommending that basic schools of nursing be placed in universities and colleges and that efforts be made to recruit large numbers of men and minorities into nursing education programs.

Burnout A state of emotional exhaustion attributable to cumulative stress.

C

Cadet Corps A government-created entity designed during World War II to rapidly increase the number of registered nurses being educated so they could assist in the war effort.

Capitation A cost management system in which a certain amount of money is paid to a provider annually to take care of all of an individual's or group's health care needs.

"Captain of the ship" doctrine A legal principle that implies that the physician is in charge of all patient care and thus should be financially responsible if damages are sought.

Caring Watching over, attending to, and providing for the needs of others.

Case management Systematic collaboration with patients, their significant others, and their health care providers to coordinate high-quality health care services in a cost-effective manner with positive patient outcomes.

Case management nursing A growing field within nursing in which nurses are responsible for coordinating services provided to patients in a cost-effective manner.

Case manager An individual responsible for coordinating services provided to a group of patients.

CCNE Commission on Collegiate Nursing Education, the accrediting arm of the American Association of Colleges of Nursing.

Centenarian A person who has reached the age of 100 or more years.

Centers for Medicare and Medicaid Services (CMS) Federal cost-containment program that establishes standards and monitors care in the Medicare and Medicaid programs. Formerly known as Health Care Financing Administration (HCFA).

Certificate of need (CON) A cost-containment measure requiring health care agencies to apply to a state agency for permission to construct or substantially add to an existing facility.

Certified nurse-midwife (CNM) A nationally certified nurse with advanced specialized education who assists women and couples during uncomplicated pregnancies, deliveries, and post-delivery periods.

Certified Registered Nurse Anesthetist (CRNA) A nationally certified nurse with advanced education who specializes in the administration of anesthesia.

Certification Validation of specific qualifications demonstrated by a registered nurse in a defined area of practice.

Change agent An individual who recognizes the need for organizational change and facilitates that process.

Chief executive officer (CEO) The senior administrator of an organization.

Chief nurse executive (CNE) The senior nursing administrator of an organization.

Chief of staff A physician in a health care facility, generally elected by the medical staff for a specified term, who is responsible for overseeing the activities of the medical staff organization.

Chronic illness Ongoing health problems of a generally incurable nature, such as diabetes.

Civil law Law involving disputes between individuals.

Clarification A therapeutic communication technique in which the nurse seeks to understand a patient's message more clearly.

Clinical coordinator See Clinical director.

Clinical director Middle management nurse who has responsibility for multiple units in a health care agency.

Clinical judgment The ability to make consistently effective clinical decisions based on theoretical knowledge, research findings, informed opinions, and prior experience.

Clinical ladder Programs allowing nurses to progress in the organizational hierarchy while staying in direct patient care roles.

Clinical nurse specialist A nurse with an advanced degree who serves as a resource person to other nurses and often provides direct care to patients or families with particularly difficult or complex problems.

Closed system A system that does not interact with other systems or with the surrounding environment.

Coalition A temporary alliance of distinct factions.

Code of Academic and Clinical Conduct Code of ethics of the National Student Nurses Association.

Code of Ethics for Nurses A formal statement of the nursing profession's code of ethics.

Code of ethics A statement of professional standards used to guide behavior and as a framework for decision making.

Cognitive Pertaining to intellectual activities requiring knowledge.

Cognitive domain Area of activity that affects an individual's knowledge level.

Cognitive rebellion A stage in the educational process wherein students begin to free themselves from external controls and to rely on their own judgment.

Collaboration Working closely with another person in the spirit of cooperation.

Collective action Activities undertaken by or on behalf of a group of people who have common interests.

Collective bargaining Negotiating as a group for improved salary and work conditions.

Collective identity The connection and feeling of similarity individuals in a particular group feel with one another; group identification.

Collegiality The promotion of collaboration, cooperation, and recognition of interdependence among members of a profession.

Commission on Collegiate Nursing Education (CCNE) The accrediting arm of the American Association of Colleges of Nursing.

Common law Law that develops as a result of decisions made by judges in legal cases.

Communication The exchange of thoughts, ideas, or information; a dynamic process that is a primary instrument through which change occurs in nursing situations.

Community-based nursing Nursing care provided for individuals, families, and groups in a variety of settings, including homes, workplaces, and schools.

Community health nursing Formerly known as public health nursing; a nursing specialty that systematically uses a process of delivering nursing care to improve the health of an entire community.

Competency Refers to the capability of a particular patient to understand the information given and to make an informed choice about treatment options.

Complementary therapies Those treatments intended to augment traditional Western medical treatments such as massage therapy or acupuncture.

Completeness An element of informed consent that refers to the comprehensiveness of the information provided.

Concept An abstract classification of data; for example, "temperature" is a concept.

Conceptual model or framework A group of concepts that are broadly defined and systematically organized to provide a focus, a rationale, and a tool for the integration and interpretation of information.

Confidentiality Ensuring the privacy of individuals participating in research studies or being treated in health care settings.

Congruent A characteristic of communication that occurs when the verbal and nonverbal elements of a message match.

Constituent Member Association (CMA) Organizational members of the American Nurses Association, such as state nurses associations or specialty nursing organizations.

Consultation The process of conferring with patients, families, or other health professionals.

Consumerism A movement to protect consumers from unsafe or inferior products and services.

Contact hour A measurement used to recognize participation in continuing education offerings, usually equivalent to 50 minutes.

Context An essential element of communication consisting of the setting in which an interaction occurs, the mood, the relationship between sender and receiver, and other factors.

Continuing education (CE) Workshops, conferences, and short courses, in which nurses maintain competence during their professional careers.

Continuous quality improvement (CQI) A management concept focusing on excellence and employee involvement at all levels of an organization.

Contracts Documents agreed upon by workers and management that include provisions about staffing levels, salary, work conditions, and other issues of concern to either party.

Copayment The portion of a provider's charges that an insured patient is responsible for paying.

Coping The methods a person uses to assess and manage demands.

Coping mechanisms Psychological devices used by individuals when a threat is perceived.

Cost containment An attempt to keep health care costs stable or increasing only slowly.

Criminal law Law involving public concerns against unlawful behavior that threatens society.

Criteria Standards by which something is judged or measured.

Critical paths Multidisciplinary care plans outlining a patient's treatments and expected outcomes, day by day.

Cross-functional team People from all parts of an organization who contribute to a particular activity and outcome.

Cross-training Preparing a single worker for multiple tasks that formerly were performed by multiple specialized workers.

Cultural assessment The process of determining a patient's cultural practices and preferences in order to render culturally competent care.

Cultural care, theory of A nursing theory focusing on the importance of incorporating a patient's culturally determined health beliefs and practices into care.

Cultural competence The integration of knowledge, attitudes, and skills that enhance cross-cultural communication and appropriate interactions with others.

Cultural conditioning The process by which a person becomes aware of and entrenched in his or her own culture's ways; culture bound.

Cultural diversity Social, ethnic, racial, and religious differences in a group.

Culturally congruent nursing care Care that incorporates knowledge, attitudes, and skills that enhance cross-cultural communication and appropriate interactions with others.

Culturally competent education Nursing education that incorporates knowledge, attitudes, and skills that enhance cross-cultural communication and appropriate interactions with others.

Culture The attitudes, beliefs, and behaviors of social and ethnic groups that have been perpetuated through generations.

Culture of nursing The rites, rituals, and valued behaviors of the nursing profession.

D

Data Information or facts collected for analysis.

Deaconess Institute A large hospital and planned training program for deaconesses established in 1836 by Pastor Theodor Fliedner at Kaiserswerth, Germany.

Decentralization An organizational structure in which decision-making authority is shared with employees most affected by the decisions rather than being retained by top executives.

Deductible The out-of-pocket amount individuals must pay before their health insurance begins to pay for health care.

Deductive reasoning A process through which conclusions are drawn by logical inference from given premises; proceeds from the general case to the specific.

Defining characteristics Signs and symptoms of disease.

Delegate To refer a task to another.

Delegation The practice of assigning tasks or responsibilities to other persons.

Demographics The study of vital statistics and social trends.

Demography The science that studies vital statistics and social trends.

Deontology The ethical theory that the rightness or wrongness of an action depends on the inherent moral significance of the action.

Dependency The degree to which individuals adopt passive attitudes and rely on others to take care of them.

Dependent intervention Nursing actions on behalf of patients that require knowledge and skill on the part of the nurse but may not be done without explicit directions from another health professional, usually a physician, dentist, or nurse practitioner.

Designer medicines Pharmacological agents developed for an individual, based on his or her genetic makeup.

Developmental theory A theory in which growth is defined as an increase in physical size and shape toward a point of optimal maturity.

Diagnosis Identification of a disease or condition.

Diagnosis-related groups (DRGs) A method of classifying and grouping illnesses according to similarities of diagnosis for reimbursement purposes.

Dietitian Bachelor's or master's degree–prepared nutrition expert who specializes in therapeutic diet preparation and nutrition education.

Differentiated practice Nursing practice at two levels, professional and technical, with differences in both educational preparation and clinical responsibilities.

Diploma program The earliest form of formal nursing education in the United States; usually based in hospitals, requires 3 years of study, and leads to a diploma in nursing.

Disaster An event or situation that is of greater magnitude than an emergency; disrupts essential services such as housing, transportation, communications, sanitation, water, and health care; and requires the response of people outside the community affected.

Disease A pathological alteration at the tissue or organ level.

Disease management A process of helping patients understand and manage their chronic conditions more effectively through phone calls, coaching and education, symptom prevention and management, and collaboration with the patient's health care provider.

Disenfranchised The state of having no power or voice in a political system.

Disseminate Publish or widely distribute scientific information, such as the findings of a research study.

Dissonance Lack of harmony.

Distance learning The process of taking classes and earning academic credit through technological means such as televised or online classes. The teacher and student may be many miles apart.

Distributed campaign A political campaign that makes extensive use of the Internet to distribute information about the candidate and to raise funds.

Documentation Written communication about a patient's condition, care, and reactions to treatments; found in the patient record/chart.

Dominant culture Mainstream culture that contains one or more subcultures.

Double effect Ethical concept encompassing the belief that there are some situations in which it is necessary to inflict potential harm in an effort to achieve a greater good.

Duty of care The responsibility of a nurse or other health professional for the care of a patient.

Duty to report The requirement, according to state law, for health professionals to report certain illnesses, injuries, and actions of patients.

E

Economic and general welfare Employment issues relating to salaries, benefits, and working conditions.

Educative instrument A tool for increasing the knowledge and power of another person.

Efficiency A criterion for successful communication that consists of using simple, clear words timed at a pace suitable to participants.

Electoral process The procedures that must be followed to select someone to fill an elected position.

Emotional intelligence Awareness of and sensitivity to the feelings of others.

Empathy Awareness of, sensitivity to, and identification with the feelings of another person.

End-of-life care Care aimed at comfort and dignity for patients who are nearing death and for their significant others.

Entrepreneur A person who envisions, organizes, manages, and assumes responsibility for a new enterprise or business.

Environment All of the many external and internal factors, such as physical and psychological, that influence life and survival.

Epidemiologist A scientist who studies the origins and transmission of diseases.

Epistemology The branch of philosophy dealing with the theory of knowledge.

Ethical decision making The process of choosing between actions based on a system of beliefs and values.

Ethics The branch of philosophy that studies the propriety of certain courses of action.

Ethnocentrism The belief that one's own culture is the most desirable.

Ethnographic research A type of qualitative research.

Euthanasia The act of painlessly putting to death a person suffering from an incurable disease; also called mercy killing.

Evaluation Measuring the success or failure of the results or "outputs," and consequently the effectiveness, of a system. It is the final step in the nursing process wherein the nurse examines the patient's progress to determine whether a problem is solved, is in the process of being solved, or is unsolved. In communication theory, it is the analysis of information received.

Evidence-based practice The use of research findings as a basis for practice rather than trial and error, intuition, or traditional methods, such as problem solving.

Exacerbation Reemergence or worsening of the symptoms of a chronic illness.

Executive branch The branch of government responsible for administering the laws of the land.

Experimental design Research design that provides evidence of a cause-and-effect relationship between actions.

Expert power Strength derived from knowledge that can influence an outcome.

Expert witness An individual called on to testify in court because of special skill or knowledge in a certain field, such as nursing.

Extended care Medical, nursing, or custodial care provided to an individual over a prolonged period of time.

Extended family A term used to describe non-nuclear family members such as grandparents, aunts, and uncles.

External degree program An alternative educational program in which learning is independent and is assessed through highly standardized and validated examinations.

External factors Values, beliefs, and behaviors of significant others that have an impact on an individual.

F

Faith community The members of a church, synagogue, mosque, or other entity who worship together and share common beliefs about religion.

Faith community nurse A specialized nurse who focuses on the promotion of health within the context of the values, beliefs, and practices of a church, synagogue, mosque, or other faith community.

False reassurance A nontherapeutic form of communication that seeks to reassure that "all will be well."

Family system The group of individuals who comprise the basic unit of family living and their interactions with one another and the larger society.

Famous trio Three famous schools of nursing founded in 1873: the Bellevue Training School, the Connecticut Training School, and the Boston Training School.

Feedback The information given back into a system to determine whether or not the purpose of the system has been achieved. A major element in the communication process.

Feminism Belief in the value and equality of women.

Fidelity An ethical principle that values faithfulness to one's responsibilities.

Flexibility A criterion for successful communication that occurs when messages are based on the immediate situation rather than preconceived expectations.

Flexible staffing A mechanism whereby nurses may work at times other than the traditional hospital shifts.

Flexner Report A 1910 study of medical education that provided the impetus for much needed reform.

Formal socialization The process by which individuals learn a new role from the direct instruction of others.

For-profit agency A health care agency established to make a profit for the owners or stockholders.

Frontier Nursing Service Founded in Kentucky in 1925, and it provided the first organized midwifery service in the United States.

Functional nursing A system of nursing care delivery in which each worker has a task, or function, to perform for all patients.

Futurist An individual who studies trends and makes predictions about the future.

G

Gatekeeper An individual, generally a primary care physician, who controls patients' access to diagnostic procedures, medical specialists, and hospitalization.

Gender-role stereotyping The practice of automatically and routinely linking specific characteristics to either males or females; also called sex-role stereotyping.

General election An election in which all registered voters may vote and may choose a candidate from any party on the ballot.

General systems theory A theory promulgated by Ludwig von Bertalanffy in the late 1930s to explain the relationship of a whole to its parts.

Generalizable Research findings that are transferable to other situations.

Generic master's degree An accelerated master's degree in nursing for people with nonnursing bachelor's degrees.

Generic nursing doctorate A doctoral degree program designed for individuals who are not already registered nurses and who possess baccalaureate degrees in other fields.

Genetic counseling Health and reproductive advice given to individuals based on their genetic makeup.

Goldmark Report A major study of nursing education published in 1923 and named *The Study of Nursing and Nursing Education in the United States.*

Governmental (public) agency An agency primarily supported by taxes, administered by elected or appointed officials, and tailored to the needs of the communities served.

Grand theory A very broad conceptualization of nursing phenomena.

Grassroots activism The involvement of a large number of people, generally widely dispersed, who are concerned about a particular issue.

Growth An increase in physical size and shape toward a point of optimal maturity.

H

Hardiness A personality characteristic that enables people to manage the changes associated with illness and to have fewer physical illnesses resulting from stress.

Health An individual's physical, mental, spiritual, and social well-being; a continuum, not a constant state.

Health behaviors Choices and habitual actions that promote or diminish health.

Health beliefs Culturally determined beliefs about the nature of health and illness.

Health care network A corporation with a consolidated set of facilities and services for comprehensive health care.

Health Insurance Portability and Accountability Act (HIPAA) Federal law, passed in 1996, designed to protect health insurance coverage for workers and their families when they change or lose their jobs.

Health maintenance Preventing illness and maintaining maximal function.

Health maintenance organization (HMO) A network or group of providers who agree to provide certain basic health care services for a single predetermined yearly fee.

Health promotion Encouraging a condition of maximum physical, mental, and social well-being.

Health promotion model A theoretical nursing model that uses illness prevention and health promotion as a basic framework.

Helping professions Professions such as social work, teaching, and nursing that emphasize meeting the needs of clients.

Henry Street Settlement A clinic for the poor founded by Lillian Wald and her colleague Mary Brewster on New York's Lower East Side.

Heterogeneous Composed of parts of differing kinds.

High-level wellness Functioning at maximum potential in an integrated way within the environment.

High-tech nursing Nursing care that involves the use of technologies such as monitors, pumps, and ventilators.

High-touch nursing Nursing care that involves the use of interpersonal skills such as communication, listening, and empathy.

Hill-Burton Act A 1946 federal law that called for and funded surveys of states' needs for hospitals, paid for planning hospitals and public health centers, and provided partial funding for constructing and equipping hospitals and health centers.

Holism A school of health care thought that espouses treating the whole patient: body, mind, and spirit.

Holistic communication Sharing both emotional and factual information and appreciating another individual's point of view.

Holistic nursing care Nursing care that nourishes the whole person—that is, the body, mind, and spirit.

Holistic nursing research Nursing research that considers the whole person—that is, the body, mind, and spirit.

Holistic values The approach to nursing practice that takes the physical, emotional, social, economic, and spiritual needs of the person into consideration.

Home health agency An organization that delivers various health services to patients in their homes.

Home health nursing Rapidly growing field of nursing in which nursing care is provided to patients in their own homes.

Homeostasis A relative constancy in the internal environment of the body.

Homogeneous Composed of parts of the same or similar kinds.

Hospice An agency that provides services to terminally ill patients and their families.

Hospice and palliative care nursing Specialized nursing care provided at the end-of-life to patients and their families in homes and residential facilities. Aimed at a comfortable and dignified death that honors the wishes of patients and loved ones.

Hospitalist Hospital-based physicians who care for patients only while they are hospitalized.

Human caring, theory of Nursing theory emphasizing the nurturing aspects of professional nursing through which curative strategies are implemented.

Human Genome Project A scientific project designed to map the genetic structure of composite human DNA, the initial phase of which was completed in 2003.

Human motivation Abraham Maslow's conceptualization of human needs and their relationship to the stimulation of purposeful behavior.

Human needs theory Theory proposed by Abraham Maslow that human motivation is determined by the drive to meet intrinsic human needs.

Human responses The problems an individual experiences as a result of a disease process.

Humanistic nursing care Care that includes viewing professional relationships as human-to-human rather than nurse-to-patient.

Humanistic nursing values The approach to professional relationships as human-to-human experiences rather than nurse-to-patient experiences.

Hypothesis A statement predicting the relationship among various concepts or variables.

I

Illness An abnormal process in which an individual's physical, emotional, social, or intellectual functioning is impaired.

Illness prevention All activities aimed at diminishing the likelihood that an individual's physical, emotional, social, and intellectual functions become impaired.

Implementation A stage of the nursing process during which the plan of care is carried out.

Incongruent Describes a confusing form of communication that occurs when the verbal and nonverbal elements of a message do not match.

Independent intervention Actions on behalf of patients for which the nurse requires no supervision or direction.

Individualized care plan A plan of care designed to meet the needs of a specific person.

Inductive reasoning The process of reasoning from the specific to the general. Repeated observations of an experiment or event enable the observer to draw general conclusions.

Inertia Disinclination to change.

Informal socialization The process through which individuals learn a new role by observing how others behave.

Informatics nurse A nurse who combines nursing science with information management science and computer science to manage and make accessible the information that nurses need.

Information technology (IT) Hardware and software used to manage and process information.

Informed consent The process of asking individuals who are scheduled to undergo diagnostic procedures or surgery or who are potential research subjects to sign a consent form once the procedures and risks have been explained and their privacy has been ensured.

Infrastructure Basic support mechanisms needed to ensure that an activity can be conducted.

Input The information, energy, or matter that enters a system.

Institutional review board A committee that ensures that research is well designed and protects the rights of human participants in the research.

Institutional structure The way in which the workers within an agency are organized to carry out the functions of the agency.

Integrative care Care that combines the best of both standard and nontraditional treatments, for example, pain control through both prescription medication and acupuncture.

Interdependent intervention Actions on behalf of patients in which the nurse must collaborate or consult with another health professional before or while carrying out the action.

Interdisciplinary team Group composed of individuals representing various disciplines who work together toward a common end.

Internal factors Personal feelings and beliefs that influence an individual.

Internalize The process of taking in knowledge, skills, attitudes, beliefs, norms, values, and ethical standards and making them a part of one's own self-image and behavior.

International Council of Nurses (ICN) The federation of national nurses associations, currently representing nurses in more than 100 countries.

Internship An apprenticeship under supervision.

Irrational belief A fixed idea that is not affected by information to the contrary.

Issues management Assisting a group to resolve a particular question about which there are significant differences of opinion.

J

Jargon Specialized vocabulary used by those in the same line of work to communicate about work-related matters.

Job hopping Moving rapidly from job to job.

Judicial branch The branch of government that decides cases or controversies on particular matters.

Justice An ethical principle stating that equals should be treated the same and that unequals should be treated differently.

K

Knowledge-based power Authority or control based on the way information is used to effect an outcome.

Knowledge technology The use of computer systems to transform information into knowledge and to generate new knowledge; expert systems.

L

Latent power Untapped strength.

Law All the rules of conduct established by a government and applicable to the people, whether in the form of legislation or custom.

Learned resourcefulness An acquired ability to use available resources in one's behalf.

Legal authority A group of people in whom power is vested by law, such as the powers vested in state boards of nursing by nurse practice acts.

Legislative branch The branch of government consisting of elected officials who are responsible for enacting the laws of the land.

Length of stay (LOS) The number of days a patient stays in an inpatient setting, such as a hospital.

Licensure The process by which an agency of government grants permission to qualified persons to engage in a given profession or occupation.

Licensure by endorsement A system whereby registered nurses or licensed practical/vocational nurses can, by submitting proof of licensure in another state and paying a licensure fee, receive licensure from the new state without sitting for a licensing examination.

Lifelong learning Continuing education and increasing knowledge throughout an individual's professional life.

Lifelong learner An individual who seeks continuing education and opportunities to increase knowledge throughout his or her professional life.

Lobby An attempt to influence the vote of legislators.

Locus of control The place an individual believes the power in his/her life resides, either within or outside of himself/herself.

Logic The field of philosophy that studies correct and incorrect reasoning.

Long-term care Care provided to individuals, such as people with Alzheimer's disease, who require ongoing assistance in the maintenance of activities of daily living.

Long-term goals Major changes that may take months or even years to accomplish.

Lysaught Report A 1970 report entitled *An Abstract for Action* that made recommendations concerning the supply and demand for nurses, nursing roles and functions, and nursing education.

M

Malpractice An act resulting in injury that occurs when a professional fails to act as a reasonably prudent professional would under specific circumstances.

Managed care A process in which an individual, often a nurse, is assigned to review patients' cases and coordinate services so that quality care can be achieved at the lowest cost.

Managed care organization (MCO) Any of a number of organizations that attempt to coordinate subscriber services to ensure quality care at the lowest cost.

Mandatory continuing education The requirement that nurses complete a certain number of hours of continuing education as a prerequisite for relicensure.

Maximum health potential The highest level of well-being that an individual is capable of attaining.

Medicaid A jointly funded federal and state public health insurance that covers citizens below the poverty level and those with certain disabling conditions; established in 1965.

Medical paternalism The attitude that health care providers know best and that "good" patients simply follow directions without asking questions.

Medically indigent Individuals and families who do not qualify for Medicaid or Medicare but cannot afford health insurance or medical care.

Medicare A federally funded form of public health insurance for citizens 65 years of age and older; established in 1965.

Members In professional associations, members may be individuals, agencies such as schools of nursing, or other associations. For example, in the ANA, the members are the state associations, whereas in the NLN, members may be either individuals or organizations.

Mentor An experienced nurse who shares knowledge with less experienced nurses to help advance their careers.

Message An essential element of communication consisting of the spoken word and/or nonverbal communication.

Metaparadigm The most abstract aspect of the structure of knowledge; the global concepts that identify the phenomena of interest for a discipline.

Metaphysics The branch of philosophy that considers the ultimate nature of existence, reality, and experience.

Middle-range theory Theory that makes connections between grand theories and nursing practice.

Milieu Surroundings or environment.

Mission The special task(s) to which an organization devotes itself.

Model A symbolic representation of a concept or reality.

Modeling An informal type of socialization that occurs when an individual chooses an admired person to emulate.

Moonlighting The practice of working a second job in addition to the regular one.

Moral development The ways in which a person learns to deal with moral dilemmas from childhood through adulthood.

Moral distress Pain or anguish of a person who unwillingly participates in perceived moral wrongdoing.

Morals Established rules or standards that guide behavior in situations in which a decision about right and wrong must be made.

Morbidity rate The incidence or occurrence of a certain illness in a particular population during a specific period of time; usually expressed as a quantity per 1000 people in a specific year.

Mortality rate The number of deaths in a particular population during a specific period of time; usually expressed as a quantity per 1000 people in a specific year.

Multidrug-resistant strains Microorganisms, such as the tubercle bacillus, that have become immune to the effects of drugs that formerly were effective against them.

Multiskilled worker Individual who has been cross-trained to perform a number of tasks formerly performed by multiple specialized workers.

Mutuality Sharing jointly with others.

Mutual recognition model A system whereby a registered nurse may be licensed in the state of residency yet practice in other states, after being recognized by them, without additional licenses.

N

NANDA-International (formerly North American Nursing Diagnosis Association) Group working since 1970 to establish a comprehensive list of nursing diagnoses.

National Council Licensing Examination for Practical Nurses (NCLEX-PN) The examination that graduates of practical nursing programs must take to become licensed to practice as licensed practical nurses (LPNs) or licensed vocational nurses (LVNs).

National Council Licensing Examination for Registered Nurses (NCLEX-RN) The examination that graduates of basic nursing programs must take to become licensed to practice as registered nurses (RNs).

National League for Nursing (NLN) National organization that seeks to advance the profession of nursing through advocacy and improving educational standards for nurses. Nonnurses may be members.

National League for Nursing Accrediting Commission (NLNAC) The arm of the National League for Nursing that accredits schools' associate degree, diploma, baccalaureate, and master's programs in nursing.

National Practitioner Data Bank (NPDB) A national clearinghouse containing reports of adverse incidents involving physicians, nurses, and other health care providers that may be useful to potential employers or patients.

National Student Nurses Association (NSNA) National organization devoted to developing leadership skills in nursing students.

NCLEX-PN National Council Licensing Examination for Practical Nurses; the examination that graduates of practical nursing programs must take to become licensed to practice as licensed practical nurses (LPNs) or licensed vocational nurses (LVNs).

NCLEX-RN National Council Licensing Examination for Registered Nurses; the examination that graduates of basic nursing programs must take to become licensed to practice as registered nurses (RNs).

Negligence The failure to act as a reasonably prudent person would have acted in specific circumstances.

Network A system of interconnected individuals; useful to develop contacts or exchange information to further a career.

NLN National League for Nursing; national organization that seeks to advance the profession of nursing through advocacy and improving educational standards for nurses. Nonnurses may be members.

NLNAC National League for Nursing Accreditation Commission; the arm of the National League for Nursing that accredits schools' associate degree, diploma, baccalaureate, and master's programs in nursing.

Nonexperimental design Research with the intent to describe or clarify a phenomenon. Not intended to test an intervention.

Nonjudgmental Describes an attitude that conveys neither approval nor disapproval of patients' beliefs and respects each person's right to his or her beliefs.

Nonjudgmental acceptance An accepting attitude that conveys neither approval nor disapproval of patients or their personal beliefs, habits, expressions of feelings, or chosen lifestyles.

Nonmaleficence The duty to inflict no harm or evil.

Nonverbal communication Communication without words; consists of gestures, posture, facial expressions, tone and loudness of voice, actions, grooming, and clothing, among other things.

Not-for-profit agency An organization that does not attempt to make a profit for distribution to owners or stockholders. Any profit made by such organizations is used to operate and improve the organization itself or to extend its services.

Nuclear family Term used to describe a mother and father and their children.

Nurse activist A nurse who works actively on behalf of a political candidate or certain legislation.

Nurse anesthetist A nurse with specialized advanced education who administers anesthetic agents to patients undergoing operative procedures.

Nurse citizen A nurse who exercises all the political rights accorded citizens, such as registering to vote and voting in all elections.

Nurse entrepreneur A nurse who engages in a business undertaking related to health care or nursing, such as owning a traveling nurse agency.

Nurse executive The top nurse in the administrative structure of a health care organization.

Nurse Licensure Compact An agreement among certain states, authorized by legislation, that they will honor licenses issued to registered nurses by other states in the compact.

Nurse manager A nurse who is in charge of all activities in a unit, including patient care, continuous quality improvement, personnel selection and evaluation, and resource (supplies and money) management. Formerly known as a head nurse.

Nurse-based practice A clinic, office, or home practice in which nurses carry their own caseloads of patients with physical and/or psychiatric needs.

Nurse-midwife A nurse with advanced specialized education who assists women and couples during uncomplicated pregnancies, deliveries, and postdelivery periods.

Nurse-patient relationship The mode of connection between a nurse and patient.

Nurse politician A nurse who runs for political office.

Nurse practice act Law defining the scope of nursing practice in a given state.

Nurse practitioner A nurse with advanced education who specializes in the health care of a particular group, such as children, pregnant women, or the elderly.

Nursing The provision of health care services, focusing on the maintenance, promotion, and restoration of health.

Nursing diagnosis A process of describing a patient's response to health problems that either already exist or may occur in the future.

Nursing goal A statement of the desired long-term or short-term outcome as a result of one or more nursing interventions.

Nursing informatics The branch of nursing that manages knowledge and data through technology with the goal of improving patient care.

Nursing information system A software system that automates the nursing process.

Nursing interventions classification (NIC) A classification system describing more than 400 treatments that nurses perform in all specialties and all settings.

Nursing orders Actions designed to assist the patient in achieving a stated patient goal.

Nursing outcomes classification (NOC) A classification system describing patient outcomes sensitive to nursing interventions.

Nursing process A cognitive activity that requires both critical and creative thinking and serves as the basis for providing nursing care. A method used by nurses in dealing with patient problems in professional practice.

Nursing research The systematic investigation of events or circumstances related to improving nursing practice.

Nursing theory A formal statement of related concepts used to explain, predict, control, and understand commonly occurring phenomena of interest to nurses.

O

Obesity A body mass index (BMI) of 30 or more.

Objective data Factual information obtained through observation and examination of the patient or through consultation with other health care providers.

Occupation A person's principal work or business.

Occupational health nurse A nurse specializing in the care of a specific group of workers in a given occupational setting.

Open-ended question An inquiry that causes the patient to answer fully, giving more than a "yes" or "no" answer.

Open posture Body position, such as squarely facing another person with arms in a relaxed position.

Open system A system that promotes the exchange of matter, energy, and information with other systems and the environment.

Organizational structure How an agency is organized to accomplish its mission.

Orientation phase The beginning phase of a nurse-patient relationship in which the parties are getting acquainted with one another.

Outcome criteria Expected results of nursing intervention.

Out-of-pocket payment Direct payment for health services from individuals' personal funds.

Output The end result or product of a system.

P

Palliative care nursing A rapidly developing specialty in nursing dedicated to improving the experience of seriously ill and dying patients and their families.

Paramedical Having to do with the field of medicine; generally used to describe ancillary workers such as emergency medical technicians.

Parental modeling A type of socialization that occurs when parents' behavior and responses to various stimuli influence a child's future behaviors and responses.

Participants The individuals who are studied in a research project.

Patient acuity The degree of illness of a particular patient or group of patients; used to determine staffing needs.

Patient advocate One who promotes the interest of patients. A nursing role.

Patient classification system (PCS) Identification of patients' needs for nursing care in quantitative terms.

Patient-centered care, also known as patient-focused care A system that emphasizes coordinating patient care to maximize patient comfort, convenience, and security.

Patient interview A face-to-face interaction with the patient in which an interviewer elicits pertinent information.

Patient Self-Determination Act Effective December 1, 1991, this law encourages patients to consider which life-prolonging treatment options they desire and to document their preferences in case they should later become incapable of participating in the decision-making process.

Patients' rights Responsibilities that a hospital and its staff have toward patients and their families during hospitalization.

Pay equity Equal pay for work of comparable value.

Peer review The process of submitting one's work for examination and comment by colleagues in the same profession.

Perception The selection, organization, and interpretation of incoming signals into meaningful messages.

Performance improvement (PI) Organizational efforts to improve corporate performance, incorporating aspects of quality management.

Person An individual—man, woman, or child.

Personal payment Direct payment for health services from individuals' personal funds.

Personal space The amount of space surrounding individuals in which they feel comfortable interacting with others; usually culturally determined.

Personal value system The social principles, ideals, or standards held by an individual that form the basis for meaning, direction, and decision making in life.

Pew Health Professions Commission One of three major national groups that in 1993 issued reports or studies of nursing education in the United States.

Phenomena Occurrences or circumstances that are observable. The singular form is phenomenon.

Phenomenological inquiry/research A qualitative research approach focusing on what people experience in regard to a particular phenomenon, such as grief, and how they interpret those experiences.

Philosophy The study of the truths and principles of being, knowledge, conduct, or nature of the universe.

Physician hospital organization (PHO) A separate corporation formed by a hospital and a group of its medical staff for the purpose of joint-contracting with managed care organizations and businesses.

Planning The third step in the nursing process, which begins with the identification of patient goals.

Point-of-care technology Information system used for entering patient data directly from the bedside.

Point-of-service organization (POS) A hybrid preferred provider organization in which the consumer selects service providers within the defined network or may go outside the network and pay a higher deductible or copayment.

Policy The principles and values that govern actions directed toward given ends. Policy sets forth a plan, direction, or goal for action.

Policy development The generation of principles and procedures that guide governmental or organizational action.

Policy outcome The result of decisions made by governmental or organizational leaders who choose a certain course of action.

Political action committees (PACs) Groups that raise and distribute money to candidates who support their organization's stand on certain issues.

Politics The area of philosophy that deals with the regulation and control of people living in society; in government, it includes the allocation of scarce resources such as health care resources.

Population The entire group of people possessing a given characteristic; for example, all brown-eyed people older than age 65.

Position paper Statement pertaining to the stance a group or organization takes on an issue; for example, the American Nurses Association's 1965 *Position Paper* advocated the baccalaureate degree as the entry level into the practice of registered nursing.

Position power Authority and control accorded to an individual who holds an important role in an organization, profession, or government.

Posttraumatic stress disorder (PTSD) An anxiety disorder characterized by an acute emotional response to a traumatic event or situation.

Power grabbing Hoarding control, taking it from others, or wielding it over others.

Power in numbers The ability of a group of people to accomplish a goal that an individual acting alone is unlikely to achieve.

Power sharing A process of equalizing resources, knowledge, or control.

Powers of appointment The authority to select the people who serve in positions such as judges, ambassadors, and cabinet officials.

Practical nurse (LPN/LVN) program A 1-year educational program preparing individuals for direct patient care roles under the supervision of a physician or registered nurse.

Preceptor A teacher; in nursing, usually an experienced nurse who assumes responsibility for teaching a novice.

Preferred provider organization (PPO) A form of HMO that contracts with independent providers such as physicians and hospitals for a negotiated discount for services provided to its members.

Premium The amount paid for an insurance policy, usually in installments.

Primary care Basic health care, including promotion of health, early diagnosis of disease, and prevention of disease.

Primary election An election in which voters who are declared members of a political party choose among several candidates of that same party for a particular office.

Primary nursing A system of nursing care delivery in which one nurse has responsibility for the planning, implementation, and evaluation of the care of one or more clients 24 hours a day for the duration of the hospital stay.

Primary source The patient is considered the primary source of data about himself or herself; in a literature review, a primary source is the original writing of a theorist or author.

Principalism Use of multiple ethical principles, such as beneficence, autonomy, nonmaleficence, veracity, justice, and fidelity, in the resolution of ethical conflicts rather than a single principle.

Private insurance Insurance obtained from a privately owned company, as opposed to public or governmental insurance.

Private practice Nursing practice engaged in by some nurses with advanced education; usually provided on a fee-for-service basis, as in most medical practices.

Privileged communications The principle that information given to certain professionals is protected and is not to be disclosed even in court.

Problem solving A method of finding solutions to difficulties specific to a given situation and designed for immediate action.

Profession Work requiring advanced training and usually involving mental rather than manual effort. Usually has a code of ethics and a professional organization.

Professional A person who engages in one of the professions, such as law, medicine, or nursing.

Professional accountabilities In the shared governance model, a basic set of responsibilities of all professional nurses regardless of practice setting.

Professional association An organization consisting of people belonging to the same profession and thereby having many common interests.

Professional boundary The dividing line between the activities of two professions. The area in which a professional person functions to avoid both underinvolvement and overinvolvement, maintaining the patient's needs as the focus of the relationship.

Professional governance The concept that health care professionals have a right and a responsibility to govern their own work and time within a financially secure, patient-centered system.

Professional outcomes The impact on a profession from political action by its practitioners.

Professional practice advocacy Includes activities such as education, lobbying, and advocating individually and collectively to advance a profession's agenda.

Professional review organization (PRO) Organizations that review Medicare hospital admissions and Medicare patients' lengths of stay.

Professionalism Professional behavior, appearance, and conduct.

Professionalization A process through which an occupation evolves to professional status.

Professional socialization The process of developing an occupational identity.

Proposition A statement about how two or more concepts are related.

Prospective payment system (PPS) A cost-containment mechanism wherein providers, such as physicians and hospitals, receive payment on a per-case basis, regardless of the cost of delivering the services.

Protocol A written plan specifying the procedure to be followed.

Provider A deliverer of health care services—hospital, clinic, nurse, or physician.

Proximate cause Action occurring immediately before an injury, thereby assumed to be the reason for the injury.

Psychomotor domain Area of activity referring to motor skills or actions by an individual; for example, learning to dance is in the psychomotor domain.

Pure science Information that summarizes and explains the universe without regard for whether the information is immediately useful; also known as "basic science."

Q

Qualitative research Research that seeks to answer questions that cannot be answered by quantitative designs and that must be addressed by more subjective methods.

Quality management See Total quality management.

Quantitative research Research that uses data-gathering techniques that can be repeated by others and verified. Data collected are quantifiable—that is, they can be counted, measured with standardized instruments, or observed with a high degree of agreement among observers.

R

Reality shock The feelings of powerlessness and ineffectiveness often experienced by new nursing graduates; usually occurs as a result of the transition from the educational setting to the "real world" of nursing in an actual health care setting.

Receiver An essential element of communication; the person receiving the message.

Reengineering Radical redesign of business processes and thinking to improve performance.

Referendum An election resulting from registered voters being asked by a legislative body to express a preference on a policy issue.

Reflection A communication technique that consists of directing questions back to patients, thereby encouraging patients to think through problems for themselves.

Reflective thinking The process of evaluating one's thinking processes during a situation that has already occurred, as opposed to evaluating one's thinking during the situation as it occurs.

Registered nurse (RN) An individual who has completed a basic program for registered nurses and successfully completed the licensing examination.

Rehabilitation services Those activities designed to restore an individual or a body part to normal or near-normal function following a disease or an accident.

Reliable Yielding the same values dependably each time an instrument is used to measure the same thing.

Remission A period of chronic illness during which symptoms subside.

Replication The process of repeating a research study as closely as possible to the original.

Research process Prescribed steps that must be taken to plan and conduct meaningful research properly.

Research question A statement, question, or hypothesis that a research study is designed to answer.

Resilience A pattern of successful adaptation despite challenging or threatening circumstances.

Resocialized The outcome of a transitional process of giving up part or all of one set of professional values and learning new ones.

Resolution A written position on an issue presented to the voting members of an association for their consideration, discussion, and vote.

Respondeat superior Legal theory that attributes the acts of employees to their employer (Latin term).

Retrospective reimbursement Insurance payment made after services are delivered.

Richards, Linda In 1873 she became the first "trained nurse" in the United States.

Risk management A program that seeks to identify and eliminate potential safety hazards, thereby reducing patient injuries.

RN-to-baccalaureate in nursing Programs enabling registered nurses who hold associate degrees or diplomas in nursing to acquire baccalaureate degrees in nursing.

Role A goal-directed pattern of behavior learned within a cultural setting.

Role model An individual who serves as an example of desirable behavior for another person.

Role strain Stress created by difficulty experienced in adjusting to a life or occupational role.

S

Salary compression A phenomenon in which pay increases are limited during an individual's career, so that the salary of a veteran nurse may be little higher than that of a recently hired novice nurse.

Sample A subset of an entire population that reflects the characteristics of the population.

School nurse Nurse specializing in the care of school-age children or adolescents and practicing in school settings.

Scientific discipline A branch of instruction or field of learning based on the study of a body of facts about the physical or material world.

Scientific method A systematic, orderly approach to the gathering of data and the solving of problems.

Scope of practice The boundaries of a practice profession's activities as defined by law.

Secondary care An intermediate level of health care performed in a hospital having specialized equipment and laboratory facilities.

Secondary source Sources of data such as the nurse's own observations or perceptions of family and friends of the patient.

Self-actualization A process of realizing one's maximum potential and using one's capabilities to the fullest extent possible.

Self-awareness Understanding of one's own needs, biases, and impact on others.

Self-care The ability to care for oneself, that is, engage in activities of daily living without assistance.

Self-insurance Coverage in which an individual or business pays for care directly rather than purchasing insurance.

Self-care model Nursing theoretical model based on the concept of ability to care for self.

Self-directed work team A method of decentralizing decision making using cross-functional groups united around common goals.

Self-efficacy A belief in self as possessing the ability to perform an activity, such as administering daily insulin.

Sender An essential element of communication; the person sending a message.

Separation of powers Under the U.S. Constitution, each branch of the federal government has separate and distinct functions and powers.

Set A group of circumstances or situations joined and treated as a whole.

Sex-role stereotyping The practice of automatically and routinely linking specific characteristics to either males or females; also called gender-role stereotyping.

Sexual assault nurse examiner (SANE) Nurse trained to collect forensic evidence and provide initial counseling following rape or other sexual assault.

Shared governance Incorporation of unit-based decision making in nursing practice models. Generic term used to describe any organization in which decision making is shared throughout.

Short-term goals Specific, small steps leading to the achievement of broader, long-term goals.

Sick role A culture's criteria that must be met before people can qualify as being "sick."

Sigma Theta Tau International (STTI) The international honor society for nursing.

Sign Outward evidence of illness visible to others, for example, a rash.

Skill mix The ratio of registered nurses to licensed practical nurses and nursing assistants in a hospital unit.

Socialization The process whereby values and expectations are transmitted from generation to generation.

Social services Services designed to assist individuals and families in obtaining basic needs, such as housing, food, and medical care.

Somatic language Language used by infants to signal their needs to caretakers—for example, crying; reddening of the skin; fast, shallow breathing; facial expressions; and jerking of the limbs.

Spelman Seminary Site of the first nursing program for African-Americans; founded in Atlanta, Georgia, in 1886.

Spiritual nursing care Care that recognizes, respects, and, if appropriate, facilitates the practice of a patient's spiritual beliefs.

Spirituality Belief in and sense of connectedness with a higher power.

Staff nurse The bedside nurse who cares for a group of patients but has no management responsibilities for the nursing unit.

Stage theory A theory that views human development as a series of identifiable stages through which individuals and families pass.

Stakeholders Individuals with an interest in an outcome or process.

Standard of care A guideline stating what the reasonably prudent nurse, under similar circumstances, would have done.

Standards of practice Formal statements by a profession of the accountability of its practitioners.

State board of nursing The regulatory body in each state that regulates and enforces the scope of practice and discipline of the members of the nursing profession.

Statutory law Law established through formal legislative processes.

Stereotypes Simplistic and preconceived image about a person or group.

Stereotyping Erroneous belief that all people of a certain group are alike.

Stress Any emotional, physical, social, economic, or other type of factor that requires a response or change.

Stressors Stimuli that tend to disturb equilibrium.

Subacute care A level of care between hospital-based acute care and long-term residential care.

Subjective data Information obtained from patients as they describe their needs, feelings, and strengths, as well as their perceptions of the problem.

Subsystems The parts that make up a system.

Supervision The initial direction and periodic inspection of the actual accomplishment of a task.

Suprasystem The larger environment outside a system.

Symptom An indication of illness felt by the individual but not observable to others, such as pain.

Synergy Combined action that is greater than that of the individual parts.

System A set of interrelated parts that come together to form a whole.

Systems theory See General systems theory.

T

Taxonomy A framework for classifying and organizing information.

Team nursing A system of nursing care delivery in which a group of nurses and ancillary workers are responsible for the care of a group of patients during a specified time period, usually 8 to 12 hours.

Technologists Personnel, such as laboratory technologists or radiological technologists, who assist in the diagnosis of patient problems.

Telehealth The practice of providing health care by means of telecommunication devices, such as telephone lines or televisions; the removal of time and distance barriers for the delivery of health care services and related health care activities through telecommunication technologies such as telephones.

Telehealth nursing The delivery of nursing care services and related health care activities through telecommunication technology, such as telephones, video conferencing, and others.

Termination phase The final phase of the nurse-patient relationship wherein a mutual evaluation of progress is conducted.

Tertiary care Specialized, highly technical level of health care provided in sophisticated research and teaching hospitals.

Tertiary source Sources of data including the medical records and health care providers, such as physical therapists, physicians, or dietitians.

Theory A general explanation scholars use to explain, predict, control, and understand commonly occurring events.

Therapeutic milieu An environment created to foster healing.

Therapist Any of several health care workers with differing educational backgrounds who work with patients with specific deficits; examples include physical therapists and occupational therapists.

Third-party payment Payment for health services by an entity other than the patient or the provider of services, such as the government or insurance companies.

Throughput The processes a system uses to convert raw materials into a form that can be used, either by the system itself or by the environment.

Tort A civil wrong against a person; may be intentional or unintentional.

Total quality management (TQM) Management philosophy and activities directed toward achieving excellence and employee participation in all aspects of that goal.

Transcultural nursing Nursing care that is based on the patient's culturally determined health values, beliefs, and practices.

Transmission In communication theory, the expression of information verbally or nonverbally.

U

Universal care Provision of health care to all people.

Unlicensed assistive personnel (UAP) Health care personnel, such as nursing assistants and home care aides, who are not themselves licensed but are supervised by licensed individuals, such as nurses or physicians.

Urbanization The process of population migration to cities.

Utilitarianism An ethical theory asserting that it is right to maximize the greatest good for the greatest number of people.

V

Valid Measuring what it is intended to measure, as in a valid test question or research instrument.

Value ethics Ethical beliefs and behaviors that arise from the character of the decision maker.

Values The social principles, ideals, or standards held by an individual, class, or group that give meaning and direction to behavior.

Ventilation The verbal "letting off steam" that occurs when people talk about concerns or frustrations.

Veracity Truthfulness.

Verbal communication All language, whether written or spoken; represents only a small part of communication.

Virtue ethics The system of ethics based on a person's natural tendency to act, feel, and judge but developed through training; ethics based on the natural traits of the decision maker.

Voluntariness The degree to which an action is brought about by an individual's own free choice.

Voluntary (private) agency An agency supported entirely through voluntary contributions of time and/or money.

Vulnerable populations Groups who are at risk and unable to advocate for themselves, such as small children, developmentally challenged individuals, the frail elderly, or the socially marginalized.

W

Whistle-blower A person who speaks out against unfair, dishonest, or dangerous practices by a company or agency. Usually an employee of that company or agency.

Whole system shared governance System in which people at all levels within the organization are included in decision making.

Woodhull Study on Nurses and the Media A comprehensive 1997 study of nursing in the print media.

Workers' compensation A federally mandated insurance system covering workers injured on the job.

Work ethic A belief on the part of an employee or group in the importance of work; an appreciation for the characteristics employers desire in employees and a commitment to exhibiting them.

Working phase The middle phase of the nurse-patient relationship, wherein goals are achieved.

Working poor Those who, although employed, are unable to earn enough to live at more than a very modest level.

Workplace advocacy Action ensuring that workers have a voice in the issues that concern them, either through collective action or through other effective means.

Yale School of Nursing The first school of nursing in the world to be established as a separate university department with an independent budget and its own dean, Annie W. Goodrich.

INDEX

A

Abels, Lori, 42
Abortion, polarization over, 223
Abstract for Action, An, 166
Abstracts, research, 284
Acceptance
  of illness, 241
  nonjudgmental, 148, 217
Accidents, child deaths due to, 16
Accountability
  challenges of, 433
  in nursing professionalism, 75
  of primary nurse, 366
Accreditation, 173-174, 375
Acronyms, avoiding, 228
Action language, 220
Active listening in holistic communication, 228
Activism. *See* Political activism
Acute respiratory distress syndrome, positioning and, 12
Adaptation
  human needs and, 296
  in Roy's conceptual model, 338-340
Adler, Mortimer, 223
Administrative law, 87
Administrative support personnel, responsibilities and
     preparation of, 360-361
Adolescence, cultural issues in, 248
Advance directives. *See also* End-of-life care; End-of-life decisions
  controversy over, 129
  defined, 104
  purposes of, 128-129
  Shiavo case and, 115
Advanced degrees, 174-177. *See also* Doctoral education;
     Master's programs
  doctorate, 175-177
  master's, 174-175
Advanced practice nurse
  Balanced Budget Act of 1997 and, 102-103
  certification of, 178-179
  federal regulations affecting, 403
Advanced practice nursing
  autonomy issues in, 24
  credentialing of, 101
  and efficiency and availability of health care, 24
  growth and categories of, 21
  issues in, 24
  specialties in, 22f
Advocacy, patient, absence of, as negligence, 96b
Aesthetics, defined, 318
African-American clinic nursing, 34-35
African-American culture, pregnancy issues and, 202

African-American nurses, 48
  numbers of, 57
  professional organizations for, 34
  in university education, 48
African-Americans
  admission to nursing programs, 32-33
  collegiate programs for, 39
  disease mortality rate differentials for, 247
  health disparities and, 123
  perceptions of health care system, 56
  population of, 57
  tuberculosis in, 34-36
Agenda for Health Care Reform, 40
Aging, impacts on nursing, 52, 55, 55f
Aging population as nursing challenge, 422-423
AIDS. *See* HIV/AIDS
Aiken, Linda, 8, 103
Alaska Natives, health disparities and, 123
Allergies
  incidence of, 15
  increase in, 425
  latex, 436
Alliance Leadership Academy, 398
Alternative therapies, 434
  types and use of, 435b
Altruism in nursing professionalism, 77
Ambulatory care settings, employment in, 6
American Academy of Ambulatory Care Nursing, 18
American Assembly for Men in Nursing, 46
American Association for the History of Nursing, 396
American Association of Ambulatory Care Nurses, 18
American Association of Colleges of Nursing
  on baccalaureate programs, 166
  Commission on Collegiate Nursing Education of, 174
  *Essentials of Baccalaureate Education for Professional Nursing
    Practice* of, 167
  Nursing Education's Agenda for the 21st Century of, 183
  white paper on differentiated practice, 432
American Association of Men in Nursing, 48
American Board for Occupational Health Nursing, 13
American Board of Nursing Specialties, 179
American College of Nurse-Midwives, 23
American Federation of Teachers, 397
American Hospital Association, Patient's Bill of Rights of, 56
American Indians. *See* Native Americans
American Journal of Nursing, 36-37
American Nurses Association, 395
  code of ethics of. *See Code of Ethics for Nurses*
  Competencies for Telehealth Technologies in Nursing of, 18
  economic and employment divisions of, 396-397
  *Educational Preparation for Nurse Practitioners and Assistants
    to Nurses* of, 165-166

Note: Entries followed by "b" indicate boxes; "f" figures; "t" tables.